The Physician Assistant Medical Handbook

The Physician Assistant Medical Handbook

Second Edition

James Brox Labus, PA-C

Concentra Medical Centers
Atlanta, Georgia

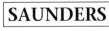

An Imprint of Elsevier

SAUNDERS
An Imprint of Elsevier

The Curtis Center
Independence Square West
Philadelphia, PA 19106

Notice

Medicine is an ever-changing field. Standard safety precautions must be followed, but as new research and clinical experience broaden our knowledge, changes in treatment and drug therapy may become necessary or appropriate. Readers are advised to check the most current product information provided by the manufacturer of each drug to be administered to verify the recommended dose, the method and duration of administration, and contraindications. It is the responsibility of the treating physician, relying on experience and knowledge of the patient, to determine dosages and the best treatment for each individual patient. Neither the Publisher nor the editor assumes any liability for any injury and/or damage to persons or property arising from this publication.

The Publisher

Library of Congress Cataloging-in-Publication Data

The physician assistant medical handbook / [edited by] James Brox Labus.–2nd ed.
    p.   cm.
    Includes bibliographical references and index.
    ISBN 0-7216-9786-0
 1. Physicians' assistants–Handbooks, manuals, etc.   I. Labus, James B.
 [DNLM: 1. Clinical Medicine–Handbooks.   2. Physician Assistants–Handbooks.
    [WB 39 P5775 2004]
    R697.P45P484 2004
 616—dc22
                                                                    2003059148

Acquisitions Editor: Thomas Moore
Production Manager: Joan Nikelsky
Editorial Assistant: Janine Kusza

For my children,
Elise and Brox:
may you achieve your potential in every way possible.

For my wife and best friend, Louise.

And to my parents Eugene and Greta Labus:
I am proud to be your son.

In Memoriam

Author James W. Becker's father,
Christian P. Becker

Author Judith E. Colver's parents,
Robert M. Lundberg and Barbara E. Lundberg

Contributors

Lisa Mustone Alexander, EdD, MPH, PAC
Associate Professor and Director, Department of Health Care Sciences,
George Washington University School of Medicine and Health Sciences,
Washington, District of Columbia
Essential Hypertension

Nancy A. Anderson, PA-C
Kaiser Permanente, Atlanta, Georgia
Casting/Splinting Techniques

James W. Becker, PA-C
Private Practice
*Appendicitis, Cholecystitis, Diverticulitis, Esophageal Disorders, Gastrointestinal
Bleeding: Lower Tract, Gastrointestinal Bleeding: Upper Tract, Hemorrhoids,
Pancreatitis (Acute)*

Katharine Breaux, MPAS, BS, PA-C
Instructor, Department of Medicine, Baylor College of Medicine; HIV
Coordinator, Department of Infectious Diseases, Houston Veterans
Affairs Medical Center, Houston, Texas
Tuberculosis

Jodi L. Cahalan, MPH, MS, PA-C
Associate Dean for Student, Alumni and Clinical Affairs, College of
Health Sciences; Director, Primary Care Physician Assistant, Physician
Assistant Program, College of Health Sciences Physician Assistant
Program, Des Moines University, Des Moines, Iowa
*Acne Vulgaris, Alopecia, Bacterial Infections, Benign Cutaneous Neoplasms,
Dermatitis/Eczema, Dermatophytosis (Fungal Infections), Cervicitis, Dysmenorrhea*

Pam Harrison Chambers, MPH, PA-C
Assistant Professor and Assistant Director, Physician Assistant Program,
Des Moines University, Des Moines; Family Practice Physician Assistant,
Lakeview Family Practice, Iowa Health Physicians, West Des Moines, Iowa
Endometriosis, Fibrocystic Breast Disease, Functional Ovarian Cysts

Judith E. Colver, MMS, PA-C
Associate Chair, Physician Assistant Studies Department, University of
Texas Health Science Center at San Antonio; Staff Physician Assistant,
Department of Family Community Medicine, University Hospital
Clinics—Downtown; Past President, Association of Family Practice
Physician Assistants, San Antonio; Chair, Public Relations Committee,
Texas Academy of Physician Assistants, Austin, Texas
*Acute Hypoxemic Respiratory Failure, Asthma, Bronchitis, Chronic Obstructive
Pulmonary Disease, Interstitial Lung Disease, Pleural Effusion, Pleurisy, Pneumonia,
Pneumothorax, Pulmonary Embolism, Sleep Apnea*

Kristine Correira, PA-C
Charleston, Massachusetts
Respiratory Arrest, Shock

R. Ellen Davis-Hall, PhD, PA-C
Associate Professor, Physician Assistant Education, University of
Nebraska Medical Center, School of Allied Health, Omaha; Physician
Assistant, Internal Medicine Consultants, Blair, Nebraska
Eating Disorders, Mood Disorders, Somatoform/Dissociative Disorders

Sue M. Enns, MHS, PA-C
Assistant Professor, Physician Assistant Department, Wichita State
University, Wichita, Kansas
Labyrinthitis, Meniere Disease, Nasal Polyps, Otitis Externa, Rhinitis, Sinusitis

Leith Audrey Fitch, BMS, PA-C
Physician Assistant, The Center for Pain Management, Atlanta, Georgia;
Georgia Association of Physician Assistants' Recent Liaison to the
Georgia Composite State Board of Medical Examiners PAAC Committee,
Atlanta, Georgia
Sprains, Strains, and Fractures

Edward Gaile, Sr., BA, BHS, PA-C
Lawrenceville, Georgia
*Congestive Heart Failure, Cor Pulmonale, Coronary Atherosclerotic Heart Disease,
Pericarditis/Pericardial Effusion, Valvular Heart Disease, Dyslipidemia*

Michaela C. Gallagher-Gonzales, PA-C
Physician Assistant, Anasazi Medical Associates, Santa Fe, New Mexico
Diabetes Mellitus, Thyroid Disorders

Ann M. Griwatz, PA-C
Physician Assistant, Emergency Department, South West Emergency
Physicians, Durango, Colorado
Adrenal Disorders, Diabetes Mellitus

William M. Hardy, PhD, MS, PA-C
Director, Post-Graduate Residency Program for PAs in Psychiatry,
University of Texas Medical Branch, Galveston; Clinical Instructor,
University of North Texas Health Science Center, Fort Worth, Texas
Dementia

Michelle L. Heinan, EdD, MS, PA-C
Interim Chair and Program Director, Department of Physician Assistant
Studies, East Carolina University, Greenville, North Carolina
*Cholecystitis, Crohn's Disease, Dyspepsia, Esophageal Disorders, Hemorrhoids,
Peptic/Gastric Ulcer Disease, Ulcerative Colitis*

Roderick S. Hooker, PhD, PA
Director of Rheumatology Postgraduate Program for Physician Assistants, Department of Veterans Affairs, Dallas, Texas; Professor, Division of Rheumatology, University of Texas Southwestern Medical Center, Dallas, Texas
Ankylosing Spondylitis, Fibromyalgia, Gout, Osteoarthritis/Osteoarthrosis, Polymyalgia Rheumatica, Rheumatoid Arthritis, Tendinitis/Bursitis

Catherine R. Judd, MS, PA-C
Clinical Assistant Professor, Physicians Assistant Program, Department of PA Studies, University of Texas Southwestern Allied Health Sciences School, Dallas, Texas
Encephalitis, Parkinson Disease, Seizure Disorders, Transient Ischemic Attack/Stroke

Keith W. Kettell, MPAS, PA-C
Department of Military and Emergency Medicine, Uniformed Services University of Health Sciences, Bethesda, Maryland
Meningitis

Nassoma King, PA-C
Physician Assistant, Winship Cancer Institute, Emory University, Atlanta, Georgia
Dyslipidemia

Mary Beth Kvanli, MPAS, PA-C
HIV Coordinator, Section of Infectious Diseases, Department of Veterans Affairs, North Texas Health Care System, Dallas, Texas
Endocarditis (Infectious), Gastroenteritis, Gonorrhea, Sepsis

James B. Labus, PA-C
Clinical Physician Assistant, Concentra Medical Centers, Atlanta, Georgia
Burns, Hyperthermia, Hypothermia, Near Drowning, Poisoning, Psychiatric Emergencies, Intracranial Neoplasm, Adjustment Disorders, Attention-Deficit Hyperactivity Disorder, Personality Disorders, Psychotic Disorders

Robert J. McNellis, MPH, PA-C
Adjunct Assistant Professor, George Washington University School of Health Care Sciences, Washington, District of Columbia; Director, Clinical Affairs and Education, American Academy of Physician Assistants, Alexandria, Virginia
Benign Prostatic Hyperplasia, Erectile Dysfunction, Prostatitis

Charlene M. Morris, MPAS, PA-C
Family Practice Physician Assistant, Glasgow, Kentucky
Infestations of the Skin, Papulosquamous Conditions, Premalignant and Malignant Skin Tumors, Vascular Conditions, Viral Disease—Vesicular, Other Viral Infections, Migraine

William A. Mosier, EdD, MPAS, LMFT, PA-C (Major-USAFR)
Assistant Professor/Intern Supervisor, Wright State University, Dayton, Ohio; Chief, Medical/Surgical PA Services, 459th Aeromedical Staging Squadron, Malcom Grow Medical Center, Andrews Air Force Base, Maryland; Director of Research, Center for the Study of Child Development, Dayton, Ohio
Dementia, Myasthenia Gravis

Nina Multak, MPAS, PA-C
Adjunct Assistant Professor, NOVA Southeastern University Health Professions Division, College of Allied Health, Physician Assistant Department, Ft. Lauderdale, Florida
Pelvic Inflammatory Disease, Uterine Prolapse, Vaginitis

Debra S. Munsell, MPAS, PA-C
Director, PA Student Educational Program, Department of Head and Neck Surgery, University of Texas–MD Anderson Cancer Center, Houston, Texas
Benign Paroxysmal Positional Vertigo, Cerumen Impaction, Eustachian Tube Dysfunction, Otitis Media, Pharyngitis, Tonsillitis

Deborah A. Opacic, EdD, PA-C
Clinical Coordinator, Physician Assistant Program, Duquesne University, Pittsburgh, Pennsylvania
Chest Tube Thoracostomy, Subclavian Line Insertion, Thoracentesis, Wound Care

Roland G. Ottley, JD, PA-C
Brooklyn, New York
Pituitary Adenoma

Jack Pike, BS, PA-C
Adjunct Clinical Assistant Professor, Physician Assistant Program, Quinnipiac College, Hamden; Physician Assistant, St. Francis Hospital and Medical Center, Hartford, Connecticut
Emergency Cricothyroidotomy, Internal Jugular Cannulation

Timothy F. Quigley, MPH, PA-C
Assistant Professor, Department of Physician Assistants, Wichita State University College of Health Professions, Wichita, Kansas
Epididymitis, Orchitis, Urethritis, Urinary Tract Infection

Charles W. Reed, MEd, MPAS, PA-C
Physician Assistant, Department of Neurology, North Texas Neurology Associates, Wichita Falls, Texas
Anemia, Bleeding Disorders, Deep Venous Thrombosis, Polycythemia Vera, Sickle Cell Disease, Heparin-Induced Thrombocytopenia, Adrenal Carcinoma, Bladder Cancer, Breast Cancer, Cervical Cancer, Colorectal Cancer, Gastric Carcinoma, Hodgkin's Disease, Leukemia, Liver Cancer, Lung Cancer, Lymphoma, Malignant Melanoma, Multiple Myeloma, Oropharyngeal Cancer, Ovarian Cancer, Pancreatic Cancer, Prostate Cancer, Renal Carcinoma, Sarcomas, Testicular Cancer, Thyroid Cancer, Uterine Cancer

M. Katherine Reynolds, BS, PA-C
Westminster, South Carolina
Multiple Sclerosis

Thomas M. Richardson, MBA, PA-C
Department of Community and Preventive Medicine, Division of
Epidemiology, University of Rochester, Rochester, New York
Arrhythmias/Dysrhythmias, Coronary Atherosclerotic Heart Disease

Sandra Lynn Roberts, MMSc, PA-C
Guest Lecturer, Physician Assistant Program, Emory University School of
Medicine, Atlanta, Georgia; Physician Assistant, Department of
Emergency Medicine, Fayetteville Medical Center, Fayetteville, Georgia;
Department of Dermatology, Dermatology Specialists of Georgia,
Newnan, Georgia; and Department of Internal Medicine and Nephrology,
Piedmont Hospital, Atlanta, Georgia
*Acid-Base Disturbances, Acute Renal Failure, Chronic Renal Failure, Electrolyte
Imbalance: Na$^+$ and K$^+$, Glomerular Disease, Nephrolithiasis, Pyelonephritis:
Upper Tract Infection, Renal and Vascular Hypertension, Tubulointerstitial
Diseases*

Mona M. Sedrak, PhD, PA-C
Associate Director of Academic Affairs, Physician Assistant Program,
Kettering College of Medical Arts, Kettering, Ohio
Peripheral Neuropathy

Rhea Sumpter, MMSc, PA, AA-C
Chief Anesthetist, Department of Anesthesia, St. Joseph's Hospital of Atlanta,
Atlanta, Georgia
Anesthesia

Paul Taylor, BS, PA-C
Instructor, Clinical Rotations, Physician Assistant Program, Emory
University School of Medicine, Atlanta, Georgia; Physician Assistant,
Departments of GYN/OB and Neonatology, Emory University, and
Department of Maternal and Child Health, Grady Memorial Hospital,
Atlanta, Georgia
Intrauterine Devices: Insertion and Removal

Diana Turner, PA-C
HIV Coordinator, Medical Service, Infectious Diseases Section, Dallas
Veterans Affairs Medical Center, Dallas, Texas
Human Immunodeficiency Virus Infection, Hepatitis (Viral), Mononucleosis, Syphilis

Pamela A. Van Bevern, MPAS, PA-C
Assistant Professor, Physician Assistant Program, Saint Louis University,
St. Louis, Missouri
Anxiety Disorders

George L. White, Jr., PhD, MSPH, PA-C
Professor and Director, Public Health Programs, Department of Family and Preventive Medicine, University of Utah School of Medicine, Salt Lake City, Utah
Cataract, Conjunctivitis, Glaucoma, Ocular Hemorrhage, Optic Neuritis, Retinal Detachment

Daniel Wood, MPAS, PA-C
Assistant Professor, Department of PA Studies, University of Texas Health Science Center at San Antonio; Physician Assistant, Family Medicine, Centro Med, San Antonio, Texas
Metabolic Bone Disorders

Preface

The Physician Assistant Medical Handbook is the first portable medical reference guide written specifically by and for physician assistants (PAs). It presents the most commonly encountered conditions in all of the major medical subspecialties, in an easily referenced format designed for quick access to specific information. Each topic is divided into definitive areas of subject matter—History, Pathophysiology, Diagnostic Studies, Differential Diagnosis, Treatment, and so on. Each of these subjects is divided in turn into relevant categories—under Differential Diagnosis, for example, the categories include Traumatic, Infectious, Metabolic, Neoplastic, and so on. These subjects and categories remain constant for all topics throughout the book. An additional feature of the *Handbook* is "Pearls for the PA"—highlighted considerations within a specific topic especially important to the PA's practice.

Now in the second edition, changes have been made to enhance the book's usefulness. Many topics have been revised to reflect major advances in both theory and management. "Preventive Considerations" and "Geriatric Considerations" have been added to provide direction in treating the entire patient. These topics are not usually found in medical reference texts, yet they are important in the comprehensive management of the patient throughout the life cycle. Also new is a chapter on common procedures that may be assigned to the PA to perform. Easy-to-follow directions and illustrations are included to augment the clinical instruction.

PAs practice in a variety of settings—academic, private, rural, and urban. "Common conditions" as such will therefore vary. Every effort has been made to include only conditions that are seen with regularity in practice. Also, the diagnosis and management of certain conditions will vary somewhat according to institutional protocols and with geographic location. To provide an accepted, up-to-date approach to each medical condition included in this *Handbook*, authors were chosen on the basis of their experience within a subspecialty. These authors helped with selection of the topics and brought a high level of expertise to coverage of their particular topic.

This book can be utilized in the didactic or clinical phase of training, in clinical practice, or in studying for the recertification examination. The format permits inclusion of in-depth information in minimal space, making the book ideal for comprehensive study as well as cursory reference. With publication of this new edition, PAs in every setting and in every phase of training should continue to find the *Handbook* a useful addition to their practice.

James B. Labus, PA-C
Atlanta, Georgia

Contents

Color plate figures follow page 72.

CARDIOLOGY

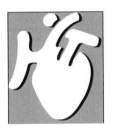

1

Arrhythmias/Dysrhythmias

Thomas M. Richardson, MBA, PA-C

DEFINITION

Arrhythmia: Any deviation in or departure from the normal sinus electrical conduction mechanism of the heart. Also called *dysrhythmia*.

HISTORY

Symptoms. The patient may be asymptomatic or may present with palpitations, dyspnea, lethargy, weakness, dizziness, chest pain, syncope, congestive heart failure (CHF), or complete hemodynamic collapse.

General. Frequently, dysrhythmias occur as a complication of an underlying illness, so a thorough review of symptoms is essential.

Age. Increase in frequency with age but may be seen in conjunction with congenital abnormalities.

Onset. Acute, paroxysmal, or asymptomatic.

Duration. Extremely variable; may last for a few seconds, hours, or days, or remain chronic.

Intensity. Variable, ranging from no symptoms to cardiovascular collapse.

Aggravating Factors. Emotional stress, caffeine, cigarette smoking, ethanol (ETOH) intake, physical activity, certain pharmacologic agents, illicit drugs.

Alleviating Factors. If relief occurs, it is usually spontaneous, but Valsalva maneuvers can be successful for some arrhythmias.

Associated Factors. Coronary artery and pulmonary disease. Congenital abnormalities.

PHYSICAL EXAMINATION

General. The physical examination rarely yields a definitive diagnosis, but it reveals the degree of hemodynamic compromise, thereby guiding the intensity and urgency of treatment. A complete and thorough examination is indicated as it may provide evidence of underlying disease and is necessary for appropriate and effective treatment.

Cardiovascular. Blood pressure (check for orthostasis and paradox) may be elevated, decreased, or absent. Tachypnea or bradypnea and elevated or decreased temperature may be noted, and arterial pulses may be present or absent. The heart rate may increase or decrease, and the rhythm may be regular, irregular, or regularly irregular.

Assessment of the jugular venous pulsation may provide clues to atrial activity.

Assessment of jugular venous distention may provide clues to volume status.

Perform precordial inspection and palpation for lifts, heaves, and dyskinetic areas.

Locate apical impulse and assess for enlargement and lateral displacement. These signs may indicate cardiomegaly.

Percussion of cardiac border may also provide evidence of cardiomegaly.

Cardiac Auscultation. Volume of S_1 and S_2 may be diminished in cases of pericardial effusion and chronic obstructive pulmonary disease (COPD). S_3 gallop may be present with CHF. S_4 gallop may be present with heart block or atrial flutter. Murmurs must be characterized in relation to possible valvular lesions.

Neurologic. Assess level of consciousness and for abnormalities suggestive of acute cerebral ischemia.

Pulmonary. Assess adequacy of ventilation and oxygenation. Auscultate for evidence of pulmonary edema or pneumothorax.

PATHOPHYSIOLOGY

Atrial Rhythms

Normal Sinus Rhythm

Normal sinus rhythm describes a regular, narrow complex rhythm that originates at the sinus node with a rate of 60 to100 beats/minute. P waves must be upright on ECG for leads II, III, and aVf. The P-R interval must be between 0.12 and 0.20 second for sinus rhythm to be diagnosed (see Fig. 1-1).

Sinus tachycardia is diagnosed when the normal sinus mechanism is present and the rate exceeds 100 beats/minute (see Fig. 1-2).

Sinus bradycardia is present when the normal sinus mechanism is present and the rate falls below 60 beats/minute (see Fig. 1-3).

Premature Atrial Contractions

Premature atrial contractions (PACs) are early atrial depolarizations originating at a focus other than the sinus node. P waves may differ in morphol-

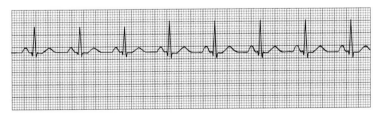

Figure 1–1. Normal sinus rhythm.

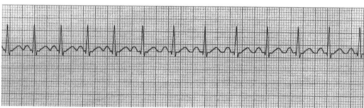

Figure 1–2. Sinus tachycardia.

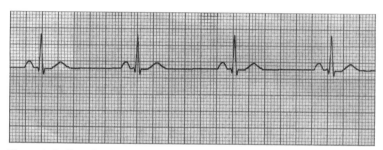

Figure 1–3. Sinus bradycardia.

ogy and axis from normal sinus rhythm. These beats are usually conducted normally, producing a normal P-R interval (see Fig. 1-4).

Supraventricular Tachycardia

The term *supraventricular tachycardia* (SVT) describes a myriad of non-sinus tachycardias originating in the atria or atrioventricular (AV) node. SVT may arise as a result of accelerated automaticity, or it may be the result of a reentrant circuit involving the AV node, a bypass tract, or even the sinus node.

SVTs are generally regular, with rates ranging from 150 to 240 beats/minute. P waves may be of nonsinus configuration or axis (P waves negative in leads II, III, and aVf). P waves generally precede the QRS complex by a normal or shortened P-R interval. P waves may also follow the QRS as a result of late retrograde depolarization of the atria; these are

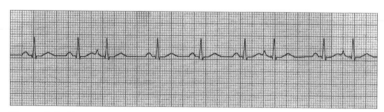

Figure 1–4. Premature atrial complexes.

known as retrograde P waves. Conduction is usually in the ratio of 1:1, but at atrial rates greater than 200 beats/minute, block may occur. The QRS complex is narrow and of normal configuration; however, aberrancy or bundle branch block may occur. In cases in which the QRS is widened or atrial activity is difficult to identify, differentiation from ventricular tachycardia (VT) may be extremely difficult.

Atrial Flutter

In atrial flutter the atrial rate varies between 250 and 350 beats/minute, producing the characteristic sawtooth flutter waves on the ECG. Ventricular rate depends on the degree of AV block present; a 2:1 ratio is most common in untreated cases. The P-R interval is usually constant and of normal length but may be short. The QRS is narrow, but aberration may occur (see Fig. 1-5). In situations in which flutter waves are not readily apparent and atrial flutter must be differentiated from SVT, carotid sinus massage may produce transient high-degree AV block, revealing diagnostic flutter waves (see Fig. 1-6).

Atrial Fibrillation

Atrial fibrillation (AF) is a chaotic atrial rhythm in which no organized atrial activity is evident on the ECG. Ventricular response is irregularly irregular, with rates typically ranging from 160 to 180 beats/minute but sometimes much lower. The QRS is usually narrow, but aberration frequently occurs (see Fig. 1-7).

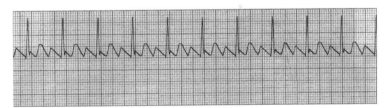

Figure 1–5. Atrial flutter.

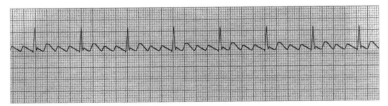

Figure 1–6. Atrial flutter with higher-grade atrioventricular (AV) block.

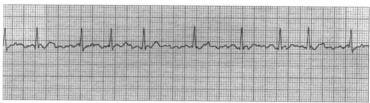

Figure 1–7. Atrial fibrillation with controlled ventricular response.

Ventricular Dysrhythmias

Premature Ventricular Contractions

A premature ventricular contraction (PVC) occurs when the ventricles are depolarized before the next expected sinus beat. As the impulse propagates through the myocardium, it does not utilize the normal conduction system; therefore, the resulting complex is wide (>0.12 second) and inconsistent in shape. Because of its ventricular origin it is not related to the normal sinus chain of events and occurs randomly, producing an irregular rhythm. PVCs may occur singly or in couplets or triplets. They may occur at regular intervals—for example, every second beat (bigeminy) or every third beat (trigeminy). PVCs may arise from a single focus (unifocal) or from multiple foci (multifocal) (see Fig. 1-8).

Ventricular Tachycardia

Ventricular tachycardia (VT) is a wide QRS tachycardia arising in the ventricle. The rate may range from 100 to 250 beats/minute. The rhythm is regular, and if atrial activity is identifiable, AV dissociation is present. At times it may be very difficult to distinguish VT from SVT with aberrancy. The following criteria, if identifiable, favor a diagnosis of VT:

1. QRS greater than 0.14 second
2. Left axis deviation
3. Presence of AV dissociation
4. A monophasic or biphasic right bundle pattern on lead V_1 tracing (see Fig. 1-9).

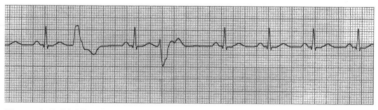

Figure 1–8. Multifocal premature ventricular complexes.

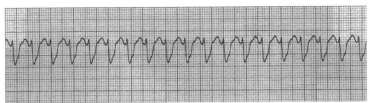

Figure 1–9. Ventricular tachycardia.

Ventricular Fibrillation

Ventricular fibrillation (VF) is a chaotic ventricular rhythm in which there is no organized complex on the ECG. It may appear as fine or coarse. VF is always a medical emergency because there is no cardiac output generated by this rhythm (see Figs. 1-10 and 1-11).

Ventricular Asystole

Asystole is the complete absence of any ventricular electrical activity. The ECG shows a flat line (see Fig. 1-12).

Atrioventricular Blocks

First Degree Atrioventricular Block

First degree AV block occurs when conduction of the atrial impulse to the ventricle is delayed at the AV node. On the ECG this appears as a prolonged P-R interval, by definition greater than 0.20 second. Otherwise the ECG is normal (see Fig. 1-13).

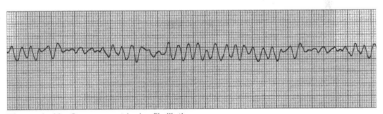

Figure 1–10. Coarse ventricular fibrillation.

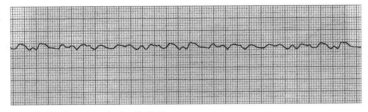

Figure 1–11. Fine ventricular fibrillation.

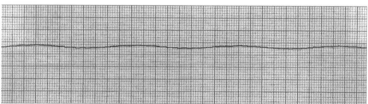

Figure 1–12. Ventricular asystole.

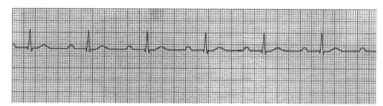

Figure 1–13. First degree AV block.

Second Degree Atrioventricular Block: Type I and Type II

Type I or Wenckebach block is characterized by a sequentially lengthening P-R interval until complete block occurs and no QRS is conducted. The cycle then usually repeats itself but may be variable. The atrial rhythm is regular, but because of variable conduction the ventricular rate is regularly irregular. QRS complexes are normal (see Fig. 1-14).

Type II ultimately results in intermittent complete block, but without lengthening the P-R interval. The atrial rhythm is regular, as is the ventricular rhythm, but because of the regular complete block the ventricular rate is less than the atrial rate. The P-R interval and QRS of conducted beats are normal (see Fig. 1-15).

Third Degree Atrioventricular Block

Third degree AV block describes complete block of electrical communication between the atria and the ventricles. The atrial rate and rhythm are

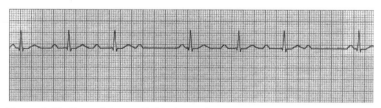

Figure 1–14. Second degree AV block: type I.

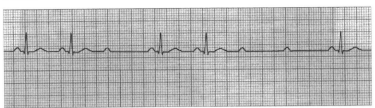

Figure 1–15. Second degree AV block: type II.

regular. If a ventricular or junctional escape rhythm develops, its timing has no relation to atrial electrical activity (see Fig. 1-16).

DIAGNOSTIC STUDIES

Laboratory

Serum Electrolytes. Evaluate for abnormalities, especially in potassium, magnesium, and calcium.

Cardiac Enzymes. Elevated cardiac enzymes—troponin, creatine kinase–MB fraction (CK-MB), lactate dehydrogenase (LDH), serum aspartate aminotransferase (AST) [formerly serum glutamic-oxaloacetic transaminase (SGOT)]—suggest myocardial infarction.

Thyroid-Stimulating Hormone (TSH). Rule out hyperthyroidism or hypothyroidism.

Toxicology and Therapeutic Drug Levels. Rule out poisoning, illicit drug use, and toxic levels as etiologic factors.

Arterial Blood Gas Analysis. Rule out hypoxemia or acid-base disturbances.

Radiology

Chest Film. Rule out cardiomegaly, CHF, pneumothorax, or primary pulmonary disease.

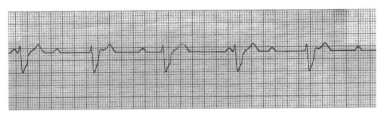

Figure 1–16. Third degree AV block occurring at level of AV node.

Cardiac Catheterization. Gold standard for assessing coronary disease. Also used for evaluation of left ventricular function, valvular and subvalvular anatomy, and intracardiac shunts.

Ventilation-Perfusion (V/Q) Scan of Lung and Spiral CT of Chest. Rule out pulmonary embolus.

Other

Holter Monitoring. Useful for documenting paroxysmal or infrequently occurring dysrhythmias. Also provides a recorded copy of the rhythm necessary for diagnosis.

Exercise Treadmill Testing. May precipitate exercise-induced dysrhythmias or reveal myocardial ischemia.

12-Lead ECG. Most useful if obtained during dysrhythmic episode, but may reveal underlying conduction abnormalities known to be associated with certain dysrhythmias or may reveal signs of other cardiac disease (e.g., ischemia, chamber hypertrophy, pericarditis).

Signal Average ECG. In patients with cardiomyopathy or recent myocardial infarction, the signal average ECG detects minute electrical variations that are known to be associated with malignant ventricular dysrhythmias.

Echocardiogram. Useful in assessing chamber size, wall thickness, myocardial contractility, valvular function, and presence of pericardial fluid—all of which in various combinations are useful in identifying any number of cardiac maladies.

Endomyocardial Biopsy. Indicated if inflammatory or infiltrative disease is suspected.

Electrophysiology Studies (EPSs). Indicated in any ventricular dysrhythmia and any atrial dysrhythmia not easily explained by a correctable cause. EPSs provide detailed information about the origin of the rhythm; thus such studies are useful both to guide therapy and to evaluate instituted therapeutic regimens.

DIFFERENTIAL DIAGNOSIS

Traumatic

Postoperative. History of cardiac surgery.

Traumatic Cardiac Contusion. History of chest wall injury; chest pain may be musculoskeletal or pericardial in origin. ECG may show changes related to myocardial injury.

Infectious

Myocarditis (Viral, Fungal, Parasitic). An inflammatory process involving the myocardium. May occur as simple upper respiratory infection and is associated with new nonspecific ECG changes, pericarditis, or dysrhythmia alone. Often undiagnosed, resulting in dilated cardiomyopathy.

Metabolic

Electrolyte Abnormality of Any Origin. Frequently asymptomatic except for rhythm disturbance. Hypokalemia and hypomagnesemia most frequently associated with diuretic use and may produce simple uncomplicated PACs/PVCs if mild, or AF or VT if severe. Hyperkalemia and hypermagnesemia most frequently associated with renal failure (acute or chronic) and may lead to bradydysrhythmias or AV block of high degree. Use of angiotensin-converting enzyme (ACE) inhibitors, potassium-sparing diuretics, and supplemental potassium can also lead to hyperkalemia.

Hyperthyroidism. AF with or without CHF may be the presenting complaint in thyrotoxicity.

Chronic Obstructive Pulmonary Disease. Primary presenting symptom is dyspnea with bronchospasm. Dysrhythmias are most commonly associated with advanced cases resulting in cor pulmonale or acute exacerbations resulting in acute hypoxia.

Cardiomyopathy (Dilated, Restrictive, Infiltrative). The most common presentation of cardiomyopathy is CHF.

Valvular Disease. Presentation varies depending on the valve involved, and discussion is found in later in this chapter.

Neoplastic
Primary or metastatic tumors may interfere with valvular or conduction system function, leading to any of numerous rhythm disturbances. Presentation is extremely variable but most closely associated with tumor location and attendant mechanical interruption of normal function.

Vascular
Pulmonary Emboli (Without Production of Mechanical Heart Failure). Chest pain, frequently pleuritic. Dyspnea is paroxysmal and may not be relieved by any maneuvers. Patient may have hemoptysis and fever. Frequent evidence of deep venous thrombosis. Chest film is normal or reveals wedged-shaped segmental density(ies).

Coronary Artery Disease. Myocardial ischemia and myocardial infarction are probably the most common underlying causes of cardiac dysrhythmias. A thorough discussion of these entities can be found later in this chapter.

Congenital
Any cardiovascular structural abnormality may predispose to dysrhythmia.

Acquired
Drug Toxicity. Many drugs have potential cardiac side effects. The most common offenders are the cardiac drugs themselves, but other medications such as tricyclic antidepressants, first-generation nonsedating antihistamines, and some prokinetic gastrointestinal drugs (Propulsid) have been shown to have arrhythmogenic properties. Illicit drugs must also be considered, especially stimulants such as cocaine and methamphetamine preparations.

Idiopathic. In some cases no underlying abnormality can be found. Presentation is frequently the dysrhythmia and its attendant symptoms. The most common example is SVT in a young athlete or paroxysmal atrial tachycardia in a normal individual.

TREATMENT

Always correctly identify the rhythm, correct any underlying abnormalities, and let clinical stability guide aggressiveness and timeliness of therapy.

Acutely, tachyarrhythmias are broken down into categories of narrow complex tachycardia and ventricular tachycardia. Assessment of the patient as stable or unstable dictates treatment. Additionally, if the patient is known to have a reduced ejection fraction, treatment may vary. Stable tachydysrhythmias typically require ventricular rate control, usually with AV node–blocking drugs. Drugs used include digitalis (loading dose of 1.0 to 1.5 mg followed by 0.125 to 0.375 mg/day, depending on age, lean body weight, and primarily renal function), calcium channel blockers, such as diltiazem (60 to 360 mg/day in divided doses three or four times a day; dosage is titrated to effect), and beta blockers. Diltiazem is also available intravenously and is bolused 0.25 mg/kg over 2 minutes, followed by a continuous infusion of 5 to 15 mg/hour, titrated to effect.

Once rate is controlled and the patient is stable, conversion to sinus rhythm may be undertaken electively—either *chemically* (quinidine gluconate 200 to 400 mg every 6 hours or glucuronate 324 to 628 mg every 8 to 12 hours, OR procainamide 250 to 1000 mg/day every 3 hours or as a sustained-release preparation every 6 hours, or 50 mg/minute intravenously up to 1000 mg, then maintenance infusion of 2 to 6 mg/minute) OR *electrically* with direct current cardioversion. If any sign of hemodynamic instability is present, direct current cardioversion (by Advanced Cardiac Life Support protocols) must be considered first line therapy. Maintenance therapy may or may not be necessary depending on the etiology of the rhythm. In cases in which conversion to sinus is not possible or maintenance of sinus rhythm is unlikely, chronic rate control is the goal.

Conversely, in acute bradydysrhythmias, the goal is to raise the effective ventricular rate either chemically (atropine, 0.5 to 1.0 mg initially, given by intravenous push, to a maximum of 2.0 mg) or electrically with pacing. In chronic conditions, medication is of no benefit and permanent pacing must be considered.

Although arrhythmias may be acute or chronic and result in minimal symptoms to full cardiovascular hemodynamic instability, for the most part, ventricular tachydysrhythmias are medical emergencies and require immediate intervention. For specific treatments and protocols refer to the Advanced Cardiac Life Support algorithms (see Figures 1-17 to 1-22) located in the appendix to this chapter beginning on page 60.

PEDIATRIC CONSIDERATIONS

Atrial

PACs occur in healthy children, as well as those experiencing digitalis toxicity or those who have undergone cardiac surgery. In children, isolated PACs generally do not cause symptoms and do not require treatment.

SVT is the most commonly occurring tachyarrhythmia in children. SVT is most often idiopathic, with an estimated 10% to 20% of cases due to underlying Wolff-Parkinson-White syndrome. If there is no evidence of hemodynamic compromise (CHF, chest pain, lightheadedness, syncope), then vagal stimulation maneuvers (carotid sinus massage, gagging, standing on head) are often effective and should be attempted first. For infants with hemodynamic compromise, conversion to sinus rhythm can often be achieved by momentarily placing a bag of ice over the baby's face to stimulate the diving reflex. For children with hemodynamic compromise, direct current synchronized cardioversion is the initial treatment of choice.

Atrial flutter occurs in children with congenital heart disease resulting in enlarged atria (e.g., mitral/tricuspid valve disease). It is also seen as a sequela of atrial surgery. Atrial flutter may occur in children with structurally normal hearts, but a high index of suspicion needs to be maintained for underlying cardiac disease. Treatment is always indicated in children.

AF is an uncommon arrhythmia in children. Most often occurs in the presence of enlarged atria or after atrial surgery. May occur in conjunction with Wolff-Parkinson-White syndrome.

Sick sinus syndrome and complete heart block may occur in children as a result of cardiac surgery or myocarditis, in association with congenital heart defects, or idiopathically. An infant whose mother has systemic lupus erythematosus is at increased risk for congenital complete heart block. Treatment is dependent on the patient's symptoms and ranges from pharmacologic intervention to the placement of a permanent pacemaker.

Ventricular

PVCs may occur in children with structurally normal hearts and should be considered a normal finding if they are uniform and are suppressed by exercise. Other common causes of PVCs are myocarditis, congenital heart disease, cardiac surgery, and drug toxicity. Additional evaluation should be conducted in children who have multiform PVCs, multiple PVCs (e.g., couplets, triplets), or PVCs that increase in frequency or are induced by exercise.

VT in children is generally associated with previous cardiac surgery. Other causes include cardiomyopathy, long Q-T syndrome, myocardial tumors, and drug toxicity. It is generally agreed that in asymptomatic patients with structurally normal hearts, treatment is unnecessary. In patients with altered hemodynamics, aggressive treatment is indicated.

VF is caused by the same factors as for VT. It is a medical emergency that necessitates immediate treatment. If the child becomes unconscious, direct current synchronized cardioversion is the treatment of choice. For the conscious child, pharmacologic treatment should begin immediately.

OBSTETRIC CONSIDERATIONS

The most common types of arrhythmias seen in pregnancy are the various kinds of tachycardias. When treatment of arrhythmias is indicated, most of the antiarrhythmic medications and electrical cardioversion can be used without danger to the fetus. One exception is the drug phenytoin, which is sometimes used for treatment of paroxysmal atrial flutter or AF or supraventricular and ventricular arrhythmias that are due to digitalis. Phenytoin is well known as a cause of congenital malformations.

Another medication that is contraindicated during pregnancy is warfarin sodium (coumadin). This drug has resulted in the "warfarin syndrome" (nasal hypoplasia, epiphyseal stippling, bilateral optic atrophy, scoliosis, mental retardation), other fetal central nervous system anomalies, spontaneous abortion, stillbirths, prematurity, and hemorrhage. If anticoagulation is indicated during the treatment of arrhythmias, the drug of choice in a pregnant patient is heparin. When heparin is used, however, there is an increased risk of maternal hemorrhage associated with the last trimester and the postpartum period.

In regard to specific arrhythmias, pregnancy in patients with AV block is well tolerated if there are no other cardiac problems. AF associated with valvular heart disease can be dangerous to both the mother and the fetus.

GERIATRIC CONSIDERATIONS

Patients of advanced age should be monitored for polypharmacy. Many drugs can interact to cause adverse events. Certain classes of cardiac drugs with antichronotropic properties—beta blockers, calcium blockers, and digitalis—are to be used in combination very cautiously. Inadvertent overdose can result, especially in those who are frail. Use of diuretics can lead to significant dehydration during periods of acute illness, potentially leading to kidney failure and higher drug levels. Electrolyte imbalance can also result, leading to arrhythmias. The use of tricyclic antidepressants in the depressed elderly should also be monitored, as overdosing can result and is difficult to treat. Fatigue and weakness are common symptoms of bradyarrhythmias and may be difficult to diagnose without careful examination of the patient. Tachyarrhythmias are often manifested as chest pain or breathlessness, as many elderly have undiagnosed coronary artery disease and do not have the functional reserves to compensate for elevated heart rates. Swift treatment is necessary.

PREVENTIVE CONSIDERATIONS

Preventive screening for arrhythmias in healthy children and adults is not recommended. A high index of suspicion is important in patients with underlying cardiac conditions who exhibit symptoms consistent with bradyarrhythmias or tachyarrhythmias.

PEARLS FOR THE PA

The ECG is the key to diagnosis, but paroxysmal arrhythmias may be missed.

A careful history, physical examination, and appropriate laboratory studies are key to establishing the etiology.

Clinical stability of the patient should always guide aggressiveness and timing of therapy.

Congestive Heart Failure

Edward Gaile, Sr., BA, BHS, PA-C

DEFINITION

Congestive heart failure (CHF) refers to that state in which abnormal circulatory congestion exists as a result of heart failure. The definition of CHF is most readily understood by considering each part of the term: *Congestive* in this context refers to the state of circulatory overload that inhibits the normal physiologic functions of tissue nutrition and elimination of metabolic waste. *Heart failure* refers to the origin or causative factor of the congestive state. Thus, CHF is a complex syndrome of cardiac structural abnormalities and functional disability that produces neuroendocrine and sympathetic nervous system responses resulting in symptomatic circulatory congestion.

HISTORY

Symptoms.   Dyspnea occurs primarily on exertion but may progress to shortness of breath at rest as heart failure becomes more severe. The worst form of dyspnea is the terrifying air hunger of pulmonary edema. Other signs and symptoms are orthopnea, paroxysmal nocturnal dyspnea, wheezing, nonproductive cough (frequently with exertion and at night), Cheyne-Stokes respirations, fatigue and weakness, night sweats, insomnia, diminished daytime urinary frequency and volume, nocturia, weight gain (subtle or sudden), peripheral edema, ascites, constipation, upper abdominal pain, cachexia, anxiety, confusion, and impairment of memory (usually in elderly with severe disease).

General.   The development of symptoms and clinical manifestations is subject to numerous factors including the patient's age, underlying cardiac lesion, extent and rate of cardiac impairment, and precipitating factors. The spectrum of symptoms and signs ranges from the mildest form, in which symptoms and cardiac impairment are produced only during marked stress, to the severe condition, in which even resting cardiac function cannot sustain life without external circulatory support.

Age.   Any.

Onset.   Extremely variable. The patient may present describing an indolent course of sporadic, few, and mild symptoms, often having no knowledge or recognized history of prior cardiac disease. Conversely, a patient may present with sudden, fulminant, life-threatening symptoms, usually with a previous history of cardiac disease but sometimes without, as in the case of sudden myocardial infarction with extensive loss of functional myocardium.

Duration.   Dependent on the state of circulatory congestion. The underlying cardiac disease/lesion may be permanent; however, the patient may avoid manifest CHF through ongoing treatment or avoidance of precipitating factors (e.g., exertion, infection, medication, noncompliance with treatment). In such cases the patient is commonly said to be in a compensated state of heart failure. Heart failure that, by virtue of a sum of signs and symptoms, produces circulatory congestion is often described as decompensated. With increasing severity (or in some cases duration) of the underlying cardiac lesion, a patient may progress to a state of constant circulatory congestion, despite avoidance of precipitating factors, that is refractory to treatment, producing what is sometimes referred to as the state of chronic CHF.

Intensity. Dependent on the degree of circulatory congestion. May be as mild as simple dyspnea on exertion or as severe as florid pulmonary edema with hypotension, acidosis, and impending circulatory collapse.

Aggravating Factors. Increasing severity of underlying cardiac disorder. Development of new cardiac lesion or condition (e.g., arrhythmia, myocardial infarction). Development of disease state affecting other organ systems (e.g., pulmonary emboli, pulmonary or systemic infection, renal failure, prostatic obstruction, liver disease, pregnancy). Development of a metabolic disorder (e.g., thyrotoxicosis). Increased workload (e.g., exertional/emotional stress, anemia, uncontrolled hypertension, arteriovenous fistula). Dietary indiscretion of sodium intake. Increased circulatory volume from intravenous fluid administration or transfusion, or drug-induced (e.g., corticosteroids, estrogen, nonsteroidal anti-inflammatory drugs [NSAIDs]). Most common aggravating factor, however, is lack of compliance with established treatment, diet, or medication, or with recommended level of exertional activity.

Alleviating Factors. Recognition of underlying cardiac disease/disorder and correction of condition if possible. Correction or elimination of external exacerbating factors: physical, environmental, or behavioral. Patients frequently alter lifestyle, diet, or exertional level (often without conscious intent) to avoid production of symptoms.

Associated Factors. Patients frequently engage in self-diagnosis and relate symptoms to other factors or disease entities (e.g., dyspnea and cough secondary to cigarette use, edema secondary to varicose veins). It is not uncommon for a patient to present with a preconceived diagnosis and give a history designed to prove it.

PHYSICAL EXAMINATION

General. General appearance is affected as the degree and chronicity of heart failure worsen. The patient with mild or early heart failure may appear normal and without distress at rest. Activity such as walking or dressing may produce dyspnea and an increase in pulse rate out of proportion to effort. Patients may be uncomfortable supine and prefer to sit or lie at an elevated angle. Jugular vein distention may be evident. Evidence of chronic, severe disease may be seen, with nondependent edema, generalized wasting, and frank cachexia.

Cardiovascular. Overall, findings may be variable from patient to patient, as the examiner may see, feel, or hear manifestations of the underlying cardiac disorder such as ectopic precordial impulses, murmurs, or dysrhythmias. The hallmark finding is the S_3 gallop sound. An S_4 gallop sound may be heard in combination with the S_3, producing a complex referred to as a summation gallop. Many forms of cardiac disorders produce CHF without cardiac enlargement, although it is frequently present.

Extremities. Ankle and pretibial edema may be seen.

Gastrointestinal. Tender or nontender hepatomegaly or ascites may be present.

Pulmonary. Moist rales may be heard on auscultation, or the chest may be dull to percussion (unilaterally or bilaterally). Cheyne-Stokes respirations may be present with severe heart failure. The patient with pulmonary edema may present with severe air hunger, anxiousness, or a sense of "impending doom."

Skin. Mild diaphoresis, mild jaundice, dusky complexion, extremity pallor and coolness, or peripheral cyanosis may be observed with various degrees of heart failure.

PATHOPHYSIOLOGY

The pathophysiology of CHF involves many variables, including structural and functional abnormalities of the heart and the homeostatic reaction of neuroendocrine and sympathetic nervous systems. Abnormality of cardiac function leads ultimately to reduced perfusion of organ systems and increased venous volume, producing circulatory congestion, which in turn prompts compensatory reactions of regulatory mechanisms.

Pathogenic entities that compromise cardiac functional ability fall into three categories:

1. Conditions that produce myocardial (muscular) failure such as idiopathic and dilated cardiomyopathy, myocarditis, metabolic/toxic disorders (beriberi, alcoholism, thyrotoxicosis), and loss of adequate muscle mass (myocardial infarction, tumor)
2. Conditions that produce mechanical abnormalities such as obstruction of blood from cardiac chambers (stenotic valvular disease, supra- or subvalvular obstruction), increased volume and workload (regurgitant valvular disease, cardiac or vascular shunts), pericardial tamponade, restrictive and hypertrophic cardiomyopathy, and ventricular aneurysm
3. Arrhythmias such as VF and cardiac standstill, extreme bradycardia and/or tachycardias, and conduction disturbances

Adaptive responses occur in neuroendocrine and sympathetic systems and are aimed at maintaining perfusion pressures of vital organs and compensating for reduced effective cardiac output. Ironically, the end result of diminished cardiac output is interpreted by the body as a reduction in total circulatory volume. This results in activation of the systemic renin-angiotensin-aldosterone and sympathetic nervous systems. Thus, neuroendocrine activation leads to an increase in the intravascular volume, whereas sympathetic responses produce increased heart rate and increased systemic vascular resistance.

DIAGNOSTIC STUDIES

Laboratory

Complete Blood Count. Usually normal but may reflect mild anemia in chronic states. Profound anemia is a possible precipitating factor. White blood cell count is elevated in infection.

Erythrocyte Sedimentation Rate. May be very low.

Serum Electrolytes. Normal in mild heart failure. In severe states, hyponatremia of dilutional origin may develop. With diuretic therapy, hyponatremia, hypochloremia, and hypokalemia are frequent. In later stages, hyperkalemia and elevated blood urea nitrogen and creatinine levels may result from reduced renal blood flow secondary to markedly low cardiac output.

Liver Function Tests. May reflect hepatic congestion with elevated bilirubin, alkaline phosphatase, lactate dehydrogenase (LDH), aspartate transaminase (AST) [formerly serum glutamic-oxaloacetic transaminase (SGOT)], alanine transaminase (ALT) [formerly serum glutamic-pyruvic transaminase (SGPT)].

Thyroid Function Tests. Usually normal; however, useful in differential diagnosis when coupled with other clinical signs and symptoms. May reflect hyperthyroid (rarely hypothyroid) state.

Arterial Blood Gas Analysis. Widely variable and dependent on severity of congestion and concomitant pulmonary disease.

Radiology

Chest Film. Cardiomegaly frequently present but not a consistent finding. Various degrees of pulmonary congestion may be present, singly or in combination: redistribution of pulmonary venous flow to upper lobes, Kerley B lines, loss of distinct margins of central and peripheral vasculature, hilar fullness (dilatation of central pulmonary veins) and clouding (edema), or diffuse cloudlike haziness of lung fields (alveolar pulmonary edema). Pleural fluid may be present either bilaterally or unilaterally (right side predominates); the radiograph may show only blunting of costophrenic angles or may reveal hydrothorax (free pleural effusion).

Other

ECG. There is no specific ECG abnormality that indicates the presence or absence of CHF. May reflect the changes of the underlying cardiac disorder (e.g., arrhythmia, myocardial infarction).

Lung Scan/Pulmonary Arteriography. Useful when presence of pulmonary emboli is suspected as an underlying cause or precipitating factor. Even with positive test results, other causes of heart failure must be considered.

Echocardiogram. Variable findings dependent on the underlying cardiac disorder. Useful in evaluating chamber sizes, wall thickness and motion, valvular integrity, ventricular function/ejection fraction, pericardial thickness, and fluid.

Cardiac Catheterization. Variable findings and limited in scope of assessing cardiac function and underlying disorder. Useful in assessing coronary disease, left ventricular function, valvular and subvalvular anatomy, and intracardiac shunts.

DIFFERENTIAL DIAGNOSIS

Traumatic
Pneumothorax.   May have history of chest injury. Paroxysmal dyspnea not relieved by change in position. Dyspnea rapidly increasing in severity and unremitting. Other possible findings: displaced trachea, chest tympany, absence of breath sounds on affected side, asymmetrical respiratory excursions of chest wall. Chest film reveals free air in thorax and lung compression.

Infectious
Pneumonia.   Febrile, productive cough with purulent sputum. May have pleuritic chest pain. Chest film more likely to show consolidation and segmental infiltrate. Laboratory tests may reflect infection with elevated white blood cell count and positive sputum and/or blood cultures.

Metabolic
Renal Failure.   Not merely prerenal azotemia. Creatinine and blood urea nitrogen levels very high, creatinine clearance very low. Urine may contain many casts and much protein.
Hepatic Disease, Intrinsic.   Hepatitis with very high values on liver function tests (enzymes). No evidence of elevated venous pressure. Edema and dyspnea usually absent. No gallop on examination.

Neoplastic
Not applicable.

Vascular
Pulmonary Emboli (Without Production of Mechanical Heart Failure). Chest pain, frequently pleuritic. Dyspnea is paroxysmal and may not be relieved by any maneuvers. May have hemoptysis and fever. Frequent evidence of deep venous thrombosis. Chest film is normal or reveals wedge-shaped segmental density(ies).

Acquired
Chronic Obstructive Pulmonary Disease.   Dyspnea in COPD more likely to develop gradually and not be relieved by reduction in body fluid volume. Bronchospasm is responsive to bronchodilator therapy. Sputum usually present. Discriminating features may be subtle, as COPD and CHF frequently are found concomitantly.

TREATMENT

Correct underlying cardiac disorder: Surgical repair of valvular lesions, shunts, ventricular aneurysm, congenital malformations. Treat arrhythmia.

Remove precipitating causes: Ensure treatment compliance, correct anemias, control hypertension, restrict sodium intake, and reduce or stop, if possible, NSAIDs, corticosteroids, estrogens.

Control circulatory congestion: Reduce cardiac workload: Reduce physical activity and lower emotional/environmental stresses. Control obesity if needed. Institute vasodilator therapy. In late, refractory stage, intra-aortic balloon pump may be indicated.

Improve cardiac contractility: Digitalis is the first-line pharmacologic agent. In severe cases, sympathomimetic agents, (e.g., dopamine, dobutamine) and phosphodiesterase inhibitors (e.g., amrinone, milrinone). If indicated, pacemaker.

Control/reduce excess fluid and sodium retention: Low-sodium diet, diuretics. In severe CHF, invasive removal of pleural effusion or ascitic fluid may be required. In refractory states, dialysis and/or ultrafiltration may be indicated.

Address neuroendocrine and sympathetic responses: Long-term management should include an angiotensin-converting enzyme (ACE) inhibitor, spironolactone, and a beta receptor–blocking agent such as carvedilol.

PEDIATRIC CONSIDERATIONS

Congenital heart disease is almost always the cause of CHF in the child, and the underlying cardiac lesion may have a latent presentation. Early recognition is essential for a favorable prognosis.

The clinical presentation of CHF in infants and children is markedly different from that in adults. In infants, a history of poor feeding, inability to nurse for extended periods of time, tachypnea and diaphoresis with feedings, poor weight gain, and wheezing or coughing may indicate CHF. Physical findings include tachycardia, tachypnea, diaphoresis, nostril flaring, intercostal retractions, dependent peripheral edema, dyspnea on exertion, orthopnea, wheezing, rales, gallop rhythm, and hepatomegaly. The presence of cardiomegaly on chest film is perhaps the most consistent finding. The causes of CHF in children are numerous and include defects that result in volume overload or pressure overload of the heart. Common volume overload defects in infants include patent ductus arteriosis and ventricular septal defects. Pressure overload is most often due to severe pulmonic or aortic stenosis or coarctation of the aorta. Primary management involves pharmacologic treatment with diuretics and digitalis.

OBSTETRIC CONSIDERATIONS

The routine management of CHF with morphine, oxygen, digitalis, rotating tourniquets, and diuretics is considered safe in the pregnant patient with CHF.

PEARLS FOR THE PA

CHF is a secondary manifestation of a primary disorder, and it is incumbent on the clinician to identify that disorder.

CHF therapy must address structural and functional abnormalities of the myocardium, reduce cardiac workload, relieve circulatory congestion, and control harmful compensatory homeostatic neuroendocrine and sympathetic nervous system responses.

GERIATRIC CONSIDERATIONS

Elderly smokers who complain of shortness of breath may be exhibiting symptoms of CHF rather than primary pulmonary disease.

PREVENTIVE CONSIDERATIONS

Compliance with treatment regimens must be emphasized. Correction of underlying contributing factors should be initiated.

Cor Pulmonale

Edward Gaile, Sr., BA, BHS, PA-C

DEFINITION

Cor pulmonale is a term that describes the pathologic effects of lung dysfunction on the right side of the heart. The definition of cor pulmonale is right ventricular dilatation, with or without hypertrophy, caused by hypertension of the pulmonary circulation due to pulmonary dysfunction. Right-sided (right ventricular) heart failure is a complication of cor pulmonale, not an essential feature of it. Excluded from the definition are pulmonary hypertension and right ventricular dysfunction due to left ventricular or congenital heart disease.

HISTORY

Symptoms. There are no specific symptoms of cor pulmonale. However, conditions that are a consequence of cor pulmonale produce symptoms that are widely variable and usually reflect the underlying pulmonary disorder or systemic venous congestion. Dyspnea at rest that is greatly exacerbated by exertion and not relieved by change in position, easy fatigability, productive and/or nonproductive cough, nonspecific chest pain, peripheral edema, upper abdominal fullness and tenderness, ascites, visible neck vein distention and wave fluctuations, and cyanosis may be present alone or in combination.

General. Because the origins of pulmonary hypertension are so diverse, there is no history particularly specific for cor pulmonale. A high index of suspicion for this disorder is indicated in any patient with pulmonary hypertension and/or any disorder causing chronic hypoxemia.

Age. Any.

Onset. Widely variable, depending on cause of right ventricular dilatation/hypertrophy from pulmonary hypertension. Clinical presentation may be acute and dramatic, as in the case of massive pulmonary embolism. Majority of cases, however, have slow, insidious development.

Duration.   Dependent on chronicity of underlying cause of pulmonary hypertension.

Intensity.   Acute cor pulmonale may be of severe, catastrophic intensity, as in the case of massive pulmonary embolism. In the remainder of cases, when cor pulmonale is present, it is tempting to measure its intensity as a function of the degree of venous congestion caused by right ventricular failure.

Aggravating Factors.   Any factor that produces or worsens pulmonary hypertension (e.g., pulmonary emboli, chronic alveolar hypoxia, exercise, polycythemia, high altitude).

Alleviating Factors.   Any factor or condition that reduces severity of pulmonary hypertension (e.g., lysis of pulmonary emboli, correction of chronic alveolar hypoxia).

Associated Factors.   Patients (and clinicians) describe aggravating and alleviating factors in terms of symptoms that are referable to the underlying pulmonary disorder or existing venous congestion.

PHYSICAL EXAMINATION

General.   Generally, physical stigmata of the underlying pulmonary disorder predominate (e.g., "blue bloater" of chronic bronchitis, "pink puffer" of emphysema). Obesity, severe kyphoscoliosis, and inspiratory and expiratory adventitious sounds are frequently present.

Cardiovascular.   In cor pulmonale with right-sided heart failure, distended neck veins that do not collapse with inspiration and prominent a and v waves may be observed.

Precordium.   Check for sternal lift from right ventricular heave, palpable S_2.

Auscultation.   Evaluate left sternal border and/or epigastrium for right-sided S_3 gallop sound. Note that quality of S_2 will be loud—booming at times—and P_2 is intensified. Listen for systolic ejection click in pulmonic region, left of upper sternum. Note any murmurs; frequently heard is the holosystolic murmur of tricuspid regurgitation located at the lower left parasternal edge, which is accentuated by inspiration. Rarely, a diastolic murmur of pulmonary valve regurgitation will be heard.

Extremities.   In acute cor pulmonale from pulmonary embolism, the patient may have evidence of deep venous thrombosis; phlebitis is frequently present. In cor pulmonale with right-sided heart failure, peripheral edema (sometimes massive) may be seen.

Gastrointestinal.   In cor pulmonale with right ventricular heart failure, hepatomegaly (occasionally pulsatile, usually tender) or ascites may be present.

Pulmonary.   In acute cor pulmonale from pulmonary embolism, the patient may not have stigmata of COPD. In such cases, appearance is one of severe anxiety, breathlessness, pallor, diaphoresis, hypotension, rapid and thready pulse, and near-collapse.

Skin.   In cor pulmonale with right ventricular heart failure, cyanosis may be evident.

PATHOPHYSIOLOGY

Increased pulmonary vascular resistance and pulmonary hypertension caused by pathologic conditions of the lung parenchyma and/or pulmonary vasculature producing increased afterload on the right ventricle, causing right ventricular dilatation with or without hypertrophy.

Cor pulmonale can be the result of an acute or a chronic condition. Acute cor pulmonale is a result of sudden, massive obstruction of the pulmonary circulation by large or multiple emboli. Chronic cor pulmonale may be caused by any of numerous long-term conditions with diverse pathophysiologic characteristics but with the common end result of producing pulmonary hypertension. For simplicity, these conditions can be separated into those that affect pulmonary vasculature and those that are (primarily) respiratory diseases. The following are examples (not all-inclusive).

Pulmonary Vasculature. Chronic, small pulmonary emboli; sickle cell thrombosis; primary pulmonary hypertension; acute respiratory distress syndrome (ARDS); toxic or particulate intravenous drug use; collagen vascular disorders; granulomatous arteritis.

Respiratory Diseases. Chronic obstructive pulmonary disease (COPD) such as chronic bronchitis or emphysema, or from cystic fibrosis. Chronic hypoventilation conditions such as severe obesity, sleep apnea syndrome, and neuromuscular weakness. Chest wall abnormalities (e.g., kyphoscoliosis). Diffuse interstitial diseases such as sarcoid, idiopathic pulmonary fibrosis, and chronic fungal infections. Also, unusual causes such as high-altitude disease (chronic mountain sickness), pulmonary resection, encroaching mediastinal tumor, and radiation injury.

DIAGNOSTIC STUDIES

Because of the diverse pathophysiologic conditions that may lead to pulmonary hypertension and cor pulmonale, the character of diagnostic studies will vary greatly. Each condition will display laboratory, radiographic, and other diagnostic study results unique to its pathologic cause and effect. Because cor pulmonale is a secondary condition due to a primary disorder, careful consideration of those entities that can lead to pulmonary hypertension is essential.

Regardless of causative condition, primary diagnostic evidence suggesting the presence of cor pulmonale may include the following.

Radiology
Chest Film. Right ventricular enlargement and filling of retrosternal space on lateral view; enlargement of main pulmonary artery and major branches, right greater than 16 mm in diameter; pruning (narrowing) of peripheral arterial vessels.

Other
ECG. Frequently normal. Presence of the so-called P pulmonale, tall peaked P waves, particularly in tracings from inferior leads (II, III, aV_F) and V_1; QRS right axis deviation frequently coupled with prominent R in V_1 to V_3, deep S in V_6, ST segment depression, T wave inversion in precordial leads.

Echocardiogram. Right ventricular dilatation and/or hypertrophy. A majority of patients have tricuspid regurgitation.

First Pass Multiple-Gated Acquisition Scan (MUGA). Reduced right ventricular ejection fraction.

Thallium 201 Scan. Thickening of free wall of the right ventricle.

Right Heart Catheterization. Elevated pulmonary artery pressures and vascular resistance, normal pulmonary capillary wedge pressure (PCWP), and wide difference between pulmonary artery diastolic pressure and PCWP.

DIFFERENTIAL DIAGNOSIS

Cor pulmonale is unique in that it is a distinct anatomic condition (right ventricular dilatation and/or hypertrophy) resulting from pulmonary hypertension caused by numerous and diverse disorders of the pulmonary system. The end result of cor pulmonale may be the production of the signs and symptoms of circulatory congestion commonly known as congestive heart failure (CHF). Differential diagnosis, then, becomes a matter of determining the origin of the symptoms of circulatory congestion (e.g., right-sided heart failure versus left-sided heart failure) while remembering that right ventricular dysfunction that is a result of left ventricular dysfunction or congenital heart disease is excluded from the definition of cor pulmonale. In summary, the diagnosis of primary right ventricular failure as a result of cor pulmonale requires the concurrence of historical, physical, and diagnostic data that implicate right ventricular dysfunction due to disease states that produce pulmonary parenchymal or vasculature abnormalities.

TREATMENT

Treatment is directed at improving the pulmonary disorder to decrease pulmonary hypertension and managing right ventricular heart failure.

Vigorous and aggressive management of the underlying pulmonary disease is required. Long-term, continuous oxygen therapy is essential to reduce hypoxic pulmonary vasoconstriction. This is in addition to any therapeutic agents or measures to improve concomitant pulmonary or systemic disease such as bronchodilators, antibiotics, pulmonary toilet, corticosteroids, discontinuance and/or avoidance of respiratory irritants, and weight reduction.

Circulatory congestion caused by right ventricular failure is managed with the therapeutic modalities used in the treatment of any form of CHF: ensuring treatment compliance, reducing sodium intake and exertional stress, weight reduction (if needed), initiation of diuretic therapy, and so forth. The use of digitalis and vasodilator therapy may be considered, although controversy remains over their long-term efficacy in right ventricular failure. In conditions causing polycythemia, phlebotomy to reduce red blood cell mass to less than 55% should be considered.

PEDIATRIC CONSIDERATIONS

Cystic fibrosis and primary pulmonary hypertension are the major pulmonary disorders leading to cor pulmonale in the pediatric age group.

Pulmonary hypertension in children is often associated with congenital heart disease, which therefore must be carefully ruled out as a potential cause. Pulmonary hypertension secondary to a congenital heart defect rarely persists if surgically corrected before 2 years of age. Occasionally, children develop pulmonary hypertension without a known causative disorder (idiopathic pulmonary hypertension). Management of children with idiopathic pulmonary hypertension primarily involves symptomatic treatment. These children develop polycythemia, CHF, and arrhythmias and require treatment for these conditions as well. Idiopathic pulmonary hypertension is progressive and irreversible. It generally has a fatal outcome within 1 year of diagnosis.

OBSTETRIC CONSIDERATIONS

In a female patient with preexisting kyphoscoliotic heart disease, cor pulmonale can develop if she becomes pregnant.

GERIATRIC CONSIDERATIONS

Conditions that may aggravate the underlying pathology increase in frequency with advancing age.

PREVENTIVE CONSIDERATIONS

Prevention of factors that aggravate or cause cor pulmonale, including prophylaxis for pulmonary emboli (heparin, platelet-inhibiting medication, sequential compression hose), recognition of polycythemia vera, recognition of symptoms at altitude, smoking cessation.

PEARLS FOR THE PA

Cor pulmonale is an anatomic disorder of the right ventricle caused by pulmonary disease.

Any patient with severe lung disease or conditions causing chronic hypoxemia, or who has evidence of pulmonary hypertension, should be evaluated for cor pulmonale.

CHF may be present in cor pulmonale; pulmonary edema is not.

Coronary Atherosclerotic Heart Disease

Edward Gaile, Sr., BA, BHS, PA-C, and
Thomas M. Richardson, MBA, PA-C

DEFINITION

A multifactorial metabolic disorder of the arteries of the heart leading to stenosis of variable degree that may lead to closure of the lumen of the artery. It is the leading cause of morbidity and mortality in North America and western Europe.

HISTORY

Symptoms. A pressure, band, viselike, burning, or crushing sensation, reported most frequently in the midsternal region. Frequently associated with radiation of the discomfort to the back, scapula, shoulder, arm, neck, jaw, or epigastric region. Patient may have slight to severe nausea, shortness of breath, or diaphoresis, or may experience vomiting.

General. Symptoms occur when the myocardial oxygen demand exceeds supply. Symptoms are most likely to occur during exertion but may occur at rest.

Age. Any; however, the risk is increased with advancing age, usually after 40 years of age.

Onset. The onset of the disease is slow and gradual, but the symptoms may be acute. Initial symptoms occur shortly before death in 25% of cases.

Intensity. Varies from a mild nagging sensation to severe crushing pain. Location of the lesion in the myocardial circulation and the degree of stenosis can play a role in the severity of symptoms.

Aggravating Factors. Any condition or event producing increased myocardial oxygen demand such as emotional upset, cold temperature, eating a large meal, exertion, and underlying medical conditions.

Alleviating Factors. Any measure that equilibrates supply and demand of the myocardium such as rest, relief of emotional stress, or correction of underlying metabolic abnormality.

Associated Factors. Risk factors include genetic predisposition, hypercholesterolemia, diabetes mellitus, advancing age, male gender, hypertension, smoking, poor diet, lower socioeconomic status, obesity, sedentary lifestyle, and residence in the southeastern United States.

PHYSICAL EXAMINATION

General. The physical examination plays a relatively small role in the diagnosis of coronary atherosclerotic heart disease (CASHD) and myocardial infarction. Pulse rate is usually rapid, but bradycardia is possible. Low-grade fever may be associated with myocardial infarction. Blood pressure may be elevated or depressed. Hypotension is an ominous sign.

Cardiovascular. Auscultate for murmurs, gallops, S_3, or signs of congestive heart failure (CHF) that may indicate myocardial dysfunction.

Pulmonary. Auscultate for rales, which may suggest CHF.

PATHOPHYSIOLOGY

CASHD is a progressive disease beginning in childhood with clinical signs and symptoms appearing in mid- to late adulthood.

Symptoms of CASHD occur when blood supply cannot meet the oxygen demands of the myocardium. This deficit may result from atherosclerotic changes due to plaque and/or thrombus within the lumen, or nonatherosclerotic changes from disorders such as collagen vascular disease, congenital anomalies, or dissecting aneurysm of the aorta or coronary artery. The normal response to increased myocardial demand is arterial dilatation. In patients with CASHD, vasodilatation may not occur, and the vessels can, in some instances, undergo vasoconstriction.

Coronary atherosclerosis is the most common cause of coronary artery disease (CAD). Atheromatous lesions are formed as follows: As low density lipoprotein (LDL) enters the endothelial cell wall, it is taken up by macrophages to form foam cells. Ruptured foam cells, along with debris from cellular death, form the lesion. The lesion can further enlarge with fissure, disruption, or thrombus formation. This may lead to complete obstruction of the vessel. Blood flow through a vessel with a fixed stenotic lesion is usually adequate until a 70% to 90% cross-sectional area of the lumen is affected. Once this is exceeded, distal flow may drop significantly during exercise or at rest. Angina is stable as long as the plaque remains stable and causes only mild to moderate obstruction. The most common cause of unstable angina is a nonocclusive thrombus on a fissured or eroded plaque. Disruption of the plaque releases aggregating platelets, which in turn contribute to continued thrombus formation and vessel compromise.

DIAGNOSTIC STUDIES

Laboratory

C-Reactive Protein/Homocysteine. Being researched for use in screening for/prediction of myocardial infarction.

Complete Blood Count/Platelets/Prothrombin Time/Partial Thromboplastin Time. Evaluate for contributing disorders such as anemia or hypercoagulable state.

Cardiac Enzymes. Cardiac isoenzymes—creatine kinase (CK), aspartate transaminase (AST) [formerly serum glutamic-oxaloacetic transaminase (SGOT)], and lactate dehydrogenase (LDH)—demonstrate staged peak elevations with myocardial infarction. CK rises within 3 to 4 hours after onset of infarction and peaks in 12 to 16 hours. AST peaks at 24 to 48 hours, and

LDH rises at 36 to 48 hours and peaks at 4 to 7 days. CK-MB is an isoenzyme specific for cardiac muscle.

Radiology
Chest Film.   Nonspecific for CASHD or angina. Aorta or coronary arteries may be calcified.

Coronary Artery Angiography.   Will show the presence or absence of lesions within the coronary arteries. It also allows measurement of left ventricular end diastolic pressure and left ventricular function.

Other
ECG.   Resting ECG is normal in 50% to 75% of patients. Q waves may be present with old or new myocardial infarctions. ST segment elevation suggests acute myocardial infarction. ST segment depression suggests ischemia, and T wave inversion suggests subendocardial injury in the corresponding area of the heart represented by the ECG leads.

Exercise Stress Test.   Evaluates the heart under increased myocardial oxygen demand. The test is limited by the patient's ability to achieve a target heart rate during progressive increments of workload, heart rate–limiting drugs, and the presence of left bundle branch block. Results of stress testing considered positive include ST segment changes, hypotensive episodes during exercise, and development of left bundle branch block, arrhythmias, or other changes during exercise (e.g., shortness of breath, diaphoresis, chest pain, early fatigue). Test may utilize thallium or other isotopes that are injected during peak exercise periods to define perfused versus unperfused areas of myocardium. The test may also involve the administration of persantine, which acts to increase oxygen demand pharmacologically and is used for patients who are unable to reach a target heart rate through exercise.

DIFFERENTIAL DIAGNOSIS

Traumatic
Chest Wall Contusion/Costochondriasis.   Pain is exacerbated or produced with any tension on the chest, bones, or muscles of the chest.

Traumatic Aortic Dissection.   History of blunt chest trauma or deceleration injury.

Infectious
Acute Pericarditis.   Pain usually occurs in younger patients and is of sudden onset, severe, and persistent and is intensified with Valsalva maneuver. Usually relieved by leaning forward and/or sitting up. Friction rub may be present on physical examination. ECG may show widespread ST segment elevation.

Pneumonia.   Produces a pleural-type pain that increases with cough or movement. Physical examination demonstrates a pleural rub or rales. Infiltrate may be seen on chest film. Sputum cultures may be positive for causative organism.

Metabolic
Hyperthrombosis. Various disorders may cause coronary artery occlusion by thrombus of red blood cells.

Neoplastic
Tumor that produces pressure, inflammation, or invasion of pericardial, pleural, muscular, or skeletal surfaces may cause chest pain. Seen on CT scan or chest film.

Vascular
Coronary Artery Spasm. Transient, nonfixed total or partial occlusion of the coronary artery lumen secondary to spasm of the smooth muscle in the artery wall.
Coronary Artery Emboli. Due to endocarditis, prosthetic valve, or left ventricular thrombus.
Pulmonary Artery Emboli. Secondary to thrombus from the left side of the heart, vegetative valves of the left side of the heart, or aortic disease.
Aortic Dissection. Due to a combination of atheromatous plaque and hypertension. Associated with a sudden onset of pain, described as "ripping" or "tearing," that radiates to the chest or abdomen.
Pulmonary Hypertension. Multiple causative disorders. Pain is due to pressure on the vascular bed.
Arteriovenous Fistula. Deep in the coronary vasculature; causes a distal vascular steal.

Congenital
Anomalous origins of the coronary arteries, arteriovenous fistula, hypoplastic or aplastic coronary arteries. Congenital abnormalities are usually discovered early in life and rarely cause chest pain in the elderly population.

TREATMENT

The goals of therapy are to alleviate immediate discomfort, limit the amount of myocardial damage, prevent further damage, and manage long-term problems.

Acute Myocardial Infarction
Sedation with anxiolytics is the first step in management.

Relieve discomfort with morphine or other analgesics. Use with caution in hypotensive patients (mean arterial pressure <65 mm Hg).

Recanalize the artery with angioplasty, atherectomy, thrombolytic agents (e.g., tissue plasminogen activator, streptokinase), or surgery.

Treat secondary conditions such as hypotension, CHF, arrhythmias, or arterial or ventricular rupture.

Unstable or Stable Angina
Relieve discomfort with analgesics (e.g., opiates).

Administer nitrates (intravenous, sublingual, transdermal, or oral), calcium channel blockers, beta blockers, or angiotensin-converting enzyme (ACE) inhibitors to re-equilibrate the supply and demand of oxygen. The goals of therapy are to keep the mean arterial pressure greater than 65 and less than 70 mm Hg, maintain the heart rate at 70 to 80 beats/minute, and prevent coronary artery spasm.

Consider intravenous heparin (1000 mL/hour after a 5000-mL bolus) with or without ECG changes.

Consider long-term, low-dose aspirin (baby aspirin) every day to reduce platelet aggregation.

PEDIATRIC CONSIDERATIONS

It is not recommended that asymptomatic children and adolescents have sports pre-participation ECGs as a part of the routine physical examination. CAD is extremely rare in this population, but distinguishing cardiac from noncardiac chest pain in this age group may be difficult. If myocardial chest pain is suspected by history, consideration should be given to familial hyperlipoproteinemia (especially adopted children), pericarditis, Kawasaki disease with coronary artery involvement, anomalous origin of the coronary arteries, arrhythmias, and obstructive cardiac lesions. ECG findings may differ in children. Initially, the findings include ST segment elevation and abnormally large Q waves that may persist for several years (Q waves may be normal). Over a period of 2 to 3 weeks the ST segment will gradually return to normal. During this time, the T wave may become inverted. Once the diagnosis is confirmed, a thorough search for the underlying disorder is performed so that effective therapy can commence.

OBSTETRIC CONSIDERATIONS

This premenopausal age group is usually protected from CAD by the presence of hormones; however, family history of dyslipidemias should be obtained. CAD leading to myocardial infarction occurs in about 1 out of 10,000 live births. Pregnant women are more susceptible to spontaneous intimal dissection, which appears as acute myocardial infarction, during or after delivery. The dissection is not associated with CAD. Consider obtaining a baseline ECG in all pregnant women who develop gestational diabetes so that there is a point for comparison if there is suspicion of the development of CAD. Recently diagnosed diabetic patients can develop significant heart disease. Patients with class I and class II heart disease (New York Heart Association classification system) rarely progress to cardiac failure while pregnant. In contrast, patients with class III and class IV heart disease should be strongly discouraged from becoming pregnant. If such a patient becomes pregnant, complete bedrest during the entire confinement is indicated. The safety of thrombolytic agents has not yet been firmly established for pregnant women. Thrombolytics should be used when clearly indicated; however, their use does carry a risk of hemorrhage in the pregnant patient.

GERIATRIC CONSIDERATIONS

CASHD incidence increases with advancing age. Often, multiple factors are involved in the accumulation of plaque and development of CAD. Risk factors should continue to be addressed regardless of age.

PREVENTIVE CONSIDERATIONS

Primary prevention remains the cornerstone of management in all patients. Screening includes blood pressure measurements, support for tobacco use avoidance/cessation, cholesterol testing (see Hypercholesterolemia: Dyslipidemia in Chapter 4), and recommendations for increased exercise and healthy diet included in every patient encounter.

Enrollment in a cardiac rehabilitation program following myocardial infarction or surgical intervention is recommended to reinforce prevention efforts and to prevent a second cardiac event. Family members are also educated about cardiac risk factors. Exercise training should begin with structured physical conditioning followed by an exercise test after 3 to 6 weeks, and then increasing exercise gradually.

There is not sufficient evidence to recommend for or against screening middle-aged and older persons of either sex for asymptomatic CAD with ECG (resting, ambulatory, or exercise). Screening asymptomatic high-risk persons is indicated when the results will influence treatment decisions. Screening asymptomatic persons is recommended for certain populations whose work affects public safety (e.g., pilots, truck drivers).

Noninvasive testing using high-speed CT has been shown to identify calcifications associated with atherosclerotic vessels and will be used more routinely as a screening tool in the future.

PEARLS FOR THE PA

The key to diagnosis is the history.

Primary preventive efforts such as smoking cessation, screening for hyperlipidemia, and encouraging exercise and healthy diet should be a part of all patient encounters.

Time equals myocardium, so confirm the diagnosis early and treat effectively.

Essential Hypertension

Lisa Mustone Alexander, EdD, MPH, PA-C

DEFINITION

Chronic condition characterized by elevation of the systolic and/ or diastolic blood pressure (>140/90 mm Hg, or marked at >170/110 mm Hg).

HISTORY

Symptoms

With *essential* hypertension: Usually none; however, the patient may complain of headaches and epistaxis with severe hypertension.

With *secondary* hypertension: Depending on the etiology, patients may have any of numerous symptoms. Renovascular hypertension should be suspected in patients who have symptoms suggestive of chronic glomerulonephritis and pyelonephritis such as recurrent hematuria. Patients suffering from aortic coarctation have no symptoms until the hypertension produces left ventricular hypertrophy. Signs and symptoms such as tremor, sweating, and pallor (suggestive of pheochromocytoma) must also be considered for establishing a diagnosis of secondary hypertension. Patients presenting with truncal obesity and purple striae should be evaluated for Cushing syndrome.

With *malignant* hypertension: An acute presentation, with symptoms of progressive renal failure, left ventricular heart failure, and stroke.

General.   Usually, patients are unaware of the condition. Risk factors associated with cardiovascular disease (e.g., smoking, obesity, high fat diet) are most often also present. Patients may have a history or symptoms of cerebrovascular or renal disease, diabetes mellitus, hyperlipidemia, or gout. Often, patients may have been treated for hypertension in the past and discontinued medication because of cost or side effects. A family history is of crucial importance, as is a dietary assessment. Psychosocial and environmental factors, especially employment, family support, and education, must also be determined. A drug history, including both prescription and over-the-counter drugs, is useful if the patient requires antihypertensive drug therapy, as there may be potential drug interactions to consider. Drug history for contraceptive use is also important to establish, as these agents may cause mild elevations in blood pressure.

Age.   Usually detected in the fourth to fifth decades of life. Men, particularly in middle age, are most commonly affected by essential hypertension. The prevalence in women increases with advancing age.

Onset.   Usually gradual.

Duration.   Essential hypertension is a lifelong condition.

Intensity.   If the disorder is treated and the patient's compliance is good, the patient's risk for cardiovascular morbidity and mortality decreases. If the condition is left untreated or the patient's compliance is poor, then the risk of target organ damage and cardiovascular morbidity increases.

Aggravating Factors. Noncompliance with medication or lifestyle modification strategies, caffeine, smoking, adrenergic stimulants (e.g., nasal decongestants or eye drops for pupillary dilatation).

Alleviating Factors. Weight loss, sodium restriction, and alcohol and tobacco avoidance all have been shown to lower blood pressure. For secondary hypertension, treatment of the underlying disorder will generally restore the patient to a normotensive state.

Associated Factors. African Americans are at greater risk to develop essential hypertension, as are elderly persons.

PHYSICAL EXAMINATION

General. An elevation in the systolic and/or diastolic blood pressure measurement on two or more readings separated by 2 minutes. Verification in the contralateral arm and with the patient sitting, lying, or standing. Arm should be supported at the level of the heart. Cuff size should be appropriate for the patient. Home readings can be taken to avoid "white coat hypertension." Height and weight measurements should also be documented.

Cardiovascular. Signs of left ventricular hypertrophy or dysfunction such as increased rate, displacement of the apical impulse, precordial heave, clicks, murmurs, arrhythmias, and the presence of S_3 or S_4 heart sounds.

Extremities. Any sign of diminished or absent peripheral arterial pulsations, bruits, and edema.

Gastrointestinal. Check for the presence of bruits, enlarged kidneys, masses, and abnormal aortic pulsation.

Head, Eyes, Ears, Nose, Throat (HEENT). Examination should look for carotid bruits, distended veins, or any enlargement of the thyroid.

Neurologic. Global assessment, with particular attention to cerebellar function.

Ophthalmologic. Check for arteriolar narrowing, arteriovenous (AV) nicking, hemorrhages, exudates, or papilledema on funduscopic examination.

PATHOPHYSIOLOGY

Essential hypertension is due primarily to increased peripheral arteriolar resistance of unknown mechanism. Secondary hypertension may or may not differ in the pathophysiology of the disease. For instance, in pheochromocytoma, hypertension is due to both increased cardiac output and peripheral resistance caused by epinephrine and norepinephrine, respectively.

DIAGNOSTIC STUDIES

Laboratory

Laboratory studies should be performed before institution of therapy. The physician assistant (PA) should always be aware of laboratory findings consistent with target organ disease.

Urinalysis. Rule out renal dysfunction or glycosuria.

Complete Blood Count. Rule out anemia before instituting therapy.

Serum Chemistry. Evaluate potassium, calcium, creatinine, uric acid, fasting blood glucose, cholesterol (both high density and low density lipoproteins), and triglycerides. Some of these tests are needed to determine cardiac risk, whereas others can rule out secondary causes of hypertension.

Plasma Renin/Urine Sodium Determinations. Evaluate for renovascular hypertension.

Radiology
Chest Film. May show cardiomegaly with long-standing hypertension, evidence of left ventricular failure, or aortic calcification.

Other
ECG. Identify rhythm or cardiac function abnormalities.
Echocardiogram. Assess left ventricular size and function.

DIFFERENTIAL DIAGNOSIS

Although the list of considerations in the differential diagnosis for hypertension can be quite lengthy, in 90% to 95% of the cases the diagnosis is that of essential hypertension. However, the PA should always consider causes of secondary hypertension such as renovascular or endocrine disorders and aortic coarctation.

Traumatic
Renal Trauma. Distant or acute; may cause renovascular hypertension.

Infectious
Repeated Urinary Tract Infections. May cause renal parenchymal disease.

Metabolic
Aldosteronism. Must be considered in patients with muscle weakness, polyuria, nocturia, and polydipsia.

Neoplastic
Pheochromocytoma. Should be suspected in patients with continuous hypertension associated with head pain, perspiration, or tremors. Elevated serum norepinephrine levels.

Vascular
Renal Artery Stenosis/Thrombosis/Arteritis. Seen on renal angiogram.

Congenital
Coarctation of the Aorta. Upper extremity hypertension associated with concomitant lower extremity hypotension.

Acquired
Drug-Induced. Especially with recreational drugs (e.g., cocaine, amphetamines), tricyclic antidepressants, ephedrine, phencyclidine, methylphenidate, and monoamine oxidase inhibitors. Estrogen preparations have also been shown to increase blood pressure.

TREATMENT

Lifestyle modifications, the keystone of nonpharmacologic therapy, should be instituted for all patients, whether or not they are treated concomitantly with pharmacologic therapy. These lifestyle changes include weight reduction, limiting alcohol intake, smoking cessation, and reduction in dietary fat and cholesterol. Pharmacologic therapy is indicated in patients with sustained (on >3 visits) elevations in the diastolic or systolic blood pressure and/or target organ damage.

Initial drug therapy for patients with mild to moderate hypertension consists of administration of a thiazide diuretic (25 mg of hydrochlorothiazide or chorthalidone) or a beta blocker. A calcium channel blocker (diltiazem 30 to 60 mg three times a day or sustained-release nifedipine 30 to 60 mg) may also be used. Patients with target organ damage may benefit from a beta blocker or an angiotensin-converting enzyme (ACE) inhibitor (captopril or enalapril). Many of these agents have synergistic effects and can be used concomitantly. Long-term clinical trials using diuretics and beta blockers have shown them to be useful and effective in controlling hypertension, as well as resulting in long-term reductions in cardiovascular morbidity and mortality.

PEDIATRIC CONSIDERATIONS

Systolic hypertension in children is a greater problem than may be suspected. Blood pressure measurements should be obtained routinely during office visits in the pediatric age group. The upper limit of normal is 110 mm Hg in children 6-10 years of age, and children aged 11-14 should have average systolic blood pressure of 120-130 mm Hg. For the patient older than 15 years of age, adult guidelines apply. Before diagnosing essential hypertension, extreme care must be taken to rule out common causes of secondary hypertension such as renal parenchymal disease, renal artery disease, and coarctation of the aorta. Management should initially focus on nonpharmacologic therapies such as weight reduction, reduced sodium intake, and regular exercise. Drug therapy should be considered if these modalities fail to lower blood pressure. Special consideration should be given to medication side effects and the potential impact of such agents on the growing child.

OBSTETRIC CONSIDERATIONS

Hypertensive patients who become pregnant should review medications with their health care provider to ensure there is no risk of teratogenic effects. Medications should be changed if necessary, but hypertension should always be treated. Blood pressure screening should be done at each visit.

Preeclampsia is acute hypertension that occurs after week 20 of pregnancy, accompanied by edema and proteinuria. Patients may be treated with medications, if necessary. Preeclampsia can also have onset post partum. Preeclampsia with seizures is called eclampsia, and necessitates delivery. The effects of hypertension on the pregnant patient and her fetus include decreased blood flow to the uterus, an increased risk of intrauterine growth retardation, and the possibility of early delivery. Therefore, the pregnancy should be carefully monitored by the use of ultrasound examination to determine the exact gestational age of the fetus. Monitoring should also include the use of nonstress test, contraction stress test, or biophysical profile beginning at gestational week 30 to ensure that the fetus is tolerating the intrauterine environment. When the pregnant hypertensive patient rests, she should be only in the left lateral recumbent position to maintain maximum uterine blood flow. Management considerations should involve self-monitoring of the patient's blood pressure at home, use of a low-salt diet, and strict abstinence from smoking and alcohol.

GERIATRIC CONSIDERATIONS

Control of systolic hypertension in this age group is imperative, as decreasing systolic pressure can prolong and improve quality of life. Single-drug therapy may not be sufficient to maintain control.

PREVENTIVE CONSIDERATIONS

Hypertension is also known as the "silent killer." Patients must be educated that lifetime treatment is required. Blood pressure measurements should be performed during every patient encounter. Treatment is instituted to avoid future complications, not to relieve the mild symptoms, if any. Ultimate vascular complications including CAD, aortic aneurysm and dissection, carotid artery disease, and peripheral arterial occlusive disease can be controlled or prevented with consistent blood pressure control and lifestyle modifications. Compliance needs to be emphasized. Contributing factors such as diabetes and hyperlipidemia must also be controlled.

Primary prevention strategies are especially important in children with a strong family history of essential hypertension.

PEARLS FOR THE PA

Essential hypertension is a chronic, lifelong condition that can be easily detected, diagnosed, and treated.

The treatment must be individualized, as certain patient populations respond better to particular drug regimens than others.

The primary goal of treatment is to reduce blood pressure, thus reducing risk for cardiovascular morbidity and mortality.

The treatment plan for all patients must include primary prevention strategies to decrease the incidence of hypertension in the general population.

Pericarditis/Pericardial Effusion

Edward Gaile, Sr., BA, BHS, PA-C

DEFINITION

Pericarditis is inflammation of the pericardium due to infection with a viral, rickettsial, bacterial, chlamydial, or fungal organism or from a noninfectious cause.

Pericardial effusion involves the accumulation of fluid in the pericardial space. The fluid accumulation may be composed of transudate, exudate, serosanguinous fluid, or frank blood.

HISTORY

Symptoms.   Severe, constant anterior chest pain is the most frequent complaint in acute pericarditis. Inspiration tends to worsen the pain, which can help distinguish between pericarditis and acute myocardial infarction. The pain can have a pleuritic component and may be referred to the neck and shoulder. The pain can also be intensified by movement and with swallowing. The onset of chest pain is typically sudden and is often accompanied by a low-grade fever and a rapid heart rate. The patient may indicate that the pain is relieved by sitting and leaning forward.

General.   A good history is essential for determining the etiology of the pericardial inflammation and must explore all elements of acute and chronic conditions as well as coexistent disease states.

Age.   Variable.

Onset.   Chest pain of gradual to sudden onset depending on the underlying cause (e.g., viral, tuberculosis, neoplastic, uremic, radiation).

Duration.   In general, symptoms of pericarditis resolve in 2 to 6 weeks. If effusion is present, surgical intervention may be necessary to achieve relief.

Intensity.   May vary from mild to severe, but is typically severe and constant.

Aggravating Factors.   Deep inspiration often aggravates chest pain.

Alleviating Factors.   Sitting and leaning forward may relieve chest discomfort.

Associated Factors.   Viral pericarditis is often preceded by an upper respiratory infection or gastroenteritis.

Coexisting disease states or conditions may be present, such as chronic renal failure, connective tissue disease, recent myocardial infarction, carcinoma, and chest irradiation.

PHYSICAL EXAMINATION

General.   The patient may be in significant distress; low-grade fever may be present. Observe/measure vital signs.

Cardiovascular. A pericardial friction rub is the classic finding in acute pericarditis. The triphasic rub can be heard, with one systolic component as the ventricles contract and two diastolic components. The early diastolic sound corresponds to ventricular filling, and the late diastolic sound corresponds to atrial contraction. The sounds are typically rough, scratchy, and high-pitched. Although variable in location, the rub can often be best heard with the diaphragm of the stethoscope at Erb's point (third left intercostal space). The intensity is also variable, but the rub may be enhanced when the patient exhales while leaning forward. The rub will decrease or resolve if a pericardial effusion develops. If the effusion creates enough pressure to cause a cardiac tamponade, cyanosis may develop along with distention of the neck veins and dyspnea. If a constrictive pericarditis develops, a pericardial "knock" may be heard in diastole, with a limitation of ventricular filling due to the constriction. Often accompanied by an elevated venous pressure and distended neck veins.

PATHOPHYSIOLOGY

Viral agents are most often implicated in acute pericarditis and include enteroviruses (coxsackieviruses A and B) and echovirus. Other viruses occasionally found include influenza, mumps, varicella, and Epstein-Barr viruses. Tuberculosis is often present in exudative pericarditis but is much less common. Rare causes include fungi, *Mycoplasma*, rickettsiae, chlamydiae, protozoa, and *Legionella pneumophila*. Often, especially in younger patients, an etiologic agent cannot be isolated. These cases are referred to as idiopathic or nonspecific pericarditis. Connective tissue disease such as systemic lupus erythematosus and rheumatoid arthritis can include pericarditis as part of the clinical picture.

Postinfarction myocardial inflammation may produce a localized fibrinous exudate with irritation of the adjacent pericardium in the early postinfarction period.

A portion of the parietal pericardium is pain sensitive where it is in close approximation with the parietal pleura at the anterior and lateral borders of the heart. The parietal pleura is also pain sensitive, which accounts for the pleuritic nature of the pain associated with acute pericarditis. The pericardium is served by the fibers from the T6 dermatome band originating from T1 to T6, which runs from the neck to below the xiphoid process. The T1 dermatome also runs down the arms. Lesions in the organs supplied by these fibers typically give rise to poorly localized pain that can radiate to the neck or shoulder.

Pericardial effusion can result as a complication of acute pericarditis due to any of the infecting organisms. It can also result from congestive heart failure (CHF), overhydration, hypoproteinemia, and neoplastic diseases. Additionally, effusion frequently accompanies uremic, radiation-induced, and idiopathic pericarditis. Bleeding into the pericardial space resulting from trauma, myocardial infarction with rupture, and aortic aneurysm or bleeding induced by a coagulation defect can also cause a pericardial effusion. The amount of fluid present in the pericardial space and the intrapericardial pressure do not correlate well. In acute cases, such as those associated with trauma, a small amount of fluid can lead to cardiac tamponade, whereas a large volume accumulated over an extended period of time can be well tolerated.

DIAGNOSTIC STUDIES

The diagnosis of pericarditis is generally presumptive; however, certain classic findings can be useful.

Laboratory
Viral Cultures. Should be done on samples taken from the pharynx and fecal material.
Acute and Convalescent Antibody Titers. On the isolated virus. A fourfold increase is confirmatory.

Radiology
Chest Film. Will show an enlarged cardiac silhouette if effusion is present.

Other
ECG. With pericarditis, will show widespread elevation of the ST segment in tracings for leads beyond those used for isolation of myocardial infarction without the characteristic reciprocal ST segment depression. Electrical alternans (seen as the heart floats back and forth relative to the surface electrodes) is a classic finding with a large effusion and a freely mobile heart.
Echocardiography. Is confirmatory, and is a sensitive, noninvasive modality to detect fluid in the pericardial space.
Pericardiocentesis. Performed for cardiac tamponade. Gram stain and culture of the fluid are performed.

DIFFERENTIAL DIAGNOSIS

Traumatic
Myocardial Contusion. Patient presents with persistent pain and antecedent trauma.
Costochondritis. Point tenderness to palpation. ECG negative.

Infectious
Pneumonia. Chest film will show infiltrate. ECG negative.

Metabolic
Myocardial Infarction. Elevation of the ST segment with reciprocal ST segment depression. Positive cardiac isoenzymes.
Cholecystitis. Pain associated with ingestion of fatty foods. ECG negative. Ultrasound study of gallbladder positive.

Neoplastic
Chest Wall/Lung Tumor. ECG negative. Chest film positive.

Vascular
Pulmonary Embolus. Significant dyspnea. Ventilation-perfusion (V/Q) scan positive.

Congenital
Not applicable.

Acquired
Psychogenic Chest Pain. All diagnostic studies are negative.

TREATMENT

Viral Pericarditis

The illness generally follows a benign, self-limited course over 3 to 6 weeks. The aim of treatment is to reduce symptoms. Analgesic and anti-inflammatory medications along with bedrest are the mainstay of therapy. Effusion usually does not develop; however, monitoring for signs of effusion and tamponade (e.g., neck vein distention, distant heart sounds, decreased arterial pressure, dyspnea), with treatment if necessary, is appropriate. The use of prednisone is controversial at present because it may add to myocardial damage.

Pericarditis with Purulent Effusion

Organisms most often implicated include staphlococci, meningococci, streptococci, gonococci, *Haemophilus influenzae*, and occasionally fungi. Drainage of the pericardial fluid via pericardiocentesis or an open surgical procedure is essential. Antimicrobial therapy is dictated by Gram stain and culture results. Infection of the pericardium with tuberculosis can manifest acutely with pericardial effusion with serosanguineous fluid and symptoms of tamponade or can evolve slowly over time and result in a constrictive pericarditis. Therapy is the same as that instituted for pulmonary tuberculosis. Surgical intervention may be necessary to free the constriction by stripping both layers of the pericardium.

Noninfectious Pericarditis

Treatment or control of the underlying condition, if possible, is mandatory.

The damage from trauma to the chest must be effectively managed emergently.

Treatment of pericarditis in a patient with uremia requires dialysis to control the underlying edema and possibly pericardiocentesis and anti-inflammatory therapy.

Radiation-induced pericardial effusion can evolve into a constrictive pericarditis.

Effusions due to neoplastic disease, systemic lupus erythematosus, and rheumatoid arthritis require treatment of the primary problem.

Anticoagulation in acute post–myocardial infarction pericarditis may be complicated by development of hemorrhagic pericardial effusion. Close observation for pericardial tamponade is essential. Steroids should be avoided for symptomatic relief in favor of aspirin and nonsteroidal anti-inflammatory drugs (NSAIDs).

Recurrent Pericardial Effusions
Occasionally, treatment of the pericardial space with a sclerosing agent to cause the two surfaces of the pericardial sac to adhere to each other is indicated to prevent relapse. However, a complication of this procedure is constriction.

PEDIATRIC CONSIDERATIONS

Pericarditis may occur in children of any age and is potentially life-threatening. Pericarditis in infants often has a viral etiology. Rheumatic fever is the most common cause of pericarditis in children. Other causes include bacterial infections, tuberculosis, cardiac surgery (postpericardiotomy syndrome), and secondary treatment with chemotherapeutic agents. Symptoms may include signs of systemic infection, chest pain, and CHF. Management is dependent on the etiology and is generally the same as in adults.

OBSTETRIC CONSIDERATIONS

In the treatment of pericarditis, the use of NSAIDs should be undertaken with caution and only when clearly indicated. Some of these drugs pose risks to the fetus that are similar to the side effects possible in the patient who is taking the NSAID. NSAIDs should not be used late in pregnancy owing to the risk of premature closure of the patent ductus arteriosus in the fetus.

GERIATRIC CONSIDERATIONS

The elderly patient is more susceptible to conditions such as myocardial infarction, carcinoma, and chest irradiation that predispose to pericarditis.

PREVENTIVE CONSIDERATIONS

Recognition and prevention of infectious disease such as upper respiratory infection and gastroenteritis are important. Appropriate immunizations

---

PEARLS FOR THE PA

A rapidly developing pericardial effusion with a small amount of fluid can cause more distress than a larger effusion that has developed gradually over time.

against common childhood illnesses are also important. General preventive strategies for myocardial infarction apply.

Valvular Heart Disease

Edward Gaile, Sr., BA, BHS, PA-C

Diastolic Murmurs

DEFINITION

Aortic regurgitation (AR): Incompetence of the aortic valve resulting in a large volume of blood flowing back into the left ventricle during diastole.

Mitral stenosis (MS): Constriction of the mitral orifice with an increase in turbulent flow across the reduced valve area.

HISTORY

Symptoms

AR. Those attributed to congestive heart failure (CHF), such as dyspnea, dyspnea on exertion, paroxysmal nocturnal dyspnea, nocturia, fatigue, and edema in later stages. Angina may develop in end-stage disease.

MS. Dyspnea on exertion is perhaps the earliest symptom. As the disease progresses, orthopnea, fatigue, and palpitations are prominent. Systemic emboli are common in patients with atrial fibrillation (AF) who are not anticoagulated.

General

AR. Most commonly due to rheumatic fever (in 75% of cases), endocarditis, and calcific aortic stenosis.

MS. True MS is almost always due to rheumatic disease. An atrial myxoma or thrombus may produce a similar murmur.

Age

AR. Often seen in the middle to older age groups when due to rheumatic disease. Traumatic AR may occur at any age.

MS. The initial rheumatic episode occurs in childhood, and the patient is asymptomatic from 15 to 25 years. Atrial thrombi and myxoma may occur at any time.

Onset

AR. Underlying condition usually evolves over many years, with insidious onset of AR. Acute AR is usually due to trauma, aortic dissection, or ongoing bacterial endocarditis.

MS. Usually gradual, with dyspnea on exertion the first symptom. Some patients develop acute decompensation with higher demands on the system as with exertion.

Duration
AR. Symptoms may develop so gradually that the patient compensates and does not present until very ill. Symptoms may not become apparent for 5 to 10 years after regurgitation begins. Survival past 2 years is low once CHF develops.
MS. Survival is limited to 10 to 12 years in untreated MS from time of symptom onset.

Intensity
AR. Mild symptoms in the early stages; often unnoticed by the affected person.
MS. Mild progression of symptoms over the prolonged disease course.

Aggravating Factors
AR. Dietary indiscretion with high sodium intake, lack of fluid restriction, noncompliance with medications (if patient has refused surgery when recommended early). Concomitant atherosclerotic heart disease with angina may decrease contractility further and hasten the development of CHF.
MS. Pregnancy, exercise, infections, and AF all can place additional burden on an overloaded left atrium and pulmonary vasculature.

Alleviating Factors
AR. Valve replacement surgery.
MS. Rest and compliance with the prescribed medical regimen are the only factors that may be of benefit to the patient.

Associated Factors
AR. When AR is due to rheumatic fever, mitral valvular disease is almost always present.
MS. Left ventricular enlargement may be present when accompanied by mitral regurgitation (MR). An enlarged left atrium is almost always present. AF is common.

PHYSICAL EXAMINATION

General
AR. Patient may be asymptomatic early on but later will appear in moderate to severe distress as symptoms of pulmonary edema develop.
MS. Patient may be asymptomatic or be confused from hypoxia associated with pulmonary edema.

Vital Signs
AR. Widened pulse pressure due to peripheral vasodilatation as a compensatory mechanism for the loss of forward flow. Diastolic pressure is often

less than 60 mm Hg. Tachycardia often present in later stages, and tachypnea reflects the degree of hypoxia.

MS. Pulse may be regular to irregularly irregular; respiratory pattern may be normal to tachypneic.

Head, Eyes, Ears, Nose, Throat (HEENT)

AR. Carotid upstroke is rapid and sharply descends. Jugular venous distention, seen later in the disease process, is associated with the development of end-stage disease and CHF.

MS. Jugular venous distention is present when right ventricular involvement has occurred as a result of pulmonary hypertension. Carotid upstroke is preserved until the right ventricle fails to fill the left atrium; biventricular failure is then apparent. Flushed cheeks and perioral cyanosis are sometimes seen.

Pulmonary

AR. May be clear to auscultation with early asymptomatic disease. Later, when CHF is present, crackles will be heard throughout the chest.

MS. Crackles throughout the lung fields are present when pulmonary edema ensues. The presence or absence of lung findings bears no relation to the degree of pulmonary hypertension.

Cardiovascular

AR. Apical impulse is displaced laterally. A high-pitched blowing decrescendo diastolic murmur is best heard along the left sternal border in the third interspace. Augmented by asking the patient to lean forward while sitting and exhale. An S_3 gallop is present in later stages, and a diastolic rumble of regurgitant blood striking the mitral valve may be present (Austin Flint murmur). An increase in the murmur can be heard with squatting and with forced expiration while leaning forward. The murmur exhibits no change with Valsalva maneuvers and decreases with deep inspiration and vasodilators.

MS. The S_1 is loudest at the apex and is the first sign of MS. The most conclusive sign of MS is an opening snap. This is a high-pitched sound occurring shortly after S_2 and is best heard at the apex. An S_3 is usually not present in MS and, if present, is of much lower pitch. The murmur of MS has a rumbling quality and is decrescendo-crescendo in pattern, occurring immediately after the opening snap. This pattern occurs as the blood volume from a filled atrium empties and is then augmented by atrial contraction. If pulmonary hypertension has developed, an accentuated P_2 may be heard, with a right ventricular heave apparent in the epigastrium. The murmur decreases with standing as the preload is reduced and increases with squatting.

Gastrointestinal

AR. Right upper quadrant tenderness of the abdomen with hepatomegaly and hepatojugular reflux may be present if biventricular failure has developed.

MS. As right ventricular dysfunction becomes more prominent, ascites, hepatomegaly, and hepatojugular reflux typically appear.

Extremities

AR. Bounding pulses are often felt distally, and capillary pulsations may be seen in the nail beds. Peripheral edema develops with the failure of the right ventricle.

MS. May be cool as cardiac output falls. Edema invariably present once right-sided failure occurs.

PATHOPHYSIOLOGY

AR. Basic hemodynamic abnormality is volume overload of the left ventricle due to the regurgitant flow of blood through the aortic valve. Initially the left ventricle can compensate with dilatation. Once maximal dilatation is achieved, the left ventricle demonstrates decreased compliance and contractility and overt signs of CHF develop.

MS. Causes an obstruction to blood flow from the left atrium to the left ventricle. This obstruction results in a volume overload in the atrium and dilatation of the chamber. The increased pressure is reflected into the pulmonary vasculature and pulmonary hypertension eventually develops. These elevated pulmonary pressures impose an unreasonable afterload on the rather thin right ventricle, and right heart failure ensues.

DIAGNOSTIC STUDIES

Laboratory. Usually noncontributory unless the patient has deteriorated and shows evidence of end-organ dysfunction.

Radiology

Chest Film

AR. Reveals a normal or enlarged cardiac shadow with elongation of the left ventricle. Aortic dilatation is not seen unless the AR is due to aortic dissection or Marfan syndrome.

MS. Reveals an enlarged left atrium and displacement of the esophagus. The left ventricle is not enlarged. Full pulmonary vasculature and peribronchial cuffing signify elevations of the pulmonary pressures. Right ventricular enlargement occurs later in the disease.

Other

ECG

AR. May suggest left ventricular hypertrophy and ST segment depression with negative T waves across the precordium.

MS. Left atrial enlargement can be seen in lead V_1 in those patients without AF.

Echocardiography

AR. Demonstrates the regurgitation and provides an estimate of the pressure gradient. Left ventricular compliance may also be estimated and other valvular abnormalities identified.

MS. Demonstration of valvular calcifications, leaflet motion abnormalities, calculation of the valve orifice, and an estimation of the gradient across the valve are helpful in determining further studies and treatment.

Cardiac Catheterization

AR. Indicated when surgery is recommended to visualize the regurgitant flow and coronary arteries. Left ventricular compliance and any other valvular abnormalities can also be demonstrated.

MS. Visualization of the coronary arteries is important before surgical correction can be attempted.

DIFFERENTIAL DIAGNOSIS

Traumatic

AR. Penetration of the leaflets or laceration of the aortic wall. Acute aortic dissection.

Infectious

AR. Bacterial endocarditis may produce a sudden acute manifestation.

MS. Almost always the result of rheumatic heart disease.

Metabolic

Thyroid Disorders and Hyperpyrexia. May but usually do not produce diastolic murmurs.

Neoplastic

AR. Myxomatous transformation of the aortic valve has become a more common cause of AR.

MS. Left atrial myxoma will produce a murmur similar to MS. Look for fever and signs of systemic embolization.

Vascular

AR/MS. Venous and arterial stenosis and/or thrombus.

Congenital

AR. Bicuspid valve and annular distention due to a variety of cardiac malformations.

MS. Usually overshadowed by any number of cardiac malformations.

Acquired

AR. Marfan syndrome, connective tissue disorders, and infiltrative diseases. Chronic hypertension.

MS. Left atrial thrombus: Look for signs of systemic embolization; tachycardia is common. With left atrial myxoma, the murmur may change or disappear with body position.

TREATMENT

AR.   In the symptomatic patient with severe AR, surgery should not be delayed. Those with mild symptomatic disease may be managed with conventional CHF therapy. Aortic valve replacement should occur before left ventricular compliance is decreased. It is important in the patient awaiting surgery that preload on the left ventricle not be reduced to the point that the left ventricle cannot maximally fill. A small reduction in stroke volume can and often does result in a severe reduction in blood pressure.

MS.   Anticoagulation is required once AF develops, and some clinicians anticoagulate all patients with MS. Diuretics are often employed during the early stages of the disease. Antibiotics are required for endocarditis prophylaxis.

Surgery should occur before pulmonary hypertension and right ventricular failure develop. Commissurotomy may be used in the younger patient if no calcifications are present. Mechanical valves are the replacement of choice except in the elderly or childbearing females.

PEDIATRIC CONSIDERATIONS

Isolated pulmonary regurgitation (PR) or insufficiency is rare in children. It generally occurs in association with an abnormal pulmonic valve and pulmonic stenosis (PS), or following treatment of PS with balloon dilatation angioplasty or surgical valvulotomy. Although most cases are mild, severe forms can occur and may result in CHF.

AR or aortic insufficiency is usually of a very mild degree. In severe AR, the left ventricle becomes dilated, eventually resulting in decreased function in some cases. Treatment of severe AR consists of aortic valve replacement.

Tricuspid stenosis (TS) is very rare in children. Tricuspid atresia (incomplete formation of the valve) does occur and will be evident early in the infant's life with CHF, cyanosis, and murmur.

MS rarely occurs in infants and children. MS does occur in adolescents and young adults as an acquired disorder secondary to rheumatic fever. Children with a documented occurrence of rheumatic fever should have a periodic cardiac assessment to rule out valvular heart disease. Treatment is similar to that for adults.

Children who are born without a right pulmonary artery or who have conditions such as atrioseptal defect, ventriculoseptal defect, or patent ductus arteriosis (left to right shunts) are at much greater risk for the development of high-altitude pulmonary edema.

OBSTETRIC CONSIDERATIONS

Aortic Insufficiency.   If the pregnant patient with aortic regurgitation also has associated CHF, conventional medical therapy is usually successful. The aortic valve may be replaced during the pregnancy if endocarditis develops or medical therapy becomes ineffective. Epidural anesthesia may be used safely.

MS. In a patient with known MS who desires to become pregnant, valvuloplasty is recommended. Otherwise, MS often worsens during the pregnancy owing to the increased cardiac output that occurs naturally during pregnancy. This leads to increased atrial pressure, which can cause pulmonary edema or AF with development of an atrial mural thrombus with possible embolization. Previously asymptomatic female patients may become symptomatic during the second trimester of pregnancy when the blood volume increases. Symptoms may abate slightly late in the third trimester, as the blood volume usually diminishes during that period.

In pregnant patients with MS, rheumatic fever prophylaxis should be given during the period of pregnancy, and subacute bacterial endocarditis prophylaxis should be administered at the time of delivery. Surgical valve repair or replacement, anticoagulation as needed (with avoidance of warfarin), and the usual cardiac regimens (digitalis, bedrest, and low-sodium diet) can be used when the condition necessitates treatment. It has also been reported that use of propranolol or atenolol relieves the symptoms.

Epidural block is the anesthetic of choice for delivery in these patients.

General Considerations
If anticoagulation is indicated, only heparin should be used. For rheumatic fever and subacute bacterial endocarditis prophylaxis, sulfonamides, ciprofloxacin, and erythromycin should be used with caution during the pregnancy; tetracycline use is contraindicated.

GERIATRIC CONSIDERATIONS

Screening using auscultation and echocardiography is indicated, especially for the patient with a history of rheumatic disease.

PEARLS FOR THE PA

AR

When a diastolic murmur is found, an echocardiogram is indicated. Any patient with AR should receive antibiotic prophylaxis against bacterial endocarditis as outlined by the American Heart Association.

MS

MS is frequently caused by rheumatic fever. The opening snap with a diastolic murmur is virtually diagnostic for MS. Operative mortality increases with decompensation; refer early once symptoms develop. It is impossible to determine the absence of pulmonary hypertension on the basis of the physical examination.

PREVENTIVE CONSIDERATIONS

Recognition and prevention of rheumatic fever. Preventive strategies for coronary atherosclerotic heart disease are indicated. Reduction in sodium intake is recommended.

Systolic Murmurs

DEFINITION

Aortic stenosis (AS): Midsystolic murmur secondary to a reduction in aortic valve area.

Pulmonic stenosis (PS): Right ventricular outflow obstruction due to pulmonic valvular abnormality.

Tricuspid regurgitation (TR): Often rheumatic in origin, TR results in ejection of blood into the right atrium during systole. Usually not an isolated lesion. Often associated with pulmonary hypertension.

Mitral regurgitation (MR): The loss of competence of the mitral valve results in blood's being forced into the left atrium during systole. As valve function gradually worsens, the left ventricle and atrium dilate to handle the increased blood volume. Ventricular wall thickness increases to maintain forward flow, and little end-diastolic pressure increase is seen until late in the course of the disease. In acute MR, the atrium and ventricle do not have time to dilate. The resultant rise in end-diastolic pressure is transmitted to the pulmonary vascular bed, and pulmonary edema ensues.

HISTORY

Symptoms

AS. Include those associated with CHF: dyspnea on exertion, paroxysmal nocturnal dyspnea, cough, fatigue, angina (in 50% to 70% of cases), syncope (in 15% to 30% of cases), sudden death.

PS. Usually right-sided heart failure predominates, with peripheral edema and occasionally syncope.

TR. In the pure form, relates to increases in the right atrial pressures. Symptoms are pain in the abdomen, bloating, change in skin color, weight gain, and edema of the ankles and legs, with dyspnea as the most prominent symptom.

MR. Depends on onset. Fatigue and dyspnea are more common over a chronic course. Progression to paroxysmal nocturnal dyspnea, orthopnea, and pedal edema signifies right ventricular involvement. Sudden pulmonary edema with mild cardiomegaly and with a sinus rhythm signifies an acute event such as rupture of chordae.

General. A full medical history needs to be obtained to rule out potentially reversible contributing factors such as thyroid disease, anemias, or recent or active systemic infections. Especially evaluate for a history of rheumatic fever.

Age
AS. In patients younger than 30 years of age, AS is almost always congenital and due to a bicuspid valve. Rheumatic disease and calcific lesions are more prominent in those of more advanced years.

PS. Almost always a disease of the young and, except in rare situations, is always congenital. The premature infant may have a stenosis-like lesion, but this is transitory.

TR. May occur at any age depending on the etiology.

MR. May occur at any age depending on the etiology.

Onset
AS. May manifest as sudden death or syncope. Dyspnea on exertion may be the only symptom in the younger population.

PS. Usually noticed shortly after birth at the first cardiac examination. When the stenosis is severe, right-sided heart failure is apparent from birth.

TR. When TR is due to rheumatic disease, onset is gradual over many years. If secondary to infective endocarditis in the intravenous drug abuser, TR will be detected during the recovery period. Gradual worsening is the rule when TR is due to a cardiomyopathy.

MR. May be insidious or acute depending on the etiology. Acute rupture is usually associated with a ruptured chorda or papillary muscle.

Duration
AS. Survival beyond 2 years is uncommon once left ventricular failure develops. Sudden death occurs in 15% to 20% of the symptomatic population and in 15% of the asymptomatic group.

TR. In an isolated form, may be tolerated for several years, especially with medical management. When TR is due to rheumatic disease, mitral involvement is often present, which will dictate the timing of operative management.

MR. When chronic, well tolerated for years without symptoms. When MR is acute, survival is poor without immediate surgical intervention.

Aggravating Factors
AS. Those activities that increase the volume load on the left ventricle, for example, excessive fluid intake and exercise. May contribute to onset of CHF. In addition, diuretic treatment for CHF may reduce preload of the left ventricle to a critical level, thereby further reducing cardiac output.

PS. Activities or habits that increase pulmonic pressures and/or demand for cardiac output (as noted for AS).

TR. Activities that worsen heart failure and stretch the right ventricle (e.g., smoking, hypercapnia) further distort the anatomy of the valve and contribute to worsened regurgitation.

MR. In chronic MR, any factor that exacerbates the symptoms of CHF (e.g., nonadherence to dietary guidelines, increased salt intake, fluid overload). The coexistence of endocarditis with an already weakened valvular structure due to rheumatic fever may produce an acute situation.

Alleviating Factors

AS. Maintaining systemic arterial pressure in an optimal range will reduce the patient's symptoms and increase functional class.

PS. Avoidance of habits/behaviors that increase pulmonary pressures.

TR. Treatment of CHF and diuresis may diminish the regurgitation. Decrease in the murmur may be heard.

MR. Treatment aimed at CHF—diuretics, digoxin, and vasodilator therapy along with dietary and fluid modification—may eliminate the need for surgery in a small percentage of patients with stable disease. The vast majority and certainly those with acute onset will require operative intervention before irreparable anatomic damage occurs.

Associated Factors

AS. When AS is due to rheumatic fever, mitral disease is almost universally present.

PS. Myxomatous tissue causing fusion of the leaflets.

TR. Mitral disease is almost always present if the TR is rheumatic in origin. Pulmonary hypertension and/or right ventricular dilatation may also be found.

MR. When MR is secondary to cardiomyopathy, TR is often present as well. Rheumatic disease may also have affected the aortic valve; this possibility should be investigated.

PHYSICAL EXAMINATION

General

AS. The patient may be young without obvious signs of CHF or older with pulmonary edema and right-sided heart failure. Vital signs: Blood pressure usually reflects the inability of the ventricle to quickly empty, and the pulse pressure is narrow. A normal rate and rhythm are more common than atrial fibrillation. Respiratory rate will reflect the degree of left ventricular dysfunction and volume overload. With a gradual course, however, the pulmonary vasculature may accept rather high levels of pulmonary hypertension before allowing the development of pulmonary edema.

PS. Symptoms of right-sided heart failure predominate; increasing weight, abdominal pain, and peripheral edema are present in later stages.

TR. Patient may be dyspneic and appear obese and/or edematous. Vital signs: May range from normal to those associated with heart failure.

MR. The patient may exhibit no outward signs of discomfort or may be in marked respiratory distress. Vital signs: May be stable or associated with a shock state depending on the etiology.

Head, Eyes, Ears, Nose, Throat (HEENT)

AS. Delayed upstroke of the carotid pulse with or without prominent jugular venous distention.

PS. Jugular venous distention may or may not be present depending on the degree of right ventricular failure. Carotid upstroke is not affected until late.

TR. Scleral icterus may be present from passive liver congestion. Jugular venous distention is prominent, often to the angle of the jaw with large V waves. Carotid upstroke not affected unless aortic disease is also present.

MR. Carotid upstroke usually brisk and short in chronic MR. Jugular venous distention not usually present unless pulmonary hypertension has developed.

Pulmonary

AS. Crackles may or may not be present.

PS. Lung fields are clear.

TR. Lung fields range from clear to filled with crackles from left-sided heart failure.

MR. Most often clear with occasional bibasilar crackles in the chronic state. When the MR is acute, crackles and rhonchi are heard throughout.

Cardiovascular

AS. S_1 is normal and S_2 is usually decreased or absent. When present, A_2 may be delayed beyond P_2 if the disease has been allowed to progress. An S_3 and S_4 may be present, reflecting the chamber dilatation. The murmur is a midsystolic, crescendo-decrescendo harsh sound usually loudest in the aortic area. Radiation may occur to the apex and the carotids. A thrill may be felt in the right second interspace and over the carotids. The apical impulse is displaced laterally owing to left ventricular enlargement. The murmur of AR will be present if the valve cannot close secondary to advanced disease The murmur increases in intensity with squatting and decreases on standing and with Valsalva maneuvers. This is in contrast to outflow obstruction due to septal hypertrophy: The murmur of asymmetrical septal hypertrophy decreases with squatting and increases on standing and with Valsalva maneuvers. The murmur is due to systolic motion of the anterior leaflet of the mitral valve against the septal wall as chamber size decreases.

PS. S_1 is clear with a split to absent P_2; an S_4 is common. The murmur is loudest at the upper left sternal border and is harsh, with radiation toward the neck. The longer the murmur, the worse the stenosis. The murmur does not radiate towards the apex. Murmur is increased with inspiration.

TR. A parasternal lift can be found with a right-sided S_3. A blowing, high-pitched murmur of variable intensity can best be heard along the left sternal border. This murmur is pansystolic and may be differentiated from MR in that it does not radiate to the axilla. The murmur is increased with squatting and inspiration and decreases with standing and Valsalva maneuvers.

MR. Point of maximal intensity (PMI) displaced laterally and inferiorly, S_1 soft, and split S_2 with a loud S_3 (except when MR is acute). The loud, blowing holosystolic murmur is best heard at the apex and radiates to the axilla. Radiation to the base may occur and may lead to confusion with AS. A flail anterior leaflet radiates to the axilla, while a flail posterior leaflet radiates to the carotids. The midsystolic click of mitral valve prolapse may also be heard. Murmur is increased with squatting, decreased with dilators, and variable with Valsalva maneuvers.

Gastrointestinal

PS. An epigastric heave of right ventricular hypertrophy may be present. If right-sided heart failure is present, hepatomegaly and ascites may be found.

TR. An epigastric lift of right ventricular hypertrophy may sometimes be felt. Hepatomegaly with pulsations and hepatojugular reflux are often found.

Extremities

PS. Cyanosis is not present. Edema may be evident.

TR. Peripheral edema is one hallmark of right-sided heart failure. This edema may extend to midthigh or the groin. Diminished peripheral pulses are indicative of coexistent left ventricular dysfunction.

PATHOPHYSIOLOGY

AS. Degeneration of the valve due to rheumatic disease or a congenitally bicuspid valve. In persons older than 70 years, sclerotic changes are seen in the tricuspid valve as well. Stenosis of the valve, whether due to rheumatic disease or a bicuspid valve, results in a pressure overload of the left ventricle. Compensation consists of left ventricular thickening and concentric hypertrophy. Continued overload causes chamber dilatation and decreased contractility. End-diastolic pressure rises and myocardial oxygen demand increases. The stenosis is deemed "critical" when the pressure in the ventricle is 50 mm Hg greater than that in the aorta during systole. This aortic valve gradient is often the decision point for the timing of surgery.

PS. Almost exclusively of congenital origin; rheumatic fever may be causative but usually must involve all the valves.

TR. In the pure form, relates to increases in the right atrial pressure, often the result of pulmonary hypertension from a failing left ventricle. Rheumatic (mitral often involved as well); right ventricular dilatation (whether due to cardiomyopathy or left ventricular dysfunction); pulmonary hypertension, trauma, or carcinoid.

MR. Congenital: May be isolated or part of other disease process (i.e., Marfan syndrome, Ehlers-Danlos syndrome). Rheumatic disease, mitral valve prolapse, chordal rupture, endocarditis, papillary muscle ischemia, and infarction and distortion of the structure due to left ventricular hypertrophy are also important causes.

DIAGNOSTIC STUDIES

Laboratory

Full laboratory analysis will augment the history and physical findings, confirming the presence or absence of reversible conditions.

Complete blood count.   Rule out anemia; elevated white blood cell count from an occult infection.

Thyroid function studies.   Rule out hyperthyroidism.

Radiology

Chest Film

AS.   Cardiomegaly with prominent left ventricle may be present. Calcification may be seen on the aortic valve.

PS.   Right ventricular enlargement may be seen in untreated cases.

TR.   Prominent great veins and right ventricular and atrial enlargement. Usually no pulmonary vascular enlargement unless left-sided heart failure also present.

MR.   With chronic disease there is an enlarged left atrium and ventricle; calcification may be present on the leaflets if MR is due to rheumatic disease. In acute MR the heart size is normal, with pulmonary edema the most striking feature.

Other

ECG

AS.   Increased voltage consistent with left ventricular hypertrophy, ST segment depression common in tracings from the left-sided leads. Intraventricular conduction delays are occasionally seen as well.

PS.   Right ventricular hypertrophy, if present, is the only associated finding.

TR.   Atrial fibrillation is almost universal.

MR.   Chronic MR causes left atrial enlargement, and most often atrial fibrillation is present. Left ventricular enlargement is clearly seen. Evidence for an infarction supports papillary muscle dysfunction. In the acute setting, normal sinus rhythm to sinus tachycardia may be the only finding.

Echocardiography

AS.   Thickened aortic leaflets with decreased mobility are present. Estimates of the valve area and the pressure gradient can also be done.

PS.   Demonstrates the severity of the stenosis and measures valve area and right ventricular chamber size.

TR.   Confirms the diagnosis and may demonstrate vegetations on the leaflets. The severity of the regurgitation can also be assessed, as well as other valvular abnormalities that may not have been apparent in the physical examination and may indicate the etiology.

MR.   Confirms the diagnosis of MR and establishes the anatomic deformity. Left ventricular function can be assessed and chamber sizes measured. During repair of the valve, transesophageal echocardiography is often used to document the success of the repair.

Cardiac Catheterization

AS.   Indicated in all younger patients and those who are symptomatic. Demonstrates the valvular defect, determines the gradient across the valve, excludes coronary atherosclerosis as the cause of angina, and assesses left ventricular compliance.

PS.   Defines the severity of the lesion by measuring end-diastolic pressure. If the pressures are high enough, the foramen ovale may be open, allowing a right-to-left shunt.

TR.   Helps to define the anatomy if other lesions are suspected and identifies the coronary artery anatomy before surgery. Usually not needed for isolated TR.

MR.   Required to confirm the diagnosis and visualize the coronary arteries. Right-sided heart catheterization may be performed at the bedside with a Swan-Ganz catheter, and the presence of a V wave on the wedge pressure tracing may help diagnose a new systolic murmur in a recent myocardial infarction.

DIFFERENTIAL DIAGNOSIS

Traumatic
Ventricular Septal Defect.   Development of a ventricular septal defect after myocardial infarction will result in a harsh murmur at the left with radiation throughout the precordium. Prompt confirmation of the diagnosis by echocardiography and rapid surgical intervention will be life-saving.

Infectious
Bacterial, Fungal, and Parasitic Vegetations on the Valvular Apparatus. Will produce murmurs in the appropriate anatomic areas.

Metabolic
Hyperthyroidism.   Usually produces a systolic murmur. Valvular disease present before the onset of hyperthyroidism will be intensified.

Neoplastic
Atrial myxomas.   Commonly produce regurgitant murmurs owing to distortion of the valves. The finding of heart failure with a normal cardiac shadow should suggest this entity in the differential diagnosis.

Vascular
Coarctation of the Aorta and Other Arterial or Venous Malformations or Stenosis.   Murmurs distributed throughout the thorax may indicate the presence of one of these.

Congenital
Patent Ductus Arteriosus, Tetralogy of Fallot, Ebstein Anomaly, and Other Congenital Defects.   All produce distinctive murmurs that vary in intensity depending on site and degree of involvement.

Acquired

Anemia and fever. Often increase demand, and a systolic ejection murmur will be heard.

Mitral valve prolapse. An important diagnosis to make because of the long-term outcome. Patients usually present for evaluation of an arrhythmia or syncope, or are referred because of the murmur. The patient is usually female, tall and thin, and complains of occasional stabbing chest pain and palpitations when questioned. The abnormality produces a click in midsystole with or without an accompanying murmur. Squatting makes the click and occasional murmur appear later in systole, whereas standing makes them occur earlier. Echocardiography confirms the diagnosis and demonstrates leaflet prolapse into the atrium during systole. Any regurgitation will also be seen at that time and can be quantified. In patients with chest pain, cardiac catheterization may be done to visualize the coronary anatomy. These patients will need prophylaxis against endocarditis. The prognosis is good for these patients, and most do not have problems. Major complications include transient ischemic attacks, arrhythmias, severe MR, and sudden death. The risk factors for prediction of these events have not been identified. Patients will need reassurance that in the majority of cases, mitral valve prolapse is benign.

TREATMENT

AS. In the symptomatic patient with severe AS, surgery should not be delayed. Those with mild symptomatic disease may be managed with conventional CHF therapy (e.g., afterload reduction and mild diuretics). Aortic valve replacement should occur before left ventricular compliance is decreased. All younger patients need valve replacement if severe stenosis is present whether symptomatic or not. It is important in the patient awaiting surgery that preload on the left ventricle not be reduced to the point at which the left ventricle cannot fill maximally. A small reduction in stroke volume can and often does result in a severe reduction in blood pressure.

PS. Balloon valvuloplasty is the treatment of choice for infants; surgery is accomplished if this fails or cannot be done. If valve replacement is required, a porcine valve is used owing to the tendency for mechanical valves to form thrombi.

TR. Patients may remain asymptomatic for years. Once symptoms develop, diuretics and digoxin may be all that are required. If TR is coexistent with MS, valve replacement or annuloplasty may be considered at the time of mitral repair.

MR. Medical treatment includes anticoagulation for patients with atrial fibrillation, prophylaxis against rheumatic fever until age 35, bacterial endocarditis prophylaxis, digitalis, diuretics, and vasodilators for those with symptoms of CHF. Surgery should be done before left- and right-sided heart failure develop. Emergent valve replacement is required for those with acute MR and pulmonary edema. In addition to intravenous diuretics and sodium nitroprusside, an intra-aortic balloon pump is often placed preoperatively to assist with afterload reduction.

PEDIATRIC CONSIDERATIONS

AS.   AS can occur at the subvalvular, valvular, and supravalvular levels. Most children are asymptomatic; however, in more severe forms, decreased exercise tolerance, chest pain, and syncope with exertion are possible. In severe AS, arrhythmia and sudden death may result. Infants may develop CHF if the degree of stenosis is severe. AS is a progressive disease. The aortic valve becomes increasingly calcified over time, resulting in a greater degree of stenosis. Owing to the progressive nature and the demand for increased cardiac output with growth, children with AS should be monitored very closely. Children with moderate to severe AS and their parents should be advised of the risk of arrhythmia and sudden death with strenuous exercise. Patients with AS should avoid all isometric exercise. Children with this condition should be counseled and advised to select appropriate recreational activities.

TR.   TR or tricuspid insufficiency is generally associated with other cardiac abnormalities that produce and elevate right ventricular pressure or dilate the right atrium, resulting in an incompetent valve. An infant who has severe TR should be evaluated for Ebstein anomaly of the tricuspid valve. Treatment consists of correcting the underlying abnormality.

MR.   MR or mitral insufficiency occurs in children and adults secondary to rheumatic fever. MR may also occur in patients with mitral valve prolapse. Children should be examined for Marfan syndrome because of the documented association of the conditions.

Other Conditions.   Children who are born without a right pulmonary artery or who have conditions such as atrioseptal defect, ventriculoseptal defect, or patent ductus arteriosis (left to right shunts) are at much greater risk for the development of high-altitude pulmonary edema.

OBSTETRIC CONSIDERATIONS

AS.   Is rarely seen during pregnancy. If it does occur, the pregnancy demands for increased cardiac output may not be met, which could lead to dyspnea, chest pain, syncope, and death. The maternal mortality rate is 17% and the perinatal mortality rate is 31%. Epidural anesthesia should be avoided during delivery, as the patient is not able to compensate for the decreases in venous return and in the systemic vascular resistance that occurs with epidurals.

MR.   This is a cardiac lesion that is usually well tolerated during pregnancy. Occasionally, however, the valve may require replacement during pregnancy. The pregnant patient with mitral insufficiency should receive rheumatic fever and subacute bacterial endocarditis prophylaxis. Epidural anesthesia can also be used at time of delivery.

General Considerations

If anticoagulation is indicated, only heparin should be used. For rheumatic fever and subacute bacterial endocarditis prophylaxis, sulfonamides, ciprofloxacin, and erythromycin should be used with caution during the pregnancy; tetracycline use is contraindicated.

GERIATRIC CONSIDERATIONS

Screening using auscultation and echocardiogram is indicated.

PREVENTIVE CONSIDERATIONS

Recognition and prevention of rheumatic fever. Preventive strategies for coronary atherosclerotic heart disease is indicated. Reduction in sodium intake is recommended.

PEARLS FOR THE PA

AS

Asymptomatic patients need prophylaxis against endocarditis. Rheumatic disease and bicuspid valves are the most common causes of AS. Sudden death cannot be predicted from the loudness of the murmur or the degree of symptoms.

PS

It is important to identify PS early before right ventricular enlargement occurs. Early valvuloplasty is highly successful, and associated risks are low.

TR

Almost never an isolated lesion; the presence of TR should prompt a search for other valvular and ventricular abnormalities.

MR

A negative history for rheumatic fever does not exclude the presence of rheumatic valve disease. If a systolic blowing murmur is best heard at the apex, an echocardiogram is indicated. In affected patients, prophylaxis against endocarditis and rheumatic fever is important. If atrial fibrillation is documented, anticoagulation is required. The incidence of embolic events is higher than that of bleeding from chronic anticoagulation. Surgery should not be delayed in the setting of acute MR or when the patient with chronic MR becomes symptomatic.

Further Reading

American Heart Association: Textbook of Advanced Cardiac Life Support. American Heart Association, Chicago, 2000.

Braunwald E, Zipes DP, Libby P (eds): Heart Disease: A Textbook of Cardiovascular Medicine, 6th ed. Philadelphia, WB Saunders, 2001.

Goldman L, Bennett JC (eds): Cecil Textbook of Medicine, 21st ed. Philadelphia, WB Saunders, 2000.

Pritchett AM, Redfield MM: Beta blockers: New standard of therapy for heart failure. Mayo Clin Proc 77:839-846, 2002.

Topol EJ: Cardiovascular Medicine. Philadelphia, Lippincott Williams & Wilkins, 1998.

Chapter 1 Appendix

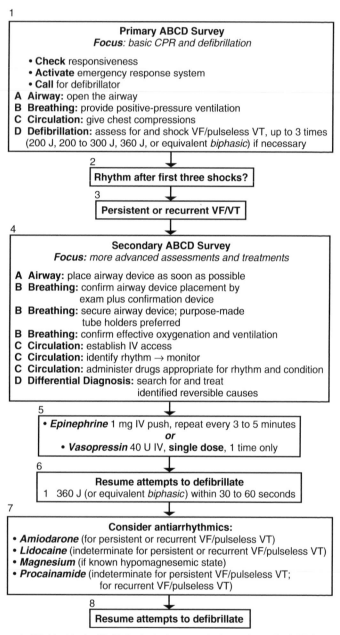

1

Primary ABCD Survey
Focus: basic CPR and defibrillation

- **Check** responsiveness
- **Activate** emergency response system
- **Call** for defibrillator
A **Airway:** open the airway
B **Breathing:** provide positive-pressure ventilation
C **Circulation:** give chest compressions
D **Defibrillation:** assess for and shock VF/pulseless VT, up to 3 times
(200 J, 200 to 300 J, 360 J, or equivalent *biphasic*) if necessary

2
Rhythm after first three shocks?

3
Persistent or recurrent VF/VT

4

Secondary ABCD Survey
Focus: more advanced assessments and treatments

A **Airway:** place airway device as soon as possible
B **Breathing:** confirm airway device placement by
exam plus confirmation device
B **Breathing:** secure airway device; purpose-made
tube holders preferred
B **Breathing:** confirm effective oxygenation and ventilation
C **Circulation:** establish IV access
C **Circulation:** identify rhythm → monitor
C **Circulation:** administer drugs appropriate for rhythm and condition
D **Differential Diagnosis:** search for and treat
identified reversible causes

5
- *Epinephrine* 1 mg IV push, repeat every 3 to 5 minutes
or
- *Vasopressin* 40 U IV, **single dose**, 1 time only

6
Resume attempts to defibrillate
1   360 J (or equivalent *biphasic*) within 30 to 60 seconds

7

Consider antiarrhythmics:
- *Amiodarone* (for persistent or recurrent VF/pulseless VT)
- *Lidocaine* (indeterminate for persistent or recurrent VF/pulseless VT)
- *Magnesium* (if known hypomagnesemic state)
- *Procainamide* (indeterminate for persistent VF/pulseless VT;
for recurrent VF/pulseless VT)

8
Resume attempts to defibrillate

Figure 1–17. Ventricular fibrillation/pulseless ventricular tachycardia (VT) treatment algorithm. (American Heart Association: Textbook of Advanced Cardiac Life Support. American Heart Association, Chicago. Reproduced with permission, *ACLS Provider Manual 2001*, © 2003, Copyright American Heart Association.)

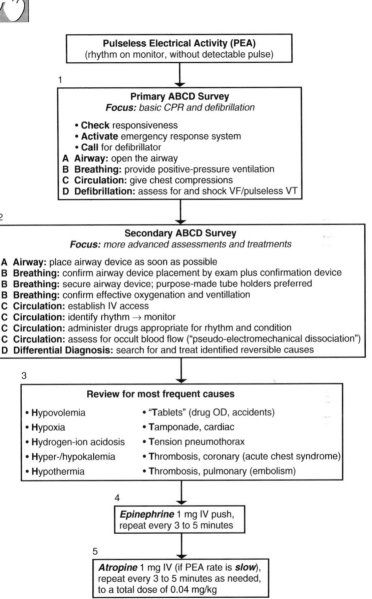

Figure 1–18. Pulseless electrical activity (electromechanical dissociation) treatment algorithm. (American Heart Association: Textbook of Advanced Cardiac Life Support. American Heart Association, Chicago. Reproduced with permission, *ACLS Provider Manual 2001*, © 2003, Copyright American Heart Association.)

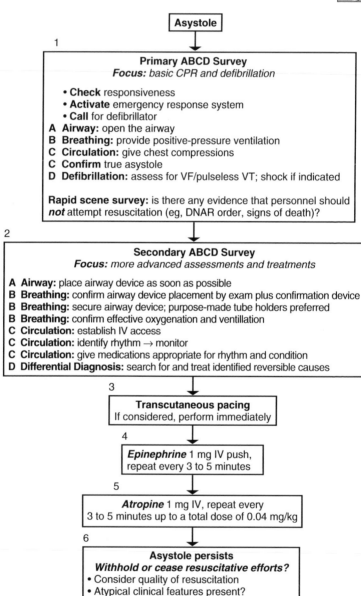

```
                        ┌─────────────┐
                        │  Asystole   │
                        └─────────────┘
                               │
                               ▼
  1
  ┌─────────────────────────────────────────────────────────────┐
  │                    Primary ABCD Survey                       │
  │              Focus: basic CPR and defibrillation             │
  │                                                              │
  │    • Check responsiveness                                    │
  │    • Activate emergency response system                      │
  │    • Call for defibrillator                                  │
  │  A  Airway: open the airway                                  │
  │  B  Breathing: provide positive-pressure ventilation         │
  │  C  Circulation: give chest compressions                     │
  │  C  Confirm true asystole                                    │
  │  D  Defibrillation: assess for VF/pulseless VT; shock if     │
  │       indicated                                              │
  │                                                              │
  │  Rapid scene survey: is there any evidence that personnel    │
  │  should not attempt resuscitation (eg, DNAR order, signs     │
  │  of death)?                                                  │
  └─────────────────────────────────────────────────────────────┘
                               │
  2                            ▼
  ┌─────────────────────────────────────────────────────────────┐
  │                   Secondary ABCD Survey                      │
  │          Focus: more advanced assessments and treatments     │
  │                                                              │
  │  A  Airway: place airway device as soon as possible          │
  │  B  Breathing: confirm airway device placement by exam plus  │
  │       confirmation device                                    │
  │  B  Breathing: secure airway device; purpose-made tube       │
  │       holders preferred                                      │
  │  B  Breathing: confirm effective oxygenation and ventilation │
  │  C  Circulation: establish IV access                         │
  │  C  Circulation: identify rhythm → monitor                   │
  │  C  Circulation: give medications appropriate for rhythm     │
  │       and condition                                          │
  │  D  Differential Diagnosis: search for and treat identified  │
  │       reversible causes                                      │
  └─────────────────────────────────────────────────────────────┘
                               │
                 3             ▼
              ┌──────────────────────────────────┐
              │    Transcutaneous pacing         │
              │ If considered, perform immediately│
              └──────────────────────────────────┘
                               │
                 4             ▼
              ┌──────────────────────────────────┐
              │  Epinephrine 1 mg IV push,        │
              │  repeat every 3 to 5 minutes      │
              └──────────────────────────────────┘
                               │
                 5             ▼
              ┌──────────────────────────────────┐
              │  Atropine 1 mg IV, repeat every   │
              │  3 to 5 minutes up to a total     │
              │  dose of 0.04 mg/kg               │
              └──────────────────────────────────┘
                               │
                 6             ▼
              ┌──────────────────────────────────┐
              │         Asystole persists         │
              │ Withhold or cease resuscitative   │
              │            efforts?               │
              │ • Consider quality of resuscitation│
              │ • Atypical clinical features       │
              │     present?                       │
              │ • Support for cease-efforts        │
              │     protocols in place?            │
              └──────────────────────────────────┘
```

Figure 1–19. Asystole treatment algorithm. (American Heart Association: Textbook of Advanced Cardiac Life Support. American Heart Association, Chicago. Reproduced with permission, *ACLS Provider Manual 2001*, © 2003, Copyright American Heart Association.)

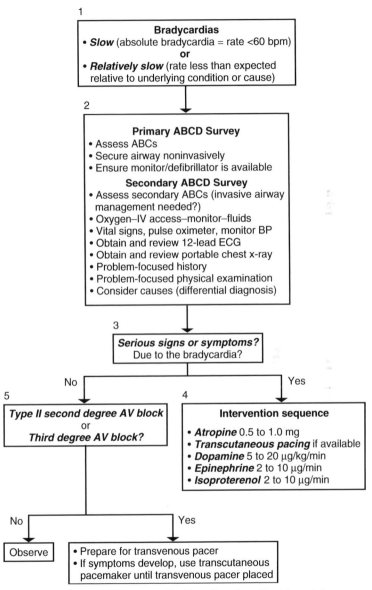

Figure 1–20. Bradycardia treatment algorithm. (American Heart Association: Textbook of Advanced Cardiac Life Support. American Heart Association, Chicago. Reproduced with permission, *ACLS Provider Manual 2001*, © 2003, Copyright American Heart Association.)

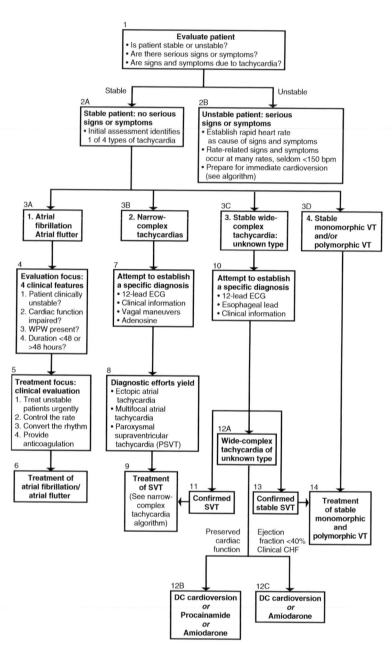

Figure 1–21. Tachycardia treatment algorithm. (American Heart Association: Textbook of Advanced Cardiac Life Support. American Heart Association, Chicago. Reproduced with permission, *ACLS Provider Manual 2001*, © 2003, Copyright American Heart Association.)

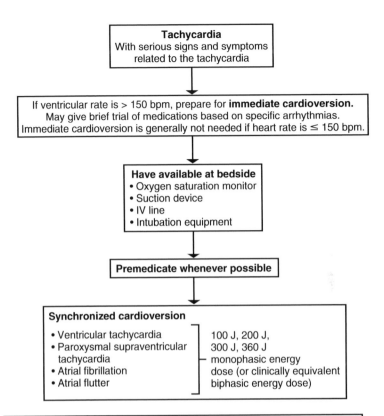

Tachycardia
With serious signs and symptoms
related to the tachycardia

If ventricular rate is > 150 bpm, prepare for **immediate cardioversion.**
May give brief trial of medications based on specific arrhythmias.
Immediate cardioversion is generally not needed if heart rate is ≤ 150 bpm.

Have available at bedside
• Oxygen saturation monitor
• Suction device
• IV line
• Intubation equipment

Premedicate whenever possible

Synchronized cardioversion

• Ventricular tachycardia
• Paroxysmal supraventricular
  tachycardia
• Atrial fibrillation
• Atrial flutter

100 J, 200 J,
300 J, 360 J
monophasic energy
dose (or clinically equivalent
biphasic energy dose)

Notes
1. Effective regimens have included a sedative (e.g., *diazepam, midazolam, barbiturates, etomidate, ketamine, methohexital*) with or without an analgesic agent (e.g., *fentanyl, morphine, meperidine*). Many experts recommend anesthesia if service is readily available.
2. Both monophasic and biphasic waveforms are acceptable if documented as clinically equivalent to reports of monophasic shock success.
3. Note possible need to resynchronize after each cardioversion.
4. If delays in synchronization occur and clinical condition is critical, go immediately to unsynchronized shocks.
5. Treat polymorphic ventricular tachycardia (irregular form and rate) as for ventricular fibrillation: see Ventricular Fibrillation/Pulseless Ventricular Tachycardia Algorithm.*
6. Paroxysmal supraventricular tachycardia and atrial flutter often respond to lower energy levels (start with 50 J).

Figure 1–22. Electrical cardioversion algorithm. (American Heart Association: Textbook of Advanced Cardiac Life Support. American Heart Association, Chicago. Reproduced with permission, *ACLS Provider Manual 2001,* © 2003, Copyright American Heart Association.)
*See Figure 1-17.

DERMATOLOGY

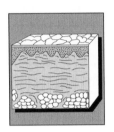

2

Acne Vulgaris

Jodi L. Cahalan, MPH, MS, PA-C

DEFINITION

An inflammatory disorder of the sebaceous hair follicle resulting in a variety of skin lesions.

HISTORY

Symptoms. Range in severity, but may include closed comedones (whiteheads), open comedones (blackheads), papules, nodules, and cysts, which are most commonly found on the face and trunk.

General. Usually unresponsive to over-the-counter (OTC) treatments.

Age. Can be seen in any age group from neonates to the elderly, but is most common in adolescents and adults in their 20s, 30s, and 40s. May occur for the first time in adults, more commonly in females.

Onset. Often in puberty, coinciding with the maturing function of sebaceous glands.

Duration. Weeks, months, or years.

Intensity. Anything from a few comedones to nodules, cysts, and scarring.

Aggravating Factors. Overaggressive cleansing of the skin; attempted mechanical removal of lesions by the patient. The roles of diet and stress as causative factors are controversial.

Alleviating Factors. Mild cases may show improvement from OTC preparations.

Associated Factors. May be caused by a variety of medications including isoniazid, medroxyprogesterone, lithium, phenytoin, iodides, and anabolic steroids.

PHYSICAL EXAMINATION

General. The patient is in no acute distress but may show signs of depression or anxiety about the lesions and/or scarring and their effect on lifestyle. Skin lesions may be readily apparent on exposed skin areas.

Skin. Any or all of the following may be noted on the patient's face and/or trunk: open or closed comedones, papules and/or pustules on erythematous bases, nodules, and cysts. Scarring from previous lesions may be present. See Figures 2-1 to 2-4 in color plate section.

PATHOPHYSIOLOGY

An increased turnover of keratin, often mediated by androgens, occurs in sebaceous glands, which leads to increased sebum production. The excess sebum, in combination with the presence of *Propionibacterium acnes,* stimulates an inflammatory response, often resulting in pustule or papule formation.

DIAGNOSTIC STUDIES

Usually none, but culture may be considered if lesions have been resistant to treatment in order to rule out fungal or other bacterial infection.

DIFFERENTIAL DIAGNOSIS

Traumatic. Not applicable.

Infectious
Folliculitis due to bacteria or fungi: Will be more widespread including extremities and involve the scalp. Pustules tend to be uniform and smaller than in acne vulgaris. No comedones or cysts.

Early impetigo: Pustules are seen but develop into weepy, crusted, maculopapular plaques and may be anywhere on the body. No comedones or cysts.

Malassezia folliculitis: Culture demonstrates *Malassezia furfur* (formerly *Pityrosporum orbiculare*). Responds to oral ketoconazole.

Metabolic
Steroid acne and *chloracne*: Are marked by known systemic or contact exposure to offending drugs or chemical. The red papulopustules may occur in small groups in limited areas or may be more widespread over the body.

Acne rosacea: Usually affects middle-aged to older adults. Inflammatory, with patchy erythema generally of the cheeks, nose, and forehead, with no significant comedones or cysts.

Neoplastic. Not applicable.
Vascular. Not applicable.
Congenital. Not applicable.
Acquired. Not applicable.

TREATMENT

Encourage twice-daily gentle cleansing of the affected skin with a mild soap.
  Topical antimicrobials are used to suppress *Propionibacterium acnes*:
    Benzoyl peroxide, 2.5%, 5%, or 10% applied twice a day after cleansing.
      Decreases inflammatory lesions and comedones, and no resistance
      develops, unlike with the other topical antimicrobials. The higher
      strengths are more effective but also more irritating to the skin.
    Erythromycin 2% or clindamycin 1% (liquid or gel) applied twice a
      day. These may be drying and are mildly irritating. Clindamycin
      also comes as a lotion, which may be better tolerated in persons
      with sensitive skin.

Other agents that may be helpful:

Topical retinoids may be added to help heal comedones and inflammatory lesions: Tretinoin 0.025%, 0.05%, or 0.1% applied once nightly. Lowest useful dose is recommended, as higher doses cause more irritation.

Adapalene 0.1% applied 1 hour before bedtime.

Tazarotene 0.05%, 0.1%: Pregnancy category X. Pregancy must be ruled out and the patient protected from pregnancy.

Systemic therapy for resistant or moderately severe acne lesions: Start one of the following antibiotics and follow up at 6 weeks. May increase dosage as needed to achieve results.

Tetracycline 500 mg twice a day is the traditional first-line drug.

Doxycycline 100 mg daily.

Minocycline 100 mg daily.

Erythromycin 500 mg twice a day.

Other oral antibiotics that may be considered are trimethoprim-sulfamethoxazole, clindamycin, and ampicillin, but because of their side-effect profiles, generally these agents are used only if others fail.

Need to treat for a minimum of 4 months before treatment failure is documented.

Isotretinoin: Indicated as first-line agent for treatment of deep and severely inflammatory acne with scarring or in resistant cases with treatment failure with other modalities. Effect is gradual and generally not noticeable during the first month. Counseling is necessary as drug is teratogenic, and all female patients must have a negative pregnancy test before therapy with isotretinoin begins, and then monthly and until at least 1 month after cessation of therapy. Must use two forms of birth control. Dosage starts at 0.5-1.0 mg/kg/day divided into twice-daily doses and can be increased up to 2 mg/kg/day. Prescriber training is required.

PEDIATRIC CONSIDERATIONS

No other specific considerations.

OBSTETRIC CONSIDERATIONS

Isotretinoin, used for first-line treatment for severe, inflammatory acne with scarring, is teratogenic. Avoid systemic therapies in patients who may be or wish to become pregnant.

GERIATRIC CONSIDERATIONS

Acne vulgaris can occur in the elderly but is most common in adolescents and young adults.

PREVENTIVE CONSIDERATIONS

Avoidance of medications such as isoniazid, medroxyprogesterone, lithium, phenytoin, iodides, and anabolic steroids.

Depression and anxiety can coexist with acne vulgaris, and this possibility needs to be addressed.

PEARLS FOR THE PA

Acne vulgaris is an inflammatory disorder of the sebaceous hair follicle resulting in a range of skin lesions.

Lesions can be treated topically or systemically.

Alopecia

Jodi L. Cahalan, MPH, MS, PA-C

DEFINITION

Hair loss in areas in which hair growth is normally seen.

HISTORY

Symptoms. Asymptomatic hair loss on the scalp or in the beard area or any other area of normal hair growth.

General. *Alopecia areata* is hair loss in round patches. *Alopecia totalis* is loss of all scalp hair and sometimes facial hair. *Alopecia universalis* indicates total body involvement.

Age. Any, but usually begins in late childhood to early teens.

Onset. Sudden to chronic.

Duration. Weeks to permanent, sometimes recycling.

Aggravating Factors. Genetic predisposition, emotional stress.

Alleviating Factors. None.

Associated Factors. Autoimmune diseases, emotional stress, thyroiditis, pernicious anemia, Addison's disease. Vitiligo may also be present.

PHYSICAL EXAMINATION

Dermatologic. Sharply circumscribed, small or large areas of hair loss with characteristic "exclamation mark" hair present peripherally, in which the pattern of hair loss is wide distally and thin proximally. No scales, underlying erythema, vesicles, or scarring should be noted. Longitudinal ridging or pitting of the nails may be present. See Figures 2-5 and 2-6 in color plate section.

DIAGNOSTIC STUDIES

Laboratory
Thyroid Function Test. May reveal hyperthyroidism or occasionally hypothyroidism as the cause of diffuse hair loss.

Rapid Plasma Reagin (RPR) Assay and Fluorescent Treponemal Antibody (FTA) Test. Rule out secondary syphilis, which may manifest with patchy hair loss.

Antinuclear Antibody Test. May be positive.

Radiology. Not applicable.

Other
Skin Biopsy. Generally unnecessary to make the diagnosis, but may be utilized to rule out other causes of hair loss. In cases of alopecia, biopsy will generally show lymphocytic infiltrates.

Culture (Including Fungal Culture)/Potassium Hydroxide Preparation and Microscopy. Rule out tinea capitis.

DIFFERENTIAL DIAGNOSIS

Traumatic
Traction alopecia: May be diffuse or sharply circumscribed. History of wearing tight braids, pigtails, or ponytail in recent past; hair loss will be localized to those sites.

Trichotillomania (mechanical pulling out of hair): Results in diffuse irregular multiple patches of loss with broken or twisted hairs, but no exclamation mark hairs are noted. History of twisting or pulling on hair is present.

Tinea capitis: Pustules and/or scaling, crusting, and "black-dot" broken hairs in bare or sparse areas are seen. Sometimes swollen, boggy, crusty lesions if hair loss is due to kerions.

Metabolic
Discoid lupus erythematosus: Erythema, heavy scale, scarring and occasional ulceration with permanent hair loss.

Male or *female pattern alopecia*: Is marked by diffuse thinning and resultant baldness at crown and/or bilateral anterior forehead scalp for males and general diffuse thinning for females. Family history common.

Neoplastic
Alopecia neoplastica: Hair loss is usually over a subcutaneous nodule, often with redness and sometimes scaling of the skin surface. This metastatic finding is most often seen with breast cancer, but may also be from primary lung tumor.

Acquired

Secondary syphilis: There may be a diffuse "moth-eaten" appearance to the hair loss.

TREATMENT

The goal of therapy is to produce hair regrowth, mainly for cosmetic reasons. Hair loss causes psychological stress, and this factor should be acknowledged. Patients with mild disease should be reassured that hair regrowth generally occurs but often takes considerable time. Those with more severe hair loss may feel more comfortable wearing a hairpiece/wig.

The following therapies may be useful:

Betamethasone dipropionate ointment 0.05% should be applied twice a day to the affected area with additional 1-inch margins surrounding area of hair loss. May try almost any other high-dose steroid ointment, with avoidance of highest-potency preparations to the face.

Anthralin, an irritant, may stimulate hair regrowth. Start at lowest concentration and may increase at three to four month intervals.

Intralesional steroids may be helpful for mild, stable disease. Systemic steroids should only be used for alopecia totalis and universalis and at low doses.

Topical minoxidil 2% has shown minimal usefulness in alopecia areata.

PEDIATRIC CONSIDERATIONS

Rare except with thyroid diseases. Hair loss in infants in the neonatal period, during the first few months of life, or following an acute febrile illness is due to the shift of hair growth from an active phase (anagen phase) to a resting phase (telogen phase) and is referred to as *telogen effluvium*. Parents should be reassured that normal hair growth will return within 6 to 12 months. Children may also present with hair loss secondary to trichotillomania, traction alopecia, or infection; as a side effect of radiation or certain drugs (cancer chemotherapeutic agents); or with alopecia areata.

OBSTETRIC CONSIDERATIONS

Many patients will notice increased hair loss post partum, which usually occurs subsequent to an actual increase in hair growth during pregnancy. For the treatment of *androgenic alopecia*, there are no known contraindications to the use of minoxidil during pregnancy.

GERIATRIC CONSIDERATIONS

Alopecia is a normal finding in many men and women in the geriatric period.

PREVENTIVE CONSIDERATIONS

Essentially none, except for avoidance and/or treatment of associated conditions such as autoimmune diseases, emotional stress, thyroiditis, pernicious anemia, Addison's disease, or vitiligo.

PEARLS FOR THE PA

Treatment begins with reassurance about the possibility of regrowth and a forewarning that initial regrowth normally begins with white hair in all age groups.

Also important is an explanation of the autoimmune/stress aspect of the disease and the variable results of most therapy.

Prognosis nearly hopeless after 5 years of loss.

Bacterial Infections

Jodi L. Cahalan, MPH, MS, PA-C

DEFINITION

Invasion of the skin, its appendages, and/or subcutaneous layer by way of thermal, mechanical, chemical, or physiologic injury and the colonization or infection with pathogenic bacteria of both aerobic and anaerobic nature. Lesions are usually due to immune system response, and purulence is present.

Bacterial skin infections are classified as follows:

Furuncles, carbuncles: Local infections of hair follicles involving single or multiple follicles, respectively.

Folliculitis: Inflammation of one or more hair follicles occurring locally or in a widespread distribution.

Impetigo: Superficial epidermal infection, generally caused by *Staphylococcus aureus* or *Streptococcus pyogenes*.

Ecthyma: Also caused by *Staphylococcus aureus* and/or *Streptococcus pyogenes*, but penetrates deeper into the epidermis than does impetigo.

Erysipelas, cellulitis: Erysipelas occurs when streptococcal infection spreads into dermal lymphatics. Cellulitis is an infection that goes into the deeper dermis and subcutaneous fat.

HISTORY

Symptoms

Furuncles, Carbuncles
Furuncle. Firm erythematous nodule affecting one hair follicle that enlarges over several days, becomes fluctuant, develops a point, and ruptures.
Carbuncle. Tender nodule, affecting several adjacent hair follicles. Larger and more painful than a furuncle.
Folliculitis. Yellowish-white pustules with a hair in the center. Often asymptomatic, but may be mildly tender or pruritic.
Impetigo. Vesicles or pustules on an erythematous base that subsequently rupture and form crusts. Cases vary in terms of number and size of lesions. May be mildly pruritic, but are generally not painful. Constitutional symptoms or fever are not generally present.
Ecthyma. Vesicles or bullae, which rupture, forming crusts with ulcerations beneath. Lesions are often tender, may be pruritic, and are generally on the lower extremity.
Erysipelas, Cellulitis. Red, warm, swollen, tender, and painful skin areas. Fevers are common. Eye may be swollen shut if affected.

General. Investigate environmental exposures or known contacts for skin injury and bacterial proximity.

Age
Furuncles, Carbuncles. Any, but more common in teens and adults than in children.
Folliculitis. Any, but especially in children.
Impetigo. Any, but most cases are in young children.
Ecthyma. Any.
Erysipelas, Cellulitis. Any, but usually in the adult.

Onset
Furuncles, Carbuncles. Sudden onset, often with progression over the next several days to involvement of more follicles over a larger area.
Folliculitis. Sudden, with few to many lesions.
Impetigo. Sudden, with one or more papules, but lesions usually develop 10-20 days after exposure to causative agent(s).
Ecthyma. Sudden, with one or more lesions.
Erysipelas, Cellulitis. Sudden but insidious.

Duration
Furuncles, Carbuncles. Days, weeks, or months until treated.
Folliculitis. Days, weeks, or months until treated.
Impetigo. Weeks or months unless treated, but generally responds quickly to treatment.
Ecthyma. Weeks or months.
Erysipelas, Cellulitis. Weeks, and can have serious complications if untreated.

Intensity

Furuncles, Carbuncles. Few local to many widespread, with only minimal systemic potential.

Folliculitis. Small, local to extensive, and widespread. Rare systemic effect.

Impetigo. Single to multiple and widespread lesions, with systemic effect possible in extensive disease.

Ecthyma. Single to multiple and widespread lesions, with systemic effect possible in extensive disease.

Erysipelas, Cellulitis. Mild to extensive local lesions, with mild to severe systemic signs common.

Aggravating Factors. Further or continued exposure to skin traumatizers, lack of treatment, uncleanliness, poor hygiene, tight clothing, immune deficiency.

Alleviating Factors. Meticulous, gentle skin cleansing, especially with antibacterials; strong, efficient immune system.

Associated Factors. Environmental exposure.

PHYSICAL EXAMINATION

General. The patient usually appears in no acute distress. Obtain vital signs including temperature to evaluate for the possibility of sepsis.

Skin

Furuncles, Carbuncles. Found everywhere there are hair follicles, but more commonly in areas predisposed to increased friction and sweating such as the upper back, chest, neck, axillae, buttocks, and groin. Inflamed, single pustules are seen with furuncles, and groups of small neighboring pustules in single region of inflammation seen with carbuncles. Carbuncles may be quite tender to palpation.

Folliculitis. Single red papules and/or pustules scattered diffusely and widely over the body anywhere there are hair follicles, especially scalp, arms, legs, axillae, trunk, and buttocks. May be seen in smaller local groups or patches (e.g., the beard area, buttocks, chest). Usually no surrounding erythema or inflammation.

Impetigo. Small red papules, vesicles, or pustules seen initially, which subsequently rupture, leaving weepy erosions, which crust. Honey-colored crusts are generally due to streptococcal infection, whereas thin, smooth crusts with varnish-like appearance are generally due to staphylococcal infection. Lesions may be solitary or multiple and exist in a wide area or grouped closely. Generally on the face or extremities of children, but may affect any location. Regional lymphadenopathy may be present.

Ecthyma. Erythematous, circular lesions, which may be moist or crusting, may occur in any location but are seen most commonly on feet, ankles, legs and thighs.

Erysipelas, Cellulitis. Local marked erythematous swellings with discrete, raised border. Seen in dry warm facial areas (e.g., ear, cheeks, nose, periorbital area in adults). Local large or small erythematous warm, tender, irregularly bordered swellings of skin and soft tissues in any area in the child or adult. Often associated with fever and listlessness. Moist serous ooze on the surface may be noted with cellulitis.

Lymphatic. All of the bacterial skin infections may cause local or regional lymph node swelling and tenderness.

PATHOPHYSIOLOGY

Furuncles, Carbuncles. Generally caused by *S. aureus*, but may also be caused by *Escherichia coli, Pseudomonas aeruginosa*, or *Streptococcus faecalis* or such anaerobes as *Peptostreptococcus, Peptococcus*, or lactobacilli.

Folliculitis. Generally caused by *S. aureus*, though it may also be caused by the fungus *Malassezia furfur* (formerly *Pityrosporum orbiculare*) or by *P. aeruginosa* in the case of hot tub, whirlpool, or swimming pool folliculitis.

Impetigo. Generally caused by *S. pyogenes* or *S. aureus*.

Ecthyma. Most commonly caused by streptococci, especially group A streptococci and *S. aureus*.

Erysipelas, Cellulitis. Most commonly caused by group A streptococci.

DIAGNOSTIC STUDIES

Generally not needed, but on occasion may be used to identify the pathogen, especially if systemic signs and symptoms are present or if the patient is unresponsive to treatment.

Laboratory
Culture with Gram Stain. Culture and stain of the lesion or discharge to identify the causative organism.

Complete Blood Count. May show an elevated white blood cell count with systemic infections.

Radiology
Not applicable.

DIFFERENTIAL DIAGNOSIS

Traumatic
Wounds. Those of the puncture or penetrating type may lead to infections with less common bacteria (e.g., *Clostridium tetani, P. aeruginosa*), which require specialized antibiotic treatment.

Inquire about tetanus inoculation status.

Infectious
Fungal kerions: Can mimic furuncles or carbuncles and the skin may even be colonized with double infection. Usually less inflammation with lesions due solely to fungal organisms, but only culture will differentiate. Most common on scalp.

Fungal/chemical folliculitis: Is differentiated by resistance to treatment, potassium hydroxide (KOH) preparations, Gram stain, and/or culture of intrafollicular matter. Causes include steroids (e.g., cortisones, androgens).

Pityrosporum orbiculare: Is the most common fungal/yeast pathogen.

Herpesvirus infection: In crusted ulcer stage can look like impetigo, but recurrent history, location, and prodrome are different.

Tularemia: Is caused by a gram-negative bacillus (*Francisella tularensis*), causing ecthyma-like ulcers, fevers, and tender lymphadenopathy. May be caused by tick bites, or may occur through rabbit handling.

Metabolic.   Not applicable.

Neoplastic.   Certain *basal cell* and *squamous cell cancers* and *metastatic lesions* to the skin may appear to be furuncles, carbuncles, abscesses, or ulcerations. Their chronic, nontender, sterile nature differentiates.

Vascular.   Not applicable.

Congenital.   Not applicable.

Acquired.   Not applicable.

TREATMENT

Furuncles and Carbuncles.   For a small number of lesions, moist heat and/or incision and drainage are usually curative. If the lesions are widespread or there is significant surrounding inflammation-cellulitis or systemic symptoms such as fever, chills, or malaise, systemic antibiotics are needed.

Dicloxacillin 250-500 mg four times a day for at least 7 days.

Clindamycin 150-300 mg four times a day for at least 7 days.

Cephalexin 500 mg four times a day for at least 7 days.

Folliculitis

Dicloxacillin 250 mg three to four times a day.

Erythromycin 250-500 mg three to four times a day. May require therapy for up to 6 weeks.

For resistant infection, ciprofloxacin 500 mg two times a day.

Avoid hot tub bathing if suspected as a cause. Avoid heat, friction, and occlusion. Keep skin clean by using an antibacterial soap; keep skin dry. Discontinue contact with oil or irritant cause.

Limited cases may be treated with topical mupirocin 2% applied once a day.

Impetigo.   If lesions are few and small, treat with topical mupirocin. Bacitracin or other topical antibiotic preparations may also be tried, but such agents are generally less effective.

Systemic antibiotics necessary for 7 to 14 days for all other cases. Any of the following may be used:

Dicloxacillin 250 mg four times a day, which is best for thick or thin crusting or bullous lesions caused by *Staphylococcus* and/or *Streptococcus,* OR

Erythromycin 250-500 mg four times a day for first-line therapy or in patients who are penicillin-allergic.

As an alternative, clindamycin 150 mg four times a day or a cephalosporin (e.g., cephalexin 250 mg four times a day) may be used.

Ecthyma
Dicloxacillin, erythromycin, clindamycin, or cephalosporin in dosages as for impetigo.

Erysipelas/Cellulitis
Penicillin V 250-500 mg four times a day for 10 days OR
Dicloxacillin 250-500 mg four times a day for 10 days OR
Erythromycin 250-500 mg four times a day for 10 days OR
Clindamycin 150 mg four times a day for 10 days OR
A first-generation cephalosporin equivalent to cephalexin 250-500 mg four times a day for 10 days

PEDIATRIC CONSIDERATIONS

Impetigo.   Superficial form of pyoderma occurring most commonly in children. Infection is characterized by classic erythematous macules that rapidly evolve into vesicles and pustules, which then rupture and form a honey-colored crust. Nonbullous impetigo most frequently suggests infection with beta-hemolytic group A streptococci or *S. aureus*. Staphylococci may represent a secondary infection. Impetigo is treated to prevent morbidity and spread to other children. Topical treatment with mupirocin (Bactroban) alone is often effective. Systemic therapy with penicillin, erythromycin, amoxicillin-clavulanate, or dicloxacillin is also effective depending on etiologic agent and sensitivities.

Bullous impetigo, caused by *S. aureus*, is mainly an infection of infants and young children. Blisters filled with clear or yellowish fluid are superficial and rupture easily, leaving a moist denuded base. In the neonate the differential diagnosis includes epidermolysis bullosa, bullous mastocytosis, herpetic infection, and early scalded skin syndrome. Obtain blood for cultures in infants or children who appear ill. Treatment can be topical with mupirocin applied three times a day. More significant infections may be treated systemically with penicillinase-resistant penicillin, cephalexin, or erythromycin.

Ecthyma.   Resembles impetigo but characterized by firm, dry, dark crust with surrounding erythema and induration. Direct pressure on lesion results in extrusion of purulent material from beneath the crust. Causative agent is usually beta-hemolytic streptococci, and systemic antibiotic therapy as for impetigo is indicated.

Perianal Streptococcal Dermatitis.   Child presents with moist, pruritic, erythematous perianal eruption associated with painful defecation and blood-streaked stools. A culture of the perianal region (and often the pharynx) will be positive for beta-hemolytic group A streptococci. Consider sexual abuse, candidiasis, pinworm infestation, psoriasis, and seborrheic dermatitis. Treat with oral penicillin or erythromycin, and reculture.

Scarlet Fever. Exanthem associated with beta-hemolytic group A streptococcal infection begins with erythematous maculopapular eruption first on the neck and in the axillae and groin and then involving the trunk and extremities. Involved skin may have the texture of sandpaper. Petechiae may occur and may be seen in a linear pattern along the major skin folds in the axillae and antecubital fossa (Pastia sign). Desquamation begins on the face toward the end of the first week and proceeds to the trunk, hands, and feet. Desquamation may continue for as long as 6 weeks.

Staphylococcal Scalded Skin Syndrome. A disease of infants and children under 10 years and caused by a group 2 phage-type *S. aureus.* Generalized erythema may or may not be preceded by prodrome of malaise, fever, and irritability due to pronounced skin tenderness. Macular eruption first involving face, neck, axilla, and groin progresses to flaccid bullae filled with clear fluid. Facial edema and perioral crusting develop. Large sheets of epidermis begin to peel away. Moist denuded areas quickly dry and heal by postinflammatory desquamation. Healing proceeds rapidly and is complete by 10 to 14 days. Treatment is with oral or parenteral semisynthetic penicillinase-resistant penicillin. Increased morbidity is associated with excess fluid loss, electrolyte imbalance, pneumonia, unstable temperature regulation, septicemia, and cellulitis.

OBSTETRIC CONSIDERATIONS

Sulfonamides, erythromycin, and ciprofloxacin should be used with caution. Tetracycline is contraindicated.

GERIATRIC CONSIDERATIONS

Trauma to the skin can occur owing to reduced sensation from a variety of systemic illnesses. Hygiene and cleanliness may be an issue for elderly patients with dementia or persons who reside in long-term care facilities.

Immune response may be blunted in the elderly.

PREVENTIVE CONSIDERATIONS

Appropriate hygiene is important to prevent bacterial infection of the skin.

PEARLS FOR THE PA

Reassure the patient that these infections are rarely dangerous in spite of the appearance and feel.

Benign Cutaneous Neoplasms

Jodi L. Cahalan, MPH, MS, PA-C

DEFINITION

Acrochordon (skin tag): A fleshy outgrowth or papilloma.

Callosities: Areas of hyperkeratosis of skin of hands or feet developing in reaction to repeated rubbing or to pressure over a bony prominence.

Dermatofibroma: Small dome-shaped, fibrous, brownish-red nodules often at sites of skin prick, puncture, or bite injury of extremities.

Hemangioma: Common vascular neoplasm of the capillary endothelium, seen most commonly on the head or neck. Most common type of tumor in children.

Keloid scars (keloids): Lesions of a hypertrophic healing response, occurring in a predisposed person, that extends beyond the original site of injury.

Lentigines (solar): Round or oval macules on the skin due to increased melanin from increased melanocytes at the epidermodermal junction. Most common on sun-exposed skin.

Lipoma: Benign tumor of adipose tissue.

Nevi (acquired melanocytic or nevocytic): A common benign skin tumor composed of melanocyte-derived nevus cells.

Pyogenic granuloma: A vascular proliferation occurring on the skin and mucous membranes.

Sebaceous hyperplasia: Prominently enlarged sebaceous glands generally occurring on the face.

Seborrheic keratosis: Benign epidermal tumor with hyperplasia of keratinocytes.

HISTORY

Symptoms
Acrochordon. Usually none, but may be accompanied by pruritus or tenderness after torsion or rubbing irritation from clothes, jewelry, or another skin surface, especially in obese persons.

Callosities. Thickened skin areas, which may become uncomfortable. In the case of a clavus (corn), there may be intense pain with walking.

Dermatofibroma. Asymptomatic dark, hard bump on lower or upper legs or arms that has often been present for months to years. Generally asymptomatic, but may be pruritic or tender.

Hemangioma. Red, purple, or bluish neoplasm occurring in infancy, usually within the first 3 to 4 weeks of life. Generally asymptomatic unless large and compressing underlying structures. Often begins as a poorly defined pink macule and then progresses to a sharply demarcated, bright red plaque or nodule.

Keloid Scars. Large overgrowth of scarring after healing of a wound or skin injury (e.g., insect bites, acne papules, skin piercing for jewelry, local surgery).

Lentigines (Solar). Painless brown spots on arms, face, legs, chest, or back, usually on sun-exposed surfaces.

Lipoma. Soft, poorly defined palpable mass, which can occur anywhere but is most commonly found on the neck, trunk, and extremities. May be small or large.

Nevi (Acquired Melanocytic or Nevocytic). Painless, flat, round brown papules found on any skin location, but most commonly on sun-exposed areas.

Pyogenic Granuloma. Fast-growing, easily injured reddish growth on skin or mucous membranes, often developing after trauma to the skin.

Sebaceous Hyperplasia. Generally a single, small, skin-colored to yellow papule with well-defined margins and umbilicated.

Seborrheic Keratosis. One or more "stuck-on"–appearing lesions, which may be pinkish, tan, brown, or black. Surface may be smooth, scaly, or velvety.

Age

Acrochordon. Usually seen in middle and old age, rarely before age 30 years, with female propensity.

Callosities. Any, but not common in childhood.

Dermatofibroma. Any, but usually adults, more often females.

Hemangioma. Any. About 20% are present at birth, with the remainder of strawberry and cavernous hemangiomas occurring within the first 2 to 4 weeks of life. Usually over age 20 for cherry angiomas.

Keloid Scars. Any age, but tend to occur before age 30.

Lentigines (Solar). Usually in later adulthood.

Lipoma. In adults, usually in the fifth to sixth decades of life; may occur in younger persons with the familial form.

Nevi (Acquired Melanocytic or Nevocytic). Peak incidence during adolescence, but may be present at birth. Remain for decades.

Pyogenic Granuloma. Any, but more common in children and young adults.

Sebaceous Hyperplasia. Adults, rarely before the age of 30; more common as age advances.

Seborrheic Keratosis. Extremely rare in children; may occur in young adults and is more common in the elderly.

Onset

Acrochordon. Gradual growth of small skin tag, with chronic increase in both size and number.

Callosities. Chronic, with repetitive rubbing, especially on the hands or over the bones of the feet.

Dermatofibroma. Noticed suddenly, but because it is asymptomatic, medical care is generally not sought until lesion has been present for quite some time. Attains maximum size after months to years and then does not change much.

Hemangioma. May be congenital or appear suddenly in early infancy.

Keloid Scars. Chronic. Overgrowth may follow healing of an injury by weeks or months, but some pruritus or irritation often persists. History of significant skin injury may be vague.

Lentigines (Solar). Chronically, occurring any time after age 30 and increasing in size and number.

Lipoma. Sudden to chronic.

Nevi (Acquired Melanocytic or Nevocytic). New lesions may develop over long periods of time.

Pyogenic Granuloma. Occurs suddenly, with rapid growth until it reaches maximum size, generally within a few weeks.

Sebaceous Hyperplasia. Gradual, chronic.

Seborrheic Keratosis. Chronic, slow-growing.

Duration

Acrochordon. Indefinite unless treatment is given or spontaneous infarction and sloughing occur.

Callosities. Indefinite, but tend to diminish as pressure and rubbing cease.

Dermatofibroma. Indefinite to permanent. Does not tend to spontaneously resolve.

Hemangioma. Fifty percent of hemangiomas fully regress by age 5 years, and 90% by age 9. If no regression occurs by age 6, then complete regression is not likely.

Keloid Scars. Indefinite, generally permanent.

Lentigines (Solar). Permanent without treatment.

Lipoma. Indefinite to permanent.

Nevi (Acquired Melanocytic or Nevocytic). Many years; fewer acquired by age 30, often fading by late adulthood.

Pyogenic Granuloma. Indefinite, long-term unless treated.

Sebaceous Hyperplasia. Permanent, long-term unless treated.

Seborrheic Keratosis. Permanent with slow growth, often with increasing pigment.

Intensity

Acrochordon. Single to numerous, widespread.

Callosities. From single, small pressure points to involvement of the entire heel or areas of the foot, or palmar aspect of hands.

Dermatofibroma. Usually single, but may be multiple.

Hemangioma. May range from single, small nodules to deeper cavernous nodules, which may be quite large. Rapidly growing lesions may cause serious complications such as obstruction of vital functions (breathing, eating), high-output cardiac failure, or Kasabach-Merritt syndrome, which leads to a coagulopathy. Cherry angiomas tend to be multiple and widespread in adults.

Keloid Scars. May range from a single, small overgrowth to widespread involvement, which may occur with multiple skin lesions, such as with acne. May be a very exaggerated overgrowth onto normal skin relative to the small size of injury.

Lentigines (Solar). Range from single, few small lesions to many, up to 1 to 2 cm in diameter.

Lipoma. May range from a single, small (1-to 3-cm) lesion to many lesions as large as several centimeters across.

Nevi (Acquired Melanocytic or Nevocytic). One lesion to several, beginning any time after birth and peaking in adolescence, to many lesions numbering 30 to 40. Lesions may flatten by 40 years of age, and many disappear by age 90.

Pyogenic Granuloma. Starts small but grows rapidly over few weeks. Easily friable, with crusting common.

Sebaceous Hyperplasia. One to many lesions, typically 1 to 5 mm in diameter, but are generally without symptoms.

Seborrheic Keratosis. One to numerous on trunk, head, extremities; does not affect the palms or soles.

Aggravating Factors

Acrochordon. Irritation from jewelry or clothes, or friction in intertriginous areas.

Callosities. Continued manual labor for hands and continued wearing of shoes that compress or rub the foot or toes.

Dermatofibroma. Further skin injury. Given that women's legs are the most common sites, repeated trauma from shaving can occur.

Hemangiomas. Patient may have difficulty eating or breathing if lesions are over the mouth or nose.

Keloid Scars. Scratching, rubbing, continued skin trauma or lesions.

Lentigines (Solar). Intense sun exposure, especially a history of sunburns.

Lipoma. Not applicable

Nevi (Acquired Melanocytic). Not applicable

Pyogenic Granuloma. Onset often follows minor trauma. Bleeds easily with minor injury. Conservative treatment often leads to recurrence of one or more lesions.

Sebaceous Hyperplasia. Not applicable

Seborrheic Keratosis. Sun damage leads to increased risk; genetic propensity.

Alleviating Factors

Acrochordon. Removal.

Callosities. For hands, cease manual labor using the hands. For feet, new, better fitting or custom-made shoes. Paring of large calluses may be helpful.

Dermatofibroma. Removal, although cosmetically the scar may be worse than the original lesion.

Hemangioma. Time necessary for regression.

Keloid Scars. Removal.

Lentigines (Solar). Appropriate treatment.

Lipoma. Removal.

Nevi (Acquired Melanocytic or Nevocytic). Time, many fade by age 90.

Pyogenic Granuloma. Removal.

Sebaceous Hyperplasia. Removal.
Seborrheic Keratosis. Removal.

Associated Factors
Acrochordon. Hereditary propensity; obesity.
Callosities. Chronic pressure and/or friction.
Dermatofibroma. Occasional history of insect bite or prick injury preceding the lesion.
Hemangioma. Hereditary predilection. Similarly located hemangiomas not uncommon in family members.
Keloid Scars. Greater predilection in dark-skinned persons, especially on the jaw line and ear lobes.
Lentigines (Solar). Familial predisposition; increasing in size and number in late years.
Lipoma. The familial form is characterized by many small lesions on trunk and extremities.
Nevi (Acquired Melanocytic or Nevocytic). No known external effects, so presumed to be of hereditary origin.
Pyogenic Granuloma. Equal in both genders.
Sebaceous Hyperplasia. Hereditary propensity, no gender propensity.
Seborrheic Keratosis. Hereditary predilection.

PHYSICAL EXAMINATION

Skin
Acrochordon. Soft, flesh-colored to brown pedunculated papule on a thin stalk of skin, ranging in size from less than 1 mm to 1 or 2 cm. Found most commonly on neck and chest and in axillae, but also common on proximal, medial thigh.
Callosities. Areas of thickened, hard, hyperkeratotic skin. Commonly found around the heels, under and around the toes, on foresoles of the feet, and over the palmar metacarpophalangeal joints of the hands. Sometimes pain on deep palpation. See Figure 2-7 in color plate section.
Dermatofibroma. Pink to brownish red, domed, firm and discrete nodule, 1 cm or less in diameter, on an extremity but rarely on palmar or plantar surfaces. Nontender and typically dimples with bilateral compression. Firm and, although fixed within the skin, is movable over subcutaneous fat. See Figure 2-8 in color plate section.
Hemangioma. Bright red macule that may be elevated and almost nodular in first 6 to 12 months. Very discrete, sharp-bordered. Located on the neck or head, but may also be found on the trunk. Deeper nodular fullness with irregular bright red and white color, or fleshy surface over deep, bruise-like reddish purple nodule, which is often compressible. Size varies from 1 to 2 cm to several centimeters for cavernous type. Cherry angiomas are red to purple, domed papules a few millimeters in diameter, found on trunk and extremities.
Keloid Scars. Thick, fibrous, fleshy, red or brown lesions seen over mature hyperplastic scars. Most common on ear lobes (after piercing), jaws

and chest, shoulder or upper back (after acne), and any site of surgery. See Figure 2-9 in color plate section.

Lentigines (Solar). Asymptomatic irregular brown macule with sharp borders ranging in size from a few millimeters to a couple of centimeters in diameter. May be roundish, oval, or square-shaped. Found on areas of chronic sun exposure.

Lipoma. Soft, subcutaneous, poorly marginated mobile mass 1 cm to many centimeters in diameter, located on the neck, trunk, or extremities. Rarely tender to pressure. Not fixed to overlying skin, which generally appears normal but is occasionally pigmented. See Figures 2-10 and 2-11 in color plate section.

Nevi (Acquired Melanocytic or Nevocytic). Classified as junctional or compound. *Junctional*: Usually darkly pigmented macules, 2 to 6 mm in diameter, with flat or slightly raised hairless borders. Occur anywhere on the body. *Compound* (intradermal): 3 to 5 mm in diameter tan, flesh-colored to reddish, moderately pigmented and slightly raised, to papillomatous. Occur with hairs on any area of body. See Figure 2-12 in color plate section.

Pyogenic Granuloma. Friable, yellow to deeply red, dome-shaped papule generally 3 to 10 mm in diameter and commonly surrounded by a collar of scales. Moist crusting on surface is easily removed, which results in oozing.

Sebaceous Hyperplasia. Small, yellow to skin-colored umbilicated, sharply demarcated papules on face. One to many in number.

Seborrheic Keratosis. Fleshy yellow, pink, tan, brown, or black, sharply demarcated, oval to round "stuck-on"–appearing raised lesion. Associated with a waxy, velvety, or scaly surface. Occurs on the trunk, head, extremities, or anywhere except the palms and soles. Single to numerous, with tendency to greater thickness and darker pigment on scalp and trunk.

PATHOPHYSIOLOGY

Acrochordon. Papule with a thin epidermis and loose collagen, with no true signs of neoplasm in dermis.

Callosities. Reactive epithelial hyperkeratosis without neoplastic change.

Dermatofibroma. Lesions contain fibroblasts, collagen, and histiocytes and may also contain hemosiderin.

Hemangioma
Strawberry Hemangioma. Early lesions show solid masses with endothelial cells. Mature lesions are less cellular and vascular spaces are more organized. Resolving lesions show fibrosis with loss of vascular space.

Cherry Hemangiomas. Small dilated vessels in superficial dermis, covered by flattened epithelium.

Keloid Scars. Thick bands of collagen.

Lentigines (Solar). Increased number of basal melanocytes with elongated rete ridges.

Lipoma. Tumor of well-circumscribed, mature adipose tissue. Always benign.

Nevi (Acquired Melanocytic or Nevocytic). All have nests of uniform nevus cells. Junctional cells are found in lower epidermis and contain melanin. Compound nevus cells are located in nests of the lower epidermis and high dermis. Melanin production is greatest in epidermal cells and decreases with depth of nevus cells, with little or none in deeper dermis components.

Pyogenic Granuloma.   Superficial, lobular mass of endothelial cells and fibroblasts.

Sebaceous Hyperplasia.   Multiple lobules of normal-appearing sebaceous gland tissue in grape-like clusters surrounding a central, large sebaceous duct, producing the umbilicated appearance.

Seborrheic Keratosis.   Hyperkeratosis in thickened epidermis with increased melanin. Melanosome macrocomplexes are found in the various cells of the skin.

DIAGNOSTIC STUDIES

Laboratory.   Not applicable.
Radiology.   Not applicable.
Other.   Biopsy should be performed on any suspicious lesion in which the diagnosis is uncertain. Biopsies can be performed by punch, excisional, or needle techniques. Acrochordon can be confused with papilloma. Nondysplastic acquired nevi can mutate into melanoma but the risk is very low. Pyogenic granuloma may be clinically similar to amelanotic melanoma.

DIFFERENTIAL DIAGNOSIS

Traumatic
Acrochordon.   May be confused with *keloid.*
Callosities.   Not applicable.
Dermatofibroma.   *Scar:* Is not as pigmented, or has a diffuse, merged border. Also, does not dimple on bilateral squeezing.
Hemangioma.   *Hematomas* and *ecchymoses:* Follow a history of contusion or injury, are more acute and self-limited, and change colors from the violaceous to blue, green, yellow, brown.
Keloid Scars.   *Hypertrophic scar:* Is overgrowth of normal healing skin that is not excessive; diminishes with time.
Lentigines (Solar).   *Postinflammatory hyperpigmentation* or *residual hemosiderin:* After bruising has a more even, consistent coloration and more diffuse border that fades lighter, especially without sun.
Lipoma.   *Hematoma:* Is more firm and dark in color, typically bluish. Sometimes tumorous isolation of fat is caused by contusion-compression injury to fatty tissue.
Nevi (Acquired Melanocytic or Nevocytic).   *Bruise:* Is diffuse and has a different color.
Hemosiderin deposit: Is also diffuse and obviously more superficial than a nevus and is always flat, even, and dark tan or brownish.
Pyogenic Granuloma.   Not applicable.
Sebaceous Hyperplasia.   Not applicable.
Seborrheic Keratosis.   Not applicable.

Infectious
Acrochordon. Not applicable.

Callosities. *Warts*: Can lead to a reactive hyperkeratosis. Pinpoint hemorrhaging commonly associated with plantar warts.

Dermatofibroma. Not applicable.

Hemangioma. *Carbuncles*: Are more pustular in nature with more inflammation and symptoms and have an acute onset with a short, self-limiting course.

Keloid. Not applicable.

Lentigines (Solar). Not applicable.

Lipoma. *Abscess*: Is usually inflamed, tender, more indurated, and fluctuant.

Nevi (Acquired Melanocytic or Nevocytic). Not applicable.

Pyogenic Granuloma. Not applicable.

Sebaceous Hyperplasia. Not applicable.

Seborrheic Keratosis. Not applicable.

Metabolic
Acrochordon. *Neurofibroma*: Is more sessile, of a larger size, and more firm and fixed.

Callosities. Not applicable.

Dermatofibroma. Not applicable.

Keloid Scars. Not applicable.

Lentigines (Solar). Not applicable.

Lipoma. Not applicable.

Nevi (Acquired Melanocytic or Nevocytic). Not applicable.

Pyogenic Granuloma. Not applicable.

Sebaceous Hyperplasia. *Xanthoma*: Is a broad, flat, whitish yellow plaque with even, discrete borders.

Seborrheic Keratosis. Not applicable.

Neoplastic
Acrochordon. *Branchial cysts*: Are usually deep purplish red and arise on the upper neck in the second or third decade of life.

Callosities. Not applicable.

Dermatofibroma. *Basal cell carcinoma*: Is usually not as pigmented, as brownish, or as firm; not as common on the legs.

Hemangioma. *Kaposi sarcoma*: Is of lymphatic endothelial origin. These lesions are violaceous or brown-red macules, papules, or nodules. Seen mostly on legs and progress proximally. Usually occur as multiple lesions and are common on face, head, and chest. Commonly associated with human immunodeficiency (HIV) virus infection.

Keloid Scars. Not applicable.

Lentigines (Solar)
Cafe-au-lait spots: Are single or multiple lesions, 1.5 cm or greater, with sharp, very finely irregular borders with an even tan color. Increased numbers associated with neurofibromatosis.

Simple lentigo: Is usually just a few millimeters in diameter, light brown to jet black. More like a junctional nevus. Onset common in childhood. Not necessarily photodistributed.

Ephelides: Are smaller freckles, 1 to 2 mm in diameter, in younger years. Occur in solar-exposed areas and fade without sun.

Lipoma. Any *malignant neoplasms, metastatic* or *other*, are more firm and less mobile or fixed.

Nevi (Acquired Melanocytic or Nevocytic)
For *melanoma* see Chapter 11, Oncology.

Dysplastic Nevus Syndrome. Familial tendency. Often with melanoma history in family or patient. Lesions tend to be more oval and larger (greater than 6 mm) than acquired nevi. They tend to have more red coloration along with color variation in single lesions. Individual lesions vary in color, size, and shape, and borders tend to meld diffusely into surrounding skin. Most prevalent on trunk and extremities and sun-exposed surfaces. May be few to over a hundred. Any new, changing or questionable lesion should be biopsied for melanoma.

Pyogenic Granuloma. *Basal cell carcinomas*: Are generally more translucent, with a more haphazard array of telangiectasias. *Amelanotic melanomas*: Are usually much slower growing, less friable, more domed, and sessile rather than pedunculated. Biopsy is the definitive diagnostic measure.

Sebaceous Hyperplasia. *Basal cell carcinoma*: Is usually larger, with translucent rolled borders and telangiectasias (tiny, fine red surface vessels). Often leave ulcerations.

Seborrheic Keratosis. *Cafe-au-lait spots*: Remain flat and even tan color, usually much larger. Increased numbers associated with neurofibromatosis. *Melanomas*: Are less distinct, with diffuse borders and more irregularity in shape, color, and elevation.

Vascular
Acrochordon. *Pyogenic granuloma* is eroded, blood red, and friable over a more widespread area.

Callosities. Not applicable.

Dermatofibroma. Not applicable.

Hemangioma. *Pyogenic granuloma*: Is more polypoid. Ulceration and inflammation are common. Affect all ages. *Arteriovenous hemangiomas*: Are bluish red papules with small nodules in adults, with thin-walled dilated veins and arteries in deeper areas. *Venous lakes*: Are violaceous, blue, small-domed papules usually of the elderly. Occur on the lips or exposed skin. Blanch completely with pressure.

Keloid Scars. *Hemangioma* and *pyogenic granuloma*: Are more reddish blue, vascular, and not as firm and generally do not occur with prior history of skin trauma.

Lentigines (Solar). Not applicable.

Lipoma. *Deep cavernous hemangiomas* or *large varicosities*: Are areas of bluish red-purple discoloration, even in subcutaneous tissue.

Nevi (Acquired Melanocytic or Nevocytic). *Hemangiomas*: Are blood-red or purple with no melanin.

Pyogenic Granuloma
Other hemangiomas: Are less sessile, less protruding, and rarely pedunculated. Also less susceptible to trauma.
Sebaceous Hyperplasia.   Not applicable.
Seborrheic Keratosis.   Not applicable.

Congenital
Acrochordon.   Not applicable.
Dermatofibroma.   Not applicable.
Hemangioma.   *Port-wine stains* (nevus flammeus): Are large, red to purple, vascular lesions associated with congenital syndromes. Cover wide, multiple-centimeter areas, usually in nerve distribution. Occur unilaterally on the face or trunk.
Lentigines (Solar).   *Congenital nevi*: Have approximately a 1% occurrence rate at birth. Raised, not macular, and often hairy, darkly pigmented.
Lipoma.   Not applicable.
Nevi (Acquired Melanocytic or Nevocytic).   *Congenital nevi*: Occur in approximately 1% of births. They are nearly always larger than other melanocytic or nevocytic nevi (1.5 cm to greater than 20 cm). The "giant" or "bathing trunk" nevi have very irregular borders and surfaces, with brown to black pigment, and tend to grow hair. Medium and smaller congenital nevi share similar characteristics but are not as grossly irregular. These nevi can undergo malignant change. Suspicious and changing lesions should be biopsied.
Pyogenic Granuloma.   Not applicable.
Sebaceous Hyperplasia.   Not applicable.
Seborrheic Keratosis.   Not applicable.

Acquired
Acrochordon.   Not applicable.
Callosities.   Not applicable.
Dermatofibroma.   Not applicable.
Hemangioma.   Not applicable.
Keloid Scars.   Not applicable.
Lentigines (Solar), Nevi.   Usually are somewhat palpable, with less discrete borders; are usually round, with some decreasing by age 40.
Lipoma.   Not applicable.

Nevi (Acquired Melanocytic or Nevocytic)
Becker's Nevi.   Are generally large, unilateral hyperpigmentations growing hair. Common on shoulders of prepubescent boys. More faint with less hair on varied body sites, usually in dermatomes of the trunk. Irregular tan macules.
Spitz Nevi.   Are sharply circumscribed, distinctive pink, orange, or red lesions. Common on face of children, but can be found elsewhere. Occur in adolescents and occasionally in adults. Characteristic histologically but are sometimes difficult to separate from melanoma. They should be excised for biopsy.

Halo Nevi. Are typical nevocytic-melanocytic nevi with a surrounding zone of depigmentation. Are benign and probably reflect attempts by immune system to eradicate.

Mongolian Spots. Are bluish black, ovoid, or roundish pigment patches. Usually occur on the sacrum of black and Asian babies. Often fade with time and are benign.

Nevus of Ota, Nevus of Ito. Both are patches of bluish melanocytosis like mongolian spots, but nevus of Ota is found unilaterally in trigeminal nerve distribution of the face. Involves the ocular structures as well as the skin. Nevus of Ito involves the neck, arm, or shoulder unilaterally. Both may be present at birth. Both more common in Asians. No treatment required.

Pyogenic Granuloma. Not applicable.

Sebaceous Hyperplasia. *Fordyce spots*: Are ectopic sebaceous glands appearing as tiny, yellow, visible but barely palpable dots, in broad groups on the lips or genitalia.

Seborrheic Keratosis. *Solar lentigo*: Is hard to distinguish early in the course but is benign. Usually not as distinctly "stuck on" in appearance and has a more uniform, smooth, tan-brown color.

TREATMENT

Acrochordon. Simple excision with scissors with or (generally) without anesthesia. Electrocautery or cryosurgery may also be used.

Callosities. Paring with surgical blade or application of keratolytics may provide temporary relief, but for long-term therapy, the mechanical irritation must be alleviated with padding, better-fitting shoes, and similar measures.

Dermatofibroma. No treatment is necessary unless symptomatic or subject to repeated trauma, or for cosmetic reasons. Excision is the most common treatment modality, but lesion will generally regrow if incompletely excised. Cryosurgery may also be used. Biopsy if there is a question about malignancy.

Hemangioma. For strawberry and cavernous hemangiomas: document location, size, and appearance and note any changes at subsequent visits. If intervention is indicated, may try intralesional triamcinolone injections at 2- to 5-week intervals. Cherry angiomas require no treatment but can be ablated with electrosurgery.

Keloid Scars. Scar revision or excision may help, but there is a significant risk of recurrence. Best to initiate early intralesional injections of triamcinolone every 3 to 5 weeks while observing for shrinkage and softening. Constant pressure by bandaging has been shown to result in some shrinkage. Silastic gel sheeting, taped over the keloid to totally cover the lesion and left in place for 12 of every 24 hours, has been beneficial.

Lentigines (Solar). Usually no treatment is required except for cosmetic purposes. Cryosurgery with liquid nitrogen, laser therapy, or bleaching agents may help.

Lipoma. Necessary only if there are nerve pressure symptoms or cosmetic or functional problems. Surgical excision can be performed in these instances.

Nevi (Acquired Melanocytic or Nevocytic). No treatment necessary, but lesions are frequently removed for cosmetic reasons or chronic irritation or are removed/biopsied if a change in lesion merits concern.

Pyogenic Granuloma. Total excision necessary to decrease chance of recurrence, although it still may return in spite of complete removal. Electrocautery may also be used. After removal, a single, crater-like scar remains.

Sebaceous Hyperplasia. For numerous unsightly lesions, isotretinoin (Accutane) may be used. Other methods that may be utilized are cryotherapy with liquid nitrogen, electrodessication, and curettage.

Seborrheic Keratosis. Removal by cryosurgery, curettage, flat excision (full-thickness or shave), or a combination.

PEDIATRIC CONSIDERATIONS

Lipoma. Rare in pediatrics. Removal can usually wait until postpartum period.

Pyogenic Granuloma. Same as in adults.

OBSTETRIC CONSIDERATIONS

Lipoma. No obstetric considerations.

Nevi (Acquired Melanocytic or Nevocytic). Moles or nevi tend to develop or change during pregnancy.

GERIATRIC CONSIDERATIONS

Not applicable.

PEARLS FOR THE PA

Acrochordon

For multiple, tiny papillomas of neck, chest, or axillae, may clip off, or apply chemical cauterant or astringent (e.g., Drysol, Monsels).

Callosities

Frequently are due to heavy labor using the hands, or to wearing tight, restrictive shoes.

Dermatofibroma

If the lesion is growing, changing, or symptomatic, keep in mind the rare dermatofibroma sarcoma, a serious malignancy.

PEARLS FOR THE PA—cont'd

Hemangioma

A conservative approach is usually safe and rewarding. Don't be quick to cut or destroy.

Keloid Scars

Be patient. High rate of recurrence after surgical intervention but rate goes down after injection series; then surgery and intralesional injection follow-up.

Lentigines (Solar)

If greater than 6 mm in diameter or irregular in size, shape, color, or elevation, consider dysplastic nevus and possible melanoma.

Lipoma

Lesions are not serious or dangerous regardless of the size.

Nevi (Acquired Melanocytic or Nevocytic)

If there is any question about the status of nevi, a dermatologic consultation is indicated.

Pyogenic Granuloma

If it fits description and has reached 1 cm across in a few weeks, treat by excision therapy: excise tangentially and send specimen for pathologic examination.

Sebaceous Hyperplasia

With reassurance, few patients require or need treatment.

Seborrheic Keratosis

Is always benign, but may be excised using cryosurgery with liquid nitrogen.

PREVENTIVE CONSIDERATIONS

Callosities. Avoid mechanical irritation, pad affected areas, use appropriate and well-fitting footwear.

Keloid Scars. Avoid piercings, aggressive treatment of acne. Obtain history prior to surgery.

Dermatitis/Eczema

Jodi L. Cahalan, MPH, MS, PA-C

DEFINITION

Atopic dermatitis: A pruritic skin condition characterized by redness, scaling, and lichenification. Cases can be acute, subacute, or often chronic. Commonly occurs in persons with a family history of asthma, hay fever, allergic rhinitis, or atopic dermatitis. All such disorders are referred to as atopy.

Contact dermatitis: Irritant contact dermatitis is a nonallergic reaction of the skin to an irritating substance; no previous exposure required. Allergic contact dermatitis occurs as a result of contact of an allergen with previously sensitized skin.

Dyshidrotic eczema (pompholyx): Chronic, recurrent, vesicular eruption of the palms, soles, and digits.

Lichen simplex chronicus: Chronic dermatitis caused by frequent and repeated rubbing or scratching.

Nummular eczema: A pruritic dermatitis characterized by coin-shaped lesions often consisting of papules, vesicles, and/or scales on an erythematous base.

Seborrheic dermatitis: Chronic, inflammatory, scaling eruption characteristically distributed in sebaceous gland areas.

HISTORY

Symptoms

Atopic Dermatitis.   Acute cases are characterized by erythema, blisters, and edema, with chronic cases showing scaling, thickening, and lichenification of the skin. Infants with infantile atopic dermatitis often present with itchy erythema of the cheeks, which develops into moist, crusted areas. Lesions may also be seen on scalp, neck, forehead, and buttocks/diaper area as well as the flexor aspects of elbows, knees, and wrists. In children, lesions appear drier and more papular, but are often seen in similar areas of the body. Pruritus is the hallmark symptom regardless of age.

Contact Dermatitis.   Burning and/or pruritus in erythematous, cracking, scaling skin. May be local or widespread.

Dyshidrotic Eczema (Pompholyx).   Small vesicles on hands and/or feet often preceded by intense pruritus. Later dry, flaking, and cracking skin with itchy, burning pain.

Lichen Simplex Chronicus.   Local isolated areas of intense pruritus that becomes pleasurable to scratch, with scratching also occurring during sleep. A raised erythematous plaque with lichenification often found at wrists, ankles, and nape of the neck and in anogenital areas, but not where scratching cannot be accomplished.

Nummular Eczema.   With acute symptoms, pruritic erythematous coin-shaped lesions that may be weeping and crusting. In the chronic stage, lesions are dry, scaling, and usually less erythematous. Lesions common on extremities, dorsum of hands and feet, and occasionally the trunk.

Seborrheic Dermatitis. Fine, white, dry scale or thick, yellowish, often greasy scales of the scalp, face, chest, and/or body folds. Pruritus or burning is common.

Age

Atopic Dermatitis. Infancy to adulthood. Majority of cases first identified in early childhood, but adult onset also possible.

Contact Dermatitis. Any.

Dyshidrotic Eczema (Pompholyx). Usually affects adults between 20 and 40 years of age. Rare before puberty or in late adulthood.

Lichen Simplex Chronicus. Adulthood, rare before puberty.

Nummular Eczema. Males affected most commonly between 55 and 65; in women, peaks from 15 to 25.

Seborrheic Dermatitis. Bimodal occurrence in infancy and adulthood. For infants, often resolves by 6 to 12 months. May begin at puberty, but adult cases most common in the third decade.

Onset

Atopic Dermatitis. Acute presentation common in younger patients, with a more gradual onset in adults.

Contact Dermatitis. Acute cases are often present within 24 to 48 hours after exposure. May be delayed with repeated exposures to mild irritants.

Dyshidrotic Eczema (Pompholyx). Sudden; each recurrence often begins suddenly as well.

Lichen Simplex Chronicus. Gradual, with increasing pruritus.

Nummular Eczema. Gradual to sudden, with single or numerous lesions in regions or clusters on legs, arms, hands, thighs, or back.

Seborrheic Dermatitis. Gradual, slow, or steady increase.

Duration

Atopic Dermatitis. Indefinite, with chronic relapses, although some infantile or childhood cases diminish by onset of adolescence or adulthood.

Contact Dermatitis. Acute contact: Days to weeks. Chronic contact: Months to years.

Dyshidrotic Eczema (Pompholyx). Recurrent attacks with symptom-free intervals of days to months, or for months to years.

Lichen Simplex Chronicus. As long as irritation is present and itch-scratch cycle continues.

Nummular Eczema. Weeks and longer, with waxing and waning periods. May resolve, only to recur in same area.

Seborrheic Dermatitis. Recurrences and remissions, especially on the scalp. Infantile form disappears and adolescent lesions disappear with time.

Intensity

Atopic Dermatitis. May range from mildly pruritic patches to edematous, weeping, and crusting lesions. May occur in one body area or may spread to cover nearly the entire body. May involve the scalp, causing hair loss.

Contact Dermatitis. Isolated and localized to generalized. Random or characteristic according to the nature of the exposure (e.g., airborne irritants involve only exposed surfaces).

Dyshidrotic Eczema (Pompholyx). Patchy lesions or generalized lesions over one or both hands and/or one or both feet.

Lichen Simplex Chronicus. Single isolated lesion to several scattered small or large plaques.

Nummular Eczema. A few regional clusters to generalized. Arms and legs are the most common sites.

Seborrheic Dermatitis. A small scale occurring on one or more of the following areas: ears, brow, eyelids, sides of nose (especially nasolabial folds), chin, chest, body folds, and trunk.

Aggravating Factors

Atopic Dermatitis. Temperature changes, emotional stress, wool contact, food/environmental allergen ingestion/contact, tight/soiled clothing. Other infections (skin and systemic).

Contact Dermatitis. Scratching or rubbing; continued contact with allergen or irritant.

Dyshidrotic Eczema (Pompholyx). Emotional stress, repeated and prolonged contact with water, chemical contactants, dryness, detergents, sensitizers (e.g., lanolin, fragrance), hyperhidrosis, and nickel ingestion.

Lichen Simplex Chronicus. Scratching and rubbing, even during sleep.

Nummular Eczema. Dryness, scratching, strong soap, hot water, emotional stress, extremes in temperature or humidity, synthetic materials, wool.

Seborrheic Dermatitis. None.

Alleviating Factors

Atopic Dermatitis. Remove allergens and minimize skin irritations including harsh soaps, hydrate skin, wear loose clothing.

Contact Dermatitis. Removal of offending contactants and treatment of lesions.

Dyshidrotic Eczema (Pompholyx). Alleviation of stress, protection from contactants or precipitants.

Lichen Simplex Chronicus. Anything that interrupts itch-scratch cycle. Long-term barrier, including during sleep.

Nummular Eczema. Skin hydration, increased humidity.

Seborrheic Dermatitis. Time, in infantile and adolescent forms.

Associated Factors

Atopic Dermatitis. Up to 50% of affected persons exhibit other allergic conditions (e.g., hay fever, asthma).

Contact Dermatitis. Numerous possible home and workplace contactants.

Dyshidrotic Eczema (Pompholyx). Found in both genders, personal or family history of atopy, increased perspiration, "type A personality."

Lichen Simplex Chronicus. Somewhat more common in females.

Nummular Eczema. Older men in dry climates. Wool and mechanical irritants.

Seborrheic Dermatitis. Greater incidence in males. Fairly common in patients with HIV infection or Parkinson's disease. Stress may play a role.

PHYSICAL EXAMINATION

Skin

Atopic Dermatitis. Acute forms occur in infancy and in childhood. Erythematous areas with small vesicles, which may be weeping. Lesions may also show scaling, cracking, and crusting. Occur on the scalp, face, and extremities (on extensor or flexor surfaces) and sometimes upper trunk and neck. Tends to spare perioral area. *Subacute*: Excoriated, lichenified papules, plaques, erosions, and crusts mainly seen on antecubital fossa, popliteal fossa, neck, and face. *Chronic*: Excoriated papules, erosions, dry and wet crusts, and fissures in thickened skin with increased skin markings (called lichenifications). Predilection for flexor areas of the arms, legs, and neck (but not axillae or groin). Also occur on the face, wrists, and dorsum of the hands and feet; often generalized.

Contact Dermatitis. Acute lesions tend to show papules and/or vesicles on an erythematous patch. Weeping serum and crusts or dry scales may also be present. Lichenified patches (dry, thickened skin with exaggerated skin lines) typical in *chronic* cases. Excoriation, due to scratching of pruritic areas, may be present. Presence of isolated lesions or regional localization is common (e.g., just top of feet, just the eyelids, back of hands, exposed surfaces). See Figure 2-13 in color plate section.

Dyshidrotic Eczema (Pompholyx). Initial presentation of pruritic, deep, grouped, small (1 to 5 mm in diameter) vesicles on the sides of the fingers, or palms and soles, which may resemble tapioca. Vesicles may coalesce into bullae. Later exhibit scaling, flaking, fissuring, and lichenification with painful erosion. Occasionally will have erythema, tenderness, and crusting of secondary infection. See Figure 2-14 in color plate section.

Lichen Simplex Chronicus. Well-circumscribed plaque of lichenified skin in round, ovoid, or linear scratch-rub pattern. Single or multiple lesions occur on the nape of neck, scalp, ankles, lower legs, thighs (medial or lateral), outer arms, vulva, pubis, or scrotum, or in perianal area.

Nummular Eczema. Coalescence of small grouped vesicles and papules that form discoid or coin-shaped plaque lesions. Occur mostly on the legs and arms but may become generalized. Common on the hands of young women. Become lichenified, dry with scaly-crusty plaques. Lesions generally on an erythematous base, but less so in chronic phase.

Seborrheic Dermatitis. White or yellowish, dry or greasy, and scaling on discrete red macules. Diffuse on the scalp. Weeping and fissuring are common with retroauricular creases and scalp involvement. Polycyclic or annular on the trunk. Predilection for scalp, beard, face (especially brow and nasolabial folds), central chest, and body folds.

PATHOPHYSIOLOGY

Atopic Dermatitis. Entire etiology is unknown, although IgE-mediated responses may play a major role.

Contact Dermatitis. Cellular, cell-mediated, or delayed hypersensitivity reaction caused by T cells after antigen contact. Tissue damage is caused by T cells and/or release of lymphokines. Spongiosis and lymphocytic infiltrates evident. Increased polymorphonuclear lymphocytes in superficial vesicles suggest a pure irritant basis.

Dyshidrotic Eczema (Pompholyx). Etiology is unknown, but with no actual sweat gland involvement, "dyshidrotic eczema" is a misnomer. Is a superficial spongiotic dermatitis.

Lichen Simplex Chronicus. Epidermal hyperplasia results as response to repeated physical trauma, causing nerve proliferation and increased touch sensation.

Nummular Eczema. Eczematous reaction pattern, often with colonization by staphylococci.

Seborrheic Dermatitis. No known cause. No organism proved, but increases of *Malassezia ovalis* (formerly *Pityrosporum ovale*) fungus and bacteria are common. Spongiotic dermatitis with neutrophils in the stratum corneum.

DIAGNOSTIC STUDIES

Laboratory

Atopic Dermatitis. None needed, as the condition is clinically apparent. Corroboration obtained by serum eosinophilia and elevated IgE in 80% of patients, but not needed to make the diagnosis.

Contact Dermatitis. Not applicable.

Dyshidrotic Eczema (Pompholyx). None; however, a negative fungal culture may help with some cases.

Lichen Simplex Chronicus. Not applicable.

Nummular Eczema. Culture if necessary to clarify differential diagnosis.

Seborrheic Dermatitis. Not applicable.

Radiology. Not applicable.

Other

Atopic Dermatitis
Skin Testing. Positive results on immediate hypersensitivity skin testing in 80% of cases. Radioallergosorbent test (RAST) in infants may elicit reaction to fish, milk, eggs, mites, grasses, or mold as causative factor. Skin testing, however, may not be helpful.

Contact Dermatitis
Patch Testing. May lead to identification of offending allergens, but only if skin is clear of sensitization in area of testing for at least 2 to 3 weeks.

Dyshidrotic Eczema (Pompholyx). Biopsy often not necessary, but may be helpful to differentiate from pustular psoriasis.

Lichen Simplex Chronicus. Not applicable.

Nummular Eczema. Biopsy to clarify differential diagnosis.

Seborrheic Dermatitis. Biopsy may help differentiate from resistant condition or disease.

DIFFERENTIAL DIAGNOSIS

Traumatic

Atopic Dermatitis. *Contact dermatitis* may be difficult to differentiate, so if condition becomes refractory to treatment, consider contact dermatitis. Usually it is in a wider range of local distributions.

Contact Dermatitis. Any skin trauma may cause a contact dermatitis.

Dyshidrotic Eczema (Pompholyx). Not applicable.

Lichen Simplex Chronicus. Not applicable.

Nummular Eczema. Not applicable.

Seborrheic Dermatitis. Not applicable.

Infectious

Atopic Dermatitis

Dermatophytosis more typical on hands and feet with scaly erythema. Positive for hyphae on KOH preparation. Unusual in infants. Sometimes the two are superimposed.

Contact Dermatitis

Dermatophytosis more common in noncontact area (e.g., under toes and feet, in groin and axillae, and under skin folds). More commonly unilateral at onset. Body lesions are typically ring lesions, round and annular with clearing, smoothing centers. Same areas for *yeast infection*; KOH testing to identify.

Yeast infection and *candidiasis* affect the same areas as for dermatophytosis, but involved skin shows beefy-red, solid patches with small red satellite maculopapules surrounding larger lesions. Sometimes have a slight whitish exudate in intertriginous area.

Dyshidrotic Eczema (Pompholyx)

In *dermatophytosis*, usually more discrete patch lesions with typical border. More inflamed. Consider id reaction for hands when cultures of scrapings from feet are positive for fungus.

Lichen Simplex Chronicus. Not applicable.

Nummular Eczema

Dermatophytosis shows positive KOH preparation and/or culture for fungus.

Herpes simplex infection has larger vesicles and less nummular, patch-like lesion.

Seborrheic Dermatitis. In *dermatophytosis* and *candidiasis,* KOH preparations and cultures are positive. Usually more circumscribed lesions with less scale, mostly on borders.

Metabolic

Atopic Dermatitis
Acrodermatitis enteropathica is an autosomal recessive condition that includes a severe eczematous dermatitis.

Wiskott-Aldrich syndrome, agammaglobulinemia, hyper IgE syndrome, and *selective immunoglobulin A (IgA) deficiency* are all rare but hard to differentiate, so if treatment fails or becomes refractory, they should be considered in the diagnosis.

Contact Dermatitis
Stasis dermatitis has slow, chronic onset and is asymptomatic, usually without contact history.

Dyshidrotic Eczema (Pompholyx). In *pustular psoriasis*, less pruritic lesions and more rapid progression to pustules.

Lichen Simplex Chronicus. In *mycosis fungoides*, more bizarre shapes, more scale possible, older people typically affected, long-term lesions, various shades of red, and less lichenification.

Nummular Eczema. In *psoriasis*, generally thicker plaques with typical silver-white heavy scale. Seen on dorsal and extensor surfaces.

Seborrheic Dermatitis. *Histiocytosis X* in infants is distinguished by its petechial component and extracutaneous and histologic features.

Neoplastic
Atopic Dermatitis. In *Letterer-Siwe disease* and *histiocytosis X* in children and *mycosis fungoides* and *Sézary syndrome* in adults, plaques become hemorrhagic and indurated. A biopsy is required.

Contact Dermatitis. Not applicable.

Dyshidrotic Eczema (Pompholyx). Not applicable.

Lichen Simplex Chronicus. Not applicable.

Nummular Eczema. In *mycosis fungoides*, biopsy may be helpful. Lesions may be more annular and less coin-like.

Seborrheic Dermatitis. Not applicable.

Vascular. Not applicable.

Congenital
Atopic Dermatitis. Not applicable.

Contact Dermatitis. Not applicable.

Dyshidrotic Eczema (Pompholyx). Not applicable.

Lichen Simplex Chronicus. Not applicable.

Nummular Eczema. Not applicable.

Seborrheic Dermatitis. In *atopic dermatitis*, affected skin is more dry and rough with lichenification later. Also mostly in flexor areas of arms, legs, less often groin or axillae.

Acquired

Atopic Dermatitis.   *Seborrheic dermatitis* often involves axillae or groin as well as scalp in infants; no positive RAST.

Contact Dermatitis.   Differentiation from *atopic dermatitis* is difficult, but atopic type usually in typical flexural distribution. With poor treatment response, consider contact type. *Contact urticaria* shows acute reddish wheal-flare with resolution in about 24 hours.

Dyshidrotic Eczema (Pompholyx)

Atopic dermatitis usually has involvement of other locations (e.g., arms, neck, legs, trunk).

Drug eruption is more widespread and inflamed.

Lichen Simplex Chronicus

Psoriasis usually shows white or silver scale and plaques, with sharper borders and less obvious lichenification markings. May be less pruritic.

Lichen planus has different distribution (e.g., wrists, hands, intraoral). Small plaques with Wickham striae, not lichenification. Surface smooth.

Chronic contact dermatitis is hard to differentiate and may lead to lichen simplex.

Nummular Eczema.   *Contact dermatitis* usually has a positive contact history and localization.

Seborrheic Dermatitis.   *Psoriasis* is indistinguishable early in course if only scalp is involved, but psoriasis usually has more discrete circumscribed plaques, especially of the scalp. Thicker white scale.

TREATMENT

Atopic Dermatitis.   The mainstay of management in patients with significantly erupted dry, lichenified skin is topical corticosteroids. Choose a medium- to high-potency ointment. Ointments more effective in this dry condition except for the thin-skin areas (e.g., face, axillae, groin.) For these areas use a low-to medium-potency, nonfluorinated ointment. These topicals should be used twice daily and are best applied after a shower or bath. For chronic and/or severe disease, parenteral corticosteroids may be necessary for short periods. For weeping and crusting lesions, soaks with Burow's solution can be utilized to remove crusts and promote healing.

An essential of correct treatment is hydration of the skin by using mild moisturizing soaps and frequent application of emollient creams, lotions, and/or oils. Avoidance of known irritants and allergens. Must stop the itch-scratch cycle. Antihistamines can be helpful for this purpose. A sedating formulation may be helpful if pruritus is severe; otherwise, a nonsedating antihistamine can be used throughout the day.

Secondarily infected cases require the use of a systemic antibiotic. Dicloxacillin, cephalexin, or erythromycin is generally used. Ultraviolet light therapy may utilize ultraviolet A, ultraviolet B, and psoralen (PUVA).

Contact Dermatitis. A topical corticosteroid applied twice a day, for up to several weeks in some cases, may be necessary. Avoidance of contactants and/or barrier protection is also necessary. Instruct the patient to use a mild soap and apply an emollient often, especially after bathing. Wet compresses applied for 20 to 30 minutes two to four times daily, especially in cases with vesicles, weeping, or crusting. For extensive dermatitis, oral prednisone in a burst and taper regimen may be helpful. Antihistamines may be of benefit.

Dyshidrotic Eczema (Pompholyx). Avoid contactants. Topical or systemic corticosteroids. Cold, wet compresses with water or Burow's solution followed by application of an intermediate-strength topical corticosteroid. Applying a barrier, such as Eucerin cream, may facilitate treatment. Severe cases may require oral prednisone 40-60 mg daily for 1 to 3 weeks with gradual taper or triamcinolone acetonide 40 mg IM. Systemic antibiotics necessary for cases with secondary bacterial infections.

Lichen Simplex Chronicus. Must interrupt the itch-scratch cycle. Topical corticosteroids may be preceded by a soak. Medium- to high-potency corticosteroids are needed, but lower dose necessary for involvement of anogenital areas (or face, although this area is rarely affected). Intralesional corticosteroids may be helpful, as is a sedating antihistamine. A barrier to prevent scratching is often necessary, even during sleep. Behavior modification training may be helpful.

Nummular Eczema. Short, lukewarm baths or showers using, at most, a mild soap followed by an emollient. For mild cases, a twice-daily application of a medium-strength steroid cream. May need to increase to a higher-potency steroid cream twice a day if no response to milder steroid or for severe cases. Extensive cases may dictate oral or intramuscular steroid use. A sedating antihistamine may help control pruritus. If secondary infection occurs, systemic antibiotics are necessary.

Seborrheic Dermatitis. Shampooing every day or two with tar, zinc, salicylic acid, or selenium sulfide shampoos is the mainstay of treatment for involvement of the scalp, which is the most common site. Shampoos should remain on at least 5 minutes to ensure penetration into scalp. A mid-potency steroid cream applied twice a day is beneficial. Low-dose steroid cream is necessary for involvement on face and intertriginous areas.

For infants, only mild (1%) hydrocortisone may be used for a limited time. Daily shampooing with baby shampoos. Keratolytic shampoo just to the affected area may be used, but only on thick scales, because toxicity is possible.

If involved skin is located on eyelids, area may be cleansed daily with baby shampoo.

In chronic disease, tar and sulfur preparations are safe and effective, but very messy.

PEDIATRIC CONSIDERATIONS

Atopic Dermatitis. Common in pediatric patients. Most will outgrow the disorder by adolescence.

Contact Dermatitis. The most common type is "diaper rash." Secondary infection with *Candida albicans* is common. Same treatment as for adult but with pediatric doses.

Dyshidrotic Eczema (Pompholyx). Not applicable.

Lichen Simplex Chronicus. None.

Nummular Eczema. Rare. Same treatment as for adult, but with pediatric doses.

Seborrheic Dermatitis. Also known as "cradle cap" in the first month of life. Avoid irritating substances, such as tars, that might get rubbed into eyes. Usually responds well to low-potency steroid creams or ointments.

OBSTETRIC CONSIDERATIONS

Potent topical steroids should be avoided; use only if expected benefit justifies potential fetal risk. Do not apply over extensive areas, in large amounts, or for prolonged periods.

GERIATRIC CONSIDERATIONS

No specific considerations.

Nummular Eczema. Males affected most commonly between 55 and 65 years of age, usually in dry climates.

PREVENTIVE CONSIDERATIONS

Atopic Dermatitis. Avoidance of aggravating factors such as temperature changes, emotional stress, wool contact, food/environmental allergen ingestion/contact, tight/soiled clothing, and infections (skin and systemic).

Contact Dermatitis. Appropriate identification and avoidance of allergen.

Dyshidrotic Eczema (Pompholyx). Avoidance of aggravating factors such as emotional stress, repeated and prolonged contact with water, chemical contactants, dryness, detergents, sensitizers (e.g., lanolin, fragrance), hyperhidrosis, and nickel ingestion.

Lichen Simplex Chronicus. Avoidance of scratching and rubbing.

Nummular Eczema. Avoidance of aggravating factors such as dryness, scratching, strong soap, hot water, emotional stress, extremes in temperature or humidity, synthetic materials, wool.

Seborrheic Dermatitis. Stress, HIV infection, and Parkinson's disease may contribute.

PEARLS FOR THE PA

Atopic Dermatitis

A lot of support and counseling–patient education required for most cases. Patient compliance is vital for control.

Contact Dermatitis

Patients frequently have a history of contact with an irritant.

Dyshidrotic Eczema (Pompholyx)

Moderate to severe cases always require systemic therapy to control. Not curable.

Lichen Simplex Chronicus

Cannot control without stopping the rubbing and scratching. Barriers are a good idea. Patting the skin, dabbing moist cloth, applying ice or creams and ointments are good, nontraumatizing, antipruritic efforts.

Nummular Eczema

Hard to differentiate among contact eczema, atopic dermatitis, and nummular eczema, but all are treated similarly and respond about the same.

Seborrheic Dermatitis

Be slow to call a scalp condition "psoriasis." Use the term seborrheic dermatitis until you are sure of the diagnosis of psoriasis—they are treated the same regardless.

Dermatophytosis (Fungal Infections)

Jodi L. Cahalan, MPH, MS, PA-C

DEFINITION

Tinea capitis: Dermatophyte (fungal) infection of the scalp and its follicles.

Tinea corporis/tinea cruris: Dermatophyte infection of the skin of the trunk, limbs, or face in tinea corporis, only the groin in tinea cruris.

Tinea pedis: Fungal infection of the skin of the feet, including toes.

Cutaneous candidiasis (moniliasis): Infection of skin, skin appendages, and/or mucous membranes with *C. albicans*.

Tinea versicolor: A superficial, asymptomatic skin infection caused by *Malassezia furfur* (formerly *Pityrosporon orbiculare*), a normal skin inhabitant.

HISTORY

Symptoms
Tinea Capitis. Scaling lesions of the scalp associated with well-defined patches of hair loss. May be asymptomatic, pruritic, or burning. Symptoms are dependent on the degree of inflammation. Lesions start small and may coalesce as they enlarge.

Tinea Corporis/Tinea Cruris
Tinea Corporis. Slowly spreading, scaly, ring-shaped erythematous lesions with central clearing found anywhere on the body.

Tinea Cruris. Same type of lesion as in tinea corporis, but is found in the groin area, but generally does not involve the scrotum.

Tinea Pedis. Lesions involving the feet, which often start between the toes, especially between the fourth and fifth digits. May appear dry and erythematous or white and macerated. May spread to sides of feet and may encompass the entire sole of the foot.

Cutaneous Candidiasis (Moniliasis). Erythematous lesions that may be papular, pustular, weepy, and tender. Most common skin areas of involvement include under the breasts, abdominal folds, groin, axillae, and rectal area. With oral candidiasis, white patches on the mucous membrane, tongue, palate, or pharynx on an erythematous base.

Tinea Versicolor. Multiple small, scaling macules most commonly seen on upper trunk, upper arms, neck, and abdomen, which are generally asymptomatic. Lesions tend to be white in tanned persons, pink or brown in light-skinned people, and hyperpigmented in dark-skinned persons. Patients may have noticed it the same season the previous year or have a history of recurrence.

Age
Tinea Capitis. Usually children, rarely adults.

Tinea Corporis/Tinea Cruris. Any, but tinea cruris more common in postpubertal males.

Tinea Pedis. Any, but not common in infants.

Cutaneous Candidiasis (Moniliasis). Any.

Tinea Versicolor. Any, but more common in adolescents and young adults.

Onset
Tinea Capitis. Subacute to chronic.

Tinea Corporis/Tinea Cruris. Sudden, with steady progression.

Tinea Pedis. Insidious to acute.

Cutaneous Candidiasis (Moniliasis). May be present at birth; otherwise, sudden.

Tinea Versicolor. Both acute and chronic.

Duration
Tinea Capitis. Chronic, weeks to months.
Tinea Corporis/Tinea Cruris. Indefinite, but with progression to new and larger growing lesions.
Tinea Pedis. Weeks to months.
Cutaneous Candidiasis (Moniliasis). Days to months.
Tinea Versicolor. Weeks, months, or even years. May disappear only to return.

Intensity
Tinea Capitis. Single, small lesion to confluent lesions involving most or all of scalp, associated with hair loss.
Tinea Corporis/Tinea Cruris. One to multiple lesions on the body with tinea corporis; may be asymptomatic or present with pruritus and/or burning. Tinea cruris exhibits single lesions to patches covering the entire groin area; significant pruritus, and may also be quite tender.
Tinea Pedis. Boggy peeling between fourth and fifth toes or all toes, patches over sole to entire "moccasin" pattern. Involves one or both feet.
Cutaneous Candidiasis (Moniliasis). Single local lesions on sites of involvement, to widespread and including systemic and internal infections. Minor and self-limiting in the otherwise healthy person.
Tinea Versicolor. Single discrete lesions in groups of large (up to 30 cm in diameter) lesions in confluent areas.

Aggravating Factors
Tinea Capitis. None.
Tinea Corporis/Tinea Cruris. Hot and humid climates, perspiration, layered or tight clothing.
Tinea Pedis. Occlusion, warmth and moisture as in hot, humid weather. Restrictive (tight) footwear, socks that may cause sweating/retain moisture.
Cutaneous Candidiasis (Moniliasis). Hot and humid conditions, tight clothing, poor hygiene, obesity, skin breakdown.
Tinea Versicolor. Heat, humidity, perspiration, poor hygiene, occlusion, adrenalectomy, Cushing syndrome, pregnancy, malnutrition, burns, corticosteroids, oral contraceptives.

Alleviating Factors
Tinea Capitis. Appropriate treatment.
Tinea Corporis/Tinea Cruris. Appropriate treatment.
Tinea Pedis. Meticulous hygiene of feet. Thorough cleansing and drying. Foot powders and appropriate treatment.
Cutaneous Candidiasis (Moniliasis). Topical treatment. Keeping area clean and dry.
Tinea Versicolor. Cooler, drier climate. Appropriate treatment.

Associated Factors
Tinea Capitis. Single, small lesion to confluent lesions involving most or all of the scalp.

Tinea Corporis/Tinea Cruris.   Animal contact, or contaminated soil.
Tinea Pedis.   Communal showering.
Cutaneous Candidiasis (Moniliasis).   Diabetes mellitus, obesity, hyperhidrosis, maceration, immune deficits, oral contraceptives, pregnancy, systemic antibiotics, systemic and topical corticosteroids, chronic debilitation, chemotherapy, carcinoma, or leukemia.
Tinea Versicolor.   Cushing syndrome or elevated cortisol from prolonged corticosteroid therapy. Skin lipids may play a role.

PHYSICAL EXAMINATION

Skin
Tinea Capitis.   Well-demarcated areas of hair loss. Remaining hairs in the area are generally broken. Surface lesion at scalp is generally scaly and may appear boggy and tender (kerion.) See Figure 2-15 in color plate section.
Tinea Corporis/Tinea Cruris.   Papulosquamous, erythematous, sharply marginated, single or multiple lesions. Early lesions generally appear as small, flat, scaly lesions that grow by increasing in diameter. Outer border may show erythematous papules or vesicles, and center may clear. Lesions are found classically on trunk and limbs, and occasionally on face for tinea corporis. Tinea cruris lesions occur in the groin and high thigh area. See Figure 2-16 in color plate section.
Tinea Pedis.   Fissuring, boggy maceration in toe webs (especially laterally), dry red scaling in local patches or in moccasin pattern of entire foot. Exhibit vesicles, pustules, and/or bullae over small or large areas with inflammation. Foul odor may be present with any, but most common with toe web disease. The vesicopustular or bullous type often has a secondary bacterial infection. With these inflammatory infections an id or dermatophytid reaction may develop on one of the hands, with a dry, scaling, vesicular eruption, or an indiscrete pruritic trunk eruption. See Figure 2-17 in color plate section.
Cutaneous Candidiasis (Moniliasis).   In diaper area, small pustules on an erythematous base. When pustules erode, scales are left at the periphery. Similar appearance in intertriginous areas, but lesions in these areas are more prone to macerate. Lesions on the penis are small papules and pustules that umbilicate. In mouth, dislodgeable white exudates or plaques on oral mucous membranes, lips, tongue; on red base membranes. See Figure 2-18 in color plate section.
Tinea Versicolor.   Sharply marginated, round lesions ranging in color from off-white to brown or pink. Lesions may be small or coalesce into large patches. Usually on upper trunk and arms and neck, but occasionally on abdomen and proximal legs. A fine superficial scaling is evident or becomes apparent with gentle scraping. No inflammation present. Rare on the face. See Figure 2-19 in color plate section.

PATHOPHYSIOLOGY

Tinea Capitis.   Most commonly caused by an infection due to *Trichophyton tonsurans,* but may also be caused by *T. mentagrophytes, T. schoenleinii* or

T. flavum, Microsporum audouinii, or *Microsporum canis*. Contact with a person, animal, or fomites contaminated with the fungus required.

Tinea Corporis/Tinea Cruris. Contact skin infection, usually with the dermatophyte *T. rubrum* or *T. mentagrophytes*.

Tinea Pedis. Skin of feet (especially between toes) and soles is invaded by dermatophytes, most commonly *T. rubrum, T. mentagrophytes*, and *Epidermophyton floccosum*. This process triggers host defensive mechanisms including hyperproliferation of skin cells and inflammation.

Cutaneous Candidiasis (Moniliasis). Stratum corneum and epidermal invasion with *candidal blastoconidia* with or without acute inflammatory cells. *C. albicans* is the most common pathogen, but *C. tropicalis* and others are possible.

Tinea Versicolor. Hyphae and spores proliferate in the skin and release phenolic compounds that lead to inhibition of tyrosinase, which inhibits epidermal melanocytes, resulting in hypomelanosis. Hyperpigmentation may be a process of hyperkeratotic lesions.

DIAGNOSTIC STUDIES

Laboratory
Fungal Cultures. Help identify specific dermatophyte or *Candida* species, although identification of a specific organism may not change therapy.
Radiology. Not applicable.

Other

Tinea Capitis
Potassium Hydroxide Preparation. Warmed on a glass slide with scrapings from lesion borders and viewed under direct microscopy; reveals hyphae, spores, mycelia of fungi.
Direct Wood's Lamp (Filtered UV Light) Examination. Fungi may glow or fluoresce green, bluish green, grayish green, or coral orange on the skin, but very few actually fluoresce.

Tinea Corporis/Tinea Cruris
Potassium Hydroxide Preparation. With scrapings from advancing borders of lesion, reveals mycelia/hyphae of fungi under direct microscopy.

Tinea Pedis
Potassium Hydroxide Preparation. Will be positive for hyphae: branching linear strands, arthrospores, or occasionally budding cells. Accomplished by placing skin scrapings on slide, applying a drop of 10% to 20% hydrogen peroxide, heating gently, and observing under microscope after about 5 minutes. Not for identification of specific organism but to verify fungal presence.

Cutaneous Candidiasis (Moniliasis)
Potassium Hydroxide Preparation. Reveals blastoconidia, hyphae, and budding spores that distinguish *Candida* species.

Tinea Versicolor
Potassium Hydroxide Preparation.   Examination of scales placed on a slide and warmed reveals a "spaghetti and meatballs" pattern of hyphae and spores.

Direct Wood's Lamp (Filtered UV Light) Examination.   Fungi may fluoresce a yellowish orange wherever the dimorphic fungus is colonizing the skin.

DIFFERENTIAL DIAGNOSIS

Traumatic
Tinea Capitis.   Not applicable.

Tinea Corporis/Tinea Cruris.   Not applicable.

Tinea Pedis.   *Pressure-rubbing* produces blisters, no lasting inflammation. No fungus demonstrable on KOH preparation. Only one or two lesions localized at rubbing sites.

Cutaneous Candidiasis (Moniliasis).   *Burns* and *blisters* will be KOH-negative and culture-negative for *Candida*. Location and history help rule out.

Tinea Versicolor.   Not applicable.

Infectious
Tinea Capitis.   *Bacterial infection* may complicate kerions and flavus and will show on culture.

Tinea Corporis/Tinea Cruris
Tinea Manuum.   The same infection of hands. *Bacterial infections* are negative for fungi by test.

Tinea Pedis
Concomitant bacterial infection very common in pustular inflammatory type of infection and needs to be treated along with fungal infection. KOH- and culture-negative for fungus if only bacterial or viral infection is present.

Herpes simplex infection produces more pain than itch sensation, and no fungus identifiable by KOH preparation or culture.

Cutaneous Candidiasis (Moniliasis).   Folliculitis may be bacterial or possibly *M. furfur* (formerly *P. orbiculare*) but negative for *Candida*. Dermatophyte may look similar, especially in the nails. Cultures differentiate.

Tinea Versicolor.   Not applicable.

Metabolic
Tinea Capitis.   Other alopecias tend to be less scaly and have negative fungal diagnostic studies.

Tinea Corporis/Tinea Cruris.   *Subacute cutaneous lupus erythematosus* is more widespread, with larger lesions, all negative by culture or KOH preparation.

Tinea Pedis. Not applicable.
Cutaneous Candidiasis (Moniliasis). Not applicable.
Tinea Versicolor. Not applicable.

Neoplastic
Tinea Capitis. Not applicable.
Tinea Corporis/Tinea Cruris. *Mycosis fungoides* may appear similar, but all lesions are negative on KOH preparation and/or fungal culture.
Tinea Pedis. Not applicable.
Cutaneous Candidiasis (Moniliasis). Not applicable
Tinea Versicolor. Not applicable.

Vascular. Not applicable.

Congenital
Tinea Capitis. Not applicable
Tinea Corporis/Tinea Cruris. Not applicable.
Tinea Pedis. Not applicable.
Cutaneous Candidiasis (Moniliasis). *Seborrheic dermatitis* is present at birth; resembles candidiasis but cultures negative.
Tinea Versicolor. Not applicable.

Acquired
Tinea Capitis. In *seborrheic dermatitis*, lesions usually less discretely circumscribed; alopecia rare. Negative fungal cultures.
Tinea Corporis/Tinea Cruris. Not applicable.
Tinea Pedis. In *dyshidrotic eczema*, no fungus on KOH preparation or culture. May occur around sides or dorsum of feet, or near the ankle.
Cutaneous Candidiasis (Moniliasis). *Leukoplakia* and *oral lichen planus* show more lace-like pattern and negative for *Candida* on culture.
Tinea Versicolor. *Vitiligo* is usually white and does not have the delicate scale of tinea versicolor or hypomelanosis of cleared psoriasis or eczemas. Does not have the same fine, demonstrable scale and differs in distribution. KOH preparation is negative.

TREATMENT

Tinea Capitis. Oral medications are required, as topical medications have difficulty penetrating into the hair follicle. Possible oral medications include terbinafine, ketoconazole, itraconazole, and griseofulvin. Topical therapies include shampoos containing ketoconazole, selenium sulfide, tar, or zinc. Treatment often takes 1 to 3 months or more and should be continued for 1 to 2 weeks after signs and symptoms resolve.
Tinea Corporis/Tinea Cruris. *Superficial* lesions may respond to topical treatment applied twice a day. Possible topical preparations include miconazole, clotrimazole, econazole, naftifine, ciclopirox, ketoconazole, sulconazole, and terbinafine. Therapy often takes 2 to 4 weeks and should be continued for 1 to 2 weeks after lesions have resolved. *Extensive* infections or nonresponsive cases may require an oral antifungal for 4 to 6 weeks at

appropriate dose per weight, given once daily with food. For adults: Ultramicrosize griseofulvin 330-375 mg/day or ketoconazole 200-400 mg/day. For children: Griseofulvin suspension at 5-10 mg/kg/day. If oral treatment is prolonged, monitor liver enzymes for possible side effects.

Tinea Pedis. Vesicular lesions may respond to wet soaks in Burow's solution for 30 minutes several times a day. In addition, infection must be treated using one of the topical antifungals as listed for tinea corporis/tinea cruris. If a secondary bacterial infection occurs, appropriate oral antibiotics will be necessary. Powders may be helpful in decreasing moisture on skin of feet, and frequent sock changes, especially after they become damp, will be beneficial.

Chronic or deep extensive infection may require ultramicrosize griseofulvin 660-750 mg orally once a day or in divided doses with food or ketoconazole 200-400 mg orally every day.

Cutaneous Candidiasis (Moniliasis)

Oral Candidiasis. Oral nystatin suspension 200,000-400,000 units three to four times daily. Swish 5 minutes and swallow; or clotrimazole troches dissolved in the mouth then swished and swallowed up to five times a day.

For perleche, use a topical cream or ointment containing nystatin, miconazole, clotrimazole, ketoconazole, econazole, or terbinafine. Clean any dentures with Peridex.

Genital Candidiasis. Use topical miconazole, clotrimazole, ketoconazole, econazole, nystatin, or terbinafine cream twice a day. In chronic infection, use oral ketoconazole 200-400 mg every day for 14 days, and repeat if necessary. Oral nystatin 500,000 units four times a day may also be used. Consider circumcision in males.

Intertriginous-Diaper Candidiasis. Use topical miconazole, clotrimazole, ketoconazole, or econazole cream twice a day; air dry affected areas, use loose clothing, and avoid plastic diapers. Absorbent powders may be helpful in decreasing moisture in the area once infection has cleared.

Tinea Versicolor. Helpful agents include the following:

Selenium sulfide 2%, overnight or daily regimens help but are associated with a high recurrence rate.

Ketoconazole 2% shampoo, lather and leave on 5 minutes, and then rinse and repeat three times.

Miconazole, clotrimazole, ketoconazole, or econazole creams are helpful once or twice daily but expensive if extended areas involved.

Oral ketoconazole 200 mg every day for 3 to 14 days; OR oral ketoconazole 200-400 mg: wait 2 hours, exercise to induce sweating, and then wait at least 1 hour before showering; repeat the process in 1 week.

PEDIATRIC CONSIDERATIONS

Tinea Capitis. Usually seen in prepubertal children. Topical antifungal agents are ineffective, and treatment with oral griseofulvin (10 mg/kg/ day) for a minimum of 6 to 8 weeks is required.

Tinea Corporis (Ringworm). Usually seen in children. Treatment is with topical antifungal agent (clotrimazole, miconazole) for 2 to 4 weeks.

Tinea Pedis. Is seen rarely in childhood but frequently in postpubertal adolescents. Atopic dermatitis may mimic tinea pedis in prepubertal children.

Cutaneous Candidiasis (Moniliasis). *C. albicans* is a common source of infection in infancy. *Candida* frequently infects the diaper area and may infect the oral mucosa, where it appears as thick, white patches on an erythematous base (thrush). An antifungal cream may be used in the diaper area. In oral thrush, a suspension of nystatin should be applied directly to the mucosa with a finger or cotton applicator. If a breastfeeding infant is seen with thrush, the mother should be questioned about symptoms of dry, reddened, painful nipples, an indication that yeast is being passed back and forth between the infant and the mother's breast.

OBSTETRIC CONSIDERATIONS

Oral medications are contraindicated in the pregnant patient. Check medication reference before instituting any therapy.

Candidiasis is more prevalent in pregnant women, commonly seen in infections of the perineum and the vagina. Pregnancy increases the glycogen content of the vaginal epithelium and promotes a greater degree of acidity. This can lead to an overgrowth of yeast. Approximately 30% to 35% of pregnant women have demonstrable yeast organisms in the vagina.

The newest antifungal medication, terconazole, is safe to use during pregnancy. In contrast, ketoconazole is contraindicated.

GERIATRIC CONSIDERATIONS

Generally no specific indications.

Cutaneous Candidiasis (Moniliasis). Contributing factors include diabetes mellitus, obesity, immune compromise, systemic antibiotics, chronic debilitation, chemotherapy, carcinoma, and leukemia, which are more prevalent in the elderly.

PREVENTIVE CONSIDERATIONS

Tinea Capitis. Not applicable.

Tinea Corporis/Tinea Cruris. Avoidance of tight clothing, perspiration, and exposure to humidity.

Tinea Pedis. Avoidance of tight footwear, and wearing socks that wick away moisture. Communal showering contributes.

Cutaneous Candidiasis (Moniliasis). Avoiding tight clothing, maintaining good hygiene.

Tinea Versicolor. To prevent proliferation of hyphae and spores, avoidance or acknowledgment of aggravating conditions such as heat, humidity, perspiration, poor hygiene, occlusion, adrenalectomy, Cushing syndrome, pregnancy, malnutrition, burns, corticosteroids, and oral contraceptives.

PEARLS FOR THE PA

Tinea Capitis

Fungal infection of the scalp. Presence of large patches of alopecia with thick, yellowish brown scutula on atrophic scarred scalp, often with erosions, is called favus.

Tinea Corporis/Tinea Cruris

Fungal infection of the skin of the trunk, limbs, face, or groin. Care should be taken with use of medium- or high-potency steroids in the groin area—indicated for short-term use only.

Tinea Pedis

Fungal infection of the feet aggravated by communal showering, occlusion, and moisture.

Cutaneous Candidiasis (Moniliasis)

Yeast infection of the skin, skin appendages, and mucous membranes. May become a systemic infection.

Tinea Versicolor

A superficial, asymptomatic skin infection caused by M. furfur (P. orbiculare), *a normal skin inhabitant.*

Infestations of the Skin

Charlene M. Morris, MPAS, PA-C

DEFINITION

Scabies: Infestation of the epidermis by *Sarcoptes scabiei*, a microscopic insect-like mite that burrows in the skin and reproduces.

Pediculosis (lice): Infestation by *Pediculus humanus capitis* (head louse), *Pediculus humana corporis* (body louse/"cootie"), or *Phthirus pubis* (pubic louse/"crab").

HISTORY

Symptoms
Scabies. Dry, red bumps with intense itch, especially at night. Affects the arms, legs, and trunk. May form impressive scrotum dermatitis.

Pediculosis (Lice)
With all forms of infestation, severe pruritus, with or without red-dot rash on body or in groin.

Pediculosis Capitis. The patient has "bugs" on the hair shafts, initially on the occipital region. May extend as the infestation progresses.

Pediculosis Corporis. Complaint of itching, especially at clothing line.

Pediculosis Pubis. Affected in groin area, may extend to communicating hairy regions.

Age
Scabies. Any, without regard to hygiene, socioeconomic status, or race.
Pediculosis (Lice). Any, but mostly school age.

Onset
Scabies. Acute.
Pediculosis (Lice). Acute with symptoms, or slow, with another person noticing the condition.

Duration
Scabies. Weeks to months until treated.
Pediculosis (Lice). Weeks to months.

Intensity
Scabies. From a few papules around hands or fingers to widespread pruritic papules of extremities and trunk. Periods of exacerbation with mild but progressive symptoms.
Pediculosis (Lice). Many mites, nits, papules, or bites, or no symptoms or signs.

Aggravating Factors
Scabies. Scratching, heat, nighttime, reinfestation.
Pediculosis (Lice). Poor hygiene, contact with infested person, or use of infected items or fomite.

Alleviating Factors
Scabies. Treatment including antipruritics.
Pediculosis (Lice). Fastidious cleaning of clothing, bedding, and living areas; appropriate treatment.

Associated Factors
Scabies. Friend or family member may have similar/same complaints.

Pediculosis (Lice). Rare in blacks; common in Latin Americans, Caribbean natives, and Caucasians. Also found in Native American Indians and persons of Asian ancestry.

PHYSICAL EXAMINATION

General
Scabies. Red, dry papulovesicles that begin at the hands, wrists, ankles, or lower legs with steady spread to wide periaxillary-shoulder area, around the waist, in the groin, and on the buttocks. Burrows or dry short-track lines with terminal papule may be noted. The mite is in the papule. The female nipple and the male penis are common sites of infestation with larger papules. Rare on face, and the face is the last area affected in children. Significant excoriation common. Purulence and inflammation are common with secondary infection. See Figure 2-20 in color plate section.

Pediculosis (Lice). Head lice mites have elongated insect-looking bodies, are small but visible, and move on the scalp and in the hair very quickly. Most common sites are behind the ears and over the occiput, but can occur anywhere on scalp in the hair. Ova attach as white nits to the base of hair shafts. Most common in girls and women.

The body louse has a larger elongated body, moves more slowly, and is found usually on the trunk and thighs of men. Nits attach to clothing seams, not hair. Bites occur as red papules and wheals, lead to excoriations and sometimes pyodermas.

The pubic louse has a wider body and looks like a small crab. They are light, almost translucent, and found in the pubic area, but may be in axillary hair, eyebrows, or eyelashes. Tan nits are readily visible on close inspection. Also leave steel-gray spots on chest, abdomen, and thighs (maculae caeruleae). See Figure 2-21 in color plate section.

PATHOPHYSIOLOGY

Scabies. Acquired by direct contact. The *S. scabiei* mite secretes enzymes that dissolve stratum corneum cells and burrows under the stratum corneum and into the epidermis to lay eggs and secrete waste. The mite and its products (ova, egg casings, and feces or scybala) are sensitizing and lead to the intense pruritus and reactive papulovesicles.

Pediculosis (Lice). Infestation is by direct contact with use of contaminated combs, brushes, clothes, beds, hats. Lice feed by biting the skin and sucking blood. This infestation may lead to allergic reactions such as eczemas and urticarias. Eggs are cemented with secretions to hair shafts as nits or to clothing (body louse). The body louse may be vector of epidemic typhus fever, relapsing fever, or trench fever. Head and pubic lice are not vectors of disease.

DIAGNOSTIC STUDIES

Laboratory. Microscopic examination for suspected louse or nit with wet preparations or dry mount.

Radiology.   Not applicable.

Other

Scabies
Potassium Hydroxide Preparation or Oil.   Viewing mites, mite parts, eggs, or feces under the microscope is diagnostic, but these are not always demonstrable.
   Skin Scraping.   Obtain scrapings of papulovesicles and/or burrows and tracks and/or scrapings recovered from under nails and smear on slide.
   Biopsy.   Rarely necessary.
Pediculosis (Lice).   Not applicable.

DIFFERENTIAL DIAGNOSIS

Traumatic.   Not applicable.

Infectious
Scabies.   *Folliculitis* is not nearly as pruritic and dry. No burrows or tracks, different locations more typical (except buttocks).
Pediculosis (Lice).   In *papular urticaria,* nits or body lice are absent.

Acquired
Scabies.   Not applicable.
Pediculosis (Lice).   *Fleas* do not stay on the body long, but bite 2 to 4 times in an area and move on and off. *Chiggers* bite several times in infested area and leave feces dots in hair or skin; involve extremities and or trunk. Any other mites "bite and run," leaving no nits or tracks or feces.

Metabolic.   Not applicable.
Neoplastic.   Not applicable.
Vascular.   Not applicable.
Congenital.   Not applicable.

TREATMENT

Scabies
Helpful agents:
   Permethrin 5% topical cream (Elimite) applied once for 8 to 12 hours
      and then washed off. May be repeated in 1 week.
   Lindane 1% cream or lotion applied for 6 hours and then washed off.
      Repeated one time a week thereafter. Should be applied everywhere
      except the face. Lindane can be used in infants but only for 2 hours
      and with care taken to avoid putting fingers in mouth.
   Crotamiton (Eurax) cream applied to entire body; repeat in 24 hours.
   Ivermectin 100-200 µg/kg once a week for 1 to 3 weeks.
Clean all linens and clothing after treatment.

Pediculosis (Lice)
OTC pyrethrin preparations: RID, A200, R&C, or permethrins such as Nix may be effective. Must treat all contacts and fomites. Lindane 1% shampoo

for head, lotion or creams for rest of body. Protect eyes, nose, mouth, and all body orifices. Apply liberally on the head and chest for head lice, entire body for other infestations. Leave creams or lotions on body overnight 10 to 12 hours; then rinse and repeat a week later. Nits should be meticulously and completely removed ("nit-picking") or combed out with special combs. Can be softened with vinegar or 3% acetic acid solution. Clothing and bedding should be hot-laundered and/or isolated in plastic bag for 3 weeks or more. Furniture should be sprayed with pyrethrins or permethrins with R&C spray. Carpets, rugs, chairs, and sofas should be vacuumed. Fomites such as brushes, combs, etc., should be isolated 3 weeks or more and super heated or frozen in freezer for 1 week. Treat all contacts concurrently. Antipruritics may be needed and helpful (e.g., topical hydrocortisone 1% with menthol 1% cream or lotion). Antihistamines, analgesics, and systemic corticosteroids may be used judiciously.

PEDIATRIC CONSIDERATIONS

Scabies. May use permethrin 5% topical cream after 2 months of age. Abuse/overuse of lindane can cause neurologic damage.

Pediculosis (Lice). Elimite is safe for infants older than 2 months. If used, lindane is applied for only 2 to 3 hours in infants, with monitoring to prevent them from placing fingers in the mouth.

OBSTETRIC CONSIDERATIONS

Scabies. Lindane can be used but with strict adherence to directions. Best to use Elimite or Eurax.

Pediculosis (Lice). Great care and monitoring using any of the topical preparations as pediculicides.

GERIATRIC CONSIDERATIONS

Scabies. Can be enountered in the elderly. May be seen in extended care facilities.

Pediculosis (Lice). Not common in the elderly.

PREVENTIVE CONSIDERATIONS

Scabies. May be spread in living conditions of close contact. Linens and clothing should also be treated.

Pediculosis (Lice). Immediate identification and treatment of affected persons. May be spread rapidly through schools and day care centers. Linens and clothing should also be treated.

PEARLS FOR THE PA

Scabies

Scabies mites have a hatch cycle of 5 to 6 days; therefore, treat again after 7 days.

Lindane, a first-line agent for scabies treatment, is an insecticide.

Pediculosis

Lice infestation. Fomites such as clothes or bedding should be laundered in hot water after each treatment. Overstuffed furniture and carpets can be treated with powder or spray pediculicide.

Ivermectin, a systemic antiparasitic preparation, may be used in severely recalcitrant cases of lice and scabies.

Papulosquamous Conditions

Charlene M. Morris, MPAS, PA-C

DEFINITION

Psoriasis: A hereditary, T cell–mediated skin disorder. Proliferative, inflammatory dermatosis manifested by red papules and chronic scaling plaques, with or without pruritus. Pustules occur in a characteristic distribution. May include an inflammatory arthritis and be related to human leukocyte antigen (HLA) B27.

Pityriasis rosea: A common inflammatory skin disease resembling an acute viral exanthem of unknown etiology. Scaling occurs in a typical pattern.

HISTORY

Symptoms
Psoriasis. Scaly, red, sometimes pruritic, thick patches, primarily on the skin of the elbows, knees, scalp, or trunk. May occur as red, pruritic, scaly skin, or slightly tender pruritic pustules of palms or soles or as chronic red dots on trunk. May be accompanied by mild to disabling arthritis.

Pityriasis Rosea. Large scaly patch, usually on the trunk, which precedes spreading lesions of dull reddish pink or tawny color on body centrally, spreading peripherally onto extremities. Asymptomatic to significant pruritus.

Age
Psoriasis. Usually adults, but up to 30% of patients may be younger than 20 years of age, especially females. Overall incidence is the same in males and in females. Rare in children.

Pityriasis Rosea. Seventy-five percent of cases occur in 10-to 35-year-old age group.

Onset
Psoriasis. Acute in small dot trunk-guttate, pustular, local, and generalized forms. Chronic in plaque forms.

Pityriasis rosea. Acute with enlarging maculopapule.

Duration
Psoriasis. Usually months to years, but weeks in some acute-onset types.

Pityriasis Rosea. Three to 10 weeks; occasionally several months.

Intensity
Psoriasis. Small single lesions or groups that occur locally in one area (e.g., genitalia, axillae) to regional lesion or groups (scalp), or generalized or universal (all of skin, nails).

Pityriasis Rosea. A few lesions to innumerable.

Aggravating Factors
Psoriasis. Minor trauma, pressure points, systemic corticosteroids, lithium, alcohol, chloroquine, intense sunlight, stress, obesity, tobacco use.

Pityriasis Rosea. Ampicillin, heat.

Alleviating Factors
Psoriasis. Mild to moderate PUVA, topical corticosteroids, stress management, hydration, lubrication, antipruritics. Other treatments, such as retinoid therapy.

Pityriasis Rosea. Sunlight, antipruritics if indicated.

Associated Factors
Psoriasis. Genetics, beta-hemolytic streptococcal infection.

Pityriasis Rosea. Winter season higher incidence, mild leukopenic lymphocytosis at disease peak.

PHYSICAL EXAMINATION

Skin
Psoriasis. Asymmetrical but bilateral salmon-red papules and plaques, with sharp margins and silver-white scale, inflamed pustules or erythrodermic, diffuse, peeling red lesions without sharp border. Lesions may be round, oval, polycyclic, or annular in discrete single lesion pattern. May also

occur in confluent large patches, serpiginous or arciform, localized, region-alized, or general as in erythrodermic–entire skin form. Nails may have pits, ridges, onycholysis, or pathognomonic yellowish spots under the nail plate. Twenty-five percent of patients have nail involvement. Alopecia is not com-mon even with the thickest of plaques. Inflammatory arthritis is most com-mon in pustular and erythrodermic psoriasis and may involve hands, feet, or joints. May cause mutilating bone erosion, osteolysis, and ankylosis involv-ing the sacroiliac, hip, and cervical areas.

Plaques are most prevalent over extensor pressure surfaces. Guttate papules are worse on the trunk. Pustular forms are mostly on the extremities and are rarely generalized. Intertriginous areas may be affected, but without thick plaques and with finer scaling. See Figure 2-22 in color plate section.

Pityriasis Rosea. A "herald patch" precedes more general eruption by 3 days to a couple of weeks. In 80% of patients this patch is the largest lesion of the exanthem. The lesions are fawn-salmon to bright red in color, are macu-lopapular, and usually have a collarette of fine scales at the margins. Lesions are typically ovoid in shape and are distributed along cleavage lines in a character-istic "Christmas tree" pattern on the back. The exanthem is usually confined to the trunk and proximal extremities. See Figure 2-23 in color plate section.

PATHOPHYSIOLOGY

Psoriasis. Probably has a multifactorial pathogenesis—hence the varied presentations and systemic involvement. Epidermal cell turnover time is decreased, probably owing to shorter cell cycle and increased cells in the dividing pool. Changes occur in keratogenous epidermal zone and in dermis with inflammation. Epidermal proteinases are elevated and also play a role. Neutrophils, lymphocytes, and monocytes are mobilized and form Munro microabscesses in the stratum corneum.

Pityriasis Rosea. Specific etiology is unproved but most widely believed to be viral. The immune system probably plays some role as well. Histopathologic changes are nonspecific but include mild acanthosis, parakeratosis, perivascular lymphohistiocytic infiltrate, and red cell extravasation.

DIAGNOSTIC STUDIES

Laboratory
Psoriasis. None needed when characteristic clinical features are present. May test for HLA-B27– associated antigen.

Pityriasis Rosea. None except to rule out conditions in the differential diagnosis.

Radiology. Not applicable.

Other
Psoriasis. Biopsy may be helpful and suggestive but not necessarily specific. Histology changes over time with acute-onset to chronic forms.

DIFFERENTIAL DIAGNOSIS

Traumatic
Psoriasis. Following skin injuries from trauma or infection, development of typical psoriatic lesions in uninvolved sites (Koebner's phenomenon) is common. Be alert to slight changes and persistent white scaling on red papules and plaques in broken skin sites from any cause.
Pityriasis Rosea. Not applicable.

Infectious
Psoriasis. *Candidiasis* mimics intertriginous psoriasis but is KOH-positive, and lesions will not resolve with psoriasis treatment and may even flare.
Pityriasis Rosea. Lesions due to *fungal cause* will be KOH- and culture-positive. In *secondary syphilis*, serologic tests will be positive.

Metabolic
Psoriasis. *Glucagonoma syndrome* is due to a malignant pancreatic islet cell tumor associated with atypical psoriasiform lesions with vesicles and erosions. Includes lesions in groin and on face and marked weight loss; anemia with histology to distinguish.
Pityriasis Rosea. Not applicable.

Neoplastic
Psoriasis. *Mycosis fungoides* mimics psoriasis, but resistant to treatment and generally less thick plaques and less silver-white scale.
Pityriasis Rosea. Not applicable.

Acquired

Psoriasis
Seborrheic dermatitis may be indistinguishable in certain sites and morphology. Usually yellower scale, especially of scalp. Responds to same treatments.
Lichen simplex chronicus may complicate psoriasis owing to pruritus and itch-rub cycle. Responds to same treatments. Encourage patient to refrain from scratching affected areas.
Psoriasiform drug eruption associated with positive history for first-time use of beta blockers, gold, or methyldopa. Clears easily with drug withdrawal and treatment.
Pityriasis Rosea. *Drug eruption* can usually be elicited by history. With *guttate psoriasis*, not only a collarette scale but may have scale over entire surface.

Vascular. Not applicable.
Congenital. Not applicable.

TREATMENT

Psoriasis
Lubrication and Desquamation. Initial and daily treatment with ointment or cream-based emollients containing 1% to 2% salicylic acid or 5%

to 10% lactic acid or 10% to 20% urea. Crude coal tar preparations for topical use are effective and have been used since the 19th century. Newer forms are better tolerated and more esthetically pleasing. Previously limited by tendency to irritate and stain. Anthralin creams are traditionally helpful, now with 30-minute contact time and increasing strengths over weeks of therapy. Effective but time-consuming and troublesome.

Corticosteroids. Corticosteroids are the most widely used therapeutic agents but can cause side effects and can be expensive and promote tachyphylaxis. Available in a wide range of potencies and absorbencies. The most potent (e.g., clobetasol, betamethasone dipropionate) should be reserved for thickest plaques in relatively small regions and not be used on face or intertriginous areas.

Middle potencies should be used for large areas in less severe conditions and short-term in the worst-affected intertriginous areas. Be alert to the risk of treating entire skin areas (e.g., erythrodermic-cortisol suppression, glucose intolerance, rarely Cushing syndrome). Risk increases with occlusion, with use of high-potency formulations, in children, and in the liver-impaired.

Ultraviolet Light Therapy. UVB and UVA exposure can be quite effective with serial exposures. UVB wave effect is enhanced after tar application (Goeckerman therapy). UVA is enhanced with 8-methoxypsoralen given topically or orally, which becomes modern PUVA. Very effective, but protective eyewear is required 8 to 12 hours after medicating orally. Systemic therapy should be used only when the risk of side effects is weighed against the benefits in long-term treatment. The response can be very helpful and dramatic in extensive involvement such as pustular or erythrodermic psoriasis. PUVA should probably be used only by specialists familiar with its use, toxicity, side effects, and drug interactions.

Other Therapies. Other treatments include the following:

Methotrexate 10 to 20 mg divided into three doses and given 12 hours apart, weekly. Oral and intramuscular forms available. Side effects include nausea, gastrointestinal upset, hepatotoxicity, and bone marrow suppression. There is a lifetime dose limit depending on liver function.

Etretinate (a retinoid) in individualized doses of 10 to 25 mg, given once daily up to three times daily, with gradual titration and adjustments to lowest effective dose. Side effects include hypervitaminosis A syndrome; adverse effects on skin, mucous membranes, and the musculoskeletal system; and elevated serum lipid levels. It is hepatotoxic, teratogenic, and embryotoxic.

Tazarotene (Tazorac) cream and gel. Apply at bedtime over no more than 20% of body surface. Category X drug in pregnancy.

Cyclosporine: In lower doses than those used for organ transplantation, helps significantly until discontinued. Psoriasis tends to return, but not in the rebound fashion seen with systemic corticosteroids. Side effects include nephrotoxicity, hypertension, hepatotoxicity, neurologic abnormalities, and an increased incidence of lymphoma. Treatment combinations are commonly used and specifically tailored to the individual patient.

Calcipotriene (Dovonex) ointment applied twice daily to affected area. Scalp solution: Apply to lesion areas; reevaluate in 8 weeks.

Pityriasis Rosea. Sunlight or UVB exposure helps control pruritus if present and may hasten lesion involution. Oral antihistamines and topical corticosteroids are also helpful if pruritus is a problem.

PEDIATRIC CONSIDERATIONS

Psoriasis. One-third of affected persons will present within the first two decades of life. Psoriasis is rare in the newborn. Commonly involved sites include scalp, knees, elbows, umbilicus, and genital area. Guttate psoriasis is a form of psoriasis seen predominantly in children. The onset frequently follows a recent streptococcal pharyngitis by 2 or 3 weeks. Initial lesions may mimic a viral exanthem. Treatment varies with age, type, and site and extent of disease. Tar preparations (enhanced by UV light) are useful. Topical corticosteroids are extremely effective but must be used with caution. Systemic steroids are typically contraindicated in childhood psoriasis. The safety of PUVA therapy has not yet been established for children. Psoriasis in infants and acute guttate psoriasis should be managed conservatively.

Pityriasis Rosea. Pityriasis rosea is most commonly seen in adolescents and children. It may be preceded by a prodrome of pharyngitis, fever, and malaise, but rarely do children report such symptoms. An annular, scaly, erythematous lesion (the herald patch) precedes the generalized eruption in approximately 80% of children. Treatment may be unnecessary. After the eruption has resolved, postinflammatory hypopigmentation or hyperpigmentation may be evident, particularly in black patients.

OBSTETRIC CONSIDERATIONS

Potent topical steroids should be avoided in the treatment of psoriasis. They should be used only when the benefit to the mother clearly justifies the risk to the fetus. If used, this group of topical steroids should not be applied over extensive areas, in large amounts, or for prolonged periods.

Etretinate and other retinoids are absolutely contraindicated during pregnancy because of their teratogenic and embryotoxic effects. These agents are sometimes used for the treatment of the pustular and erythrodermic forms of psoriasis. Beginning medications during menstruation or after a negative pregnancy test is recommended. Avoidance of pregnancy during retinoid therapy is mandatory.

GERIATRIC CONSIDERATIONS

Psoriasis. Long-term psoriatic arthritis may be present.

Pityriasis Rosea. No specific considerations.

PREVENTIVE CONSIDERATIONS

Psoriasis. Avoidance of aggravating factors such as minor trauma, unrelieved pressure points, systemic corticosteroids, lithium, alcohol, chloroquine, intense sunlight, stress, obesity, tobacco use.

Pityriasis Rosea. Ampicillin and heat will exacerbate symptoms.

PEARLS FOR THE PA

Psoriasis

Scaly, red, sometimes pruritic, thick patches, primarily on skin of the elbows, knees, and trunk. Hereditary inflammatory disorder. Care should be taken with all medications used owing to potential side effects.

Pityriasis Rosea

In most cases, reassurance of the patient that the condition is benign and self-limited is adequate management.

Premalignant and Malignant Skin Tumors

Charlene M. Morris, MPAS, PA-C

DEFINITION

Actinic keratosis: A sharp outlined growth on sun-exposed skin with tan or clear scale on an erythematous base. May become nodular. Some potential for malignant degeneration.

Basal cell carcinoma: A malignant epithelial tumor with potential for local invasion and destruction. Small metastatic risk. Most common human malignancy with approximately 500,000 new cases annually. Variants include nodular, superficial, morpheaform, pigmented, and infiltrative.

Squamous cell carcinoma: A malignant tumor arising from keratinocytes, generally occuring in sun-exposed areas of older people.

Malignant melanoma: The neoplastic transformation of melanocytes in the epidermis (in situ and biologically benign) that spreads to the dermis and may metastasize. More rapid horizontal growth in superficial spreading melanomas and more rapid vertical growth in nodular melanoma.

HISTORY

Symptoms
Actinic Keratosis.   Dry, rough, warty, scaly lesion on the head or arms.

Basal Cell Carcinoma.   Chronic sore or bump that is generally painless, bleeds easily, seems to heal, and yet never resolves completely. Usually occurs in sun-exposed areas.

Squamous Cell Carcinoma.   Lesions are chronic ulcers or open, changing, hard bumps on exposed surfaces. Painless until late stages.

Malignant Melanoma.   New or old pigmented skin lesions that change in size, shape, color, or elevation and may itch or bleed easily.

Age
Actinic Keratosis.   Middle age and upward.

Basal Cell Carcinoma.   Forties and greater. Occasionally seen in the teens, twenties and thirties if history of extensive childhood sun exposure, especially with sun burns.

Squamous Cell Carcinoma.   Over forty, increasing incidence into old age.

Malignant Melanoma.   Median age at diagnosis is the mid-40s.

Onset
Actinic Keratosis.   Chronic.

Basal Cell Carcinoma.   Insidious and chronic.

Squamous Cell Carcinoma.   Insidious over months.

Malignant Melanoma.   Months to years.

Duration
Actinic Keratosis.   Permanent or malignant degeneration.

Basal Cell Carcinoma.   Permanent.

Squamous Cell Carcinoma.   Indefinite; without treatment, continues to invade surrounding tissues.

Malignant Melanoma.   Steady, progressive growth or changes.

Intensity
Actinic Keratosis.   Single lesion to many.

Basal Cell Carcinoma.   Single lesions, from a few millimeters to a few centimeters in diameter. Sometimes multiple lesions in various stages of slow growth and development.

Squamous Cell Carcinoma.   Single, isolated lesion to a few scattered discrete tumors. From small, superficial to large, deep lesions with potential to metastasize.

Malignant Melanoma.   One or two primary lesions, rarely multiple.

Aggravating Factors
Actinic Keratosis.   Significant sun exposure, expecially burns before age 20 in lightly pigmented persons. Renal transplantation.

Basal Cell Carcinoma. Extensive sun exposure, especially sunburns in childhood, fair skin color, and, less frequently, x-ray therapy, thermal injury, or inorganic arsenic exposure.

Squamous Cell Carcinoma. Extensive sun exposure, especially with burns, prior burn scars, chronic ulcers, discoid lupus lesions, prior x-ray skin damage, industrial carcinogen oils, and tar exposure.

Malignant Melanoma. UV sunlight exposure. Intermittent burning exposures are more important than cumulative or chronic exposure time. Environmental exposure to carcinogens. A viral factor is hypothesized.

Alleviating Factors

Actinic Keratosis. Good sun protection: use of sunscreen with sun protection factor (SPF) of 15 or greater, wearing protective clothing and hats, sun avoidance.

Basal Cell Carcinoma. Prevention from birth, with sunblock and clothes to protect light-colored skin.

Squamous Cell Carcinoma. Exposure factor avoidance.

Malignant Melanoma. Sunlight protection, avoidance of sunburns, and early detection.

Associated Factors

Actinic Keratosis. Family history of skin cancers.

Basal Cell Carcinoma. Not applicable.

Squamous Cell Carcinoma. Seen predominantly in males, except on lower legs, where it is more common in women. Fair-complexioned individuals more prone.

Malignant Melanoma. Phenotypic factors associated with melanoma include light skin; blond or red hair; blue, green, or gray eyes; and family history of melanoma. Presence of melanocytic nevi nears 100% if the patient has dysplastic nevus syndrome and family history of melanoma in two or more first-degree relatives.

PHYSICAL EXAMINATION

Skin

Actinic Keratosis. Erythematous macule with overlying clear or tan scale. Easier to palpate than visualize, on face, bare neck, dorsal surfaces of hands and arms, bare scalp, and occasionally the upper chest and back. Evaluate all areas of increased sun exposure. Some lesions may have thicker cutaneous horn–like or nodular surface. See Figure 2-24 in color plate section.

Basal Cell Carcinoma. On long-term sun-exposed skin. Almost 80% are found on the head and neck. Trunk and extremities are the next most common sites. Appear as translucent-opal papules and nodules with rolled borders and telangiectasias. They often have depressed or ulcerated centers or appear as flatter, broader, rough, plaque-like lesions with fine rolled borders. Some have blue, black, or brown pigmentation. Sometimes almost dry and scaly-like. Occasionally a yellowish to waxy, translucent, indurated, deeper plaque, with barely perceptible elevated surface and with diffuse borders. See Figure 2-25 in color plate section.

Squamous Cell Carcinoma. Indurated papule, plaque, or nodule with adherent keratotic scale. Often eroded, crusted, and/or ulcerated on exposed areas, especially the lip, top of ear, head, neck, and dorsum of the hands and arms. May also occur in old burn scar or irradiation sites. All typically present without distinct margins. See Figure 2-26 in color plate section.

Malignant Melanoma. The lesion appears as a pigmented macule, flattened papule, plaque, and/or nodule. May be a new lesion or a recently changing lesion. Haphazardly marked color variegation with two or more of the following: black, brown, pink, red, whitish gray, and blue. Borders are irregularly irregular, often with a notch. The mean diameter is 1 to 2 cm, but may be as small as 2 mm. The risk of metastasizing is greater with lesion size larger than 6 mm and with more vertical growth. More commonly found on the upper back and legs or under nails in both genders, the face in females, and anterior trunk in males. Dark-skinned persons may develop acral lentiginous melanomas on palms, soles, or genitalia. Bathing suit areas generally spared. See Figure 2-27 in color plate section.

Lymphatic
Malignant Melanoma. Evaluate for lymphadenopathy.

PATHOPHYSIOLOGY

Actinic Keratosis. Hypertrophic damaged keratinocytes and thickened dry stratum corneum. Sometimes overlaid with a hyperkeratosis column.

Basal Cell Carcinoma. Proliferation of basaloid cells in dermis with palisading hyperchromatic nuclei. One variant has increased pigment in the melanocytes and melanophages. In another, the morphology has increased strands of basaloid cells in a thickened fibrous stroma.

Squamous Cell Carcinoma. Anaplastic groups of atypical epithelial squamous cells proliferating in strands in the epidermis, dermis, and/or subcutaneous tissue. Cells are of irregular shape and size and have large nuclei and variable keratinization.

Malignant Melanoma. Melanocytes reside in the basal layer of the epidermis and synthesize melanin. Melanin is important in protecting against DNA damage from UV rays. Neoplastic transformation occurs in these cells and they are able to produce their own growth factors and develop autonomous growth. Four growth patterns are noted in malignant melanoma. The most common type, occurring in 60% of melanomas, is the superficial spreading pattern. It is usually an irregularly pigmented macule with one or more areas of nodularity. Nodular melanoma accounts for 15% to 30% of melanomas. It is usually deeply pigmented (bluish black) and raised. It is most common in men and is more aggressive and faster growing than the superficial spreading type. Lentigo melanoma accounts for 5% to 10% of melanomas and is usually a facial lesion occuring in Caucasian women. It has a low risk to metastasize. The acral lentiginous type is seen on the palms, soles, and nail beds. It is a rare type, accounting for only 2% to 8% of melanomas in Caucasians, but for 35% to 60% of melanomas in dark-skinned patients. Ulceration is commonly observed in this type.

DIAGNOSTIC STUDIES

Laboratory.   Not applicable.
Radiology.   Not applicable.

Other

Actinic Keratosis
Biopsy.   If advanced or nodular, and a question of malignant degeneration.

Basal Cell Carcinoma
Biopsy.   Punch, incisional, or deep tangential type.

Squamous Cell Carcinoma
Biopsy.   Any isolated, keratotic, eroded, ulcerating papule, plaque, or nodule that is 6 to 8 weeks old or older to rule out carcinoma.

Malignant Melanoma
Biopsy.   Excisional biopsy of complete lesion whenever possible.

DIFFERENTIAL DIAGNOSIS

Traumatic
Actinic Keratosis.   *Wounds* should resolve in less than a month.
Basal Cell Carcinoma.   *Wound ulcers* heal in days to weeks, and rarely have characteristic raised, rolled borders.
Squamous Cell Carcinoma.   *Wounds* should resolve in less than a month.
Malignant Melanoma.   *Wounds* should resolve in less than a month.

Infectious
Actinic Keratosis.   Not applicable.
Basal Cell Carcinoma.   *Infectious papules, plaques, nodules* have more inflammatory response, are more distinct, may radiate heat, and heal.
Squamous Cell Carcinoma.   *Infectious papules, plaques, nodules* have more inflammatory response, are more distinct, may radiate heat, and heal.
Malignant Melanoma.   *Infectious papules, plaques, nodules* have more inflammatory response, are more distinct, may radiate heat, and heal.

Metabolic
Actinic Keratosis.   *Ichthyosis* or dry scaling will be more widespread and diffuse, without small isolated lesions.
Basal Cell Carcinoma.   Not applicable.
Squamous Cell Carcinoma.   *Diabetic ulcers* occur on lower legs and are more distinct, wide, and deep without the papules or nodularity.
Malignant Melanoma.   Not applicable.

Neoplastic
Actinic Keratosis.   Not otherwise applicable.

Basal Cell Carcinoma. Not otherwise applicable

Squamous Cell Carcinoma
Bowen's Disease (Squamous Cell Carcinoma in Situ). A hyperkeratotic erythematous patch or plaque with sharp demarcation of a few millimeters to several centimeters in diameter. Lesion does not change for years in spite of most treatment for the papulosquamous conditions for which it is most commonly mistaken. A 3% to 5% chance of evolving to frank carcinoma.

Erythroplasia of Queyrat. A carcinoma in situ. A bright red, velvety plaque on the penis of older men, particularly the uncircumcised.

Bowenoid Papulosis. A fleshy, flat, rough-topped papule of the external genitalia of men and women. Is a squamous cell carcinoma in situ and often mistaken for condyloma acuminatum.

Keratoacanthoma. A rapid-growing epidermal neoplasm of purported benign, self-healing nature, but difficult to differentiate from squamous cell carcinoma even histologically. Typically occurs on sun-exposed area, is 1 cm or larger, and appears as a domed, rolled-border, reddened, fleshy papulo-nodule with central invagination or umbilication having a large keratin plug. Treat as for squamous cell carcinoma.

Malignant Melanoma. Not otherwise applicable.

Vascular
Actinic Keratosis. Not applicable.
Basal Cell Carcinoma. Not applicable.
Squamous Cell Carcinoma. *Venous* or *arterial ulcers* are more eroded from the surface downward without papule or nodularity. Become larger.
Malignant Melanoma. Not applicable.

Congenital
Actinic Keratosis. Not applicable.
Basal Cell Carcinoma. *Nevi* are more concentric, uniform, and symmetrical without ulceration; rare umbilication.
Squamous Cell Carcinoma. Not applicable.
Malignant Melanoma. *Cafe-au-lait spots* remain even-colored, tan macules. *Black hairy nevi* may be precursors to melanoma (5% risk), so they must be followed, and changing areas biopsied. *Nevi of melanocytic type* are possible melanoma precursors, and changes in size, shape, color, or elevation dictate need for evaluation. With *other pigmented nevi*, no change over lifetime equals low risk for melanoma especially all under 6 mm in size.

Acquired
Actinic Keratosis. Small lesions of *nummular eczema* are larger and more inflamed, have flaky dry scale, and are not as adherent.

Basal Cell Carcinoma
Fibrous papule may be whitish and clear but not with rolled border and without telangiectasias. Firm superficial, smaller, and uniform. *Trichoepitheliomas* are fleshy papules that do not ulcerate.

Seborrheic keratosis has "stuck-on" appearance, no rolled borders, and no central depression or ulcerations.

Squamous Cell Carcinoma.   Not applicable.

Malignant Melanoma.   Not applicable.

TREATMENT

Actinic Keratosis.   Based on presence of tenderness, cosmetic effect, and malignant potential:

  Liquid nitrogen cryosurgery without anesthesia OR

  Electrodessication and currettage with anesthesia OR

  Topical 5-fluorouracil twice a day for 3 to 4 weeks

May be individualized in patients with sensitive skin to daily or every-other-day usage. Recalcitrant dermatoses may require 10 to 12 weeks of therapy.

  Biopsy thick, advanced lesions to rule out squamous cell skin cancer.

Basal Cell Carcinoma.   Multiple modalities exist for treatment including electrodessication and curettage, deep cryosurgery, CO_2 laser destruction and curettage, excision, and occasionally x-ray therapy. If aggressive clinicopathologic features exist, or if lesion is located in strategic (i.e., cosmetic) areas (e.g., nose area, ear, near eyes), consider micrographic surgery. With microscopic accuracy the tumor is excised in toto with little normal tissue. Permanent cure is obtained in 95% to 100% of cases. The other measures reach 90% to 95% cure rates with initial treatment. Biopsy verification is indicated before any of these methods is used.

Squamous Cell Carcinoma.   Based on size, location, and level of invasion. Aggressive biologic or deep invasive histologic tumors should be removed by excision or micrographic surgery. Superficial, small, and early in situ forms can be destroyed by electrodessication and curettage or laser. Irradiation and cryosurgery can be effective as well.

Malignant Melanoma.   Deep, wide, complete excision. If lesion is less than 0.5 mm thick, then excise with less than a 2-cm margin beyond the lesion border. If lesion is greater than 0.5 mm thick, then excision margins should be up to 3 cm beyond lesion borders. Elective lymph node dissection is controversial; most clinicians advocate waiting for signs or palpability to remove regional nodes.

  Single-agent or combination chemotherapy may be used in metastatic disease but yields low overall complete response rates. Melanoma vaccines are being evaluated and may be promising in severe, advanced disease.

  Lesions should be staged. To properly stage the lesion, determine width and depth, and to establish the prognosis, the entire lesion should be excised. If anatomic structures would be injured or function jeopardized by biopsy procedure in cases with low probability of malignancy, use a deep incisional biopsy.

  Consider oncology referral.

PEDIATRIC CONSIDERATIONS

Malignant melanomas are uncommon in childhood and appear as pigmented nodules with variegated colors within a single lesion. Melanomas arising in congenital pigmented nevi, which are present in approximately 1% of newborn infants, account for most melanomas of childhood. Giant congenital nevi (>20 cm) are associated with leptomeningeal melanocytosis and a predisposition to development of malignant melanoma (incidence of 6% to 10%, with half developing by age 5). Early total excision is treatment of choice. The best approach to medium-size (1.5 to 20 cm in diameter) and small (<1.5 cm) congenital nevi is less clear, but excision prior to adolescence is strongly recommended.

Prolonged exposure to strong sunlight during childhood and adolescence is recognized as a predisposing factor in the development of basal cell and squamous cell carcinomas. Anticipatory guidance should be provided to parents regarding the use of sunscreens and sunblocks.

OBSTETRIC CONSIDERATIONS

Although pregnant women may present with prognostic features worse than those in nonpregnant controls, this does not equate with a more severe prognosis.

PEARLS FOR THE PA

Squamous Cell Carcinoma

If any question, biopsy or refer. Non–solar exposure–related squamous cell carcinomas have more potential to metastasize (as high as 30%).

Malignant Melanoma

It is important to excise the entire lesion, if possible, to determine the prognosis. Diagnostic features summarized by ABCDE:

> *Asymmetry—not the same appearance from one section to another*
>
> *Border—irregular, with scalloped edges*
>
> *Color—variegated, with different shades of brown, black, gray, and white.*
>
> *Diameter—greater than 6 mm*
>
> *Elevations—usually present, with distortion of the geography; best viewed with side-lighting*

GERIATRIC CONSIDERATIONS

Those persons with long-term sun exposure should undergo regular examinations for skin changes that may suggest skin cancer. Inquire about occupations and recreational activities that may have led to prolonged sun exposure. Presentation generally begins in the mid-40s and becomes more prevalent with age.

PREVENTIVE CONSIDERATIONS

SLIP, SLAP, SLOP: Slip on a shirt, slap on a hat, and slop on suntan lotion.

Actinic Keratosis.   Sunscreens (with SPF15 or higher) and/or protective clothing for lengthy or intense sun exposure should be used as prevention.

Basal Cell Carcinoma.   Prevention is important. Preventing sunburn, especially before age 5, and treating actinic keratosis minimize the risk.

Vascular Conditions

Charlene M. Morris, MPAS, PA-C

DEFINITION

Urticaria/angioedema (hives): Cutaneous reactivity manifested by transient wheals and transudation of fluid from small cutaneous vessels. Usually involves pruritus and may be triggered by immune, immunoglobulin E (IgE), and nonimmune hypocomplementemic as well as physical factors. *Urticaria* is a vascular reaction in the epidermis. *Angioedema* is the same vascular reaction occurring deeper, in the dermis and subcutaneous layers. There are more than seven types of urticaria/angioedema.

HISTORY

Symptoms.   Transient wheals, welts, hives. Pruritus, pain with walking (when the feet are involved), flushing, burning at the various involved sites.

General.   May have systemic symptoms in a minority of cases (e.g., wheezing [in cholinergic urticaria], fever [especially in serum sickness], hoarseness, stridor, dyspnea, arthralgia). These symptoms may develop rapidly into anaphylaxis.

Specific irritants include stroking the skin or other means of pressure in dermographism. Cold contact or cold submersion in cold urticaria. Sun exposure for minutes to reactive skin in uncommon solar urticaria. Heat, emotional stress, or exercise in cholinergic urticaria. Any repetitive rubbing (e.g., drying the back) or any mechanical vibrations in vibratory angioedema. Persistent pressure to feet, buttocks, or palms in pressure urticaria. Minor trauma or no detectable irritants may precede flare episode of hereditary angioedema. Third trimester of pregnancy leads to pruritic urticarial papules and plaques of pregnancy in some. Contact penetration or ingestion of offending drugs or food, inhalant allergens, infection, bites of insects or arthropods, internal disease, and psychogenic stress factors trigger allergic urticaria and angioedema. Water contact in aquagenic urticaria.

Age. Any.

Onset. Acute within minutes to hours, or chronic over hours to days.

Duration. Hours; with transient recurring flares. Acute flares last less than 30 days. Chronic flares occur over 30 days to months.

Intensity. Localized, regional or generalized.

Aggravating Factors. Specific irritants (see under General).

Alleviating Factors. Avoidance of offending trigger factors.

Associated Factors. Familial propensity. Systemic disease, infections, and emotional stress may exacerbate the condition.

PHYSICAL EXAMINATION

Skin. Multiple wheals and papules, 1 to 2 mm in diameter, located on the trunk and extremities in cholinergic type. Small, 1-cm wheals to large 8-cm edematous plaques on the trunk or extremities, including hands and feet, face, lips, tongue, and ears. Skin-colored enlargement of eyelids, lips, and tongue is common in angioedema. Other lesions are pink to red, with larger lesions having a pale central halo-like area. The lesions are roundish, oval, arciform, annular, polycyclic, serpiginous, and bizzare in pattern shapes. They are arranged in annular, arciform, linear, local, or wide areas including pressure and exposed areas depending on the type of urticaria. See Figure 2-28 in color plate section.

PATHOPHYSIOLOGY

Biologically active materials from mast cells and/or basophilic leukocytes sensitized with IgE antibodies cause acute urticaria. Mediators cause increased venule permeability; some cases are related not to immunologic factors but to nonimmunologic factors such as drugs, compounds capable of histamine release, or physical agents including trauma. Activation of the complement system plays a role in type III immune complexes involved in serum sickness urticaria and that of connective tissue–vascular disease. Histamine H_1 and H_2 receptors are both involved, and the histamine release leads to the erythema, wheal-flare, and pruritus.

DIAGNOSTIC STUDIES

Laboratory
Chemistry Profile. Used as a baseline.
Complete Blood Count with Differential. Used as a baseline.
Erythrocyte Sedimentation Rate. Elevated in inflammatory conditions.
Hepatitis Profile/Functional C_1 Esterase Screening. Used as a baseline.

Radiology.   Not applicable.

Other.   Ultrasound examination for early diagnosis of bowel involvement. If abdominal pain is present, this may indicate edema of the bowel.

DIFFERENTIAL DIAGNOSIS

Traumatic
Traumatic wheal-flare is reproducible with physical factor contact (e.g., ice, heat, pressure, stroking).

Infectious
Secondary syphilis will give positive result on rapid plasma reagin (RPR) assay or Venereal Disease Research Laboratories (VDRL) test.

Streptococcal infection/candidiasis will have positive smears or cultures.

Metabolic
Cholinergic urticaria is provoked by exercising or sweating.

Neoplastic
Not applicable.

Vascular
Vasculitides will show more petechial, purpuric, or dark purple lesions. In *urticaria perstans*, a feature of necrotizing vasculitis, hive-like lesions are not transient but persistent; other features are nodules and necrotic ulcers.

In *erythema nodosum*, typically indurations of subdermal nodules are tender and not as transient.

In *erythema multiforme*, classic iris target lesions of palms, soles, hands, feet, forearms, elbows, mouth, lips, eyes, and penis. Lungs affected 30% of the time.

Each of the foregoing is a reactive vascular condition caused by idiopathic factors, infections, or drugs.

Congenital.   Not applicable.
Acquired.   Not applicable.

TREATMENT

Anaphylaxis and hereditary angioedema may lead to life-threatening laryngeoedema and require appropriate emergent care. Acute and chronic urticarias generally diminish with time regardless of the etiology.

First-line treatment is elimination of etiologic factors such as chemicals or drugs. Second-line treatment includes an H_1 antihistamine such as hydroxyzine HCl 25-50 mg two to four times a day in adults or a nonsedating H_1 blocker such as fexofenadine, cetirizine, or loratadine 1 tablet every 12 to 24 hours. If there is no response, an H_2 blocker may be added such as cimetidine 400 mg three times a day or 800 mg at bedtime in adults or ranitidine 150 mg twice a day.

If unsuccessful, an H_1 blocker from a different class may be selected. Cyproheptadine is the most effective in cold urticaria two to four times daily.

Next add doxepin 25-75 mg at bedtime (adults). If no response, add pseudoephedrine 30 mg every day.

Prednisone, in a dose of 40-60 mg every day for 2 weeks and tapered to 10 to 20 mg every other day before stopping, may be required in severe disease. Remember, even the worst cases will probably resolve in a few months.

PEDIATRIC CONSIDERATIONS

Vascular disorders occur in 20% to 40% of newborns. They may occur as isolated defects or be confined to the skin, or they may be a feature of various syndromes.

The *"salmon patch"* is the most common vascular lesion of infancy. Common sites include the nape of the neck ("stork bite"), upper eyelids, and glabella. Ninety-five percent of those appearing on the eyelids or glabella disappear within the first year, and 50% of those found on the neck resolve spontaneously. *Port-wine stains*, dark red or purple macules present at birth, appear unilaterally on the side of the face or an extremity. A port-wine stain on the face in the distribution of the ophthalmic branch of the trigeminal nerve, or associated with hemihypertrophy of the side of the face, should suggest Sturge-Weber syndrome. If this lesion is found over an extremity and in combination with bony and soft tissue hypertrophy and venous varicosities, Klippel-Trenaunay-Weber syndrome is implied.

Strawberry hemangiomas are bright red, raised, and well circumscribed. Most are not present at birth but appear within the first 2 months. The most common sites include the face, scalp, and thorax. Often the lesions represent a mixture of capillary and venous elements. Hemangiomas grow rapidly during the first 6 months and most do not enlarge after 12 months. A spontaneous process of involution then begins, and 50% resolve by age 5, 90% by age 9, and the rest by adolescence. No treatment is generally necessary. Mild complications include ulceration and pyoderma. More serious complications can occur when platelet trapping within the lesion results in thrombocytopenia (Kasabach-Merritt syndrome) or when location or size compromises vital structures (e.g., airway obstruction, visual obstruction).

Cavernous hemangiomas are more deeply situated lesions and appear more diffuse and ill defined. They are cystic and firm, and the overlying skin may appear bluish in color. Rarely do these tumors impinge on vital structures, but if involvement of underlying structures is suspected, appropriate radiologic studies should be performed.

OBSTETRIC CONSIDERATIONS

No specific indications.

GERIATRIC CONSIDERATIONS

No specific indications.

PREVENTIVE CONSIDERATIONS

Avoidance of known irritants such as drugs (evaluate for side effects), cold, sun exposure, heat, emotional stress, repetitive rubbing, pressure, foods, inhalants, infections, insect bites, water.

It is imperative to identify the cause, as life-threatening anaphylaxis can develop.

PEARLS FOR THE PA

Life-threatening anaphylaxis can develop in urticaria/angioedema.

From 70% to 90% of cases of chronic urticaria are idiopathic.

Use of histamine H_1 plus H_2 blockers provides additive effect.

Viral Disease—Vesicular

Charlene M. Morris, MPAS, PA-C

DEFINITION

Herpes simplex: Skin or mucous membrane infection, marked by vesicles on red base caused by herpes simplex virus (HSV) and *Herpesvirus hominis*. Exists in acute and recurrent forms.

Herpes zoster (shingles): Reactivated, self-limited infection of latent varicella-zoster virus in one or two nerve roots, inflaming the related sensory nerves. Manifested by eruption in a dermatomal pattern on the skin unilaterally, never crossing the midline.

Varicella (chickenpox): Acute, primary infection of the skin with varicella-zoster virus. Previously common exanthem of the childhood diseases.

Hand-foot-and-mouth disease: Contagious skin infection caused by enterovirus/coxsackievirus A 16 or enterovirus 71. Typically affects the mouth and/or hands and feet.

HISTORY

Symptoms

Herpes Simplex.   Prodrome of itch, tingle, and/or burning at the infection site. Painful group of blisters on intraoral surfaces, lips, or face. Primary episode may include headache, fever, and tender swollen glands in the region of infection. These symptoms are less common in the recurrent setting. With *herpes genitalis*, symptoms include severe pain, itching, dysuria, mucoid discharge, and tender inguinal lymph nodes.

Herpes Zoster (Shingles). One-to 4-day prodrome with fever, headache, malaise. Pain and paresthesias (itching, tingling, burning) ipsilateral to rash appearance site. Unilateral, painful blisters with red bases in a narrow pattern. Regionally enlarged, tender lymph nodes.

Varicella (Chickenpox). Widespread pruritic papules, clear vesicles, and crusts together in any area of head, mouth, trunk.

Hand-Foot-and-Mouth Disease. Bright red-ringed papules, vesicles, ulcers in mouth, dysphagia. Red macules, papules, and grayish white vesicles of hands and feet. May have malaise and low-grade fever with a sore throat.

Age

Herpes Simplex. Children as young as 1 to 5 years of age, but incidence peaks rapidly after 15 years of age and slows by age 30 for primary disease.

Herpes Zoster (Shingles). Any, but more than 60% of cases in over-50 age group. Less than 10% under 20 years.

Varicella (Chickenpox). Any, but more common in childhood. Neonates can acquire the infection from mothers.

Hand-Foot-and-Mouth Disease. Infants and children.

Onset

Herpes Simplex. Acute, with tingling, stinging prodrome for a few hours to 1 to 2 days in over 50% of patients for primary or recurrent disease. Infectious contact occurs 2 to 20 days before active signs of infection. Neurologic pain may precede each recurrence.

Herpes Zoster (Shingles). Acute prodromal pains, paresthesias that are followed by skin lesions in approximately 4 days.

Varicella (Chickenpox). Acute after up to 14-day incubation. The patient remains asymptomatic for a few days before the outbreak. Viral prodrome is common, with fever, myalgia, chills, arthralgias up to 3 days before; symptoms may continue up to a few days after eruptions.

Hand-Foot-and-Mouth Disease. Acute with oral lesions. Incubation is 3 to 5 days.

Duration

Herpes Simplex. Acute, self-limited for 2 weeks or more in primary and 10 days or less in recurrent episodes. Less if treated with antiviral medications.

Herpes Zoster (Shingles). Prodrome and skin lesions in 4 days, vesicles to pustules in 3 to 4 days, crusts by tenth day, and resolution in most by 3 weeks. Postherpetic pain that lasts 2 months to many years can occur, especially in older patients.

Varicella (Chickenpox). One to 3 weeks.

Hand-Foot-and-Mouth Disease. Self-limited, 7 to 10 days to healing. Less if treated with antiviral medications.

Intensity

Herpes Simplex. One herpetiform (cluster) to a few lesions in primary disease; one or two lesions with recurrent disease. Recurrences average 2 to 3 times per year for oral herpes (herpes labialis) and 4 to 8 times per year for genital herpes.

Herpes Zoster (Shingles). Most typical is many vesicular groups, on red bases, over one or two dermatomes unilaterally. Occasionally occur in one or two groups, especially in young patients.

Varicella (Chickenpox). Subclinical with few to no lesions, or generalized with full body and mucous membrane involvement.

Hand-Foot-and-Mouth Disease. A few to a mouthful of painful erosions and few, several, or many red-based gray vesicles of toes, fingers, palms, and soles.

Aggravating Factors

Herpes Simplex. UV irradiation, fever, systemic illness, emotional stress, fatigue, trauma, menses, pregnancy all known to reactivate the virus.

Herpes Zoster (Shingles). Compromised cellular immunity. Physical and mental stressors.

Varicella (Chickenpox). Immunocompromise, secondary bacterial infection, varicella pneumonia (rare), encephalitis, and Reye syndrome (in children who have taken aspirin during the course of disease). Heat hastens outbreaks.

Hand-Foot-and-Mouth Disease. Epidemics due to enterovirus 71 occasionally are associated with central nervous system disorders (aseptic meningitis, polio-like paralysis, and encephalitis). Children younger than 3 years may also get a maculopapular rash in the diaper area, including the buttocks.

Alleviating Factors

Herpes Simplex. Analgesics, antipyretics, antipruritics, compresses with boric acid solution or Burow's solution, mupirocin, or Polysporin ointment.

Herpes Zoster (Shingles). Corticosteroids, nonsteroidal anti-inflammatory drugs (NSAIDS), narcotics, Burow's solution compresses, and acyclovir.

Varicella (Chickenpox). Varicella vaccine. Antipruritics, antipyretics, Burow's solution compresses, topical antibiotics, and for severe or complicated disease, antiviral medications.

Hand-Foot-and-Mouth Disease. Symptomatic therapy.

Associated Factors

Herpes Simplex. Immunocompromised patients will have more severe or disseminated outbreaks. HSV infection is known to lead on occasion to erythema multiforme in 7 to 14 days, following herpetic infection.

Herpes Zoster (Shingles). Immunocompromise such as with acquired immunodeficiency syndrome (AIDS) and leukemia, Hodgkin's disease, and other malignancies; also immunosuppressive drugs and corticosteroids.

Varicella (Chickenpox). Communicable. Possibly causes developmental deformities with congenital infection in first trimester of pregnancy. Most fetal infection resolves without residua.

Hand-Foot-and-Mouth Disease. Limited epidemics seen in warmer months.

PHYSICAL EXAMINATION

General

Herpes Simplex
Primary Infection.   Swollen tender regional lymph nodes. Clusters of vesicles on red base in oral cavity on any mucous membranes or on dry lips or skin of face. Occasionally any other area of the skin including fingers (herpetic whitlow) lasting up to 6 weeks for type I infection. Type II infection appears as 10 to 15 papules progressing to red-based vesicles, to erosions, to grayish white ulcers on any area of male or female genitalia. Neonates can acquire the disease from mothers by vaginal delivery. See Figure 2-29 in color plate section.

Recurrent Infection.   Fewer clustered vesicles or ulcers, may be 10% of those seen in primary genital disease. Less prominent swollen, tender adenopathy, sites of which will be close to or include area of the primary infection. Less recurrence of mucosal oral disease or whitlow.

Herpes Zoster (Shingles).
Unilateral, palm-sized groups of vesicobullae on raised inflamed base over dermatome. Vesicles may become purpuric, necrotic, and crusty, and leave scars. Can occur in the ophthalmic distribution of the trigeminal nerve and result in infections and complications in the eye. Regional lymph nodes are enlarged and tender. Possible but rare in the mouth or vagina.

Varicella (Chickenpox).
Single, small, widespread lesions progressing rapidly through papular stage to vesicles and pustules. Typically followed by umbilication and crusting. Successive crops of vesicles erupt for 4 to 5 days and become crusted by 1 week. It is not uncommon to have three successive crops of lesions, so that any area of skin will manifest all stages of the disease at the same time. May occur anywhere on the body. See Figure 2-30 in color plate section.

Hand-Foot-and-Mouth Disease.
Widespread or densely grouped red-ringed vesicles, 2 to 8 mm in size. Progress quickly to painful denuded erosions on any intraoral membranes, including tongue, hard palate, and buccal mucosa. Red macules progress to gray vesicles with a red ring. The skin lesions follow the oral lesions and are found on the sides and dorsum of the fingers, toes, hands, and feet, and may be on the soles and palms.

PATHOPHYSIOLOGY

Herpes Simplex.   The virus enters at mucous membrane or injured skin site by contact with infected person, most commonly at the mouth or genitalia for adults. The virus replicates in epidermal and dermal cells and is transported to the neuronal nucleus and can spread distally to additional skin sites. Also, by unknown means, the virus enters a lifelong latent stage in the nuclei of neural ganglia. Periodic reactivation then leads to the recurrent episodes of infection and skin–mucous membrane manifestation or replication. Viral shedding is possible in the crust stage.

Herpes Zoster (Shingles).   Varicella-zoster virus, during varicella infection, clinically or subclinically invades the sensory nerves and migrates to the neural ganglia and becomes latent until some event reactivates the virus (e.g., immunosuppression, malignancy, trauma). The infection travels along the sensory nerve, causing inflammation, pain, and a vesicular eruption.

Varicella (Chickenpox). Very contagious virus acquired by direct contact with infected person who has varicella (by inhaling infected airborne droplets) or by direct contact in those with herpes zoster. Virus replicates in skin, causing the typical vesicular eruption that progresses to crusting. Contagion persists from 2 days before first crop of eruptions until all the lesions are crusted. The virus migrates along axons to become latent in nerve ganglia and, if later reactivated, causes herpes zoster (shingles).

Hand-Foot-and-Mouth Disease. Highly contagious virus that directly invades the skin or migrates to the skin after direct contact with infected person. Colonizes the bowel and spreads by fecal-oral route.

DIAGNOSTIC STUDIES

Laboratory

Herpes Simplex
Viral Cultures. Performed by deroofing of vesicles and scraping from the base of an open lesion.
Blood Titers. Assay for antibody for HSV to immunoglobulin G (IgG) and immunoglobulin M (IgM). Effective to identify acute and latent disease.

Herpes Zoster (Shingles)
Viral Culture. Confirm diagnosis if indicated.
Varicella (Chicken pox). Viral culture, if indicated.

Hand-Foot-and-Mouth Disease
Viral Culture. Virus retrievable from vesicular fluid, throat secretions, and feces.

Radiology. Not applicable.

Other

Herpes Simplex
Tzanck Preparations. Performed by deroofing vesicle, scraping the base, smearing on slide, and allowing to air dry. Giemsa stain is performed to look for giant multinucleated epithelial cells.
Tissue Culture. This is the best confirmatory test, but it takes up to 3 days and is not available in all laboratories.

Herpes Zoster (Shingles)
Tissue Culture. Takes longer than for HSV. May aid in diagnosis.
Varicella (Chickenpox). Tzanck preparation or tissue cultures verify. Usually not necessary.
Hand-Foot-and-Mouth Disease. Not applicable.

DIFFERENTIAL DIAGNOSIS

Traumatic
Herpes Simplex. *Burn blisters* have no prodrome and have appropriate history.
Herpes Zoster (Shingles). Not applicable, only as a possible reactivation trigger.
Varicella (Chickenpox). Not applicable.
Hand-Foot-and-Mouth Disease. Not applicable.

Infectious

Herpes Simplex
In *coxsackievirus infection*, usually isolated vesicles on hands, on feet, and in mouth; not clustered.
In *syphilis*, generally larger, single ulcers without significant pain and not recurrent. RPR assay positive.
Lesions of *chancroid* enlarge from primary pustule and are raggedly irregular, culture-positive for bacteria (*Haemophilus ducreyi*). Lymph nodes suppurate and drain.
Lymphogranuloma venereum is a painless papule, pustule, or ulcer of penis, but with large, double lymph node involvement in groin. Cultures positive for virulent strain of *Chlamydia trachomatis*.
Herpes Zoster (Shingles). *Zosteriform herpes simplex with neuralgia* is difficult to differentiate, but HSV grows quickly on tissue culture, and condition can recur.
Varicella (Chickenpox). In *eczema vaccinatum*, history, usually in atopic patient, with known recent vaccination or exposure to the vaccinated person with cowpox vaccine for smallpox. Rare, as only the military may be using vaccine.
Hand-Foot-and-Mouth Disease. In *herpetic gingivostomatitis* and *herpangina*, the pronounced red ring around the lesion is absent. Less common on hard palate.

Metabolic
Herpes Simplex. Not applicable.
Herpes Zoster (Shingles). Not applicable.
Varicella (Chickenpox). Not applicable.
Hand-Foot-and-Mouth Disease. In *aphthous stomatitis*, usually few lesions and less painful and without the bright red ring around lesion.

Neoplastic. Not applicable.

Vascular
Herpes Simplex. Not applicable.
Herpes Zoster (Shingles). In *necrotizing vasculitis*, distribution is not dermatomal and is bilateral.
Varicella (Chickenpox). Not applicable.

Hand-Foot-and-Mouth Disease.   Not applicable.

Congenital
Herpes Simplex.   Not applicable.
Herpes Zoster (Shingles).   In *varicella infection in infants,* the mother has a history of gestational varicella.
   Varicella (Chickenpox).   Not applicable
Hand-Foot-and-Mouth Disease.   Not applicable.

Acquired
Herpes Simplex.   In *Behçet's disease,* usually has oral and genital ulcers, yellow rather than white ulcer; surface coagulum. Large lesions of genitals, usually the scrotum, are deeper and heal with scars. Negative cultures or tests.
   In *Crohn's disease,* bowel disease a major part of the history. Negative HSV culture. Genital and oral ulcers are more granulomatous.
Herpes Zoster (Shingles).   Not applicable.
Varicella (Chickenpox).   In *folliculitis infections* or *oil contact,* lesions have no significant stages; only papulopustule.

Hand-Foot-and-Mouth Disease
Erythema multiforme is more diffuse and bullous than sharp red erosions of hand-foot-and-mouth disease. More localized to gums and buccal mucosa.
   Drug reaction such as to sulfa medications is associated with history of medication use.

TREATMENT

Herpes Simplex
VALACYCLOVIR (Valtrex): Varying doses dependent on creatinine clearance. For otherwise healthy patients >18 years of age:
   Herpes progenitalis, primary episode: 1 g every 12 hours for 10 days.
   Herpes progenitalis, recurrent: 500 mg every 12 hours for 3 days.
   Herpes progenitalis, prophylaxis: 500 mg/day; reevaluate after 1 year.
FAMCYCLOVIR (Famvir): Varying doses dependent on creatinine clearance. For otherwise healthy patients >18 years of age:
   Herpes progenitalis, primary episode: 250 mg three times a day for 7 to 10 days.
   Herpes progenitalis, recurrent: 125 mg twice daily for 5 days.
   Herpes progenitalis, prophylaxis: 250 mg orally, twice daily; reevaluate after 1 year.
   Herpes, recurrent in HIV infection: 500 mg twice daily for 7 days.
ACYCLOVIR (Zovirax)
   Herpes progenitalis, primary episode: 200 mg five times a day for 10 days.
   Herpes progenitalis, prophylaxis: 400 mg twice daily or 200 mg three to five times a day; reeevaluate at 12 months.

Recurrences are common after cessation of prophylaxis therapy but with less frequency.

Acyclovir may be used in children at 200 mg four times a day for 5 days. In children weighing more than 40 kg, dosing is the same as for adults.

For *herpes labialis*:

Pencyclovir 1% cream applied every 2 hours while patient is awake for 4 days; begin at earliest sign of symptoms.

For *herpetic whitlow*:

Acyclovir 400 mg three times a day for 10 days OR

Valacyclovir 1000 mg twice daily for 10 days OR

Famciclovir: 250 mg PO three times a day for 5 to 10 days.

Herpes Zoster (Shingles)

Antiviral medications are given as early as possible in course of infection for maximal effect on symptoms and duration:

Acyclovir 800 mg five times daily for 7 to 10 days for *zoster*; 800 mg four times daily for 5 days for *varicella* (for children, 20 mg/kg four times a day for 5 days; for children >40 kg, same as adult dose)

OR

Valacyclovir 1000 mg three times a day for 7 days OR

Famciclovir 500 mg PO three times a day for 7 days.

ALL WITH OR WITHOUT gabapentin 300 mg daily on day 1, 300 mg twice daily on day 2, 300 mg three times a day on day 3 up to 1.8 g per day total dose. Dose adjusted in renal disease.

OR

Prednisone 30 mg PO twice daily for 7 days, then 15 mg PO twice daily for 7 days, then 7.5 mg twice daily for 7 days.

Prednisone may reduce symptoms and minimize the development of postherpetic neuralgia. Care should be taken with prednisone use in immunocompromised persons, as it can lead to dissemination of the disease.

For disseminated disease or in severely immunocompromised patient:

Acyclovir 10 mg/kg IV every 8 hours for 10 days.

For *analgesia*, NSAIDs or narcotics are used to relieve symptoms.

Burow's solution (aluminum sulfate, calcium acetate) compresses applied 15 to 30 minutes three or four times a day, followed by antibiotic ointment, may speed healing.

Varicella (Chickenpox)

For severe or complicated disease in adults, use antiviral medications as just outlined. Otherwise, use supportive care including antipruritics and antipyretics. Do not use salicylates in children under 14.

Varicella-zoster immune globulin (VZIG) may be used in high-risk patients exposed to chickenpox or zoster. Ideally administered within 96 hours, protection continues for 3 weeks. May be repeated, if necessary.

Burow's solution (1:40) compresses can be applied for 15 to 20 minutes three or four times daily for symptomatic relief.

Treat secondary bacterial infection with systemic antibiotics as directed (see Bacterial Infections earlier). It is important to treat the symptoms to minimize pruritus with attendant scratching, excoriation, and scarring.

Hand-Foot-and-Mouth Disease. Symptomatic only, with analgesics, acetaminophen, topical xylocaine viscous, and diphenhydramine elixir swished and swallowed. Hospitalization may be required for supportive care in severe cases.

PEDIATRIC CONSIDERATIONS

Herpes Simplex Virus Infection. Maternal infection with HSV type 2 (and occasionally type 1) during pregnancy or parturition is associated with intrauterine infection and, more commonly, neonatal disease. It is characterized by disseminated viremia with multisystem involvement or may be localized to the brain, skin, eyes, or oropharynx. Signs may be present at birth, but vesicles may appear up to 7 days after birth. Mortality is high in neonates with systemic infection.

In infants and children, 60% of HSV infections appear as gingivostomatitis, almost always due to type 1 HSV. The primary episode often appears in infants younger than 6 months. Presenting symptoms include irritability, salivation, refusal to eat, foul odor, and fever (often with temperatures of >103° F). It can last 7 to 14 days and is self-limited. Symptomatic and supportive therapy is important. In infants, stomatitis may lead to severe dehydration, shock, electrolyte imbalance, and hypoproteinemia. For older children, local analgesics (viscous lidocaine or benzocaine lozenges) may help. Cold fluids or semisolid foods may be tolerated when other food is refused.

On the skin, the lesion consists of groups of vesicles on an erythematous base. These rupture, scab, and heal within 7 to 10 days. In children the vesicles may become secondarily infected and in that case only, antibiotics are useful.

Viral Exanthems. In the pediatric age group numerous viral infections exist that are associated with dermatologic manifestations. A variety of different patterns are seen in these viral exanthems including a generalized maculopapular eruption that mimics measles (morbilliform), petechial eruptions, vesiculobullous eruptions, scarlet fever–like eruptions (scarlatiniform), and oral eruptions. These disorders include measles, rubella, erythema infectiosum, roseola infantum, varicella, and many others. A more complete discussion is beyond the scope of this book, and the reader is referred to textbooks on pediatric infectious diseases for further information.

Aspirin, as an antipyretic, should not be used in the pediatric age group.

Varicella (Chickenpox) Vaccine. When varicella vaccine is given at approximately 1 year of age, the seroconversion rate is 97%. In children older than 13 years at time of first immunization, only 78% achieve immune status, but a second dose gives a seroconversion rate of 99%. Postvaccine varicella incidence is no more than 15%. The varicella vaccine also provides relative protection from developing cutaneous herpes zoster later in life.

Acyclovir is approved for use in children older than 2 years.

OBSTETRIC CONSIDERATIONS

Herpes Gestationis.   An autoimmune condition that occurs during pregnancy and the postpartum period. It is a pruritic condition involving vesicles on normal-appearing and erythematous skin. Lesions usually first appear on the abdomen. There is an associated possibility of up to 30% fetal mortality rate, and an increased incidence of premature deliveries. High-potency topical steroids and diphenhydramine may be of help. Usually, oral prednisone is needed to adequately treat the condition throughout the pregnancy.

Herpes Simplex Virus.   HSV infection complicates 1% to 2% of all pregnancies. The main risk of infection posed to the fetus from a mother with primary HSV infection occurs during delivery: If a mother is experiencing a primary active outbreak (attack), a vaginal delivery creates a 50% chance of HSV transmission to the baby. This leads to the recommendation of delivery by cesarean section if the woman has genital herpetic lesions present. Up to 60% of women delivering infected infants may be asymptomatic, and 1% to 2% of all women (pregnant and nonpregnant) chronically shed the virus in saliva and genital secretions. Women can also carry an active herpes infection of the cervix and have no symptoms. Infants delivered vaginally to mothers with active recurrent HSV infection had an approximately 8% risk of transmission of the infection. There is also an approximately 12% infection rate in fetuses with intact amniotic membranes.

HSV infection in the neonate is often catastrophic, with an approximately 50% mortality rate. Therefore, serologic testing and clinical observation are recommended. Maternal primary HSV infection has also been found to increase the risk of prematurity and intrauterine growth retardation.

Acyclovir and valacyclovir are both pregnancy category B. Use should be limited to severe life-threatening maternal primary HSV infections. Disseminated maternal infection is more likely in a woman who is pregnant.

Herpes Zoster.   In contrast to chickenpox, maternal herpes zoster seldom poses a risk of congenital infection to the infant.

Varicella.   Pregnant women who are at all unsure of their immune status in regard to varicella should avoid persons with varicella infections. If a pregnant woman does develop varicella, the frequency of congenital infection is rare. If it does occur, however, the fetus can develop a syndrome of limb hypoplasia, chorioretinitis, cutaneous scars, cataracts, cortical atrophy, and microcephaly.

If a mother contracts chickenpox immediately before or shortly after delivery, the infant can then be administered varicella-zoster immune globulin.

GERIATRIC CONSIDERATIONS

Herpes zoster is more frequently encountered in persons older than 50 years of age. Herpes simplex and herpes zoster are aggravated by immunocompromise and systemic illness, which is more common in the elderly.

PREVENTIVE CONSIDERATIONS

Herpes simplex is a sexually transmitted disease. Appropriate precautions such as barrier contraception are indicated for prevention.

Varicella vaccine is extremely effective if given at 1 year of age (see Pediatric Considerations). Children who receive the varicella vaccine are much less likely to develop chickenpox or zoster.

PEARLS FOR THE PA

Herpes

Herpes simplex occurs unilaterally, in a dermatomal distribution, and may affect the genitals, oral mucosa, and skin. Lymphadenopathy may also occur.

Herpetic whitlow is an HSV infection manifestation in the nailbed, often associated with professions dealing with close body contact with others, such as dentistry, medical assisting/nursing, and cosmetology.

Antiviral medications should be started within 72 hours of outbreak for best results.

Both valacyclovir and famciclovir dosages must be adjusted for renal insufficiency.

With recurrent infections, maintenance dose antiviral medications may prevent breakthrough.

Varicella (Chickenpox)

Not uncommon to notice the three stages of the lesions occurring simultaneously.

Tzanck preparation does not differentiate herpes simplex from herpes varicella.

Hand-Foot-and-Mouth Disease

Self-limited, contagious infection caused by enterovirus (coxsackievirus) A 16 or enterovirus 71.

Other Viral Infections

Charlene M. Morris, MPAS, PA-C

DEFINITION

Measles (rubeola): Infection with paramyxovirus, an RNA virus related to the canine distemper virus. Was previously common in childhood, but the numbers of cases dropped off significantly in the mid-1960s after a nationwide immunization program.

Roseola (exanthem subitum): Viral exanthem that is thought to be due to human herpesvirus 6; one of the most common childhood diseases.

Erythema infectiosum (fifth disease): Infectious exanthem caused by a parvovirus.

Rubella (German measles): A mild viral infection with mild illness and an exanthem of pink discrete and confluent macules.

Molluscum contagiosum: A poxvirus group DNA virus infection of the epithelium. Molluscum contagiosum virus (MCV) I and MCV II identified as the cause.

Warts (verrucae): Epithelial cell infection from inoculation with human papillomavirus (HPV). Most common cutaneous infection. Occurs on any skin or mucosal surface. Classified by causative HPV strain and appearance and location. Classified as common warts (verruca vulgaris), flat warts (verruca plana), plantar warts (verruca plantaris), and genital warts (condyloma acuminatum). Common warts and genital warts are the most common varieties encountered.

HISTORY

Symptoms

Measles (Rubeola). Viral upper respiratory infection (high fever, respiratory congestion, sore throat, cough, and conjunctivitis) precedes a red papular rash that spreads to cover entire body, by 2 to 4 days.

Roseola (Exanthem Subitum). Three to 5 days of high fever, followed by body rash. Mild irritability or malaise possible with mild respiratory symptoms.

Erythema Infectiosum (Fifth Disease). Rare prodrome of low-grade fever, malaise, and headache. Rash on extremities and bright red cheeks. From 5% to 15% of children may have sore throat, coryza, and abdominal and joint pain. Arthritis is a common adult complaint.

Rubella (German Measles). Prodrome consists of lymph node enlargement of the postauricular, posterior, cervical, and other nodes. The patient may complain of sore throat, malaise, fever, headache, cough, and eye pain, which precedes a rash of the face that spreads downward.

Molluscum Contagiosum. Painless, pearly papules on any area of skin. Sometimes involved area reddened, excoriated from scratching, and spreading.

Warts (Verrucae)

Common Warts. Hard, rough papules on hands, elbows, fingers, and knees. Painless except that some palmar lesions with pressure are tender. Small and large with thickening.

Flat Warts. Asymptomatic, slightly raised, flat-topped, flesh-colored or pinkish brown, small lesions on face, hands, and occasionally knee areas or lower legs.

Plantar Warts. Small, firm depressions or callused firm plaques or discrete, papules on the sole of the foot. May be very tender with pressure, especially with bilateral squeeze.

Genital Warts. Asymptomatic genital/perianal papules or cauliflower masses.

Age

Measles (Rubeola). Childhood, now most common in those who have not been immunized.

Roseola (Exanthem Subitum). Six months to 3 years. Over half of cases seen in children younger than 1 year.

Erythema Infectiosum (Fifth Disease). Usually children, but occasionally an adult.

Rubella (German Measles). Was previously common in children; now most common in those who have not been immunized.

Molluscum Contagiosum. Children of any age, adults.

Warts (Verrucae)

Common Warts. School-age children, decreasing incidence in young adults especially after age 25 years. Periungual warts occur at any age.

Flat Warts. Young children, males in beard skin area, or young women on lower legs.

Plantar Warts. Typically ages 5 to 25 years, but seen at any age.

Genital Warts. Young adults, occasionally young children from parental inoculation or sexual abuse.

Onset

Measles (Rubeola). Acute, with prodrome after 1-week incubation. Next to appear are Koplik spots on buccal mucosa during the prodrome. An exanthem rash appears at 4 to 7 days, with some overlap, to an average 7 to 10 days.

Roseola (Exanthem Subitum). Acute, with 3 to 5 days of fever. May indicate exposure to infected person about 1 week earlier.

Erythema Infectiosum (Fifth Disease). Acute, with red cheek patches.

Rubella (German Measles). Acute, with prodrome illness. Symptoms and rash develop quickly, beginning on the face. Fifteen-to 21-day incubation.

Molluscum Contagiosum. Acute eruption of a few lesions.

Warts (Verrucae)

Common Warts. Sudden appearance of small papule(s).

Flat Warts. Sudden, with several lesions.

Plantar Warts.   Small papule acutely with growth and callus formation, in a progressive steady fashion.
Genital Warts.   Sudden appearance of one or more lesions.

Duration
Measles (Rubeola).   Seven to 10 days.
Roseola (Exanthem Subitum).   High fever for 3 to 5 days; rash within 2 days, which lasts for 1 to 3 days.
Erythema Infectiosum (Fifth Disease).   Extremity and possible body rash within 4 days of cheek eruption. Lasts days to weeks and may reappear after apparent resolution. Triggered by temperature, sunlight, or emotional, exertional, or other factors.
Rubella (German Measles).   The rash fades in about 3 to 4 days.
Molluscum Contagiosum.   Up to 2 years without treatment. Single lesions come and go over several months.

Warts (Verrucae)
Common Warts.   Weeks, months, years.
Flat Warts.   Weeks, month.
Plantar Warts.   Months to years.
Genital Warts.   Months, with recurrences possible for years.

Intensity
Measles (Rubeola).   From several morbilliform areas about the head and centrally to involvement of most skin areas.
Roseola (Exanthem Subitum).   Fever, with temperatures of 103° to 104° F possible, that resolves when rash appears on neck and trunk.
Erythema Infectiosum (Fifth Disease).   Bright red cheeks and papules on extremities. Evolve into reticulate lacy patterns and may spread to the trunk. May wax and wane for days to weeks.
Rubella (German Measles).   No prominent rash to confluent morbilliform or scarlatiniformlike rash. Involves face, trunk, and extremities.
Molluscum Contagiosum.   Children: 5 to 100 papules. Adults: 5 to 30 papules. Immunocompromised persons: Hundreds or thousands.

Warts (Verrucae)
Common Warts.   Single lesion to discrete, scattered lesions that may number several to many.
Flat Warts.   Always multiple discrete lesions, close-set groups to several groups, wide-set.
Plantar Warts.   One, few, or numerous.
Genital Warts.   Single, isolated lesion to several confluent masses to near total coverage of genitals or anus.

Aggravating Factors
Measles (Rubeola).   Malnutrition.
Roseola (Exanthem Subitum).   Pharyngitis and adenopathy may also be present, with upper respiratory infection–type symptoms.

Erythema Infectiosum (Fifth Disease). None.
Rubella (German Measles). None.
Molluscum Contagiosum. Depressed cell-mediated immunity.

Warts (Verrucae)
Common Warts. Trauma, pressure, and skin breakage injury sites. Autoinoculation.
Flat Warts. Skin trauma, leg shaving, face shaving. Autoinoculation.
Plantar Warts. Pressure trauma.
Genital Warts. Highly contagious.

Alleviating Factors
Measles (Rubeola). None or symptomatic treatment.
Roseola (Exanthem Subitum). Only acetaminophen for fevers.
Erythema Infectiosum (Fifth Disease). Temperature extremes, especially heat.
Rubella (German Measles). Symptomatic prodrome treatment.
Molluscum Contagiosum. Enhanced cellular immune mechanism treatments.

Warts (Verrucae)
Common Warts. Occasionally resolve spontaneously with time. Hypnosis or "charming" possibly effective in susceptible patients.
Flat Warts. "Tincture of time" may resolve many.
Plantar Warts. "Tincture of time."
Genital Warts. Sometimes spontaneous resolution or no recurrence.

Associated Factors
Measles (Rubeola). Pneumonia is present in half of patients, and otitis media is common. Less common are encephalitis, myocarditis, and croup-like condition. Conjunctivitis can be significant, especially in light-sensitive patients.
Roseola (Exanthem Subitum). Enanthem of pink discrete papules on uvula and soft palate possible. Rare complications include febrile seizures, encephalitis, and thrombocytopenic purpura.
Erythema Infectiosum (Fifth Disease). Sunlight exposure, heat, emotions, exercise.
Rubella (German Measles). Severe infection of fetus acquired transplacentally causes developmental abnormalities in the first trimester. Most common in the spring. Arthritis occasionally occurs, mostly in adults and females.
Molluscum Contagiosum. Sexual activity with infected person. Autoinoculation common. Immunologic factors. Incubation 4 to 8 weeks on average, but is variable.

Warts (Verrucae)
Common Warts. Kuebner's phenomenon positive. Immunosuppression or compromise.
Flat Warts. Kuebner's phenomenon. Immunocompromise.
Plantar Warts. Autoinoculation.

Genital Warts. Immunocompromise. In 1% of cases or more, lesions are common warts.

PHYSICAL EXAMINATION

General

Measles (Rubeola). Pharyngitis, conjunctivitis, splenomegaly, adenopathy, fever, occasional otitis media, and pneumonia are present in 50% of cases.

Roseola (Exanthem Subitum). Fever, with mild respiratory infection signs, pharyngitis, or mild adenopathy, or no findings.

Erythema Infectiosum (Fifth Disease). Most patients are otherwise well. Adults may have symptoms of arthritis.

Rubella (German Measles). Mild fever, arthritis, and arthralgia most common in women. Patients may have features of an upper respiratory infection.

Molluscum Contagiosum/Warts. Patients generally appear normal.

Skin

Measles (Rubeola). Red, discrete papules that become confluent and form the typical morbillifom rash beginning on the head and/or neck and spreading over the body. Koplik spots on buccal mucosa; tiny white or gray dots on inflamed base. See Figure 2-31 in color plate section.

Roseola (Exanthem Subitum). After fever, a pink maculopapular 2- to 5-mm-lesion rash develops. It is diffuse on the neck and trunk. Fades within 3 days. See Figure 2-32 in color plate section.

Erythema Infectiosum (Fifth Disease). Bilateral, fiery red cheek patches or plaques. Within 4 days, a papular rash becomes evident on the arms and possibly the legs. Evolves into a reticulate, lacy pattern and may spread to the trunk. Occasional exanthem of rose-colored pinpoint macules (Forscheimer spots) and/or petechiae of the soft palate. See Figure 2-33 in color plate section.

Rubella (German Measles). Pink, discrete macules of the face that spread rapidly to involve the trunk and extremities. Lesions can be absent in up to 40% of infected patients or appear morbilliform or scarlatiniform. See Figure 2-34 in color plate section.

Molluscum Contagiosum. Pearly, flesh-colored, white, or reddened papules, sometimes translucent, with a white bead molluscum body visible in papule. Asymptomatic and smooth surfaced. Round, oval, or hemispherical, from a few to several millimeters in diameter. A central umbilication is pathognomonic. Occasionally will exhibit significant inflammation. May become larger in size or be furuncle-like. In children, 5 to 100 papules occur on the extremities, face, and upper trunk. In otherwise healthy adults, 5 to 30 papules may be present on inner thighs, pubis, and genitalia. Sometimes occur on the mucosal epithelieum in children and adults.

Warts (Verrucae)

Common Warts. Hyperkeratotic papules ranging from 1 mm to a few centimeters in diameter. Occur on the extremities (especially hands and knees). Lesions appear round and skin-colored with pathognomonic central black dots (thrombosed dermal capillaries). Common on nail borders or under nail edges. Occasionally exhibit filiform 1-mm bases; are several millimeters long, isolated, or arising from hyperkeratotic papule on face, neck, or genitalia. See Figure 2-35 in color plate section.

Flat Warts. Flesh-colored or pinkish brown flat-topped papules, a few millimeters in diameter. Smooth surface compared with vegetative surface of other warts. Round, oval, polygonal, or linear in shape owing to induction by physical trauma. Found on face, hand, dorsal surfaces, and shins.

Plantar Warts. Occur at points of pressure (e.g., under toes, under metatarsal heads, or heel, areas where footwear presses chronically). Appear as flesh-colored punctate depressions, shiny papules, or crowded confluent plaques, or deep thick plaques. Most develop a thick hyperkeratotic covering early. Tenderness, sometimes marked, with pressure.

Genital Warts (Due to Human Papillomavirus). Skin-colored, pink or red pin-head papules or cauliflower-like excrescences. Soft and filiform or sessile. Occur as single or clustered lesions on penile frenulum, corona, glans, prepuce, meatus, or shaft or on scrotum or perianally in males; on labia, clitoris, or perineum, in vagina, and on perianal areas in females.

PATHOPHYSIOLOGY

Measles (Rubeola). The paramyxovirus enters the respiratory system and incubates for approximately 1 week; then acute infection is manifested as the respiratory prodrome. Koplik exanthem and skin exanthem demonstrate syncytial giant cells, dyskeratosis, spongiosis, and parakeratosis.

Roseola (Exanthem Subitum). Simple viral pathology.

Erythema Infectiosum (Fifth Disease). Respiratory tract is invaded by single-stranded DNA parvovirus after contact with infected person.

Rubella (German Measles). Papillomorbilliform body eruption involving the trunk initially, caused by infection with rubella virus. White blood cell (lymphocytes) infiltrates (inflammation) in the skin layers.

Molluscum Contagiosum. Poxvirus DNA invades the epidermal cells, interacts, and transforms into papular enclosed cores or molluscum bodies, which are globules of viral protein and transformed epithelial cells.

Warts (Verrucae). Mucosa or cutaneous epithelium becomes infected with human papillomavirus (HPV), a double-stranded-DNA papovavirus. Acquired by direct contact with infected person or possibly from sloughed, infected epidermal cells. As name implies, humans are the only reservoir of HPV. Inoculation is through open skin, and infection spreads in part by autoinoculation. Infection is somewhat dependent on cell-mediated immunity and susceptibility of host. Incubation and latency periods are unknown but, with condyloma, studies suggest a 3-month average. Approximately 60 HPV types have been identified.

DIAGNOSTIC STUDIES

Laboratory

Measles (Rubeola)

Clinical presentation is generally sufficient for diagnosis. Koplik spots are pathognomonic.

Acute and Convalescent Serum.   Hemagglutination antibodies rise fourfold.
Complete Blood Count.   Leukopenia and lymphopenia common.

Erythema Infectiosum (Fifth Disease)
The red cheek pattern with lacy arm-leg rash is an easy diagnosis.
IgM or IgG Assay for Detection of Parvovirus.   Is available at selected laboratories, but rarely required.

Rubella (German Measles)
Hemagglutination-Inhibition.   Fourfold rise in IgG to rubella titer is diagnostic. Acute infection evident if rubella-specific IgM is positive.
Molluscum Contagiosum.   Not applicable.
Roseola (Exanthem Subitum).   Not applicable.
Warts (Verrucae).   Usually easy to diagnose by clinical presentation. Southern blot hybridization analysis is definitive test for DNA virus and HPV typing. Rarely required.

Radiology

Measles
Chest Film.   May reveal pneumonia.

Other

Molluscum Contagiosum
Microscopy.   Excision of a molluscum body "pearl" is performed. Examination of its contents will show viral protein and epithelial cells.
Shave Biopsy.   Diagnostic and curative.

Warts (Verrucae)
Microscopy.   Pare the hyperkeratotic surface and view.
Biopsy.   Identifies verrucae, but not HPV.

DIFFERENTIAL DIAGNOSIS

Traumatic
Roseola (Exanthem Subitum).   In *heat rash*, no fever prodrome, and wider areas of distribution.
Erythema Infectiosum (Fifth Disease).   In *child abuse (slapping)*, child will not have extremity-body lacy rash.
Warts (Verrucae).   Not applicable, except it may lead to Koebner's phenomenon.

Infectious
Measles (Rubeola).   *Other exanthems* do not show Koplik spots and morbilliform rash.
Roseola (Exanthem Subitum).   *Other exanthems* do not typically follow 3 to 5 days of fevers and limited rash areas.

Rubella (German Measles). With *other exanthems,* rashes vary enough, as does pattern of spread. IgG- and IgM-specific antibodies confirm suspicions.

Molluscum Contagiosum. In *folliculitis-furunculosis,* no umbilications or viral molluscum core. More often tender.

Warts (Verrucae). *Condylomata lata* tend to be flat and not papillomatous but vegetative in appearance. Also are darkfield- and RPR assay–positive if due to *secondary syphilis.* Patients with condylomata acuminata may need RPR assay.

Metabolic
Not applicable.

Neoplastic

Molluscum Contagiosum
Basal cell carcinoma is hard on palpation, with telangiectasias and rolled borders, but not typical umbilication.

Keratoacanthoma has a firm keratin central plug and is larger than most molluscum lesions. No molluscum bodies.

Warts (Verrucae). *Bowenoid papulosis* shows red or hyperpigmented small papules, sometimes tiny with flat tops. Isolated lesion to many on genitalia. Histologic features of squamous cell carcinoma in situ, although behaves as a benign lesion. Caused by HPV 16. Associated with cervical neoplasia in infected patients and sexual contacts.

Vascular
Not applicable.

Congenital
Warts (Verrucae). *Epidermodysplasia verruciformis* is a rare, autosomal recessive condition, in which persons are predisposed to many HPV-type infections. These begin in childhood with patches of lesions on the trunk and arms. Thirty percent will develop squamous cell carcinoma, usually in sun-exposed areas, with tumors arising in third decade of life.

Acquired
Roseola (Exanthem Subitum). In *reactive allergic rash,* generally some pruritus and more prominent rash.

Erythema Infectiosum (Fifth Disease). *Lupus* is rare in children and will not show extremity rash. Will not spontaneously resolve in days to weeks.

Warts (Verrucae). *Calluses* will have no black-dot capillaries after paring. No underlying discrete lesion. Skin lines not usually disrupted throughout thickness.

TREATMENT

Measles (Rubeola). Nonspecific. Supportive care. Treat secondary infection as outlined in Bacterial Infection. Protect exposed patients 1 year of age and under with immune serum globulin. Susceptible persons should receive live measles vaccine.

Roseola (Exanthem Subitum). None, symptomatic for fever. Reassurance.

Erythema Infectiosum (Fifth Disease). None.

Rubella (German Measles). None, but vaccination provides effective protection. Upper respiratory infection–like prodrome is treated symptomatically.

Molluscum Contagiosum. Cure is dependent on removal, mechanical destruction, or chemical drying out of the infected epithelial cells in the lesion and molluscum body. *Adults* may be treated with curettage removal, cryotherapy (with liquid nitrogen), trichloracetic acid (50% to 80% concentrate applied; avoid contact with uninvolved skin), and taping or application of salicylic acid preparations (e.g., Duofilm,Occlusal). In *children*, cryosurgical liquid nitrogen (painful), salicylic acid preparations (e.g., Duofilm, Transversal, Transplantar patches, Occlusal), cantharidin (with caution, as major blistering can occur), excision, electrocautery, or laser surgery (likely to scar and is more costly, so best avoided for this viral infection) can be used.

Warts (Verrucae). No reliable cure. Treatment is generally aimed at destruction, but with modalities designed to minimize morbidity and scarring, as many recur or new ones erupt. Try not to cause nail deformity in periungual wart treatment, and avoid plantar scars, which can be painful to walk on for a lifetime. This conservative approach is especially important because many warts will resolve in up to 2 years.

   Liquid nitrogen cryosurgery is the most widely used for single or few lesions, but is painful.

   Topical salicylic acid, in acrylic vehicle (Occlusal) or in plasters (Mediplast) or gel patch (Transversal-Transplantar), may be effective alone or in combination with lactic acid (as in Duofilm) and is painless.

   Formalin may help eradicate plantar and flat warts, can be used on facial lesions, and is mostly painless.

   Bleomycin and alpha-interferon injected intralesionally are effective. Painful necrosis may develop with bleomycin.

   Tretinoin applied daily can help flat warts.

   Systemic retinoids may help in immunosuppressed patients with infection and those with epidermodysplasia verruciformis.

   Immunotherapy, after sensitization to dinitrochlorobenzene, can be successful in creating an allergic reaction in the wart area, which may lead it to resolve. Some concern for mutagenicity.

   Podophyllin 20% to 25% applied weekly and 50% or stronger trichloroacetic acid are effective in treatment of genital warts.

   Electrosurgery, excision, laser destruction are used as a last resort for warts and for large, widespread condylomata.

   Hypnosis and "charming" have shown positive effect on warts.

   Blenderm tape or duct tape can be applied to each lesion overnight to soften, which is abraded the next day with a pad-like substance or "Buf Puf."

   Laser ablation is very effective if warts do not resolve with medical therapy.

PEDIATRIC CONSIDERATIONS

Never use aspirin as an antipyretic.

Erythema Infectiosum (Fifth Disease). Once the rash has appeared, the patient is probably no longer contagious and can attend school.

Viral Exanthems. In the pediatric age group, numerous viral infections exist that are associated with dermatologic manifestations. A variety of different patterns are seen in these viral exanthems including a generalized maculopapular eruption that mimics measles (morbilliform), petechial eruptions, vesiculobullous eruptions, scarlet fever–like eruptions (scarlatiniform), and oral eruptions. These disorders include measles, rubella, erythema infectiosum, roseola infantum, varicella, and many others. A more complete discussion is beyond the scope of this work, and the reader is referred to textbooks on pediatric infectious diseases for further information.

Molluscum Contagiosum. A common cutaneous viral infection acquired by direct contact with an infected person or contaminated fomites. Removal of the papule with a dermal curet is curative but painful and frightening to infants and children. Careful application of cantharidin to the central umbilication is less traumatic and usually successful. Recurrences are common.

Warts (Verrucae). Children and adolescents have the highest incidence of all types of warts. Condylomata acuminata can be transmitted with or without sexual contact. However, in prepubertal children, be suspicious of sexual abuse.

OBSTETRIC CONSIDERATIONS

Measles (Rubeola). Isolate infected patients from pregnant or other hospitalized patients.

Erythema Infectiosum (Fifth Disease). Can cause hydrops fetalis if pregnant woman is infected.

Warts (Verrucae). Systemic treatments are not appropriate in pregnancy.

Rubella (German Measles). Congenital rubella infection is a devastating disease that can occur in infants born to mothers infected in the first trimester of pregnancy. The infection causes congenital malformations of the ophthalmologic, cardiac, and neurologic systems as well as tissue inflammation and damage, intrauterine growth retardation, and increased possibility of spontaneous abortion. Often, therapeutic abortion is recommended in the early stages of pregnancy if there has been maternal rubella infection in the first trimester. It is unclear if passive immunization of the woman at the time of infection helps to modify the congenital sequelae. Rubella vaccination with live attenuated virus is contraindicated in pregnant women.

GERIATRIC CONSIDERATIONS

No specific indications.

PREVENTIVE CONSIDERATIONS

Measles, mumps, and rubella are now rare because of immunizations. Condylomata acuminata can be transmitted sexually, so barrier protection is recommmended.

PEARLS FOR THE PA

Measles (Rubeola)

Upper respiratory infection precedes a red papular rash. Koplik spots are pathognomonic.

Roseola (Exanthem Subitum)

High fever is followed by a rash, diffuse on the head and neck, that fades in 3 days.

Erythema Infectiosum (Fifth Disease)

Self-limited condition manifested by bright red cheeks. Arthritis is a common adult complaint.

Rubella (German Measles)

Prodrome of lymph node enlargement of the postauricular, posterior cervical, and other nodes, followed by a rash on the face that spreads downward.

Molluscum Contagiosum

A poxvirus group DNA virus infection of the epithelium. Transmitted by sexual contact and autoinoculation and affected by immunologic factors.

Warts (Verrucae)

Many warts will resolve in approximately 2 years.

Further Reading

Dunihoo DR: Fundamentals of Gynecology and Obstetrics, 2nd ed. JB Lippincott, Philadelphia, 1992.

Thompson LW, Brinckerhoff L, Slingluff CL: Vaccination for melanoma patients. Curr Oncol Rep 2:292, 2000.

Saenz-Badillos J, Brady MS: Pregnancy-associated melanoma occurring in two generations. J Surg Oncol 73:231, 2000.

Murphy JL: Physician Assistant Prescribing Reference: Available at http://www.prescribingreference.com

Morris CM: What is the risk of herpes zoster following varicella immunization? Available at http://www.medscape.com/Medscape/PhysicianAsst/AskExperts/2001/10 @Refs:Sams WM, Lynch PJ: Principles and Practice of Dermatology, 2nd ed. New York, Churchill Livingstone, 1996.

Frankel DH: Field Guide to Clinical Dermatology. Philadelphia, Lippincott, Williams & Wilkins, 1999.

Anderson PC, Malaker KS: Managing Skin Diseases. Baltimore, Williams & Wilkins, 1999.

Arndt KA, Wintroub BU, Robinson JK, LeBoit PE: Primary Care Dermatology. Philadelphia, WB Saunders, 1997.

Epstein E: Common Skin Disorders. Philadelphia, WB Saunders, 2001.

Baltrani VS: Clinical features of atopic dermatitis. Immunol Allergy Clin North Am 1:22, 2002.

Kristal L, Klein PA: Atopic dermatitis in infants and children. Pediatr Clin North Am 4:47, 2000.

Elewski BE: Tinea capitis: A current perspective. J Am Acad Dermatol 1:42, 2000.

Lesher JL: Oral therapy of common superficial fungal infections of the skin. J Am Acad Dermatol 6:40, 1999.

EMERGENCY MEDICINE

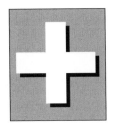

3

Burns

James B. Labus, PA-C

DEFINITION

Burn: A disruption in the normal integrity and biologic function of the skin from a thermal source, noxious chemicals, electrical current, or radiation.

HISTORY

Symptoms. The patient presentation varies depending on the etiology of the burn injury (i.e., thermal, electrical, chemical, or radiation), the depth of the injury (superficial, deep, or full-thickness), and the presence or absence of an inhalation injury.

General
Obtain a detailed history of the injury including type of burn, conditions of exposure, physical environment, associated injury, and medical history.

Thermal Injuries. Thermal injury is the classic burn injury from flame, steam, or scalds from hot liquids. Scald injuries often show a "high water mark," with a pattern of injury consistent with the history. Inhalation is more common with fires occurring in a closed space and with associated injury or intoxication that decreases level of consciousness.

The presence of an inhalation injury is one of the leading mediators of mortality and morbidity in thermal trauma. Direct thermal injury of the airway rarely occurs below the vocal cords because of the capacity of the upper airway to cool inspired air. Direct burn injury above the vocal cords causes edema that can lead to total airway occlusion if left untreated.

If a thermal injury occurs inferior to the vocal cords, the cause is steam inhalation. Smoke inhalation is the inspiration of the products of combustion and can be thought of as injury to the lung. Carbon monoxide (CO) poisoning is a classic associated injury in this setting, as CO displaces oxygen from the hemoglobin molecule. Symptoms of CO intoxication are those of alterations in mental status due to hypoxemia. Signs that may indicate that a patient may have suffered smoke inhalation include burns from fires occurring in an enclosed space, burns about the face, and carbonaceous sputum. The other chemical associated with asphyxiation is hydrogen cyanide. Hydrogen cyanide is formed with the burning of polymers (i.e., some plastics).

Chemical Burns. Chemical burns occur following alkali or acid exposure, with the degree of tissue damage determined by the concentration of the offending agent and the length of exposure. Often seen in occupational and agricultural exposures as well as with domestic violence.

Chemical burns typically affect exposed areas of the body (face, eyes, extremities). The average burn size is usually small, and mortality rate is lower than for other burn types. However, wounds may take longer to heal.

The initial injury may appear to be mild, but more significant findings may appear over time. Systemic effects of the chemical are also possible.

Electrical Injuries. In many cases the most difficult type of burn injury to initially treat. Cardiac disturbances are commonly associated with the initial injury. There is often occult tissue damage between the entry and exit wounds, which makes underestimation of the size of the injury a common (and sometimes) fatal mistake. Accumulations of hemoglobin and myoglobin in the kidney can lead to acute renal failure unless vigorous volume resuscitation is instituted. Associated multisystem injuries are often present and should be vigorously sought during the initial evaluation. Exposures to voltage of 600 volts or more are considered high-voltage injuries.

Radiation Injuries. Radiation injury is seen most commonly in the setting of solar radiation exposure (sunburn) and with use of external beam radiation in the treatment of neoplasms. Sunburns should not be trivialized, especially if more than 20% of the body surface area (BSA) is involved.

Age. Overall, burns occur with the greatest incidence in childhood up to the fourth decade of life. Young children and the elderly suffer more scald-type burns. Electrical burns occur in young children, adolescents, and persons who work with electricity.

Mortality is greater in the elderly. Persons considered to be at high risk for burns are children younger than 10 years of age, adults older than 50, and those with underlying medical conditions.

Onset. Acute to subacute.

Duration. Skin integrity may worsen in the hours to days following injury with thermal, chemical, or radiation injuries. Electrical burns may result in delayed tissue breakdown.

Intensity. Mild with superficial wounds to severe and life-threatening with full-thickness wounds.

Aggravating Factors. Continued exposure to the noxious agent or to the heat source. Failure to remove clothing, jewelry, or other materials/objects that may retain heat.

Alleviating Factors. Prompt treatment; removal of the noxious agent; analgesics.

Associated Factors. Multisystem trauma, substance abuse, and child abuse all must be suspected. Upper airway or pulmonary injury is a possibility if the burn occurred in a smoke-filled environment. Occult injuries.

PHYSICAL EXAMINATION

General. All burn-injured patients should be monitored for level of consciousness. Any alteration in mental status may indicate hypovolemia, severe inhalation injury, head trauma, intoxication, or other underlying medical conditions. Burn wounds do not bleed. If the patient is experiencing significant blood loss, search for associated underlying injuries. In cases of electrical burn, examine for both entry and exit wounds. The exit wound should be near where the patient was in contact with a conductive surface.

Burns are categorized according to depth of tissue penetration by the offending agent.

Partial-thickness/superficial burns/first degree burns: Injury is confined to the superficial elements of the dermis. Wound is red, moist, swollen, and painful. The usual course is spontaneous healing, usually in about 7 days.

Partial-thickness/deep/second degree burns: These injuries are divided into superficial partial-thickness (SPT) and deep partial-thickness (DPT) burns. In SPT burns, the epidermis and the superficial (papillary) layer of the dermis are affected. There is skin blistering but good perfusion of the dermis (intact capillary refill). Healing should occur in 2 to 3 weeks. In DPT burns, the burned area extends into the deep (reticular) layer of the dermis, damaging hair follicles and sweat and sebaceous glands. The skin may be blistered and appears yellow or white. Capillary refill and sensation are impaired. Healing (with scar formation) takes about 21 days to 2 months.

Full-thickness/third degree burns: These injuries are characterized by cellular injury that involves the entire epidermis and dermis. Wound is pearly white or black and charred. Small coagulated blood vessels may be visible through the surface of the wound. Injury site is painless to pinprick/touch. These wounds have lost the capacity to regenerate skin tissue, and skin grafting will be needed for final wound closure.

Burns that extend through the skin into deep tissues (subcutaneous tissue, muscle, and bone): These injuries are life-threatening. Amputation of the affected area or extensive reconstructive surgery is required. These are sometimes referred to as fourth degree burns.

Evaluate the extent of BSA involved by applying the "Rule of Nines" (see Fig. 3-1 for adult chart and Fig. 3-2 for pediatric chart). All body parts of the adult are assigned a percentage of total circumferential BSA based on multiples of nine. For smaller burns, use the patient's hand size as 1% to calculate the area of the burn.

Cardiovascular. Cardiovascular collapse may occur as a result of hypovolemia secondary to translocation of plasma volume from the intravascular to the extravascular spaces.

Extremities. Evaluate the adequacy of distal neurovascular status. Continue regular monitoring of distal pulses. With full-thickness circumferential injuries to the limbs, monitor for evidence of compartment syndromes, which can develop secondary to swelling beneath the surface of the wound. Remove all clothing and jewelry from the extremities. Continue to evaluate the extremities for delayed thrombus formation, especially with electrical injuries.

Gastrointestinal. Paralytic ileus and gastric dilatation may be present in patients with large burns.

Neurologic. Note initial mental status and any focal neurologic abnormality that may be due to associated injury. Neurovascular status distal to the burn should be evaluated; this aspect of management is especially important in electrical injury.

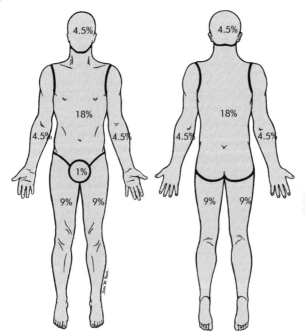

Figure 3–1. Rule of nines: Adult. Calculating the extent of body surface area (BSA) involved by the burn. (From Hockenberry M, Wilson D, Winkelstein ML, Kline, NE. Wong's Nursing Care of Infants and Children, 7th ed. St. Louis, Mosby, 2003, p 1228.)

Pulmonary.   On the initial survey, the airway patency and respiratory competence must be evaluated. The patient may require intubation. Perform a thorough pulmonary examination, especially in cases in which inhalation injury is suspected. Indications for inhalation include carbonaceous sputum production and expiratory wheezing. Bronchoscopy may be indicated.

Skin
Thermal Burns.   With flame burns, carbonaceous debris is usually present, and the burn lesions will be somewhat irregular in both shape and distribution of the body parts affected.

Chemical Burns.   The degree of tissue damage is determined by the concentration of the offending agent and the duration of exposure.

Electrical Burns.   Characterized by a usually small entry wound and one or more separate exit wounds. A "blowout" effect may be seen, in which the burn lesion is surrounded by a flash burn, as a small flash is often given off as the electrical current exits the body.

Radiation Burns.   Erythema affecting the exposed areas of skin.

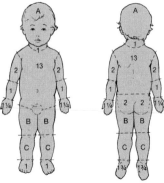

RELATIVE PERCENTAGES OF AREAS AFFECTED BY GROWTH

AREA	BIRTH	AGE 1 YR	AGE 5 YR
A = ½ of head	9½	8½	6½
B = ½ of one thigh	2¾	3¼	4
C = ½ of one leg	2½	2½	2¾

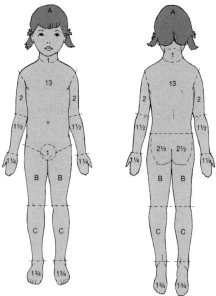

RELATIVE PERCENTAGES OF AREAS AFFECTED BY GROWTH

AREA	AGE 10 YR	AGE 15 YR
A = ½ of head	5½	4½
B = ½ of one thigh	4½	4½
C = ½ of one leg	3	3¼

Figure 3–2. Rule of nines: Pediatric. Calculating the extent of body surface area (BSA) involved by the burn. (From Thibodeau, GA, Patton, KT. Anatomy & Physiology, 4th ed. St. Louis, Mosby, 1999, p 176.)

PATHOPHYSIOLOGY

Burn Shock

One of the early causes of burn mortality is cardiovascular collapse due to hypovolemia. Burn shock is due to a loss of plasma volume from the intravascular to the extravascular spaces. At the time of the burn injury there is a loss of the normal integrity of the capillary beds. This capillary injury is maximal in the body part burned but occurs to a significant degree throughout the body. The capillary instability results in a loss of plasma volume from the intravascular spaces to the extravascular tissues, manifested by gradually increasing edema. The loss of intravascular volume can be profound; for example, with a 40% BSA burn, up to 75% of the total circulating plasma volume can be lost within the first 24 hours. The resulting hemoconcentration causes a cascade of pathophysiologic effects that can lead to cardiovascular collapse.

The skin is composed of a superficial epidermal layer and the deeper dermis. The skin has several functions: it prevents fluid loss, provides a barrier to the environment, maintains body temperature, allows for sensory perception, and serves as an excretory organ.

The skin is thicker in the palms of the hand and soles of the foot and on the upper part of the back. Skin thickness changes throughout life. Early and late in life, the skin is thinner. Damage to skin cells occurs at temperatures greater than 113° F (45° C).

Etiology-Associated Findings

Thermal Injury. Pulmonary injury from inhalation causes bronchospasm, obstruction, and atelectasis. Acute respiratory distress syndrome (ARDS) may result. These symptoms are due to damage of the endothelial cells, mucosal edema of the distal airways, and reduced surfactant activity.

Chemical Injury. May cause injury in addition to the primary burn. Thermal injury (from compounds that produce heat), allergic reaction, and systemic effects all can occur,

Electrical Injury. The passage of current through the body heats tissue. The effects of the heat are vascular spasm, neurologic injury, and muscle cell death. Disruption of the electrical activity of the heart is more common with electrical shock that traverses the body.

DIAGNOSTIC STUDIES

Laboratory

Complete Blood Count. Increased hematocrit due to hemoconcentration and loss of plasma volume. Normal to slightly increased white blood cell count in the acute phase.

Electrolytes. Increased potassium, especially in the setting of extensive cellular distribution in electrical injuries. Measure blood urea nitrogen (BUN)/creatinine levels to establish baseline values, and monitor regularly for renal status, especially in electrical injury.

Serum Myoglobin and Creatine Kinase (CK). Evaluate for muscle damage, especially with electrical burns.

Arterial Blood Gas Analysis. Normal to near-normal Po_2 does not exclude the presence of an inhalation injury or CO poisoning. Patients often will have a metabolic acidosis as burn shock progresses. Increased carboxyhemoglobin levels suggest inhalational injury.

CO Level. As indicated for inhalation injury.

Urinalysis. The presence of hemoglobin or myoglobin in the urine is indicative of lysis of red blood cells or severe muscular damage (especially noted in electrical injuries). Vigorous volume resuscitation must be instituted to clear these products from the renal system.

Toxicology Screen. Mandatory in all trauma patients.

Radiology

Chest Film. Often nondiagnostic initially in the presence of an inhalation injury.

Other Radiographs. Other radiologic studies may be indicated depending on the history of events surrounding the injury and the likelihood of associated injuries.

Other

Bronchoscopy. The only way to define the presence of an inhalation injury. The airway is inspected for the presence of carbonaceous material or swelling around the cords. If these findings are present, the patient should be intubated to prevent swelling that can lead to airway occlusion.

ECG. Imperative, especially in electrical injury to evaluate for arrhythmia. ECG monitoring should be used in any patient who has sustained a high-voltage injury, demonstrates cardiac signs and symptoms, or has experienced a loss of consciousness.

DIFFERENTIAL DIAGNOSIS

As burns are due to an acute, traumatic injury, the concept of differential diagnosis does not apply.

TREATMENT

Prehospital

It is imperative to establish the airway, initiate fluid resuscitation, and stop the burning process by removing the patient from the heat source and removing clothing or metal objects (e.g., jewelry, belt buckles) that may retain heat.

Consideration is given for pain relief; the burn wound is protected with a clean, dry sheet; and the patient is transported to the appropriate facility.

Airway

If the airway is found to have evidence of direct thermal injury, intubation is the only means by which to ensure that the airway will remain patent as edema formation progresses. Intubation is also indicated for significant facial or neck burns, respiratory distress, progressive hoarseness, or altered mental status. Burns to the neck and chest may lead progressively to restrictive respiratory compromise.

Ventilation
If high CO levels are found, the patient will require 100% humidified O_2.

Intravascular Volume Resuscitation
Large-bore peripheral intravenous lines inserted through nonburned areas, if possible, are necessary to deliver plasma volume resuscitation fluids. All burn-injured patients with skin involvement of greater than 20% BSA are at risk for significant plasma volume loss and require fluid resuscitation.

The timetable for fluid replacement begins from the time of the burn injury, not the time of arrival at the emergency department. The calculated hourly volume is used as a guide to fluid resuscitation, and the well-hydrated burn-injured patient should be voiding about 1 mL/kg/hour. A Foley catheter is inserted to assist with measurement of fluid output. Monitor for the development of pulmonary edema or ARDS due to inhalation injury or from large quantities of fluid administered.

Wound Care
In the acute phase the primary goal of wound care is to stop the burning process. The patient should be disrobed. Noxious materials should be lavaged from the surface of the burn wound. Protective isolation is helpful as long as it does not isolate the patient from necessary care. The application of topical antibiotics or dressings should be deferred until the patient has been stabilized, surveyed for associated injuries, and transferred for definitive wound care. The wound is wrapped with a moist, saline-soaked dressing. If the burn area is large, monitor for hypothermia.

Analgesia
All analgesics should be administered intravenously in small, frequent doses. Because of edema formation, intramuscular injections have uncertain absorption. Anxiolytic medication may be considered.

Antibiotics
Withhold intravenous antibiotics. Giving antibiotics initially will only help to select out resistant organisms.

Tetanus Prophylaxis
Tetanus prophylaxis should be given to all burn patients.

Escharotomy
If compartment syndromes are present, escharotomy is indicated. An incision is made on the medial and lateral aspects of the burned extremity, and can be extended out into each digit if necessary.

Gastric Decompression

Burn-injured patients are at risk for the development of stress ulcers, necessitating the use of gastric decompression through a nasogastric tube (on low intermittent suction) and the use of antacids.

Etiology-Associated Components of Treatment

Chemical Injury. The key principle of treatment is to stop the burning process. All liquid chemicals should be copiously lavaged from the surface of the burn wound with tap water. The application of neutralizing agents is mentioned only to be condemned. Powdered chemicals should be brushed off the patient before lavage is instituted.

Electrical Injury. It is imperative to prevent injury to rescuers by using safety measures at the scene of the injury. The power source should be turned off whenever possible. Suspect formation of rhabdomyolysis after electrical injury. Monitor myoglobin in the urine. Treat myoglobinuria with urinary alkalization: Add 44-50 mEq of sodium bicarbonate to each liter of intravenous fluid.

Radiation Injury. Radiation therapy injuries are usually fairly discrete and can be easily treated by a hiatus in exposure.

Sunburn. If more than 20% BSA is involved, plasma volume replacement may be appropriate, as would special wound care considerations.

PEDIATRIC CONSIDERATIONS

BSA calculations differ in infants and toddlers (see Fig. 3-2). Be aware of the possibility of child abuse or neglect. One indication may be burn injuries that are not consistent with the history offered by the parent. Burn injuries are more common in this age group, and the skin is thinner than in a healthy adult.

OBSTETRIC CONSIDERATIONS

Obstetric consultation and fetal monitoring are required. Spontaneous pregnancy termination is possible with large burns. The requirements for fluid replacement are greater than those typical in a nonpregnant patient. Initial management of burn-injured patients includes monitoring of respiratory and hemodynamic status. Management in a pregnant patient should be no different in regard to assessment and remediation of respiratory defects.

Electrical shock injuries are a special consideration, as amniotic fluid is an exceptionally efficient conductor of electricity. Pregnant patients should be closely observed with fetal monitoring or fetal heart tones. Obstetric consultation is mandatory.

GERIATRIC CONSIDERATIONS

Any patient older than 50 years of age and those with underlying medical problems are considered high-risk patients. The skin of a geriatric patient is thinner than that of a healthy adult.

PREVENTIVE CONSIDERATIONS

The following precautions are important in preventing burn injuries.

Gasoline and other flammable liquids should be kept away from heat sources.

Cigarettes/lighters and matches should be used safely (not in bed) and kept away from children.

Hot water heaters should be set at the lowest possible setting (<125° F recommended) to prevent scalds.

When involved in recreational activities such as camping, be aware of safety rules for fire and electricity and apply them. Have a means of communication in case of injury.

Household prevention of electrical injury includes capping unused sockets with plastic caps, inspecting extension cords, and unplugging cords and electrical devices when not in use. Restrict a child's access to small metal objects that can go into sockets. Ground fault interrupters can be installed in circuits that are in close proximity to household water sources.

Chemicals should be stored in appropriate containers and out of reach of children. Do not mix chemicals.

Use sunscreen when going outdoors. Limit exposure to the sun.

PEARLS FOR THE PA

Burn wounds do not bleed; if bleeding is present, look for associated injuries.

The condition of the upper airway cannot be determined by any means other than fiberoptic bronchoscopy.

Ice applied to the burn wound surface will only lead to hypothermia and further injury.

Give all analgesics intravenously.

Hyperthermia

James B. Labus, PA-C

DEFINITION

Heatstroke is a potentially fatal medical emergency that develops secondary to malfunctioning thermoregulatory mechanisms. *Heat exhaustion* is a milder form of hyperthermia and can occur prior to heatstroke. *Heatstroke is a medical emergency.*

Heat edema may occur in the first days after exposure to a new hot environment. Patients may present with mild swelling of the hands and feet.

Prickly heat is a rash that affects covered areas of the skin. It is caused by an acute inflammation of the sweat ducts. The rash is pruritic, erythematous, and maculopapular. The primary risk is secondary infection.

Heat sycope is a condition in which the patient may transiently lose consciousness as a result of postural hypotension. This phenomenon is due to the body's response to heat of peripheral vasodilatation accompanied by volume depletion.

Heat cramps are involuntary cramping of the muscles occurring during or after strenuous exercise. Usually affects the calf muscles. It is secondary to electrolyte loss and volume depletion.

HISTORY

Symptoms

Heatstroke. Temperature may be above 105° F (40.5° C). The presence of mental status changes (confusion, irritability, hallucinations, coma) is the primary factor differentiating between heatstroke and heat exhaustion. The patient may present with ataxia or seizure. Anhidrosis may be present but is not a consistent feature. Initial symptoms include headache, dizziness, nausea, vomiting, muscle cramps, concentrated urine.

Heat Exhaustion. Temperature can be normal to 104°F (40°C). Mental status is normal. The patient may complain of malaise, dizziness, headache, weakness, nausea, vomiting, myalgias, or muscle cramps.

General. Hyperthermia typically occurs on hot, humid days in susceptible persons. It can be divided into exertional and nonexertional types. Nonexertional hyperthermia occurs in persons with impaired thermoregulatory mechanisms (as in chronic illness, medication use, and the extremes of age—the elderly and infants). Exertional-type hyperthermia occurs in any age group and affects persons who may have intact homeostasis but perform significant physical activity, (usually) in hot and humid climates.

Age. Any, but more frequent in both the young and the elderly populations. Young, otherwise healthy athletes are at risk.

Onset. Rapidly progressive, within hours.

Duration. Hours.

Intensity. Initially mild; however, severe central nervous system symptoms rapidly develop. There is up to an 80% mortality rate with heatstroke.

Aggravating Factors. Hot, humid weather, physical exertion, chronic disease, medications, alcohol consumption, and obesity; dehydration.

Alleviating Factors. Hydration and cooling. Acclimatization to a new hot, humid environment over the course of about 1.5 weeks. Physical conditioning.

Associated Factors. Anhidrosis; diaphoresis may be seen in rapidly progressive heatstroke secondary to exertion.

PHYSICAL EXAMINATION

General.   With heat exhaustion, temperature may be normal. With heat-stroke, temperatures greater than 105°F (40.5°C), hypotension, tachycardia, and respiratory depression.

Cardiovascular.   May have sinus or supraventricular tachycardia, or peripheral vasodilatation.

Neurologic.   May have confusion, disorientation, generalized seizures, focal deficits, or coma.

Pulmonary.   Tachypnea progressing to bradypnea.

Skin.   Hot and dry. Diaphoresis may be present or absent.

PATHOPHYSIOLOGY

Any condition that increases internal heat generation or impairs thermoregulatory mechanisms can lead to heat-related illness.

The body's normal response to a hot environment is hypothalamic stimulation of the autonomic nervous system. This results in decreased vasomotor tone, increased blood flow to the skin (with an increased heart rate to maintain perfusion), and sweating. Medications or conditions that decrease heart rate, prevent peripheral vasodilatation, affect the hypothalamus, or increase metabolic rate can impair the normal cooling mechanism.

The body loses (or gains) heat through the following mechanisms:

Radiation: The body generates heat that is lost to the environment.

Convection: The loss of surrounding body heat to the air (or heat gain if temperature of the air is greater than body temperature).

Conduction: The shift of heat from a warm to a cooler surface, such as from the body to the ground, air, or water. Water is 25 times more conductive than air.

Evaporation: The conversion of a liquid (sweat) to a gas, resulting in heat loss. Humidity blocks evaporation, leading to heat retention. Likewise, dehydration will not allow for adequate sweat response.

DIAGNOSTIC STUDIES

Laboratory
Complete Blood Count with Differential
Elevated white blood cell count with infectious process.

Chemistry Profile.   Evaluate for evidence of volume depletion; potassium and magnesium levels are variable. Hypernatremia with low to absent fluid intake. Liver function may be abnormal with primary liver disease, causing the altered mental status. Blood urea nitrogen (BUN)/creatinine may be abnormal, with acute tubular necrosis and renal failure due to hyperthermia.

Prothrombin Time/Partial Thromboplastin Time/INR. Look for prolongation (patient with hyperthermia may develop disseminated intravascular coagulopathy).

Urinalysis. Rule out infection and rhabdomyolysis.

Blood Culture. Differentiate from infectious process.

Toxicology Screen. Rule out contributing factor of medication use/abuse.

Radiology

CT/MRI. Studies of the brain as needed to rule out primary neurologic cause of the mental status changes.

Chest Film. As a baseline and used to evaluate for primary pulmonary conditions contributing to the elevated temperature. Pulmonary edema is a potential complication of fluid rescuscitation.

Other

Lumbar Puncture. As needed to differentiate from infectious process.

ECG. May show tachycardia, ST segment or T wave changes, premature ventricular contractions, or arrhythmias.

DIFFERENTIAL DIAGNOSIS

Traumatic

Head injury can be differentiated by history. The injury, whether remote or acute, may involve the hypothalamus.

Infectious

Primary infection of any system may cause fever.

In *meningitis*, may see nuchal rigidity, Brudzinski and/or Kernig signs, leukocytosis with a shift, positive results on cerebrospinal fluid cultures.

In *sepsis*, positive results on blood cultures.

Metabolic

In *epilepsy*, history of generalized or focal seizure.

In *diabetic ketoacidosis*, history of diabetes; patient may have "fruity" odor of ketones on the breath, hyperventilation, mental status changes.

In *thyroid storm*, abnormal thyroid function studies.

Neoplastic

With *hypothalamic tumors*, positive CT study/MRI scan of brain.

Vascular

With *stroke*, history of transient or permanent neurologic deficit, positive CT study/MRI scan of brain.

Congenital

Not applicable.

Acquired

With *medication use/abuse* of phencyclidine, cocaine, amphetamines, anticholinergics, and salicylates; alcohol withdrawal.

TREATMENT

Heat Exhaustion

Immediately cool the patient by moving to shade, providing oral hydration, applying ice packs to the groin, axilla, and neck. Remove clothing as appropriate. Spray the patient with water to enhance cooling using evaporation. Volume and electrolyte replacement in the emergency department (ED) as needed.

Heatstroke

On the scene, rapid cooling measures as listed above should be employed. The patient should however, be kept on NPO status. Cooling should be continued during transport.

In the ED, the patient should be immersed in cool water. This technique is relatively contraindicated if the patient may require cardiac monitoring and/or defibrillation. During cooling, the extremities should be massaged to prevent vasoconstriction. Body temperature should be monitored and cooling discontinued when patient's temperature is lowered to 101° F (38.5° C).

Oxygen and intravenous fluid therapy (with normal saline or Ringer's lactate given at 250 mL/hour) should be started, cardiac monitoring instituted, a Foley catheter placed, and serial monitoring of core temperature (via rectal or esophageal probe or Foley catheter) performed. Consider central venous pressure catheter as needed.

Iced gastric lavage via nasogastric tube should be used only if the airway is protected.

Prior abdominal surgery is a relative contraindication to cooling using peritoneal lavage.

If all other measures fail at reducing temperature, cardiopulmonary bypass may be considered.

PEDIATRIC CONSIDERATIONS

The pediatric patient is more prone to hyperthermia because of increased intrinsic heat production and decreased ability to sweat. Malignant hyperthermia, inherited as an autosomal dominant trait, usually occurs initially in childhood. Clinical suspicion of malignant hyperthermia should be raised for children with fever of unknown etiology, muscle cramps, and increased creatine kinase values.

OBSTETRIC CONSIDERATIONS

Cooling using peritoneal lavage is relatively contraindicated.

GERIATRIC CONSIDERATIONS

Rapid fluid replacement may lead to pulmonary edema. The geriatric patient is more prone to hyperthermia because of impairment of thermoregulatory mechanisms. Cardiovascular, neurologic, and peripheral vascular disease and the use of multiple medications that modify these systems, as well as obesity, physical deconditioning, and reduced production of sweat, all contribute to the increased incidence of hyperthermia.

PREVENTIVE CONSIDERATIONS

The following precautions are recommended to prevent heat-related illness.
Climate conditions should be checked and appropriate provisions made, especially for persons engaging in strenuous work or exercise and those who are predisposed to hyperthermia.
Social services for chronically ill and elderly (e.g., access to air conditioning, fans) can reduce the burden of suffering during heat waves.
Workers, athletes, and military personnel should be given time for acclimatization prior to significant physical exertion.
Know the effects of medications required for primary medical conditions.
Hydration should be immediately available during work/activity in hot, humid weather conditions.

PEARLS FOR THE PA

History is the key to the diagnosis of hyperthermia.

Initiate treatment as soon as a diagnosis is suspected, as delay in cooling can lead to organ damage.

Hypothermia

James B. Labus, PA-C

DEFINITION

A disorder secondary to impaired intrinsic thermoregulatory capability or to exposure to frigid environments.
Mild hypothermia results when body temperatures are between 98.6° F (37° C) and 91.4° F (33° C); *moderate hypothermia*, when temperatures are

between 89.6° F (32° C) and 80.6° F (27° C); *severe hypothermia*, when temperatures are less than 78.8° F (26° C).

HISTORY

Symptoms. Presentation varies, with symptoms becoming more severe as hypothermia worsens. Patients initially present with shivering, peripheral vasoconstriction, and mild impairment of fine motor skills (e.g., dysarthria, ataxia), mild mental status changes, tachypnea, tachycardia, blood pressure elevation, nausea, and/or fatigue.

As hypothermia becomes moderate, shivering gives way to muscular rigidity; the patient is obtunded and may lose consciousness; hypotension, bradycardia, and low respiratory rate are present; pupils may be dilated; the patient may inappropriately undress; a metabolic acidosis may be noted; and there is an increased risk for dysrhythmia (especially ventricular fibrillation).

As hypotension becomes severe, the patient may appear to be deceased. In the comatose patient, cranial nerve responses (e.g., corneal/oculocephalic) and deep tendon reflexes may be absent; spontaneous movements are undetectable; pulmonary edema, apnea, acid-base abnormalities, severe hypotension, coagulopathy, and increasing bradycardia and dysrhythmias leading to asystole may be findings; and the risk of developing ventricular fibrillation is considerable.

General. Obtain a full medical history for contributing conditions such as hypothyroid, hypoadrenal, hypopituitary, or hypoglycemic states. Alcohol abuse, neurologic damage (hypothalamic), septicemia, significant skin disease or injury (barrier loss), and iatrogenic factors (cold fluid replacement) may also contribute to or cause hypothermia.

Age. Most common in the very young or old, especially in those patients with serious preexisting medical conditions.

Onset. The usual scenario is fairly rapid cooling in the setting of immersion or accidental exposure to a harsh environment. Chronic hypothermia can also develop, especially among the elderly in poor housing conditions.

Intensity. Ranges from mild symptomatology to coma and death.

Aggravating Factors. Consumption of intoxicants, chronic coexisting illnesses.

Alleviating Factors. Dry clothing, isometric exercises, warm liquids.

Associated Factors. None.

PHYSICAL EXAMINATION

General. Obtain core body temperature using an esophageal thermometer or high rectal probe. Check to make sure that the thermometer will measure very cold temperatures.

Observe the patient for shivering. Obtain vital signs to evaluate for cold-related hypertension, respiratory depression, and tachy-/bradycardia and dysrhythmia.

Fully examine the patient for coexisting injuries.

Cardiovascular. Auscultate for dysrhythmia. Palpate for peripheral as well as central pulses (pulse may be very weak). Palpate for a minimum of 1 minute, as there may be extreme bradycardia.

Lungs. Auscultate for pulmonary edema.

Extremities. Examine for frostbite.

First degree: Redness (may have blue appearance), swelling, decreased sensation.

Second degree: Surface blistering with swelling.

Third degree: Full-thickness skin damage that may extend to muscle and/or bone. May have a black appearance.

Neurologic. Perform a mental status examination. When possible, assess fine motor skills. Assess speech for dysarthria. Gait examination may reveal ataxia. Although the patient may appear essentially brain dead, aggressive treatment is indicated.

Skin. Evaluate for bruising, as coagulopathies may be present.

PATHOPHYSIOLOGY

The body loses (or gains) heat through the following mechanisms:

Radiation: The body generates heat that is lost to the environment. Insulating clothing and a hat can prevent this type of heat loss.

Convection: The loss of surrounding body heat to the air. Cold, unblocked wind can be responsible for this type of heat loss.

Conduction: The shift of heat from a warm to a cooler surface such as from the body to the ground, air, or water. Water is 25 times more conductive than air, so it is imperative to stay dry.

Evaporation: The conversion of a liquid to a gas via the skin (sweat) or exhaled air, resulting in heat loss.

The response of the body to mild hypothermia is to produce and retain warmth (e.g., shivering, elevation of blood pressure). As hypothermia progresses, there is a slowdown of organ systems (e.g., slowed respirations, hypotension) that reduces the utilization of oxygen.

Cardiac output drops progressively as hypothermia worsens. Heart rate drops owing to slowed atrioventricular (AV) nodal conduction, and the risk of arrhythmias increases. As core temperature approaches 86° F, the myocardium becomes increasingly irritable, which can lead to life-threatening ventricular fibrillation. Blood pressure remains fairly stable owing to increased peripheral vascular resistance, unless the hypothermia is severe.

Decreasing core body temperature depresses renal blood flow and glomerular filtration. The term "cold diuresis" is used to describe the volume loss that may be seen in these patients.

There is a fluid shift from the intravascular space to the extravascular space. This shift can lead to embolus/thrombus formation. Also, platelets are inhibited at cold temperatures, causing an increased risk of bleeding.

If the patient has been taking liver-metabolized medication, the levels may accumulate during the period of hypothermia. Pancreatitis may also develop.

DIAGNOSTIC STUDIES

Laboratory
Complete Blood Count. Examine for the presence of hemoconcentration; elevated white blood cell count is an indicator of concurrent illness.

Serum Chemistry. Evaluate for blood urea nitrogen (BUN)/creatinine, sodium and potassium abnormalities associated with renal dysfunction. Glucose may be abnormal as a result of comorbid diabetes mellitus.

Arterial Blood Gas Analysis. Respiratory acidosis is frequently present owing to hypoventilation.

Thyroid Function, Serum Cortisol, Serum Calcium. Hypothyroidism, hypopituitarism, and adrenal insufficiency are metabolic conditions that alter thermoregulation and must be sought in the early workup.

Toxicology Screen. Ethanol and drug overdoses are common comorbid conditions.

Amylase/Lipase. May be elevated with pancreatitis.

Radiology
Chest Film. As indicated to rule out pulmonary edema or pneumonia.
CT/MRI of the Brain. If a hypothalamic cause is suspected.

Other
ECG. Continuous ECG monitoring is imperative, as myocardial irritability and dysrhythmias are commonly seen. Presence of Osborne waves (widened QRS complexes with a J point deflection) is a classic electrocardiographic finding.

DIFFERENTIAL DIAGNOSIS

Traumatic
With *spinal cord lesions*, history of traumatic event; progressive or obvious quadraparesis, paraparesis, or hemiparesis.

Infectious
In *sepsis*, positive blood cultures, presence of fever.

Metabolic
In *hypothyroidism*, abnormal thyroid function studies.

In *hypopituitarism*, pituitary neoplasm seen on CT/MRI, history of pituitary or skull base tumor, abnormal levels of prolactin, adrenocorticotropic hormone (ACTH), growth hormone, or thyroid-stimulating hormone.

In *adrenal insufficiency*, abnormal ACTH, emotional lability, hyponatremia.

In *uremia*, elevated BUN/creatinine; may have a history of acute or chronic renal failure.

In *hypoglycemia*, depressed serum glucose.

In *Wernicke's encephalopathy*, abnormal findings on neurologic examination. May have abnormal CT/MRI of brain.

Neoplastic
With *hypothalamic lesion*, abnormal CT/MRI of brain.

Vascular
With *intracranial vascular events*, acute onset, may have severe headache or focal neurologic findings; abnormal CT/MRI of brain.

Congenital
Not applicable.

Acquired
With *intoxication*, history of use/abuse. Positive toxicology screen.
 Hypothermia Following Major Surgery. History of recent general anesthesia.
 Hypothermia Following High-Volume Intravenous Resuscitation. History of such.

TREATMENT

Mild Hypothermia
Treatment strategies can take the form of passive or active rewarming. Passive rewarming is generally considered the safest modality.
 Remove all clothing and apply dry clothing, warm blankets, or forced warm air system.
 Give warmed intravenous fluid (98.6°F [37° C] to 105.8°F [41°C]) or oral fluid, but avoid caffeinated beverages.

Moderate Hypothermia
Rewarm the patient using the foregoing techniques, but insulate the patient from both above and below. Warm packs applied to the groin, axilla, and neck may be used.
 Handle the patient as gently as possible to avoid precipitating ventricular fibrillation. Keep the patient in a reclining position to prevent orthostatic blood pressure changes. Do NOT massage the extremities. Administer oxygen. If the patient is intubated, avoid overinflating the cuff with cold air, because the cuff will inflate further as the air in the cuff warms and may obstruct the endotracheal tube.
 Use normal saline for intravenous resuscitation. Do not use lactated Ringer's, as the cold liver cannot metabolize lactate.

Severe Hypothermia
Active rewarming may be implemented with profound hypothermia and/or cardiopulmonary arrest using warm gastric, colonic, mediastinal, or peritoneal lavage, heated oxygen administration, and hemodialysis
 For the patient in cardiopulmonary arrest, use cardiopulmonary resuscitation (CPR) with EXTREME caution, as CPR can prove fatal if ventricular fibrillation is initiated. Central and peripheral pulses may be weak and difficult to palpate.

If pulses are absent for at least 1 minute of palpation, consider CPR, as electromechanical dissociation can also occur.

Treat and correct underlying medical conditions, and consider thiamine supplementation if alcohol abuse is thought to be a contributing factor.

PEDIATRIC CONSIDERATIONS

No specific indications. If the hypothermia is due to cold water immersion, see "Near Drowning."

OBSTETRIC CONSIDERATIONS

No specific indications.

GERIATRIC CONSIDERATIONS

The geriatric patient is more prone to hypothermia because of increased likelihood of concurrent medical illness, use of medications, and impaired thermoregulatory mechanisms.

PREVENTIVE CONSIDERATIONS

The following precautions are recommended for the prevention of hypothermia.

PEARLS FOR THE PA

Survival following hypothermia is possible even in patients who show little signs of life on presentation. A patient is not dead until he or she is warm and dead.

Be aware of the possibility of underlying medical conditions, intoxication, or trauma as the root cause of the patient's hypothermia.

Observe the patient for possible hypotensive episodes once rewarming is under way. These episodes are thought to be due to increasing amounts of peripheral blood returning to the heart, overwhelming cardiac capacity.

Hypothermia can occur in ANY environment.

Climate conditions should be checked and appropriate provisions made.

Layer clothing if cold weather is likely.

Do not venture onto unknown frozen ponds or lakes.

Social services for chronically ill and elderly are important during cold weather periods.

Be prepared in ANY environment, as hypothermia can occur even in the summer (especially with immersion in water).

Near Drowning

James B. Labus, PA-C

DEFINITION

A disorder characterized by hypoxemia, with or without aspiration, following submersion in fresh or salt water.

HISTORY

Symptoms. Alteration in mental status, tachypnea, wheezing, cyanosis, hypothermia, laryngospasm.

General. Prolonged submersion in fresh or salt water is frequently associated with use of motor or recreational vehicles, boating, or shallow water diving accidents. Entry of water into the upper airway results in laryngospasm. From 10% to 20% of near-drowning episodes occur without direct aspiration, but the victim presents with hypoxemia secondary to persistent laryngospasm. In aspiration events, the extent of injury is dependent on the amount of water inhaled.

Age. Any, but primarily in the first or second decades. Incidence of 90,000 episodes/year, with a 5:1 male-to-female ratio. The elderly are also at increased risk.

Onset. Rapid.

Duration. Postimmersion symptoms may occur 24 to 48 hours after the event.

Intensity. Varies. Following rescue, the patient may be awake and alert, or may be comatose, with severe cardiopulmonary dysfunction.

Aggravating Factors. Coexistent multisystem trauma (e.g., spinal cord injury).

Alleviating Factors. Early intervention, correction of hypoxia.

Associated Factors. Often occurs in the setting of multisystem trauma. Cervical spine injuries may be present (e.g., in diving injuries). Substance abuse and child abuse are frequently encountered.

PHYSICAL EXAMINATION

General. Patient presentations range along a continuum from mild respiratory and cardiovascular abnormalities to cardiovascular arrest and coma. Core body temperature is recorded to evaluate for hypothermia. Observe for dyspnea, tachypnea, or use of accessory muscles of respiration.

Cardiovascular. The patient may experience cardiac arrest owing to prolonged hypoxemia.

Neurologic. Mental status changes (e.g., confusion, lethargy) due to hypoxemia or direct neurologic trauma (e.g., head or spinal cord injuries) may be noted. Definitive mental status evaluation should be performed after hypothermia is corrected. Cervical spine should be palpated for tenderness in diving injuries to evaluate for potential injury.

Pulmonary. Persistent laryngospasm is a common occurrence and must be ruled out by careful airway inspection in the immediate resuscitative period. Auscultation may reveal wheezing, rales, or rhonchi. Tachypnea and cyanosis are common. Symptoms consistent with pulmonary edema.

PATHOPHYSIOLOGY

Laryngospasm is due to entry of water into the upper airway. From 80% to 90% of near drowning episodes are associated with aspiration. The extent of pulmonary injury is dependent on the amount of water aspirated.

The immediate, life-threatening events after a near drowning episode are respiratory failure and ischemic neurologic injury. Underwater, involuntary breathing occurs at a point determined by the Po_2 or Pco_2. This involuntary breath leads to aspiration of water and subsequent emesis. If laryngospasm develops, the glottis closes and prevents aspiration. Both aspiration and laryngospasm lead to hypoxia.

Pulmonary exposure to both seawater and fresh water washes surfactant from the alveoli. This loss leads to atelectasis, ventilation-perfusion mismatch, and breakdown of the alveolar-capillary membrane.

Aspiration of material from the water such as bacteria, algae, sand, particulate matter, emesis, and chemical irritants can further injure the lungs.

Noncardiogenic pulmonary edema may occur from aspiration, surfactant loss, inflammatory contaminants, and cerebral hypoxia.

DIAGNOSTIC STUDIES

Laboratory

Complete Blood Count. Used as a baseline. Can indicate an infectious process early or late in the course.

Prothrombin Time/Partial Thromboplastin Time. Use as a baseline to note any coagulopathies.

Pulse Oximetry. An effective means to continuously monitor therapy.

Electrolytes.   Serum sodium and chloride usually show minor changes regardless of the salt content of the water aspirated.

Arterial Blood Gas Analysis.   A profound metabolic acidosis is common, as are hypoxia and hypercarbia. Serial arterial blood gases are utilized to assess the adequacy of airway and ventilatory support.

Toxicology Screen.   For ethanol and drugs. Frequently associated with near drowning episodes, especially those occurring in persons with altered neurologic function.

Radiology

Chest Film.   Appearance consistent with noncardiogenic pulmonary edema. May be normal initially.

Cervical Spine Radiographs.   Especially if the patient was diving, to rule out fracture.

Skeletal Survey.   Indicated if multiple trauma is suspected.

Abdominal Radiographs.   May show gastric dilatation.

Other

ECG.   May show supraventricular tachycardia due to hypoxia, acidosis, or cardiac arrest.

DIFFERENTIAL DIAGNOSIS

As near drowning is due to an acute, traumatic event, the concept of differential diagnosis does not apply.

TREATMENT

Rapid cautious rescue to prevent injury to or drowning of rescuers.

Spinal precautions should be undertaken, especially with diving incidents.

Cardiopulmonary resuscitation should begin immediately. Supplemental oxygen should be started in all patients. Transport all patients to the emergency department for evaluation.

Clues to the presence of a spinal injury include paradoxical respirations, flaccid limb(s), priapism, unexplained hypotension, and bradycardia.

Inspect the upper airway to rule out laryngospasm. Maintain an adequate airway, with intubation if necessary, especially if the signs of hypoxemia are present. Maintenance of the airway will reduce the likelihood of gastric dilatation or aspiration of gastric contents. Intubated patients should be placed on an FIO_2 of 100%.

Positive end-expiratory pressure ventilation may be required to ensure adequate gas exchange.

Nasogastric tube (on low intermittent suction) may be placed to decompress gastric dilatation and to prevent aspiration of gastric contents.

A Foley catheter is placed to guide fluid management.

Monitor oxygen saturation, acid-base status, and volume status.

Treat associated/underlying injuries, hypovolemia, hypothermia, hypoglycemia.

Central venous catheters should not be used because of the risk of ventricular fibrillation.

Cardiac monitoring and appropriate cardiac support are indicated, in accordance with the Advanced Cardiac Life Support guidelines.

Hypothermia can occur with even brief periods of immersion. It is treated with warmed intravenous solutions and oxygen. Core body temperature must be monitored.

Prophylactic use of antibiotics or corticosteroids is not indicated.

Disposition

If there is no evidence of significant submersion, consider discharge of the patient.

If the patient is asymptomatic or has mild symptoms after a significant near drowning episode, observe for several hours for development of symptoms.

If the patient has mild to moderate hypoxia that can be corrected by oxygen therapy, hospital admission is indicated until hypoxia resolves and there are no complications.

In patients who require intubation and mechanical ventilation, the prognosis generally depends more on the neurologic status than on the direct pulmonary injury. However, serious aspiration pneumonia or progressive, irreversible lung injury can also occur.

PEDIATRIC CONSIDERATIONS

A majority of infant drownings occur in the bathtub.

In children, 40% to 90% of drownings occur in swimming pools, 75% of which occur during supervision.

The diving reflex, manifested by slowed heart rate and shunting of blood preferentially to the brain and heart in response to cold water submersion, is more prominent in the young patient.

Patient survival has been documented with submersions of up to 40 minutes.

Resuscitative measures should be aggressively attempted despite an initially bleak presentation.

OBSTETRIC CONSIDERATIONS

No specific indications.

GERIATRIC CONSIDERATIONS

The potential for falls in and around water should be appreciated, and appropriate measures taken to prevent falls. Providing nonslip surfaces in bathtubs is a consideration.

PREVENTIVE CONSIDERATIONS

Alcohol and drugs are associated with 25% to 60% of drownings. Personal flotation devices (PFDs) were not used in about 75% of drownings associated with boating.

Swimming lessons, boating safety classes, water safety lessons, wearing PFDs in or around water, discouraging alcohol and drug use, installing childproof fencing around pools, wearing wetsuits to prevent hypothermia when in the water, and proficiency in basic cardiac life support all are important considerations to prevent drowning.

PEARLS FOR THE PA

In cases of near drowning, a high index of suspicion needs to be maintained for multisystem trauma or substance abuse.

Hypothermia and near drowning are closely related, and hypothermia needs to be recognized and immediately treated.

Rule out persistent laryngospasm in the early resuscitative period.

Poisoning

James B. Labus, PA-C

DEFINITION

The ingestion of a noxious substance in such volume as to result in interference with normal biologic function.

HISTORY

Symptoms. Depending on the offending agent, symptoms may involve any organ system. Nausea, vomiting, diarrhea, headache, dizziness, blurred vision, stupor, paresthesias, seizures, respiratory distress, diaphoresis, anhidrosis, and rash are common.

General. Routes of administration include inhaled, ingested, absorbed via the skin or mucous membrane, and injected. Exposure can occur in the workplace or home, during recreation, or with prescribed medications.

Though often difficult, it is important to identify the substance involved. Question the patient, family, or friends about access to potential poisons. Have someone (police, fire, or rescue personnel or social worker or family member) search the scene for empty drug or alcohol containers. It is essential to know as accurately as possible the quantity of the ingestant and the time of the ingestion.

Age. Approximately 50% of poisonings involve children younger than 5 years of age; 5% involve children 6 to 12 years; 5% involve teenagers; and 40% involve adults.

Onset. Depends on substance.

Duration. Depends on substance.

Intensity. Depends on substance.

Aggravating Factors. Intentional poisoning is associated with higher morbidity rates than those for accidental poisoning. Preexisting health problems (e.g., those affecting the liver and kidneys) can interfere with the elimination rate of the poison and the toxic effects.

Alleviating Factors. Early intervention.

Associated Factors. Mental illness, traumatic injury with altered mental status.

PHYSICAL EXAMINATION

General. Undress and inspect the patient. Fully examine the patient, as findings may vary greatly with different poisons/medications. Observe for cyanosis, flushing, excessive diaphoresis, signs of associated injury, marks suggesting repeated injections, bruising (coagulopathy). Check the patient's clothing and person for any hidden medications, but use caution for hidden needles.

Abdomen. Auscultate for hypoactive/hyperactive bowel sounds; palpate for tenderness. Distended bladder suggests urinary retention.

Extremities. Check for tremor or fasciculations.

Heart. Auscultate for tachy/bradycardia, arrhythmia.

Head, Eyes, Ears, Nose, Throat. Examine the pupils for reactivity; assess extraocular movements for nystagmus, Examine the oropharynx for hypersalivation or dryness

Lungs. Auscultate and percuss for pulmonary edema, pneumonia, respiratory depression.

Neurologic. Note the level of consciousness. Examine the cranial nerves; test coordination and cerebellar function; evaluate muscle tone, cognition, and ability to ambulate.

PATHOPHYSIOLOGY

Depending on drug, the normal physiologic mechanisms of any organ can be disrupted.

DIAGNOSTIC STUDIES

Laboratory
Toxicology Screens. On gastric fluid, serum, and urine to identify the substance.
Electrolytes. Evaluate for abnormality.
Liver Function Tests. Assess baseline function and evaluate for likely degree of damage.
Arterial Blood Gas Analysis. Assess adequacy of ventilation.

Radiology. Not applicable.
Other. Not applicable.

DIFFERENTIAL DIAGNOSIS

Traumatic
Head injury can be differentiated by history and CT/MRI of the brain.

Infectious
In *meningitis*, may see nuchal rigidity, Brudzinski and/or Kernig signs, leukocytosis with a left shift, positive cerebrospinal fluid.

In *gastrointestinal infections*, no history of toxic ingestion; negative toxicology screen.

Metabolic
In *epilepsy*, history of seizure; negative toxicology screen.

In *schizophrenia*, at-risk patient; negative toxicology screen.

In *depression, mania*, at-risk patient; negative toxicology screen.
Neoplastic. Not applicable.
Vascular. Not applicable.
Congenital. Not applicable.

Acquired
In *depression*, patient may have a history, may be seeking help. Do not discount the possibility of intentional overdose.

TREATMENT

Immediately support cardiovascular and respiratory systems.

Whenever possible, have course directed by the regional poison control center.

For the patient who arrives in the emergency department unresponsive and with an unknown history, consider beginning oxygen, naloxone, 50% dextrose in water, 100 mg thiamine (in adults).

It is important to rid the patient of the poison. Mechanisms to remove the poison are:

Brush or wash external chemicals. Remove clothing that contains the chemical.

Induce vomiting for ingested poisons as appropriate. Vomiting can be induced using ipecac at a dose of 15 mL for children and 30 mL for adults. If the patient does not vomit after 30 minutes, the dose may be repeated.

Another, more invasive measure is orogastric lavage.

Bind the poison in the gut lumen. Binding of poison can be done using activated charcoal. This method is used when vomiting is contraindicated. A cathartic such as magnesium citrate may be administered with the charcoal to increase passage. Bowel irrigation can also be considered using polyethylene glycol by mouth or via nasogastric tube.

Enhance elimination from the body. If a substance is injected or cannot be bound in the stomach or intestines, it must be neutralized or elimination must be enhanced. When appropriate, the urine can be alkalized using intravenous sodium bicarbonate. It is imperative to monitor potassium levels while using this technique.

Hemodialysis may be necessary if a poison is rapidly absorbed by the intestine or is injected. It is used for rapid elimination in select cases.

See Appendix "Symptoms and Treatment of Specific Poisons" for management of overdose with specific drugs.

PEDIATRIC CONSIDERATIONS

Children may have different tolerances and reactions to various medications. Treatment should be withheld pending consultation with the regional poison control center (PCC). Prevention is the key to management, as children are more at risk for accidental poisoning.

OBSTETRIC CONSIDERATIONS

Initial management of poisoning should remain the same as in the non-pregnant patient. Naloxone (Narcan) has been proved to be safe and effective in the management of narcotic overdoses in the pregnant patient. Elevated alcohol intake ("alcohol poisoning") throughout a pregnancy can lead to fetal alcohol syndrome. This usually affects children born to mothers who drink more than six alcoholic beverages per day during the first trimester.

Cocaine use in a pregnant woman, particularly in large amounts, can cause sudden fetal death, premature delivery, small for gestational age infant, asymmetrical fetal growth, mental retardation, premature rupture of membranes, and many other organ and organ system defects.

The following chemical compounds have been implicated as having profound effects on fetal well-being. Organic mercury compounds can cross the placenta. The fetus then may develop congenital cerebral palsy, mental retardation, and other defects secondary to mercury concentration in the fetal central nervous system. Lead has also been found to cause growth retardation and central nervous system abnormalities in the fetus as well as increased chance of spontaneous abortion and stillbirth. Ethylene oxide, formaldehyde, methylene chloride, and CO may pose potential reproductive hazards.

GERIATRIC CONSIDERATIONS

The elderly patient is at risk for multiple medical problems that require multiple medications. Close attention to drug interactions is imperative. Poisons should be kept in well-marked, appropriate containers, separate from medications and food.

PREVENTIVE CONSIDERATIONS

The following precautions are recommended for the prevention of poisonings.

The poison control center telephone number should be immediately available at all phones.

Teach children about the dangers of poisons and to stay away.

Supervise children.

Avoid drug interactions by noting and researching other medications a patient may be taking. Check and balance systems are available in many pharmacies.

Patient identification should be checked prior to giving any medication.

Use labels on medications, and drug information sheets should be provided to the patient.

Store poisons in proper containers/places. Do not use food containers for poisons.

Light should be turned on when giving or taking medication to avoid potential mix-up.

Do not call medication "candy," as it may confuse children. It is best not to take medication in front of children.

Protective clothing should be used at home and at work as directed.

Do not mix products, to avoid creating untoward reactions.

Do not burn fuels or charcoal or operate gasoline-powered engines in confined spaces.

Cabinets containing medications or poisons should be locked.

Know the names of plants in your yard and house.

Be aware of medicines that visitors may bring into the home, and keep them secured.

Fuel-burning appliances should be professionally installed and inspected annually.

Check the house for lead-based paints.

PEARLS FOR THE PA

Diagnosis of poisoning should be suspected in anyone with unexplained symptoms and physical signs related to the gastrointestinal, respiratory, cardiovascular, and/or central nervous systems associated with drug intoxications.

Supportive therapy should be instituted immediately, even before drug identification.

The history of the drug type and dose taken is often unreliable.

Approximations should be overestimations (i.e., assume an empty pill bottle means that the patient ingested the contents of a full pill bottle).

Contact the regional poison control center for management guidance.

Look for signs of trauma and venous track marks.

Psychiatric Emergencies

James B. Labus, PA-C

DEFINITION

A *psychiatric emergency* is an acute pathologic cognitive/behavioral response to known intrapersonal or interpersonal (e.g., shame, guilt, abandonment, rejection) stressors. This maladaptive thought/behavior occurs in response to emotional changes that precipitate an acute situation requiring immediate intervention.

Emergencies are manifested as threatened or actual suicide attempt, substance abuse, domestic violence, violence outside the home, homelessness, and exacerbation of chronic mental illness.

The most common psychiatric emergencies are those associated with depression, mania, schizophrenia, and substance abuse.

HISTORY

Symptoms. Suicidal ideation and/or homicidal ideation in response to affective disorder, usually depression/anxiety or mania, and occasionally compounded by psychosis (paranoia or command hallucinations for self-destruction).

General

Presentation is usually through self-referral or family/friend but can be through the legal system All presentations require serious intervention because they occur either immediately before or after a destructive attempt.

Inquire about life changes, marital status, financial changes, family changes and support, family history of suicide/violence, past suicide attempts (plan and intent), anniversaries of significant events (positive and negative), medical history (physical condition), mental health, psychiatric history, religious beliefs, impulsivity, or other self-destructive behavior. Obtaining this information is dependent on a relationship of trust.

Patients may show signs of self mutilation. These patients may have had a past suicide attempt and/or a psychiatric history. For violence, determine the cause of the violence. If there is a break with reality (hallucinations), hospitalization is required. The cause of the violent behavior (if based in reality) may be able to be rectified.

Age. Peak incidence for suicide in men is age 45 and for women, age 55. The older the patient, the more serious the intent. Psychiatric emergencies are rare before the age of 12 years. Adolescents are an at-risk group and require special care (see Pediatric Considerations section).

Onset. Usually immediate in response to intrapersonal loss or interpersonal loss (significant life change, loss of self-esteem, or loss of loved one).

Duration. Maladaptive behavior will persist until effective intervention has occurred or a destructive attempt is made.

Intensity. Acute; intervention always requires a psychiatrist, with probable psychiatric hospitalization.

Aggravating Factors. Intoxication, cognitive impairment, chronic pain, single relationship status, unemployment, social isolation, medical illness.

Alleviating Factors. Early intervention, supportive family/friends, psychotherapeutic relationship.

Associated Factors. Concurrent psychiatric disorders (e.g., psychosis/paranoia), substance abuse, noncompliance with medical regimens for chronic disease. Single, nonmarried, divorced, and widowed persons and those in poor physical health have higher suicide rates.

PHYSICAL EXAMINATION

General. Physical symptoms will vary in relation to the underlying psychopathology. Most common is depression with psychomotor retardation, unkempt appearance, agitation, and coexisting medical problems. Monitor vital signs to evaluate for undisclosed ingestion of toxins (overdose or poisons) or underlying medical conditions.

Neuropsychiatric. Approach the patient in a nonthreatening manner.

Subtle incorporation of the mental status examination into the interview is essential. Look for/assess eye movements, eye contact, pupil reactions, tics, involuntary movements, speech pattern, and motor function for intoxication or overdose. Observe gait, muscle strength, and tone. Monitor alertness and orientation. Evaluate insight to rule out delusional systems. Memory, concentration, and decisiveness are impaired by depression. Judgment impaired by helplessness, hopelessness, and negative thought processes will be detrimental to the outcome of a psychiatric emergency.

Cardiopulmonary. Evaluate for possible pulmonary disease (hypoxia) and heart disease that may be masking as anxiety.

Neurologic. A comprehensive examination needs to be performed to look for focal findings that suggest a primary neurologic disorder.

PATHOPHYSIOLOGY

Etiologic determinants are as varied as the psychopathology underlying the emergency. Common psychologic determinants are associated with major affective disorders (unipolar and bipolar depressions, schizophrenic-affective disorders, and organic affective syndromes). The comorbidity of drug/alcohol dependence is common in the psychiatric emergency. The heritable component of these comorbid factors gives rise to the common prevalence of suicide and homicide within the family histories.

Decreased serotonin levels have been associated with suicide.

DIAGNOSTIC STUDIES

Laboratory
Toxicology Screen. For urine/serum drug levels of prescribed and non-prescribed medications.

Complete Blood Count. Rule out infectious process associated with an elevated white blood cell count.

Electrolytes. Rule out hyponatremia, hypokalemia/hyperkalemia. Elevated blood urea nitrogen and creatinine levels in renal damage.

Thyroid Function Tests. Evaluate for hypothyroidism/hyperthyroidism.

Liver Function Tests. Rule out hepatic dysfunction.

Megaloblastic Anemia Panel. Rule out nutritional deficiency states.

Radiology
CT/MRI of the Brain. As indicated and when possible (may require sedation) to rule out primary neurologic process.

Other
ECG. Rule out underlying cardiac abnormality.

Pulse Oximetry. Rule out hypoxia.

Psychologic
Once the patient is stable, evaluation with the Hamilton, Becks, Zung, or Wechsler test may be helpful in documenting underlying affective disorders and the degree of cognitive impairment.

DIFFERENTIAL DIAGNOSIS

Any physical condition that can lead to anxiety, depression, or behavioral change can appear as a psychiatric emergency. Generally, with medical conditions, the changes are acute, and there is no history of a previous psychiatric illness or symptoms; also, they can occur in older persons with a history (or risk) of a medical condition, substance abuse, or focal neurologic finding.

Traumatic

Head trauma, acute or remote, can cause behavior changes.

Infectious

In *mononucleosis*, patients are usually febrile and have lymphadenopathy and a positive Monospot test result.

In *hepatitis*, patients may have hepatomegaly, jaundice, and a positive hepatitis profile.

In *meningitis*, patients are usually febrile and have nuchal rigidity, Brudzinski and/or Kernig signs, and positive cerebrospinal fluid cultures.

In *encephalitis*, patients may have focal neurologic signs, a history of viral illness, or a positive CT/MRI scan.

Metabolic

In *hypothyroidism*, a positive thyroid profile.

In *electrolyte imbalance*, abnormalities found on serum chemistry evaluation.

In *diabetes mellitus*, history of diabetes, elevated serum glucose.

Hypoxia can cause severe anxiety. Sedation of the affected patient will worsen the hypoxia.

Neoplastic

With *malignant or benign neoplasms* of the brain, will have a positive CT/MRI. Other neoplasms will be seen on radiographs and may also cause electrolyte disturbances.

Vascular

In *cerebrovascular disease*, acute onset, positive CT/MRI of brain, and/or focal neurologic findings.

Myocardial infarction may cause significant anxiety.

Acquired

Substance abuse may be the cause of the behavior or may coexist with a psychiatric condition. Toxicology screen should be performed on all patients with behavior change.

Congenital

Not applicable.

TREATMENT

Based on clinical experience and judgment, the diagnosis of a psychiatric emergency is determined by the immediacy of the threat to the life and health of the patient and/or others. All such conditions must be taken seriously, even in the apparently insincere or manipulative patient. The intent or motive of the patient experiencing the emergency may be hidden or masked in a delusional system. Concurrent drug/alcohol dependency may compound the difficulty of the diagnostic process. Psychotic episodes and post-traumatic stress syndrome flashbacks threatening physical harm to self or others must be treated as emergencies.

First, secure the emergency situation for the patient and others by removing all weapons, toxins, and hazards. If the patient is psychotic, delusional, intoxicated, or severely agitated, restraint may be necessary before further evaluation and treatment can be done. Emergency medical treatment takes precedence over any psychiatric assessment if there is even a remote possibility of a toxic ingestion or medical complication. A confidential and noncritical environment is essential. Time, understanding, and a supportive, accepting attitude are conducive to a favorable outcome. Involve the treatment team by referring the patient to a psychiatrist, calling the supervising physician, consulting with the patient's therapist or counselor, and maintaining rapport with family/friends. Many communities have intervention teams highly trained in this process. Never leave the patient unattended. Disposition is dependent on multiple factors requiring the involvement of the psychiatrist. Hospitalization, voluntary or involuntary, is required when the risk of harm to the patient or others is high. Twenty-four-hour-a-day support is required regardless of the setting (hospital or home). Outpatient therapy may be considered depending on family and social support group, degree of threat, presence/absence of a means to carry out threat, and impulsivity.

Pharmacotherapy is usually required with antidepressants, antipsychotics, or sedatives.

Sedatives should be precribed by health care professionals with experience. Dosing is based on the degree of agitation, coexisting medical problems, and availability of resuscitative measures.

Sedatives include:
  Diazepam (Valium)
  Lorazepam (Ativan)
  Haloperidol (Haldol)
  Chlorpromazide (Thorazine)
  Close observation for respiratory disturbance must be maintained when giving sedatives.

PEDIATRIC CONSIDERATIONS

Psychiatric emergencies (suicide/homicide) are rare in childhood (<12 years of age). This maladaptive behavior seldom develops until after early adolescence. There may be suicidal or near-suicidal gestures with developing childhood depressions. Thus, thorough evaluation of serious accidents or accident-prone behavior is indicated. Suicide is more prevalent in children with unstable family life.

Risk factors for youth suicide include prior suicide attempts, aggressive behavior in boys older than 12 years of age, substance abuse history, depression with withdrawal, a history of running away or current pregnancy in girls, and suicidal ideation. Hospitalization is warranted in these cases. Prior to discharge, a comprehensive plan involving continued treatment, medications, and home, school, and social support is put into place.

OBSTETRIC CONSIDERATIONS

Postpartum psychosis may result in suicide or infanticide. Close observation should be undertaken for the development of this condition. The postpartum period may be when underlying psychoses or other mental conditions become apparent. The patient may have had a history of psychiatric illness, which worsens after delivery.

GERIATRIC CONSIDERATIONS

Older patients are more serious in their intent and more often successful in suicide attempts. Anxiety- and depression-causing medical conditions are more prevalent in the elderly. Therefore, a full medical history and evaluation should be undertaken, especially with an acute mental status change.

PEARLS FOR THE PA

Never leave the patient unattended.

No matter how subtle or passive, take all psychiatric emergencies (e.g., threats, gestures, ideation) seriously.

Do not dismiss or overlook subtle suicidal/homicidal ideation or comments expressed during physical examinations, yearly check-ups, or routine medical follow-up.

Always rule out primary medical conditions causing the symptoms. Do not assume that the suicidal/homicidal patient can be monitored or discouraged. Good treatment requires stabilization, thorough assessment, appropriate referral/consultation, and proper disposition.

PREVENTIVE CONSIDERATIONS

Suicide is preventable. Recognition of the risk, taking the patient seriously, inquiring about depression, and taking a psychiatric history all are beneficial. Appropriate intervention during the crisis period may help to avoid dangerous and fatal consequences.

Always involve the treatment team (psychiatrist, supervising physician, therapist, social worker).

Respiratory Arrest

Kristine Correira, PA-C

DEFINITION

A premorbid condition in which there is insufficient transfer of oxygen and/or inadequate elimination of carbon dioxide resulting in the patient's inability to respire.

HISTORY

Symptoms.   The patient is unable to breathe spontaneously.

General.   The patient may have a history of specific allergies causing respiratory symptoms, neuromuscular injury, or chronic pulmonary disease.

Age.   Any.

Onset.   Depending on precipitating factors, can be sudden or gradually progressive.

Duration.   Respiratory arrest may be sustained for only a matter of minutes before tissue damage develops, leading to death.

Intensity.   Severe and incapacitating.

Aggravating Factors.   Depending on the circumstance, may be aggravated by foreign body inhalation, exposure to an irritant or allergen, chemical exposure, or neuromuscular injury. People with chronic pulmonary disease are particularly susceptible to arrest with the onset of fulminant pulmonary infection.

Alleviating Factors.   Opening and securing a patent airway. Ventilation and oxygenation.

Associated Factors.   Can develop from many underlying causes (e.g., airway obstruction, drowning, stroke, smoke inhalation, drug overdose, trauma, infection, allergy, anaphylaxis, chronic pulmonary disease).

PHYSICAL EXAMINATION

General.   The patient may be unconscious.

Vital Signs. Respiration is essentially absent. If seen soon after onset of respiratory arrest, patient may still have a measurable blood pressure and heart rate.

Head, Eyes, Ears, Nose, and Throat. Look for signs of trauma. Depending on duration of anoxia, may see anisocoria and/or nonreactive pupils. Look for upper airway obstruction. May see neck vein distention if patient has not already progressed to circulatory collapse; observe for displaced trachea.

Neurologic. A complete neurologic examination must be performed as soon as possible after the patient's respirations have been supported, to rule out cerebral injury.

Pulmonary. Breath sounds will be absent; assess stability of rib cage. Look for signs of trauma.

Skin. Look for signs of trauma or venous track marks. May see cyanosis or diaphoresis.

PATHOPHYSIOLOGY

The mechanisms that can lead to respiratory arrest are hypercapnic and nonhypercapnic failure.

1. Hypercapnic failure (usually secondary to hypoventilation; Pco_2 is elevated, Po_2 is normal or decreased). This can occur in patients with normal lungs who have a structural chest wall abnormality or neuromuscular disease. This is also seen in patients with chronic lung disease (e.g., emphysema or asthma) who cannot adequately eliminate carbon dioxide.
2. Nonhypercapnic failure (usually secondary to oxygenation failure; Po_2 is decreased, Pco_2 is normal or decreased). This can develop in patients with ventilation-perfusion mismatch, hemoglobin abnormalities, interstitial lung disease, impaired oxygen uptake by the tissues (e.g., in cyanide poisoning).

DIAGNOSTIC STUDIES

Priority must be placed on opening and maintaining an airway, then ventilating and oxygenating the patient.

Laboratory
Arterial Blood Gas Analysis. Must be performed initially and repeated every 15 minutes to assess adequacy of ventilation.

Complete Blood Count. Look for evidence of infection or hemoglobin abnormality.

Carbon Monoxide Level. For patients with a history of fume or smoke inhalation.

Toxicology Screen. Rule out overdose/poisoning.

Radiology
Chest Film.   Indicated for all patients.
Cervical Spine X-ray Study.   If upper airway obstruction is suspected.
May show foreign body, displaced trachea, edema affecting the airway.

Other
ECG.   If any trauma or possibility of underlying cardiac disease, cocaine
use, or suspected pulmonary embolism.
Ventilation-Perfusion Scan, Chest CT, or Angiogram.   These studies will
detect pulmonary embolism.

DIFFERENTIAL DIAGNOSIS

Traumatic
With *head, airway*, or *chest injury*, history of trauma, including electrical
injury or lightning strike.

Infectious
Pneumonia can be differentiated on the chest film.
    In *meningitis*, may see nuchal rigidity, Brudzinski and/or Kernig signs,
leukocytosis with a shift to the left, positive cerebrospinal fluid cultures.
    In *sepsis*, positive blood cultures.
Metabolic.   Not applicable.

Neoplastic
In *lung cancer*, mass seen on radiograph or CT scan of the chest.

Vascular
    In *stroke*, positive neurologic findings and/or positive CT/MRI scan of
the brain.
    In *pulmonary embolism*, positive ventilation-perfusion scan, CT scan, or
pulmonary arteriogram.
Congenital.   Not applicable.

Acquired
With *airway obstruction*, may have history of aspiration.
    With *smoke inhalation*, history of smoke inhalation, may have associated
burns.
    With *drug overdose*, positive toxicology screen.
    With *allergy leading to anaphylaxis*, may have a history of allergy causing
respiratory symptoms.
    In *asthma*, history of asthma.
    In *chronic pulmonary disease*, may have history of pulmonary disease
and/or positive radiograph or CT scan of the chest.

TREATMENT

Immediately clear the airway and provide mask-to-mouth or bag-valve-mask resuscitation. Endotracheal intubation should be performed as soon as possible by the most skilled person available. Once the airway is secured, provide adequate ventilatory support.

Cricothyroidotomy or tracheostomy is an alternative means to obtain an airway. See Chapter 19, "Procedures," section "Emergency Cricothyroidotomy."

Define and treat the underlying cause.

Closely monitor urinary output, cardiovascular function, and respiratory function.

PEDIATRIC CONSIDERATIONS

Children younger than 2 years of age are susceptible to rapid deterioration in pulmonary function after only modest insult. Respiratory conditions are by far the most common nontraumatic cause of severe pediatric illness.

OBSTETRIC CONSIDERATIONS

Respiratory arrest resuscitation should include the standard management steps of clearing the airway, carrying out endotracheal intubation, and administering supplemental oxygen according to Advanced Cardiac Life Support guidelines.

With *respiratory distress*, maternal hypoxia must be recognized and treated promptly. The effects of maternal hypoxia can be profound; often fetal distress will result as indicated by a decrease in fetal heart rate variability and number of accelerations as well as episodes of fetal bradycardia (rate of less than 110 beats/minute). Traumatic conditions resulting in maternal hypoxia such as pneumothorax, tension pneumothorax, and flail chest are treated in the manner as for the nonpregnant patient.

Pregnancy induces changes in the pulmonary system that can lead to dyspnea, physiologic hyperventilation, and possible atelectasis. In response to these changes, pregnant patients have chronic, compensated respiratory alkalosis.

During administration of oxygen, the patient should be in the left lateral decubitus position to facilitate effective oxygen circulation, as uterine pressure on the inferior vena cava can cause sequestering of a significant percentage of the circulating blood volume.

GERIATRIC CONSIDERATIONS

Any patient with a long pack-year history of smoking can be presumed to have some degree of chronic obstructive pulmonary disease (COPD). Even elderly patients who have never smoked have decreased tidal volume and lung compliance as a part of aging. Thus, geriatric patients in general are at a greater risk of respiratory arrest from underlying pulmonary disease.

PREVENTIVE CONSIDERATIONS

Any strategy that prevents conditions that lead to respiratory arrest, of which there are many, will reduce its incidence.

PEARLS FOR THE PA

Once ventilation and oxygenation are supported, the clinician must attempt to define and treat the underlying cause.

Cardiac arrest rapidly follows untreated respiratory arrest.

Irreversible neurologic damage is the inevitable sequela of delayed treatment of respiratory arrest.

Shock

Kristine Corriera, PA-C

DEFINITION

An acute clinical syndrome mediated by a severe underlying perfusion deficit and resultant multisystem organ dysfunction. Shock can be divided into three broad categories: hypovolemic, cardiogenic, and distributive. Distributive shock includes the common conditions of septic shock and anaphylactic shock, described later on, and the less common conditions of toxic shock syndrome (TSS), adrenal crisis, and neurogenic shock.

Hypovolemic shock: An acute clinical condition secondary to an acute loss of circulating intravascular volume. Symptoms occur when 20% to 25% of total intravascular volume is lost.

Cardiogenic shock: Hypoperfusion due to decreased myocardial performance, leading to multiorgan system dysfunction. The vast majority of these cases are due to myocardial infarction. The mortality rate from cardiogenic shock approaches 75%.

Distributive shock: Hypoperfusion due to a drop in systemic vascular resistance, usually with normal or increased cardiac output.

Septic shock: Sepsis is due to the hematogenous spread of viruses, fungi, parasites, and most commonly, gram-negative bacteria. Be aware that "sepsis" and "septic shock" have been poorly defined in the past and thus represent a range of clinical presentations. *Septic shock* is currently defined as sepsis with hypotension and inadequate tissue perfusion despite fluid resuscitation.

Anaphylactic shock: Shock due to rapid hemodynamic compromise caused by an allergic reaction to medications, venoms, foods, or other potentially noxious substances.

HISTORY

Symptoms

Hypovolemic. Alterations in mental status from confusion to coma. Hypotension, tachypnea, tachycardia.

Cardiogenic. The clinical manifestations are dependent on the underlying cause of pump failure, concurrent illnesses, compensatory mechanisms, and the extent of end-organ dysfunction.

Distributive. Clinical manifestations are dependent on the underlying cause of the loss in vascular tone.

Septic. Patients with septic shock will have fever, chills, and general malaise along with symptoms relating to the site of infection (pneumonia, urinary tract, abdominal organ).

Anaphylactic. Patients will usually (though not always) give a history of an exposure followed by symptoms ranging from mild to dramatic and rapidly fatal. Urticaria, flushing, and angioedema are the most common findings. Hypotension with peripheral vasodilatation and capillary instability are common features. Cardiovascular effects combined with respiratory symptoms of laryngeal edema, tachypnea, and bronchospasm are the major pathophysiologic events.

General

Hypovolemic. Usually encountered in the setting of multisystem trauma or major thermal injury, although dissecting aortic aneurysm may be the cause. Closed head injuries are *never* the cause of hypovolemic shock (although scalp injuries may contribute), as the cranial vault will not allow for enough blood loss to lower the hematocrit before death ensues due to herniation.

Cardiogenic. The vast majority of these cases are due to myocardial infarction. A history of coronary atherosclerotic heart disease is often present. The mortality rate from cardiogenic shock approaches 75%. It is often difficult to separate out cardiogenic from septic shock in the early stages. The elderly, especially those with chronic illnesses or conditions such as cirrhosis, diabetes, disseminated cancer, or transplantation with associated immunomodulation, are particularly at risk, as well as those patients who have recently undergone invasive medical procedures. Other causes include cardiac contusion, tension pneumothorax, cardiac tamponade, arrhythmias, congestive heart failure, acute valvular dysfunction, cardiomyopathies, and pulmonary embolus.

Distributive

Septic. Usually occurs in patients with a past medical history significant for chronic disease, corticosteroid therapy, antineoplastic agents, immunosuppressive therapies, and recent invasive procedures. Genitourinary infections are common sources, especially when indwelling catheters have been in place, and following instrumentation. Other common sources include pneumonia (especially in intubated patients), perforated viscus, intra-abdominal abscess, biliary tract infections, cholangitis, and presence of an intravenous line.

Anaphylactic. Most commonly caused by parenteral antibiotic administration, especially of penicillins and cephalosporins, intravenous radiocontrast, and hymenoptera stings (which cause an injected exposure). *Anaphylaxis* is a loosely defined term. Some clinicians use the term only for severe reactions, whereas others consider milder reactions (such as those that occur with intravenous radiocontrast) as anaphylaxis, even though fatalities are rare. It may mimic the presentation of a severe asthmatic episode or may be confused with primary cardiogenic shock from myocardial infarction.

Age

Hypovolemic. Can occur in any age group; however, the greatest incidence is in the first four decades of life.

Cardiogenic. Most common after the fourth decade of life.

Distributive. Can occur in any age group

Onset

Hypovolemic. Rapid.

Cardiogenic. Gradual to rapid.

Distributive. With infectious etiology, onset is gradual, whereas in other types of shock, onset is rapid, with anaphylaxis occurring within 1 hour of exposure (or minutes if severe).

Duration

Hypovolemic/Cardiogenic. If unchecked, can rapidly lead to death.

Distributive. All forms can lead rapidly to cardiovascular collapse. Anaphylaxis in its severe form is rapid and dramatic.

Intensity. Life-threatening.

Aggravating Factors. Concurrent chronic illnesses or conditions such as cardiac disease, cirrhosis, diabetes, disseminated cancer, or transplantation, as well as recent invasive procedures and corticosteroid, chemotherapeutic, and immunosuppressant therapies.

Alleviating Factors. Immediate resuscitative measures including high-flow oxygen and supportive measures aimed at normalization of vital signs.

Hypovolemic. Controlling bleeding, maintaining the airway, repleting volume loss. Place patient in Trendelenburg position.

Cardiogenic. Determine the etiology and treat appropriately.

Distributive. Aggressive fluid resuscitation is indicated for all forms of distributive shock.

Septic. Immediate institution of broad-spectrum antibiotic therapy. Determine the etiology and treat appropriately.

Anaphylaxis. Treat immediately with epinephrine, parenteral diphenhydramine, and histamine H_2 blockers (cimetidine, ranitidine). Also treat with corticosteroids but not with the same priority.

Associated Factors. Concurrent medical conditions must be addressed after vital functions are stabilized, as they may contribute to, or complicate, long-term management.

PHYSICAL EXAMINATION

General
Three stages of shock can be identified:

Compensated, when the patient's body systems maintain blood pressure and perfusion.

Decompensated, when compensatory mechanisms are overwhelmed, leading to hypotension and hypoperfusion.

Irreversible

Prognosis is best when intervention occurs while the patient is still in compensated shock but signs are subtle. Confusion or irritability, tachycardia, cool and pale skin, and delayed capillary refill all are signs of compensated shock—but note that patients in compensated distributive shock may have warm extremities with bounding pulses, although still tachycardic.

Hypovolemic. Depending on the amount of blood lost, the patient can present in no apparent distress, or can be tachycardic, tachypneic, or hypotensive, or can have mild to marked mental status changes and be near death.

Cardiogenic. The patient will often exhibit alterations in mental status from anxiety to coma. The patient may have been complaining of chest discomfort.

Distributive. As with other forms of shock, the patient presents with hypotension, tachycardia, and tachypnea, along with alterations in mental status ranging from confusion to coma. Unlike in other forms of shock, the patient with distributive shock (or a precursor to it) may have warm extremities with bounding pulses and an increased pulse pressure.

Septic. The patient may be febrile or hypothermic. The septic source may not be immediately obvious.

Anaphylactic. Patient presents with a range of symptoms from rash to complete cardiovascular collapse. In the initial stages, this clinical condition may be difficult to distinguish from cardiogenic shock or asthmatic crisis.

Cardiovascular
Cardiogenic. Tachycardia, hypotension, dyskinetic apical cardiac impulse, a new third or forth heart sound, or a new murmur of mitral regurgitation, possibly indicative of papillary muscle dysfunction. Jugular venous distention is often present.

Distributive
Septic. Tachycardia with hypotension (<90 mm Hg) due to loss of intravascular tone. Cardiac output is usually elevated.

Anaphylactic. Hypoexemia and hypotension may lead to dysrhythmias and inadequate coronary arterial perfusion.

Gastrointestinal

Distributive
Anaphylactic. Nausea, vomiting, cramping, abdominal pain, diarrhea.

Neurologic

Distributive
Septic. Alterations in mental status ranging from slight to profound. Seizures may occur, especially with sepsis from meningitis, or with anaphylaxis.

Anaphylactic. Symptoms range from anxiety to coma, with convulsions in advanced stages.

Pulmonary
Cardiogenic. Tachypnea, pulmonary crackles.

Distributive
Septic. Tachypnea with moist rales or crackles if pulmonary infection is present.

Anaphylactic. Hoarseness, tachypnea, wheezing.

Renal
Distributive. Oliguria due to inadequate renal perfusion.

Skin
Cardiogenic. Cool, moist, pale and dusky.

Distributive
Septic. Skin and extremities are warm and well perfused during sepsis, becoming pale, dusky, cool, and moist as shock sets in.

Anaphylactic. Skin changes are the most common manifestation of anaphylaxis, including flushing, urticaria, pruritus, and angioedema.

PATHOPHYSIOLOGY

Hypovolemic
Patient presentation can best be understood by utilizing the American College of Surgeons' Advanced Trauma Life Support nomenclature for describing the degree of intravascular volume loss.

Class I hemorrhage—loss of <800 mL of blood: No appreciable clinical symptoms in a normal, otherwise healthy person. Normal physiologic processes will replace this volume within 24 hours.

Class II hemorrhage—loss of 800 to 1500 mL of blood: This represents a 15% to 30% loss of total circulating volume. Symptoms include tachycardia, tachypnea, and decrease in pulse pressure. Neurohumoral compensatory mechanisms include increased peripheral vascular resistance, tachycardia to maintain cardiac output, and increased cardiac contractility to maintain a near-normal systolic blood pressure. Mild mental status changes may be apparent.

Class III hemorrhage—loss of 1500 mL of blood or greater: Potentially life-threatening, 30% to 40% loss of total intravascular volume. Symptoms include tachypnea, tachycardia, mental status changes, and a significant fall in systolic blood pressure. Patients with this degree of blood loss will require vigorous volume replacement and transfusion therapy.

Class IV hemorrhage—loss of more than 40% of total blood volume: Exsanguination that is immediately life-threatening. The patient is markedly tachycardic.

Note that hypovolemic shock may also be caused by severe gastrointestinal losses and burns.

Cardiogenic

Cardiac shock is a syndrome of hypoperfusion and severe end-organ dysfunction. The vital organs most affected are the heart, brain, and kidneys. The autoregulation mechanisms of the brain fail to compensate as mean arterial pressure drops below 60 mm Hg. Perfusion deficiencies lead to alterations in mental status ranging from confusion to coma. As the shock state worsens, cardiac function is negatively affected as systemic hypotension worsens coronary perfusion. With failure of the myocardium comes an increase in left ventricular end-diastolic pressure, with the development of pulmonary edema and impaired gas exchange. The resultant hypoxemia further negatively affects myocardial performance, thus setting up a downward spiral of hemodynamic instability. As mean arterial pressure falls, the glomerular filtration rate drops, with oliguria being a common clinical manifestation.

Distributive

Pathophysiology depends on the etiology.

Septic shock is a hyperdynamic cardiovascular state exhibiting a high cardiac output, normal cardiac filling pressures, and low systemic vascular resistance. Endotoxemia causes severe alterations in capillary permeability, allowing for intravascular volume depletion and septic shock. Sepsis causes significant multisystem organ damage including hepatic dysfunction with clotting abnormalities and pulmonary microvascular damage leading to acute respiratory distress syndrome (ARDS).

Anaphylactic shock is an antigen-antibody reaction, usually immunoglobulin E–mediated, that causes the release of physiologically active substances, such as histamine, leukotriene B$_4$, platelet-activating factor, and prostaglandins. These substances can cause increased capillary permeability, vasodilatation, dysrhythmia, and pulmonary vascular and bronchial constriction.

DIAGNOSTIC STUDIES

General Note: The immediate treatment of the patient suffering from shock proceeds according to physical findings, and the initiation of immediate life-saving measures should not be delayed while awaiting laboratory or radiographic data.

Distributive.   No laboratory studies are indicated for anaphylactic shock. But because of the many and diverse causes of other types of distributive shock and their sequelae, extensive diagnostic studies are required.

Laboratory

Complete Blood Count
In *hypovolemic shock*, counts are initially normal during loss of intravascular blood volume. After crystalloid fluid resuscitation, significant decrease in hemoglobin and hematocrit occurs. Leukocyte count usually normal at this time.

In *cardiogenic shock*, the complete blood count helps rule out underlying anemia or septic foci (with an elevated white blood cell count.)

In *distributive shock*, white blood cell count elevation is a consistent finding in septic shock. Platelet count increases as an acute phase reactant and then decreases with disseminated intravascular coagulation (DIC).

Electrolytes.   Examine creatinine and blood urea nitrogen (BUN) levels for adequacy of renal function. Hyperkalemia may occur in burn-injured patients or may contribute to cardiogenic shock. Hyponatremia or hypernatremia can occur from gastrointestinal losses. Hypokalemia may occur from excessive diarrhea as well as acidosis (from bicarbonate losses).

Toxicology Screen.   Mandatory for all trauma patients.

Arterial Blood Gas Analysis and Lactate Level.   In *septic shock*, patients will develop metabolic acidosis from anaerobic metabolism. Serum lactate levels are prognostic: The higher the lactate level, the more severe the shock and the worse the prognosis.

Cardiac Isoenzymes.   In *cardiogenic shock*, serial specimens should be sent for isoenzyme assay to examine for myocardial cell injury.

Pan-Cultures (Blood, Urine Sputum, Stool).   In *septic shock*, used to identify the septic source.

Radiology
Chest Film and Kidney-Ureter-Bladder (KUB) and Cervical Spine Series.
In cases of *hypovolemic shock*, indicated as part of a survey for potentially life-threatening injury in a trauma patient.

In *cardiogenic shock*, the chest film is examined for signs of pulmonary edema, tension pneumothorax, and pericardial effusion.

In *septic shock*, the chest film can identify occult pneumonia.

Ultrasonography. If a biliary infection is the suspected source of septic shock.

CT. In *septic shock*, abdominal CT if intra-abdominal or retroperitoneal sources of infection are suspected.

CT of the brain with signs of increased intracranial pressure, or if an intracranial source of infection is suspected (from recent intracranial surgery, recent sinusitis, or otitis).

Urinalysis. In *septic shock*, examine urine for the presence of bacteria and leukocytes.

Clotting Studies: Prothrombin Time, Partial Thromboplastin Time, Platelets, Bleeding Time. In *septic shock*, evaluate for coagulopathies.

Other

ECG. In *cardiogenic shock*, evidence of ST segment changes suggestive of myocardial ischemia and/or bradydysrhythmias and tachydysrhythmias.

In *anaphylactic shock*, dysryhthmias are common, with potential T wave inversions, heart block, and other electrophysiologic disturbances.

DIFFERENTIAL DIAGNOSIS

Shock is an acute clinical entity caused by a multiplicity of factors. Therefore, the concept of differential diagnosis as such does not apply.

TREATMENT

General

Airway. Always secure the airway before any other treatment.

Breathing. High-flow oxygen for all shock patients. Ventilatory support as needed.

Hypovolemic

In the setting of multisystem trauma or major burn injury, all patients who present in shock are hypovolemic until proven otherwise. The initial treatment should follow Advanced Trauma Life Support guidelines, which specify a rational and deliberate approach to initial resuscitation.

Circulation. Be sure all obvious external sources of bleeding are controlled. An initial fluid challenge is delivered to the patient. This is a bolus of 1 to 2 L of Ringer's lactate solution or normal saline that is rapidly infused via short, large-bore, peripheral intravenous lines. This volume infusion serves as both a treatment and a diagnostic modality.

Responses to Fluid Challenge. Patients can be categorized according to the nature of their response to the fluid challenge:

1. Rapid responders: Patients who demonstrate sustained hemodynamic stability in response to the initial 2-L bolus have lost no more than 20%

of their total intravascular volume. No further special fluid replacement maneuvers are necessary, and the global patient evaluation can continue.

2. Transient responders: It is common for patients to initially respond to the initial fluid bolus and then drift back into a hypotensive state. This response is usually indicative of continued active bleeding. Continued vigorous volume resuscitation is required, and preparations should be made for the administration of whole, cross-matched blood. These patients need to be made ready for rapid surgical intervention to control further blood loss.

3. Nonresponders: In these patients there is no hemodynamic response to the initial volume replacement. Immediate surgical intervention is required to control hemorrhage. Continued vigorous crystalloid volume resuscitation is required, and consideration should be given to the delivery of type O, Rh-negative blood if type-specific blood is not available.

Cardiogenic
Circulation. To reverse hypotension (systolic blood pressure <90 mm Hg), crystalloid fluid volume resuscitation combined with the titrated delivery of inotropic support is required. Dopamine in doses up to 10 mg/kg/minute can increase myocardial contractility, renal blood flow, and peripheral vascular resistance.

In patients with an established diagnosis of myocardial infarction, immediate cardiac catheterization with angioplasty and thrombolytic therapy may be beneficial.

In patients with severely compromised cardiac status, intra-aortic balloon pump therapy may be indicated.

Distributive
Circulation. Provide crystalloid volume in 500-mL-bolus increments to restore intravascular volume. End points of fluid therapy would be a normal blood pressure, pulmonary wedge pressure 15 to 18 mm Hg, and a central venous pressure in the range of 12 to 16 mm Hg.

Inotropic support in the form of dopamine 10 mg/kg/minute may be necessary to ensure adequate hemodynamics but only after adequate (administration of 4 or more liters) fluid resuscitation.

In *septic shock*, empiric therapy with broad-spectrum antibiotics, adjusted for renal function, should be administered AS SOON AS POSSIBLE. Surgical, percutaneous, or open drainage of abscesses should be performed as soon as possible to manage the septic burden.

In *anaphylactic shock*, give epinephrine 3-5 mg by the subcutaneous (if the patient is not in extremis), intravenous, endotracheal, intravenous, or sublingual route; may need continuous infusion for refractory shock. Also give an antihistamine—either diphenhydramine (H_1 receptor blocker) 25-50 mg IM or IV or cimetidine (H_2 receptor blocker) 300 mg IM or IV; both may be given PO in milder reactions. Inhaled beta agonists such as albuterol will treat bronchospasm.

Anaphylactic reactions are also usually treated with parenteral or oral corticosteroids. These agents treat bronchospasm and skin manifestations of anaphylaxis but do nothing for cardiovascular effects; thus, they are not of a high priority in severe reactions. Some clinicians use corticosteroids to prevent a recurrent reaction (one that occurs after the short-lived medications listed previously have cleared the patient's system), even though the incidence of these subsequent manifestations are unknown and they are usually mild when they do occur.

PEDIATRIC CONSIDERATIONS

The clinical manifestations of blood loss are far more dramatic in children than those seen in adults. For this reason, monitoring hemoglobin and hematocrit is crucial in the developing child.

Sometimes it is difficult to distinguish supraventricular tachycardia from tachycardia secondary to fever, dehydration, and sepsis in infants. In general, a heart rate less than 200 beats/minute represents sinus tachycardia and therefore is likely to be due to infection or dehydration.

GERIATRIC CONSIDERATIONS

Geriatric patients have diminished cardiac, pulmonary, and vascular capacities; as a result, compensatory mechanisms are more easily overwhelmed. Thus, shock can develop more quickly and with less insult than in younger patients.

Note: Low-normal blood pressure in an elderly patient with a history of hypertension could represent *compensated shock*.

Shock states cause cardiovascular stress; thus, a cardiac evaluation (ECG, cardiac enzymes) should be performed.

Administering epinephrine to a geriatric patient greatly increases the risk of inducing a myocardial infarction. It should be used only in the case of severe, life-threatening anaphylaxis.

OBSTETRIC CONSIDERATIONS

In the first-trimester obstetric patient, fluid and electrolyte replacement is essentially the same as in the nonpregnant patient. For patients in their second and third trimesters of pregnancy, the management of hypotension and its effects on the health of the fetus warrants careful review. Decreased uterine blood flow due to maternal hypovolemia can result in fetal distress or even death. The signs of actual or impending stress are often manifested only by decreases in fetal heart rate variability and accelerations or bradycardia. Early signs of fetal distress may be the first clinical indication of an unsuspected maternal hemorrhage—an important consideration, because a pregnant trauma patient can lose up to 30% to 35% of her blood volume before she displays any clinical signs. Owing to the physiologic changes of a larger blood volume and increased vascularity of the uterus during pregnancy, the potential for significant and even catastrophic blood loss is present.

The pregnant patient with suspected shock should be closely monitored via maternal blood pressure and urinary output and fetal heart rate. The patient should be placed in the left lateral decubitus position, if possible, or at least should have a small pillow or blanket placed under her right hip to avoid exacerbating the hypotension. Intravenous fluid replacement should be approximately three times the estimated fluid loss. Ringer's lactate solution is preferred; however, other crystalloids can be used. Large amounts of normal saline solution should be avoided if possible, owing to the possibility of causing hyperchloremia in both mother and fetus. If blood or blood products are needed, a pregnant woman will need at least 25% more blood than a nonpregnant woman of similar size. The blood should be typed and cross-matched to avoid Rh factor problems. If blood is needed early in the resuscitation, type O Rh-negative blood should be used. If indicated, military antishock trousers can be used as long as the abdominal compartment is not inflated. Volume expanders should be avoided, because they are not as effective as crystalloid solutions in improving and maintaining fetal oxygenation. Vasopressors should be a therapeutic modality of last resort owing to the possibility of compromised uteroplacental blood flow.

PREVENTIVE CONSIDERATIONS

Hypovolemic shock is commonly caused by hemorrhage occurring as a result of trauma. General injury prevention strategies (wearing seat belts, using car seats, for example) will reduce the sequelae of accidents.

Cardiogenic shock is most commonly a result of cardiovascular disease, so employing cardiac disease prevention strategies will reduce its incidence.

Elderly or immunocompromised patients with any signs of infection should contact their primary care provider before sepsis and septic shock set in.

Patients with a history of anaphylaxis should be given a prescription for at least one epinephrine autoinjector to keep close at hand in case of exposure to an offending allergen.

PEARLS FOR THE PA

The causes of shock are classified as hypovolemic, cardiogenic, and distributive; septic shock and anaphylactic shock are by far the most common forms of distributive shock.

Signs of compensated shock can be subtle (confusion, irritation, tachycardia, tachypnea, cool and pale skin) but are important to recognize, as interventions are most effective during this stage.

Continued

PEARLS FOR THE PA—cont'd

In distributive shock (or immediate precursor conditions), the patient will present with warm extremities and bounding pulses.

The findings on physical examination guide the initial treatment of shock.

Central venous lines are inappropriate for initial volume replacement.

Administer antibiotics and, if required, perform surgical drainage AS SOON AS POSSIBLE *for patients with sepsis and septic shock.*

Hemoglobin and hematocrit will be normal prior to crystalloid administration in a patient with hemorrhagic hypovolemic shock.

Closed head injuries are never a cause of hypovolemic shock.

Consider supraventricular tachycardia in a pediatric patient with a heart rate of 200 beats/minute.

Inotropes are never a substitute for vigorous volume resuscitation.

Further Reading

Auerbach PS, Donner HJ, Weiss EA: Field Guide to Wilderness Medicine. Philadelphia, Mosby, 1999.

Labus JB, Lauber AA: Patient Education and Preventive Medicine. Philadelphia, WB Saunders, 2001.

eMedicine Journal> Emergency Medicine> Allergy and Immunology: Anaphylaxis. Available at http://www.emedicine.com/emerg/topic25.htm

eMedicine Journal> Emergency Medicine> Infectious Diseases: Shock, Septic. Available at http://www.emedicine.com/emerg/topic533.htm

eMedicine Journal> Medicine, Ob/Gyn, Psychiatry and Surgery> Critical Care: Shock, Distributive. Available at http://www.emedicine.com/med/topic2114.htm
http://www.ameriburn.org/

www.cdc.gov/ncipc/factsheets/poison_prevention.htm

ENDOCRINOLOGY

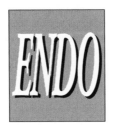

4

Adrenal Disorders

Ann Griwatz, PA-C

DEFINITION

Clinical manifestations of adrenal disorders are those related to excessive or insufficient hormone production.

Addison disease is due to adrenal gland damage causing aldosterone, adrenal androgen, and cortisol deficiency.

Cushing syndrome is secondary to overproduction of cortisol, mineralocorticoid, catecholamine, and adrenal androgens.

Pathologic states also include adrenal masses found incidentally on imaging studies. Often these tumors are not associated with endocrine pathology. These states can have overlapping features.

Symptoms

Adrenal Insufficiency.   Weakness, weight loss, anorexia/nausea/vomiting, abdominal pain, hypotension with dehydration, salt craving, diarrhea, constipation, syncope, vitiligo. When insufficiency is primary and adrenocorticotropic hormone (ACTH) levels are high, hyperpigmentation of skin, nails, palmar creases, mucous membranes is seen.

Adrenal Excess.   Truncal obesity, muscle wasting, weight gain, weakness, hypertension, hirsutism, amenorrhea, purpuric striae (commonly abdominal), easy bruisability, acne, osteoporosis, proximal myopathy, edema, palpitations, headaches, polyuria, polydipsia, diaphoresis, and susceptibility to infection. Emotional variability can result in depression, confusion, and even psychosis.

General.   The symptoms may be insidious in onset. New weight gain or loss, glucose intolerance, or hypertension may indicate glucocorticoid, mineralocorticoid, or catecholamine excess. Patients with pheochromocytomas and carcinoid tumors usually have a longer clinical course and exhibit typical cushingoid features. Inadequate adrenal hormone production often appears as mild chronic fatigue or may not be noted until a stressful event (e.g., myocardial infarction/failure, pneumonia) precipitates a crisis.

Secondary insufficiency states can occur following cessation of exogenous steroid use. Alternatively, excess use of steroids can induce a Cushing syndrome.

Age/Incidence.   Primary adrenal insufficiency is uncommon and can occur at any age, affecting men and women equally. Secondary, iatrogenic states can also occur at any age. Excess states associated with pituitary-dependent adrenal hyperplasia are most common in adults in the third or fourth decade of life.

Onset.   Gradual to acute.

Duration.   Months to years.

Intensity.   Asymptomatic to acute crisis.

Aggravating Factors

Adrenal Insufficiency. Stress, illness, trauma, hemorrhage, surgery, or dehydration. AIDS and cytomegalovirus (CMV) infection regularly induce adrenal abnormalities. Certain medications often can potentiate adrenal insufficiency states: rifampin, ketoconazole, megestrol acetate (Megace), phenytoin, and opiates.

Adrenal Excess. Medical illness requiring high-dose steroid therapy (systemic lupus erythematosus, organ transplantation). Use of beta blockers in the presence of pheochromocytoma may cause an increase in blood pressure. Other illnesses (e.g., lung cancer) can trigger the sudden manifestation of Cushing syndrome.

Alleviating Factors

Adrenal Insufficiency. Correction of underlying medical illness, replacement of hormone.

Adrenal Excess. Tapering of hormone replacement or removal of adrenal tumors.

Associated Factors

Adrenal Insufficiency. Mineralocorticoid (aldosterone) insufficiency may be severe enough to cause hypotension, salt loss, or hyperkalemia. Severe dehydration, hyponatremia, and hyperkalemia are cardinal signs of severe mineralocorticoid insufficiency, suggesting primary adrenocortical insufficiency.

Adrenal Excess. Endocrine excess from the adrenal gland may be due to pheochromocytoma causing hypertension, or a carcinoid tumor causing diarrhea and flushing. If a pituitary adenoma causes ACTH secretion (Cushing disease), bilateral adrenal hyperplasia may result.

Secondary hyperaldosteronism (not due to adrenal tumor) may occur with renal artery stenosis, diuretics, volume depletion, or ectopic ACTH secretion.

Overt diabetes mellitus (DM) occurs in almost 20% of persons with adrenal excess; it is suspected that adrenal excess states predispose them to develop DM.

PHYSICAL EXAMINATION

General

Adrenal Insufficiency. May exhibit noticeable weight loss.

Adrenal Excess. Patient may have obvious signs: truncal obesity, moon facies, buffalo hump, hirsutism, extremity muscle wasting, acne, emotional lability.

Cardiovascular

Adrenal Insufficiency. Hypotension may be present secondary to cortisol or mineralocorticoid deficiency.

Adrenal Excess. Hypertension may be seen with mineralocorticoid, glucocorticoid, or catecholamine excess.

Extremities
Adrenal Insufficiency. Increased pigmentation.
Adrenal Excess. Muscle wasting and fungal infections in nails or skin are seen in Cushing disease.

Head, Eyes, Ears, Nose, Throat
Adrenal Insufficiency. Oral mucosa may be hyperpigmented.
Adrenal Excess. Cataracts may be seen with cortisol excess.

Genitourinary
Adrenal Insufficiency. Axillary and pubic hair may be less prominent than normal in females owing to a lack of adrenal androgens.
Adrenal Excess. *Candida* infections with Cushing disease.

Neuropsychiatric
Adrenal Insufficiency. Asthenia.
Adrenal Excess. Depression, labile emotions, psychosis with high cortisol levels.

Skin
Adrenal Insufficiency. Hyperpigmentation of the palmar creases, fingernails, elbows, knees, buccal mucosa, areolae, and nipples (due to elevated ACTH levels).
Adrenal Excess. Striae, acne, hirsutism, easy bruisability, and thin skin all are seen owing to elevated glucocorticoid levels.

PATHOPHYSIOLOGY

Adrenal Insufficiency
Idiopathic adrenal atrophy, usually due to autoimmune damage to the adrenal gland, is the most common cause of primary adrenal insufficiency (in approximately 80% of cases). Other causes include surgery, congenital adrenal hyperplasia, medications (metyrapone, ketoconazole, opiates, rifampin, aminoglutethimide), tuberculosis, heparin therapy, trauma, metastatic carcinoma, familial adrenal insufficiency, fungal infections, sarcoidosis, complications of AIDS, or CMV necrotizing adrenalitis. Rare genetic mutations can cause primary adrenal insufficiency in infancy or childhood and even later, in adulthood.

With secondary adrenal insufficiency, the cause is lack of ACTH due to pituitary or hypothalamic dysfunction. Pituitary suppression after exogenous steroid intake is the most common cause of ACTH deficiency.

Pituitary insufficiency will result in a lack of ACTH, thus leading to cortisol insufficiency but not mineralocorticoid insufficiency (mineralocorticoid system will still be intact because this system does not require ACTH, and the renin-angiotensin system can continue to stimulate aldosterone release).

Only a few weeks of high-dose glucocorticoid administration can result in prolonged adrenal insufficiency.

Adrenal Excess

The hypercortisolism supports fat distribution associated with the development of the classic moon facies, buffalo hump, and truncal obesity. This is associated with hyperinsulinemia and insulin resistance.

Hypercortisol states are most commonly due to prolonged, high-dose exogenous glucocorticoids prescribed for the treatment of asthma or inflammatory rheumatoid disease.

Cushing syndrome refers to clinical presentations of cortisol excess. Cushing disease, a rare disorder, is specifically due to an ACTH-producing pituitary tumor yielding high glucocorticoid levels and adrenal hyperplasia. Adrenal tumors, ectopic ACTH production, and bilateral nodular hyperplasia all may cause Cushing syndrome. Mineralocorticoid excess may be primary (as with adrenal adenoma or hyperplasia) or secondary (as in renovascular diseases or high renin states). High levels of glucocorticoids have a mineralocorticoid effect. Pheochromocytoma is a rare endocrine tumor that may cause hypertension due to catecholamine excess.

DIAGNOSTIC STUDIES

Laboratory

Serum Cortisol.   Upper limit of normal: in the morning, 25 µg/dL; in the evening, 10 µg/dL. Highest level is in the morning (ACTH surge due to circadian rhythm) and the lowest level in the late afternoon. Level is increased in stress and with elevated ACTH.

24-Hour Urine Cortisol.   High in Cushing syndrome, with levels greater than 120 µg/24 hours.

ACTH level.   Upper limit of normal: 50 pg/mL. May be elevated in approximately 50% of patients with Cushing disease. The level varies in the day, with the highest level in the morning and the lowest level in the evening. This circadian rhythm may be lost in Cushing disease, with stress, and during hospitalization.

Serum Sodium.   Normal: 136-144 mEq/L. May be low in glucocorticoid deficiency. May be slightly elevated or high normal with mineralocorticoid excess.

Serum Potassium.   May be low with mineralocorticoid excess (less than 3.5 mEq/L) and elevated with adrenal insufficiency (greater than 5.0 mEq/L).

Serum Bicarbonate.   May be elevated with mineralocorticoid excess (greater than 25 mEq/L) causing metabolic alkalosis.

Plasma Aldosterone.   Normal: supine 1-16 ng/dL, upright 4-31 ng/dL, with a normal serum potassium. May be elevated with mineralocorticoid excess from tumor, usually in conjunction with hypokalemia and low renin.

Suppression of aldosterone (with sodium infusion) or stimulation (upright posture) may be useful.

Plasma Renin Activity. Normal: supine 0.15-2.33 ng/mL/hour, upright 1.13-3.95 ng/mL/hour. Low with volume expansion, aldosterone-producing tumor, and hyperkalemia. Elevated with volume depletion, reninoma, hemodynamically significant renal artery lesion, and hypokalemia.

Plasma 18-Hydroxycorticosterone. Normal: less than 80 ng/dL. Elevated in most cases of unilateral adrenal tumor in conjunction with postural decrease in aldosterone level.

Urinary 17-Hydroxcorticosteroids. May be elevated in glucocorticoid excess states, e.g., Cushing disease/syndrome, excess ACTH or corticosteroid therapy. May be deficient in glucocorticoid deficiency states, e.g., Addison disease, pituitary deficiency of ACTH secretion, administration of potent corticosteroids.

Pheochromocytoma Studies
Check with the laboratory before ordering the studies for the use of proper preservatives and list of foods or medications that may interfere with the results.

24-Hour Urine for Total Catecholamines
Normal: at 0 to 12 months of age, less than 20 µg/24 hours; at 13 months to 5 years, less than 40; at greater than 5 to 15 years, less than 80; at older than 15 years, less than 100.

24-Hour Urine for Fractionated Catecholamines
NOREPINEPHRINE
Normal: less than 85-100 µg/24 hours.
EPINEPHRINE
Normal: less than 25-30 µg/24 hours.

24-Hour Urine for Vanillylmandelic Acid
Both less sensitive and less specific than metanephrine or catecholamine assay. Normal: 2-7 mg/24 hours.

24-Hour Urine for Metanephrine
Normal: less than 1.3 mg/24 hours.

Radiology
CT/MRI. To localize adrenal or pituitary tumors or used in diagnosing bilateral adrenal hyperplasia.

Nuclear Medicine Contrast CT with [^{131}I]Metaiodobenzylguanidine (MIBG). Indicated to visualize pheochromocytoma when biochemical confirmation is inadequate, or to localize extra-adrenal pheochromocytomas.

Other
Stimulatory Tests. Used to rule out Addison disease. Procedure is to infuse synthetic ACTH (cortosyntropin 250 µg or 0.25 mg) and obtain baseline and 1-hour cortisol levels. The cortisol should be double baseline or

reach a serum level of greater than 18 µg/dL (495 nmol/L). If primary adrenal insufficiency is present, ACTH will be elevated; if autoimmune disease exists, antiadrenal antibodies will also be present. If the level is low (less than 18 µg/dL), the diagnosis of primary insufficiency (Addison disease) is confirmed. Secondary adrenal insufficiency can be distinguished by measuring aldosterone levels from the same blood sample. In primary adrenal insufficiency the aldosterone increment will be subnormal.

Suppression Tests.   Used to diagnose mineralocorticoid tumors. Attempt renin suppression (renin stimulates aldosterone release) by volume expansion in the supine position (saline infusion) and obtain serum aldosterone level. To diagnose Cushing disease, perform an overnight dexamethasone suppression test. The patient is given 1.0 mg of dexamethasone orally between 11 PM and midnight. As early as 8 AM, obtain a cortisol level (normal is less than 5.0 µg/dL). If it is high, then Cushing disease or the syndrome may be present. False positives are seen in patients with active alcoholism, depression, obesity, and acute psychologic or physiologic stress. After confirming high cortisol levels, continue workup with evaluation of cortisol suppressibility with a dexamethasone suppression test: 2-day low-dose (0.5 mg/6 hours for 48 hours), or high-dose (6 mg/6 hours for 48 hours). ACTH secretion is measured to determine whether the excess cortisol is due to pituitary versus adrenal pathology (pituitary causes will suppress cortisol, whereas adrenal causes will not). In normal subjects, ACTH secretion will be suppressed and urinary free cortisol levels will decrease to less than 50% of pretreatment level in the low-dose test. In patients with Cushing disease, pituitary ACTH secretion is resistant to suppression from the low dose, so urinary cortisol levels will not decrease as expected. When Cushing disease is present, the high-dose test will yield a reduced urinary free cortisol (50%) from patient's baseline, because it is dependent on pituitary ACTH.

DIFFERENTIAL DIAGNOSIS

Traumatic
Adrenal trauma with hemorrhage may cause adrenal insufficiency.
  Pituitary trauma may cause adrenal insufficiency.
  With *trauma-associated stress*, high cortisol levels may be present.

Infectious
Adrenal infection may cause adrenal insufficiency.
  In *sepsis*, high cortisol levels may be present.

Metabolic
Bartter syndrome is an uncommon metabolic disorder associated with high renin, high aldosterone, and hypokalemia without hypertension.

  Neoplastic.   Not otherwise applicable.

Vascular
Renal artery stenosis can cause high renin with a secondary rise in aldosterone.

Congenital

Multiple endocrine neoplasia II or *III* may be associated with pheochromocytoma.

Acquired

Exogenous cortisol intake may cause cortisol excess symptoms.

With *stress*, high cortisol levels may be present acutely or chronically.

TREATMENT

Adrenal Insufficiency

Cortisol Deficiency

Acute cortisol deficiency potentially causing cardiovascular collapse can be treated with prompt intravenous steroid delivery of a bolus of 100 mg hydrocortisone sodium phosphate or hydrocortisone sodium hemisuccinate in an infusion of 5% dextrose in 1 L of normal saline, followed by a continuous infusion of hydrocortisone to be modified as patient improves over hours to days with steroid replacement adjusted to maintenance levels, with mineralocorticoid resumed if needed.

Chronic treatment involves replacement with exogenous glucocorticoids to achieve physiologic levels. Longer-acting steroids such as prednisone 5.0-7.5 mg/day, given at bedtime, or hydrocortisone 20-25 given every morning and 10-12.5 given at bedtime. Adjust doses according to weight. Patients need education regarding the risks of discontinuing therapy and should wear medical ID bracelets.

In the setting of surgery, acute illness, or trauma, the steroid dosage should be temporarily increased.

Primary Mineralocorticoid Insufficiency

Replacement of mineralocorticoid (not if ACTH deficiency is the only abnormality) with fludrocortisone 0.05-0.15 mg/day if salt intake is adequate (150-200 mmol/day). Check for hyperkalemia, hypertension, and edema formation and adjust regimen accordingly.

Adrenal Excess

Cortisol Excess

Treatment depends on etiology of the excess. Initially, supplement with potassium and high protein intake. In suppression therapy patients need education about the risks of discontinuing treatment and the importance of a slow taper to allow endogenous corticosteroid production to resume. If symptoms are severe, blocking steroid secretion is feasible with medications such as aminoglutethimide 250 mg two or three times a day, ketoconazole 400 mg/day increasing to a maximum of 1200 mg/day, or metyrapone 2-4 g/day (as adjunctive therapy).

If pituitary tumor is seen on MRI, a transsphenoidal exploration of the pituitary is performed to remove the adenoma. Laparoscopic surgery can be performed to remove adenoma or carcinoma. Despite surgery, the majority of patients with adrenal carcinoma die within 3 years. Lungs or liver metastasis commonly occur. Adjuvant radiation therapy may be indicated for residual tumor.

Primary medical treatment of adrenal carcinoma is administration of mitotane, an isomer of the insecticide DDT. Begin with 0.5 g three to four times a day, gradually increasing to tolerability, typically around 6 g daily. Higher doses may be necessary though gastrointestinal and neuromuscular toxicity almost always occurs. The result is a medical adrenalectomy. Mitotane is a cytotoxic drug that is selective for glucocorticoid-secreting cells in the adrenal cortex; it may also affect the zona glomerulosa and extra-adrenal tissue producing the same. Urinary and plasma cortisol levels must be measured to determine mitotane efficacy.

Mineralocorticoid Excess
Surgery, usually laparascopic, if tumor is present.

Medical therapy with spironolactone initially at 25-100 mg/8 hours, with a taper once blood pressure and potassium are normalized. Chronic therapy in men is often limited by untoward side effects including gynecomastia, decreased libido, and impotence.

Amiloride or spironolactone can also be used. Hypertension secondary to idiopathic adrenal hyperplasia is usually not responsive to bilateral adrenalectomy.

Pheochromocytoma
Surgical excision of the lesion is essential, preceded by α-adrenergic blockade with phenoxybenzamine 10 mg/12 hours, at least 10 to 14 days before surgery. Increments of 10 mg/12 hours, for at least 10 to 14 days are usually added every few days until the blood pressure is controlled and stable. Paroxysmal variations in blood pressure can be managed with oral prazosin or intravenous phentolamine. Generous salt intake concomitantly will preserve adequate plasma volume.

PEDIATRIC CONSIDERATIONS

If hypertension, obesity, or striae are present in the pediatric age group, need to exclude Cushing syndrome, mineralocorticoid excess, and pheochromocytoma.

If hypokalemia is present, need to exclude Cushing syndrome, metabolic enzyme deficiency, and mineralocorticoid excess.

If the patient presents with short stature, obesity, early puberty, virilization, or early acne, need to exclude cortisol excess and androgen excess state such as congenital adrenal hyperplasia.

OBSTETRIC CONSIDERATIONS

Adrenal Insufficiency

Addison disease is rare in pregnancy. In some cases, pregnancy can occasionally lead to the development of adrenal insufficiency. The disorder is difficult to detect, as many of the symptoms (e.g., chronic fatigue, weakness, weight loss, anorexia, increased skin pigmentation, hypoglycemia) are symptoms also attributable to pregnancy. Continued weight loss, nausea, and vomiting should alert the clinician to the possibility of adrenal insufficiency. Infants born to mothers with adrenal insufficiency are normal and almost never exhibit evidence of adrenal supression.

Adrenal Excess

Pregnancy rarely occurs in patients with adrenal hyperfunction, as oligomenorrhea or amenorrhea is present in 75% of cases. If a patient does become pregnant, increased fetal loss and premature labor are possible. However, neonatal adrenal insufficiency rarely occurs as a result of adrenal hyperfunction in the mother.

If adrenal hyperfunction develops in a pregnant patient, the underlying cause is usually an adrenal tumor. The dexamethasone supression screening test, which is used in many cases to aid in diagnosis, is not useful in the pregnant patient owing to elevated levels of transcortin and corticosteroid-binding globulin, which elevate plasma cortisol levels.

If adrenalectomy is chosen as treatment, the patient has an improved chance of delivering a normal infant.

GERIATRIC CONSIDERATIONS

Chronic illness requiring medication use is more common in the elderly population. Always consider medications as the cause of adrenal insufficiency or excess.

PREVENTIVE CONSIDERATIONS

Abrupt cessation and excess use of exogenous steroids can cause symptoms of adrenal disease. Use steroid medications as indicated, and taper the dosage when and if they are to be discontinued.

Diabetes Mellitus

Ann M. Griwatz, PA-C, and Michaela C. Gallagher-Gonzales, PA-C

DEFINITION

Diabetes mellitus (DM) is a group of chronic metabolic disorders characterized by chronic, abnormal metabolism of glucose and lipids resulting in hyperglycemia and hyperlipidemia.

Diabetes is categorized as type 1 and type 2. Type 1 DM, previously known as insulin-dependent diabetes mellitus (IDDM) or juvenile-onset diabetes, is hyperglycemia due to absolute insulin deficiency attributed to autoimmune- or viral-mediated pancreatic beta cell destruction.

Type 2 DM, previously known as non–insulin-dependent diabetes mellitus (NIDDM), is a hyperglycemic condition secondary to inadequate insulin production and/or insulin resistance.

HISTORY

Symptoms

Type 1 DM. Symptomatic hyperglycemia: polyuria, polydipsia, polyphagia, weight loss, and fatigue. Glucosuria-induced osmotic diuresis leading to dehydration. Hyperglycemia causes blurred vision and nausea/vomiting and leads to frequent fungal or bacterial infections. Diabetic ketoacidosis (DKA) is not uncommon. DKA is rare in type 2 DM.

Type 2 DM. Asymptomatic until glucose is high. Often manifests like type 1 DM with symptomatic hyperglycemia: polydipsia, polyuria, polyphagia, blurred vision, pruritus, recurrent skin and vaginal infections (fungal and bacterial), paresthesias, and obesity. Glucosuria-induced osmotic diuresis leading to dehydration.

General

Type 1 DM accounts for about 10% to 20% of all cases of DM. Type 2 DM accounts for 80% to 90% of the cases.

Obtain a full and complete history of risk factors and complications in known and new diabetics. Estimate the control the patient has from self-monitoring of blood glucose, and assess the patient's understanding of the disease and how dietary and eating patterns affects glucose. Ask about the level of physical activity and whether a diabetic educator or nutritionist is involved. Inquire about burning sensation of feet (possible neuropathy), blurred vision, thirst, polyuria, erectile dysfunction, and occurrence of hypoglycemic episodes.

Age

Type 1 DM. Usually develops in childhood or adolescence but may begin at any age.

Type 2 DM. Generally affects persons older than 40 years of age but more often seen in overweight, physically inactive children and teens.

Onset

Type 1 DM. Typically gradual, but 20% to 30% of patients will present acutely with DKA

Type 2 DM. Gradual development of postprandial hyperglycemia, prior to the elevation of fasting glucose, often several years prior to symptoms.

Duration

Type 1 DM. Lifelong. May have some C-peptide and may be able to use oral medications until insulin exhausted.

Type 2 DM. Progressive loss of beta cell function. May eventually need insulin.

Intensity

Types 1 and 2 DM. Usually mild, but may be incapacitating at any stage of illness. Acute onset requires intensive treatment.

Aggravating Factors

Types 1 and 2 DM. Dietary indiscretion, physical illness, lack of exercise, trauma, noncompliance with insulin or medical regimen, certain medications (e.g., thiazide diuretics, phenytoin, prednisone). Patients with type 1 DM should be careful not to exercise excessively as their insulin is exogenous, so they are at unique risk for hypoglycemia

Alleviating Factors

Type 1 DM. Tight control of hyperglycemia with proper insulin regimen and dietary compliance. Maintaining hemoglobin A_{1c} (Hgb A_{1c}) below 7% of total hemoglobin minimizes complications.

Type 2 DM. Weight loss, dietary compliance, exercise, and medical compliance. Maintaining Hgb A_{1c} below 7% minimizes complications.

Associated Factors

Type 1 DM. Metabolic alkalosis can occur. Patients often have a compromised immune response and hypertension.

Complications of diabetes are macrovascular—strokes, myocardial infarction (MI), and peripheral vascular disease—and microvascular—retinopathy, nephropathy, neuropathy, and predisposition to infections.

The risk for MI with diabetes is equal to that in a nondiabetic patient who has already had a coronary event.

Type 2 DM. Hypertension, hyperlipidemia, compromised immune response, and atherosclerosis leading to silent coronary artery disease. Diabetic nephropathy occurs in less than a third of the patients; symptoms are similar to those seen with type 1 DM.

PHYSICAL EXAMINATION

General. Type 1 DM patients are typically lean, whereas type 2 DM patients are generally overweight. Postural hypotension indicates a depleted plasma volume in type 1 DM, secondary to diuresis occurring in the body's attempt to unload the excess glucose. Obesity (usually localization of fat deposits on the upper segments of the body) and mild hypertension are common in type 2 DM.

Cardiovascular. Evaluate for heart murmurs, abdominal bruits, decreased peripheral pulses particularly in the lower extremities.

Head, Eyes, Ears, Nose, Throat. Funduscopic examination should be performed to evaluate for cataracts, hemorrhages, microaneurysms, exudates, changes in vessel caliber, and cotton-wool spots.

Neurologic. Evaluate sensation using all modalities including touch, temperature, proprioception, and vibratory sense; all are decreased in patients with peripheral neuropathy.

Skin. Eruptive xanthomas on the eyelids and flexor surfaces of limbs and buttocks are not uncommon. Erythematous, violaceous plaques on the anterior surfaces of the lower legs due to necrobiosis lipoidica diabeticorum are rare. It is not uncommon to see brownish atrophic lesions in the pretibial regions. Candidal infections can produce edema, erythema, and papular rash in intertriginous regions of the vagina, breasts, and axillae and between the fingers. Examine the feet for onychomycosis, tinea pedis, and ulcers.

Thyroid. Size, presence of nodules.

PATHOPHYSIOLOGY

Type 1 DM

Patients with type 1 DM are genetically predisposed (95% of patients possess human leukocyte antigen (HLA)-DR3 or -DR4, or both) to autoimmune destruction of pancreatic beta cells. Clinical onset of type 1 DM may occur years after this autoimmune process begins. Only 10% to 12% of patients diagnosed with type 1 DM have first-degree relatives who carry the same diagnosis. Concordance rate among monozygotic twins is about 50%. Type 1 DM is a response triggered by the development of antibodies to the serum islet cell cytoplasmic antibodies and islet cell surface antibodies (grossly equal numbers of antibodies to glutamic acid decarboxylase and insulin are found). Viral etiology is suspected, with the development of Type 1 DM after viral infections seasonally. Beta cell damage may result from cytokines.

Although the presentation of type 1 DM may be acute (with DKA), declining C-peptide levels may be seen up to 8 years prior to the diagnosis of diabetes. From 80% to 90% of the insulin-secreting beta cells must be destroyed before hyperglycemia develops. Circulating insulin is virtually absent within a year of onset of diabetes as a result of the absence of endogenous secretion; despite the presence of insulinogenic stimuli, plasma glucagon level is elevated.

Type 2 DM

Impaired insulin secretion, peripheral insulin resistance, and increased hepatic glucose production characterize type 2 DM. DKA is rare, although nonketotic, hyperglycemic-hyperosmotic coma (NKHHC) can develop. Adults are most commonly affected, although adolescents and children can develop type 2 DM. The majority of these patients have an element of tissue insensitivity to insulin irrespective of their weight. Insulin resistance is aggravated by the aging process and abdominal visceral obesity, with a postreceptor defect and decreased insulin binding to plasma membrane receptors. Commonly a state of hyperinsulinemia exists early in the disease, although ultimately patients have insulin levels below those of normal persons at similar levels of glycemia. Genetic predisposition plays a similar role in the incidence of type 2 DM; concordance rate among monozygotic twins is greater than 90%.

Weight loss can lead to a state of normoglycemia. Diet and exercise, with or without oral medication, can treat type 2 DM effectively, though sometimes episodic or chronic insulin management is required to correct severe hyperglycemia and NKHHC. Previous reference to type 2 DM as "non–insulin-dependent DM" is no longer accurate owing to the need for insulin in many cases.

DIAGNOSTIC STUDIES

Laboratory

Urinalysis.   Glucosuria and ketonuria are frequently seen.

Fasting Blood Glucose.   A fasting (greater than 8 hours) blood glucose level (BG) of 126 mg/dL or higher on more than one occasion establishes the diagnosis in patients. Symptomatic hyperglycemia (e.g., polyuria, polidipsia) plus a random BG of 200 mg/dL or greater is also sufficient to make a diagnosis of DM. Diagnosis based on these criteria should be confirmed on a subsequent day. BG between 110 and 125 indicates impaired glucose tolerance (IGT), a state that tends to precede type 2 DM. Normoglycemia is defined by glucose levels of 65-109 mg/dL.

Oral Glucose Tolerance Test (OGTT).   Used if fasting glucose levels are borderline for diagnosis and clinical suspicion is high. Diagnosis of type 2 DM is established by a blood glucose level greater than 200 mg/dL, 2 hours after a 75-g glucose load. Diagnosis is IGT if 2-hour post-load glucose is 140-199 mg/dL; normoglycemia is defined as a glucose level below 140 mg/dL.

Glycosylated Hemoglobin (Hgb A_{1c}).   Indicates the degree of control over the previous 12 weeks. Goal is 7.0% or less for fewer complications. (The American Society of Clinical Endocrinologists recommends A_{1c} of less than 6.5%.) With very tight control, risk of hypoglycemia is greater. The A_{1c} is not used for diagnosis, but if elevated on screening it prompts more careful evaluation to diagnose diabetes. Monitor twice a year if DM is controlled (7.0 or less), more frequently (every 3 months) if it is not. An A_{1c} greater than 8.0 prompts a change in diabetes management

Serum Insulin Level.   May be elevated in some type 2 DM patients. Using an insulin sensitizer such as metformin can help to normalize insulin in prediabetic and diabetic states.

C-Peptide.   An indicator of the patient's ability to produce insulin, indicating whether oral medicines would be effective. Evaluate in a fasting state after initially high glucoses have been controlled.

Blood Urea Nitrogen (BUN)/Creatinine Levels.   Are frequently elevated in diabetic nephropathy. After approximately 5 years, patients with type 1 DM develop albuminuria not associated with other urinary tract disease. This indicates impending end-stage renal disease within 3 to 20 years.

Lipid Profile.   Elevated fasting triglycerides (250 mg/dL) and decreased high-density lipoprotein cholesterol (35 mg/dL) are frequently seen in type 2 DM patients.

Vitamin B_{12} and Folate.   Deficiency implicated in neuropathy. Maintain in mid-normal range (around 500 mg). Monitor if giving metformin, which can interfere with the absorption of vitamin B_{12}. If levels are lower than desired, supply vitamin in injection form followed by oral supplementation (to maximize effect).

Radiology.   Not applicable.

Other
ECG.   Frequently normal but may show evidence of ischemia (T wave inversion, ST segment elevation) in patients with microvascular disease; patients are often without chest pain or other relevant symptoms of ischemia.

DIFFERENTIAL DIAGNOSIS

Traumatic
Not applicable, although glucose may be elevated from stress.

Infectious
With *asymptomatic urinary tract infection* (UTI) or *vaginitis* due to *Candida*, polyuria may be present. Usually differentiated as UTI by the presence of

pyuria, bacteriuria, or a positive urine culture. UTIs frequently lead to an exacerbation of DM, especially if untreated.

Metabolic

In *diabetes insipidus*, patients present with polyuria and polydipsia. No evidence of hyperglycemia or glucosuria; normoglycemia.

In *Cushing syndrome*, abnormal results on dexamethasone suppression test or an increased 24-hour urinary free cortisol (greater than 100 mg/24 hours); CT scan may reveal adrenal neoplasm.

In *renal tubular disease/benign renal glucosuria*, glucosuria without hyperglycemia.

In *hypothyroidism/hyperthyroidism*, abnormal thyroid function studies.

In *cirrhosis*, elevated values on liver function studies, history of hepatitis or alcohol abuse.

In *pancreatitis*, elevated serum amylase and lipase. May have history of alcohol abuse or cholelithiasis.

Neoplastic

With *pheochromocytoma*, elevated plasma catecholamines, 24-hour urine metanephrine or vanillylmandelic acid; CT scan may reveal neoplasms of the adrenal medulla.

With *glucagonoma* of pancreatic alpha cells, positive CT scan of pancreas. *Adrenal neoplasm* will be seen on CT of the abdomen.

Vascular

In *anemia*, decreased hemoglobin and hematocrit. May have nutritional deficiency.

Congenital

With *hypoglycemia in the neonate* when gestational diabetes is present in the mother, affected children may have an increased incidence of obesity when they have reached teen years and an increased risk of DM.

Acquired

In *depression*, history of anhedonia, sleep disturbance, disturbed appetite, decreased libido.

Medication-induced hyperglycemia may be caused by steroids, sympathomimetic drugs, niacin/nicotinic acid, thiazide diuretics, phenytoin, pentamidine, minoxidil, hormones containing high-androgenic progesterones, megestrol acetate, protease inhibitors, interferons, and growth hormone.

TREATMENT

The major goals of management are normalization of blood glucose levels, prevention of microvascular and macrovascular complications, and helping

the patient achieve as normal lifestyle as is possible. These goals are achieved by the following measures:
- Patient education
- Diet
- Exercise
- Oral hypoglycemic agents, including insulin secretagogues
- Insulin

Specifics for each aspect of treatment follow.

Patient Education
A team approach (provider, certified diabetic educator, and nutritionist) to treatment is crucial. Patient and family members need to understand the treatment plan with 100% clarity.

Diet
The goals of dietary management are slightly different in type 1 DM and type 2 DM patients.

Type 1 DM
An American Diabetic Association (ADA) diet stresses the major goal of calorie restriction as a means of achieving or maintaining ideal weight. Also, it is essential to match the time and level of insulin intake to the caloric intake (less than 10% saturated fat). This includes a restriction of fat intake to less than 35% of total calories and reduction of cholesterol intake to less than 300 mg daily. Carbohydrates can be ingested liberally (as much as 60% of total calories) as long as refined and simple carbohydrates are avoided as snacks. Percentage of total calories from protein should be 15% to 20%. Saccharin and aspartame are noncaloric sweeteners, while sorbitol and fructose are caloric sweeteners, none of which alter the glycemic control. Carbohydrate counting can be instituted, covering the number of grams eaten with rapid-acting insulin in a ratio of 1 unit to 10 to 20 grams of carbohydrate.

Type 2 DM
For the obese patient, weight reduction by calorie restriction and low fat intake. Address the cardiovascular risk factors of hypertension and dyslipidemia. Low-calorie diets and modest weight reduction often lead to measurable reduction of glycemia. Long-term weight reduction is rare. Increased intake of dietary fiber is encouraged to improve glycemic control and correct lipid abnormalities. Exercise reduces hyperglycemia and insulin resistance.

Exercise
Asymptomatic cardiac changes occur at younger ages in both type 1 and type 2 DM patients. Exercise tolerance cardiac testing should be done for both groups at 35 years of age. Also indicated is close monitoring for other

microvascular complications including nephropathy and albuminuria, retinopathy, peripheral vascular disease, and neuropathy. Vigorous exercise is contraindicated in untreated proliferative retinopathy. Moderate-intensity aerobic exercise three to four times a week for 30 to 45 minutes is beneficial. Exercise helps to reduce insulin resistance, lowers glucose, increases the sense of well-being, and aids in weight loss when combined with reduced caloric intake. It also enhances insulin absorption. Insulin is more rapidly absorbed when injected into a limb that is exercised, which can result in hypoglycemia.

Oral Hypoglycemic Agents
Insulin Secretagogues (e.g., Sulfonylureas)
Used in patients with type 2 DM when diet and exercise fail to normalize blood glucose level. Sulfonylureas work best when administered before a meal, as they increase the postprandial insulin output from the pancreas. These agents are contraindicated in patients with a sulfa allergy. Second-generation agents (glyburide, glipizide) are safer than older agents because of their shorter half-life, lower incidence of associated hypoglycemia and drug interactions, and ability to be excreted in the bile in patients with renal disease. Capable of causing hypoglycemia and some weight gain. Because the major side effect is hypoglycemia, patients should be started on the lowest effective dose with the dosage increased every 1 to 2 weeks until the maximum effective dosage is reached.

First-Generation Sulfonylureas:
Chlorpropamide (Diabinase): 100-750 mg given orally every day

Second-Generation Sulfonylureas:
Glyburide (DiaBeta, Micronase, Glynase Prestab): 1.25-20 mg given every day or twice a day
Glipizide (Glucotrol): 2.5-40 mg given every day or twice a day
Glucotrol LR: 5-10 mg every day, maximum of 20 mg daily; maximum doses should be split in doses twice a day
Glimepiride (Amaryl): 1-4 mg daily, maximum of 8 mg per day

Amino Acid Derivative Insulin Secretagogue:
Nateglinide (Starlix): 120 mg at 1 to 30 minutes prior to meals, three times a day

Biguanides
Metformin (Glucophage) works for patients with type 2 DM by reducing insulin resistance and decreasing hepatic gluconeogenesis. It is effective for monotherapy with very low risk of hypoglycemia and weight gain. Metformin also has a lipid-lowering effect and can be used to good benefit with sufonylureas. Gastrointestinal side effects are common but often temporary and can be prevented if these agents are taken with meals. Metformin is contraindicated in patients with renal or hepatic disease.

Metformin (Glucophage): 500 mg usually twice a day, up to 2550 mg a day, in two or three divided doses

Combination Biguanide and Sulfonylurea
Glyburide + metformin (Glucovance): 1.25/250-20/2000 mg in a single dose (with low doses) or divided doses (with higher doses)

Alpha-Glucosidase Inhibitors
An adjunctive agent for use in patients with type 2 DM. It delays carbohydrate absorption in the small intestine, thereby reducing the incidence of postprandial hyperglycemia. Gastrointestinal side effects are common and often temporary and can be avoided if the drug is taken with meals.

Miglitol (Glyset): 25-100 mg three times a day with first bite of meals

Acarbose (Precose): 25-100 mg three times a day with first bite of meals

Thiazolidinediones
Troglitazone reduces insulin resistance in skeletal muscle and may preserve pancreatic beta cell function. Moderate reduction in hyperglycemia and triglycerides can be achieved with this drug, which can be used for monotherapy or in conjunction with metformin, insulin, or sulfonylureas. Side effects include hepatotoxicity.

Rosiglitazone (Avandia): 4-8 mg/day in a single dose

Pioglitizone (Actos): 15-30 mg once daily, maximum of 45 mg/day

Metiglinides
Repaglinide (Prandin): 0.5-4 mg within 30 minutes of meals two to four times daily

Insulin
Indicated for all patients with type 1 DM and for type 2 DM patients in whom glucose is inadequately controlled by diet, exercise, and oral hypoglycemic agents.

Species Sources
Human insulin is now available in synthetic preparations and is the favored choice owing to less antigenicity compared with animal insulins. Animal insulin preparations include beef and pork insulins and a combination of the two.

Types of Insulins
Rapid-acting insulins: lispro (Humalog) or aspart (NovoLog); onset at 15 minutes, duration 3 hours. Used at mealtimes on a sliding scale and in insulin pumps. Less postprandial hypoglycemia than with regular insulin. Taken immediately prior to a meal. Do NOT use at bedtime; may cause nighttime hypoglycemia.

Regular insulin: onset at 0.5 hour, peak at 1 to 5 hours, duration 24 hours. More likely to be associated with hypoglycemia than the rapid-acting insulins. Taken 30 minutes before meals.

Isophane (NPH—neutral protamine Hagedorn) or zinc suspension: onset at 1 to 3 hours, peak at 6 to 12 hours, duration 18 to 24 hours. May be added to oral regimen when A_{1c} is insufficiently controlled.

NPH/aspart/lispro mixtures (75/25 or 70/30 mixtures of NPH and aspart): intended to provide extended and short-term (postprandial) control of glucoses. Do NOT use at bedtime; may cause nighttime hypoglycemia.

A "24-hour-acting insulin," glargine (Lantus), has been developed; its action resembles continuous insulin infusion. This longer-acting insulin has an onset of action at 1.5 hours and duration of at least 20.5 hours. Glargine has no true peak onset and should prevent nocturnal hypoglycemia. Start low dose at bedtime; adjust dose upward by 1 unit every night until fasting blood glucose is in target range. If switching over from previous insulin regimen, begin at 70% of previous total insulin dose and adjust upward. Glargine should be used with rapid-acting or short-acting insulin (e.g., lispro) before meals. Or may consider adding to an oral agent regimen. Long-term safety of glargine remains to be established.

Dosing Considerations

Intensive insulin treatment for type 1 diabetes involves multiple daily injections or the use of an insulin pump and frequent self-monitoring of glucose. It involves considerable patient education about diet, specifically on carbohydrate counting and self-management. The insulin regimen is designed to emulate the normal secretion of insulin in a nondiabetic individual. Formulas are provided to guide the patient in choosing insulin doses based on dietary carbohydrate consumption and the individual's response to the fast-acting insulin.

Trials of inhaled, nasal spray, and transdermal insulin are ongoing, as well as studies of the effectiveness of islet cell transplantation.

Patients receiving insulin self-monitor blood glucose before breakfast, lunch, and dinner; at bedtime (urine glucose measurements have decreased specificity); and when symptomatic. The results of these levels form the basis for adjusting the insulin dosage. Insulin sites should be rotated on a daily basis. The most efficient sites for absorption are the anterior abdominal wall, anterior thighs, and posterior arms. It is crucial to clean the injection site and to avoid areas of inflammation, scarring, and lipoatrophy.

The frequency of monitoring for type 2 diabetes is dictated by the level of control, with more frequent monitoring done when the A_{1c} indicates need for tighter control. Intensive insulin therapy produces better control in type 1 diabetics. The Diabetes Control and Complications Trial has shown reduced complications with good control, with hemoglobin A_{1c} of 7.0 or below.

If insulin needs to be added to the oral regimen, it can begin with the BIDS regimen (*b*edtime *i*nsulin, *d*aytime *s*ulfonylureas or other oral agents). Begin with small dose at bedtime; adjust according to FBS readings. As beta cell function deteriorates, oral agents become less likely to control glucose levels, and other insulin is added as the oral agents are discontinued (NPH or glargine at bedtime). Consider giving NPH at suppertime if use at bedtime causes early morning hypoglycemia.

The dosage requirement for subcutaneous insulin is decided on an individual basis. In general, adults require less insulin (0.6-0.8 U/kg/day) than adolescents (1-1.5 U/kg/day). Insulin dosages are most commonly divided into two or three injections (one injection 20 to 30 minutes before breakfast, dinner, and often bedtime). Usually these injections include a combination of regular plus NPH insulin. Regular insulin will prevent large fluctuations in the blood glucose concentration that result from absorption of carbohydrates from the morning and evening meals. The morning NPH insulin dosage will be active for the noon meal. If adequate, the evening dose of NPH will act throughout the night to maintain suppression of glucose production by the liver.

As a general rule, one-half of the total daily insulin dose (TDD) is given in the morning and one-quarter before dinner and the last quarter before bed. This is frequently subdivided into two-thirds intermediate-acting insulin and one-third short-acting insulin for the morning dose. The dinner dose is further divided into one-sixth short-acting insulin and one-sixth intermediate-acting insulin substituted for the one-third short-acting insulin dose component.

Common Schedules for Insulin Administration
- Two-thirds of total daily dose of NPH and regular insulin (70/30 or similar proportion) in the morning, with the last third before evening meal.
- NPH and regular insulin in the morning, with regular insulin before dinner and NPH insulin at bedtime.
- Regular insulin at each meal, with semilente at bedtime.

Management of Early Morning Hypoglycemia
- Dawn phenomenon is more common in type 1 DM patients than in type 2 DM patients. This refers to a morning rise in plasma glucose concentration with associated rise in ketones that occurs in response to a surge of cortisol and growth hormone, inducing hepatic gluconeogenesis. Diagnosis is established by normal blood glucose level at 3:00 to 4:00 AM and hyperglycemia at 8:00 AM.
- Somogyi effect occurs in patients with type 1 DM, who develop nocturnal hypoglycemia (diagnosis is established by having the patient check blood glucose level at 4:00 AM), which stimulates counterregulatory hormones that produce high blood glucose levels by 7:00 AM.

Waning of circulating insulin levels is the most common cause of morning hyperglycemia.

COMPLICATIONS OF DIABETES MELLITUS AND THEIR TREATMENT

Complications of diabetes mellitus are as follows.

Diabetic Ketoacidosis

DKA is an insulin-deficient, catabolic, hyperglycemic state with overproduction of counterregulatory hormones and dehydration. It results from severe insulin deficiency and osmotic diuresis and is manifested by severe dehydration and alterations in mental status. Physiologic attempts to reduce hyperglycemia induce excess loss of sodium, potassium, and water; this is accompanied by acidosis secondary to hepatic ketone release, causing a metabolic acidosis with subsequent respiratory compensation.

Common etiologic factors for DKA are infection, myocardial infarction, inflammation, poor compliance with medications, surgery, stress, medications (pentamidine, steroids), hormonal changes (pre-ovulation), and trauma. Clinical manifestations include polyuria, polydipsia, orthostatic hypotension, hyperventilation (Kussmaul respirations), tachycardia, fever, and lethargy. Patients often have the characteristic fruity odor of ketones on the breath. Nausea, vomiting, and abdominal pain (may resemble acute abdomen) are common. Laboratory findings in DKA include hyperglycemia (glucose greater than 250 mg/dL), presence of ketones in the blood and/or urine, arterial pH range between 6.8 and 7.3, and an anion gap metabolic acidosis. Patients are treated as follows:

Fluid Replacement. The usual fluid deficit is 0.1 L/kg. Fluid replacement should begin promptly, even before laboratory results have been received. Normal saline (0.9%) is used initially unless the patient is elderly or has a history of congestive heart failure (CHF), in which case 0.45% NaCl is substituted. Give at rate of 1 L/hour for the first 2 to 3 hours, 250 to 500 mL/hour for the next 12 hours. Monitor electrolytes, glucose, ketones, and fluid status. After about two hours of fluid replacement, potassium supplement (10 mEq/L/h) is probably needed if serum K+ is less than 5.5 mEq/L, ECG and serum creatinine are normal, and there is urine output. If the serum K+ is less than 3.5 mEq/L, administer potassium at 40-80 mEq/L/h or give bicarbonate. Continue above until acidosis is resolved and serum glucose concentration drops below 250 mg/dL; change intravenous fluid to $D_{5.45}$ NaCl to protect against excessive osmotic shifts of fluids into the cerebral tissues.

Insulin. Intravenous insulin, 10- to 20-unit bolus of Regular insulin, followed by 5-10 units/hour administered in saline. (500 units Regular in 1 L normal saline to equal 0.5 unit/mL.) Monitor serum glucose hourly for the first 2 hours, then every 2 to 4 hours. Increase insulin dose by 2- to 10-fold if no improvement noted at 2 to 4 hours. When the serum glucose level approaches 250-300 mg/dL, decrease the insulin dosage to 2-3 units/hour and continue this dose until adequate fluid replacement has been achieved and metabolic acidosis has been resolved. The patient can then be restarted on the normal daily insulin regimen.

Investigate for myocardial infarction or other causes of the condition.

Metabolic Acidosis (pH<6.9). Sodium bicarbonate is not favored unless the patient is severely acidotic from sepsis, lactic acidosis. If serum bicarbonate is 6 mEq/L or less or the pH is 7.10 or less (or both), bicarbonate should be given in a sufficient amount to raise the bicarbonate concentration to 10-12 mEq/L.

Monitoring of Therapy. Heart rate, blood pressure, respiratory rate, and mental status should be recorded every 30 to 60 minutes. Serum potassium and bicarbonate, as well as the anion gap and an ECG, should be monitored every 1 to 2 hours. Blood glucose should be monitored hourly by fingersticks. A decrease in the anion gap or an increase in plasma bicarbonate indicates that ketogenesis has been inhibited. Initiate longer-acting insulin when patient is taking food orally.

Complications of Diabetic Ketoacidosis. Complications of DKA include cerebral edema, cardiac dysrhythmias, shock, myocardial infarction, venous thrombosis, and acute pancreatitis.

Nonketotic Hyperglycemic-Hyperosmolar Coma (NKHHC)

State of extreme hyperglycemia (glucose greater than 600-1000 mg/dL), acidosis (pH 7.3 or greater), hyperosmolarity (serum glucose greater than 350 mOsm/L), severe dehydration, prerenal azotemia (uremia); and absence of ketones to mild hyperketonemia. This results in altered mental status, nausea, vomiting, orthostatic hypotension, evidence of dehydration (dry mucous membranes, poor skin turgor), possible seizures, and increased risk of death. This condition is precipitated by a stressful event such as infection, surgery, poor medical compliance, cerebrovascular accident, or myocardial infarction. Alternatively, it can be the presenting condition in a patient with yet undiagnosed type 2 DM. NKHHC can also be induced by peritoneal or hemodialysis, tube feeding, or large intravenous glucose loads. The patient is often elderly and dehydrated from lack of fluid intake or impaired thirst drive.

Treatment. The guidelines for therapy are essentially the same as for diabetic ketoacidosis with the exception of bicarbonate therapy. Hyperosmolality, volume depletion, and free water deficit are more severe in NKHHC. Mortality is also greater in NKHHC. Fluid replacement should be carefully monitored; if it is too rapid, the patient's neurologic function can worsen. Potassium supplement is dictated by and should be adjusted to reflect the improving levels. Insulin therapy is usually necessary. Patients in NKHHC are also more sensitive to insulin than in DKA, requiring smaller doses. Start with 5-10 units followed by 3-7 units/hour continuous infusion. When plasma glucose is at or below 13.9 mmol/L, glucose should be added. Subsequently, insulin is decreased to 1-2 units/hour. Insulin should continue until the patient is taking food orally and shifted to a subcutaneous insulin regimen.

Hypoglycemia

Can occur in any diabetic from a variety of causes. Commonly, a hypoglycemic event occurs after a skipped meal or unusual physical exertion, during menstruation, and with errors in insulin administration (such as giving inappropriate amounts of insulin) or with overdose of an oral agent. Non–drug-induced hypoglycemia can also be caused by hypothyroidism, hypopituitarism, fasting, exercise, severe liver or renal disease, insulin receptor antibodies, islet cell adenoma/carcinoma, mesenchymal tumors, autoimmune disease in nondiabetics, or Addison disease. Medications that can exacerbate hypoglycemia include alcohol, insulin, sulfonylureas, pentamidine, disopyramide, salicylates, and beta blockers, particularly propranolol.

Not all patients with severe hypoglycemia will have autonomic symptoms of palpitations, diaphoresis, nervousness, hunger (attributed to increased sympathetic activity and epinephrine release, particularly those with autonomic dysfunction). Instead, they may experience only neuroglycopenic symptoms of visual changes, irritability, tremor, fatigue, hunger, stupor, light-headedness, paresthesias, or cognitive impairment, or syncope and coma. Some patients experience glucose unawareness, or asymptomatic episodes of hypoglycemia. This may be a maladaptation to previous episodes of hypoglycemia. Strict avoidance of hypoglycemia may reverse the unawareness.

Treatment. Treatment includes ingestion of simple carbohydrates (15 g for a blood glucose of 50-60 mg/dL: 4 oz of fruit juice or regular soda, 1 cup milk, 2 tablespoons of raisins, or 3 glucose tablets). When oral treatment is not reasonable, 1 ampule (50 mL) of $D_{50}W$ is given intravenously. This can be followed by a second ampule or continuous intravenous glucose (usually $D_{50}W$ at 100 to 125 mL/h), depending on the response. For more severe symptoms when patient is less responsive, 1 mg glucagon given by intramuscular injection or honey or glucose gel or jelly in the cheek can be used. Patients who are susceptible to attacks may carry a 1-mg ampule of glucagon for a quick subcutaneous or intramuscular injection followed by oral glucose administration.

Hypertension

The goal of blood pressure control is a pressure of 130/80 mm Hg, and normal blood pressure of 120/70 mm Hg is ideal. Antihypertensive therapy is the treatment of choice. Angiotensin-converting enzyme (ACE) inhibitors are the first-line agents in diabetics. (Do not use in pregnancy). Angiotensin receptor blockers can be used in patients who experience a cough with ACE inhibitors. Thiazide diuretics can affect glucose control. Other choices include calcium channel blockers and beta blockers.

Hyperlipidemia

Statins are more effective in achieving control of hypercholesterolemia. Triglycerides respond to better control of glucose levels (when hyperglycemia is present), to fibrates (gemfibrozil and fenofibrate), and to niacin. A combination of a statin and a long-acting niacin is available for mixed hyperlipidemia. The concomitant use of statins and fibrates increases the risk of myalgias and rhabdomyolysis. Monitor creatine kinase (CK) and muscle symptoms if using together.

Renal Impairment

Obtain a nephrology consultation for patients with creatinine concentrations over 3.5 mg/dL, especially if elevating rapidly. General guidelines are to establish shunt access at creatinine concentrations of 5-6 mg/dL and to start dialysis at 10 mg/dL.

PEDIATRIC CONSIDERATIONS

Diabetes mellitus is the most common childhood endocrine disorder. The predominant form affecting children is type 1 DM. Other forms of diabetes in childhood are uncommon and usually associated with obesity, pancreatic disease (e.g., cystic fibrosis), or a few rare syndromes.

Most children with diabetes are diagnosed early, with the classic symptoms of polyuria and polydipsia. Weight loss of several weeks' duration due to dehydration and calorie loss from glucosuria may be noted. Other common complaints include enuresis in a previously toilet-trained child, fatigue, weakness, and listlessness. Rarely does a child present with severe DKA. If it occurs, there is risk for cerebral edema in children with new-onset diabetes and DKA. If headache starts, give mannitol, 0.5-1 g/kg IV of 20-25% solution.

Serum glucose must be evaluated to exclude glucosuria secondary to a renal tubular defect. An oral glucose tolerance test is rarely necessary in children. A random blood glucose level greater than 200 mg/dL or a fasting blood glucose greater than 126 mg/dL on two occasions is diagnostic.

In patients who do not have ketosis at diagnosis, the presence of anti-islet or anti-insulin antibodies is 90% diagnostic for type 1 DM. For a newly diagnosed nonketoacidotic diabetic, hospitalization is usually not necessary as long as family members receive adequate education and the child is carefully monitored when insulin treatment is begun.

Diabetic education for the patient, family, and caregivers is of utmost importance, including hypoglycemic symptoms and treatment of complications, home monitoring of glucose levels and urine ketone monitoring, and administration of medicines and management of diet, stress, and exercise. Wearing "medical alert" tags should be encouraged.

Synthetic human insulin is recommended for children with newly diagnosed type 1 DM (use of beef- or pork-based preparations can result in insulin antibody formation). Dosage depends on the age and weight of the child and whether any endogenous insulin is still being produced, as well as on the presence of ketonuria. A newly diagnosed diabetic requires a dose of 0.5-0.1 unit/kg/day by subcutaneous injection. In children younger than 5 years of age, in the absence of ketonuria, lower doses of insulin (0.2-0.5 unit/kg) may be adequate. Established diabetics usually require 0.7-1.0 unit/kg/day. In an obese child or during adolescence, the dose usually increases to 1.3 units/kg/day.

Twice-daily injection of a combination of regular insulin plus an intermediate-acting (NPH) insulin is recommended to approximate the physiologic insulin release in a nondiabetic state. Approximately two-thirds of the total dose is usually given before breakfast and the other one-third before dinner. Careful adjustment of the total daily insulin dose must reflect response patterns documented by blood glucose testing over several days.

Many children with newly diagnosed diabetes exhibit a "honeymoon" phase, in which the initial dose of insulin will need reduction (to as low as 0.5 unit/kg) to keep glucose levels within normal range. This phase eventually stops as beta cell destruction continues, and the patient becomes completely insulin dependent. The child with diabetes will eventually need to learn to self-administer insulin, approximately around 10 years of age. Insulin pens may be easier for the child to handle. Insulin pumps are successfully used in children.

Dietary management of diabetic children includes a consistent balanced diet with age-appropriate calorie intake and consistent meal schedule. Children require approximately 1000 calories plus 100/year of age daily. Fat intake should be restricted to approximately 30% of total calories. Carbohydrates should account for 55% to 60%, and the remainder should be derived from protein. The diet should contain complex carbohydrates, and the use of refined sugar and simple carbohydrates should be minimized. Cholesterol and intake of saturated fats should be reduced. The daily eating pattern (both meals and snacks) should remain consistent in time and intake. Younger children usually have three meals and three snacks a day. Breakfast and lunch should each account for approximately two-tenths of total daily calorie intake, dinner three-tenths, and snacks (mid-morning, mid-afternoon, bedtime) each one-tenth. Older children often omit the mid-morning snack, and these calories may be added to breakfast or lunch.

Referral to a nutritionist is an important component of diabetes management. Patients should consult with a nutritionist twice a year.

Regular aerobic exercise should be encouraged to foster a sense of well-being, promote social interaction, maintain proper weight and blood pressure, and improve glucoregulation and lipid metabolism. The benefits of exercise outweigh the risks of hypoglycemia during and following exercise. An additional carbohydrate exchange for every 30 minutes of exercise consumed 30 minutes before activity may prevent hypoglycemic reactions.

Hypoglycemia (insulin reaction) is the most commonly encountered complication. It occurs suddenly, with the common symptoms being tremor, weakness, headaches, decreased alertness, hunger, sweating, restlessness, and behavioral changes. If hypoglycemia is left untreated, central nervous system glucopenia may result in confusion, loss of consciousness, and seizure. Concentrated simple sugar such as 2 to 3 small candies or a nondietetic soft drink should be given. If a meal is not anticipated within an hour, a complex carbohydrate and fat/protein-containing snack should be consumed. Subcutaneous glucagon, 0.5 mg for a child or 1.0 mg for an adolescent, should be given if the patient is unresponsive or unable to swallow.

Check urine ketones in hyperglycemia with glucose over 250 mg/dL and during illness. If moderate or marked ketonuria is present, the patient should seek treatment. A dose of regular insulin equivalent to 10% to 20% of the total daily dose should be administered subcutaneously every 3 hours until the urine ketones are significantly reduced or negative. Drinking juices and other fluids should be encouraged. If Kussmaul respirations, fruity or acetone odor to the breath, or other signs of metabolic acidosis develop, the patient should be evaluated in a medical facility immediately.

Monitor Hgb A_{1c} every 3 months. The child's growth, neurologic functioning, social interactions, and response to the disease, as well as control of glucose levels, should be evaluated. Query about any diabetic complications such as peripheral neuropathy, visual changes, and so on. Maintain growth charts at each visit. With every visit, monitor blood pressure and peripheral pulses and perform funduscopic and neurologic examinations.

Yearly laboratory studies should include urinalysis, blood urea nitrogen (BUN), creatinine, cholesterol, triglycerides, thyroid antibodies, and thyroid-stimulating hormone. A 24-hour urine collection for microalbumin and creatinine clearance should be done to assess for proteinuria. An annual referral for an ophthalmologic examination is recommended.

OBSTETRIC CONSIDERATIONS

There are two categories of diabetes mellitus that can occur in the pregnant patient; chronic DM and gestational diabetes. There is a 9% to 12% occurrence of gestational diabetes and less than 1% incidence of type 1 DM. In gestational diabetes insulin requirements increase, as can resistance, leading ultimately to hyperglycemia.

Prior to a planned pregnancy, optimize glucose control in the diabetic patient. In nondiabetic patients, screening for diabetes is performed at 28 weeks; DM developing during pregnancy needs the same attention to strict control. Initially in the pregnancy there is increased insulin sensitivity, and hypoglycemia risk exists for type 1 (particularly with hyperemesis gravidarum), so control can be eased to just above A_{1c} levels of 7.0%, but in the second and third trimesters insulin resistance increases, and the dose of insulin needed in type 1 diabetics may double.

All obstetric patients should be screened for glucose intolerance. Borderline or latent diabetic conditions may become clinically apparent when the patient becomes pregnant owing to an alteration in glucose tolerance brought on by pregnancy.

Criteria for Gestational Diabetes

Fasting glucose of greater than 125 mg/dL or postprandial or random glucose greater than 200mg/dL

50-g glucose solution challenge: glucose greater than 140 mg/dL. (If greater than 130 mg/dL, proceed to 3-hour glucose tolerance test.)

100-g glucose tolerance test: perform fasting after 3 days of unrestricted carbohydrate diet (positive is meeting or exceeding two values; if only one is positive, repeat in one month).

Fasting glucose of 95 mg/dL or greater

1-hour glucose: 180 mg/dL

2-hour glucose: 155 mg/dL

3-hour glucose: 140 mg/dL

Gestational Diabetes Treatment

Exercise and diet with carbohydrate restriction. Insulin if fasting glucose levels are greater than 95 mg/dL or 2-hour postprandial glucoses are greater than 120 mg/dL. Oral medications are contraindicated, as is the use of ACE inhibitors. Serial ultrasound examinations are used to evaluate for possible macrosomia. Recommend restriction of weight gain

A mother with diabetes is at increased risk of developing pregnancy-induced hypertension, preeclampsia, chronic hypertension, hyperglycemia, glucosuria, hydramnios, urinary tract infections, pyelonephritis, and antepartum and postpartum infections. There is also the possiblilty of progression of retinopathy and nephropathy, and of the development of DKA at a lower glucose than when the patient is not pregnant. Infants are at risk for congenital defects, macrosomia, prematurity, and respiratory distress syndrome. During the perinatal period there is the possibility of the infant's manifesting hypoglycemia, hypocalcemia, hyperbilirubinemia, polycythemia, intrauterine fetal demise, and/or renal vein thrombosis. The overall neonatal mortality rate is 1% to 5%. Thyroid disorders are more frequent following the pregnancy (thyroiditis and hypothyroidism).

Insulin therapy needs to be instituted if the fasting blood sugar is greater than 105 mg/dL or if the 2-hour oral glucose tolerance (ingestion of 75-g oral glucose load) test level is greater than 155 mg/dL. The patient should be monitored closely via the fasting and 2-hour postprandial plasma glucose, and intermittent Hgb A_{1c} throughout the pregnancy. Ultrasonographic surveillance should be done at regular intervals during the first two trimesters and every 2 to 4 weeks during the third trimester to screen for the development of fetal macrosomia, anomalies, and developing polyhydramnios. At 15 to 19 weeks of gestation, maternal serum alpha-fetoprotein assay should be done to screen for neural tube defects. Maternal weight gain is recommended at 25 to 35 pounds. Episodes of ketoacidosis should be avoided altogether because of its association with lower intellectual function in the child and possible death. The patient should also have a comprehensive ophthalmologic test every trimester owing to the increased incidence of diabetic retinopathy during pregnancy.

The newly diagnosed diabetic patient should also receive a baseline ECG and undergo determination of 24-hour urine protein and creatinine clearance. Time of delivery must be precisely chosen to avoid the possibility of respiratory distress versus profound glucose alterations in the fetus. The patient must be maintained in a euglycemic state during labor and delivery.

Insulin therapy is recommended over oral hypoglycemic agents, including metformin (pregnancy category B) and the sulfonylureas (depending on the agent, categories B and C).

GERIATRIC CONSIDERATIONS

The elderly often have an altered sense of taste, poorly fitting dentures, decreased mobility, depression or apathy, and financial issues and may have cognitive impairment. All of these may affect compliance, dietary and medical. Patients need to understand the need to eat, particularly when taking sulfonylureas; taking these agents without food can lead to hypoglycemia and resultant risks of confusion and falls.

PREVENTIVE CONSIDERATIONS

Screen patients who are overweight and sedentary, with family history of diabetes, or history of gestational diabetes. Syndrome X or the dysmetabolic state (obesity, hypertension, hypertriglyceridemia, low levels of high-density lipoprotein [HDL], impaired fasting glucose) is a risk factor for development of diabetes.

If the fasting glucose levels are above 95-100 mg/dL, or the 2-hour postprandial glucoses (after a meal with carbohydrate) are above 140, counsel the patient to become more physically active and to lose weight by caloric restriction, especially with fats and, to an extent, carbohydrates. Utilize a diabetic educator or a dietician/nutritionist to assist with dietary management.

Compliance and tight control of serum glucose is important to prevent complications of the disease. A teaching aid: Compare the body with a favorite car you want to preserve to become a classic. You will wax it more often, change the oil, bring it in for tune-ups, and lovingly care for it to have it carry you around in style. The body with diabetes needs the same care, and it will get you where you want to go just fine, with care.

PEARLS FOR THE PA

Only 10% to 20% of diabetics are afflicted with type 1 DM.

Fasting blood sugar of 126 mg/dL or higher on more than one occasion establishes the diagnosis.

The two major goals of management are normalization of blood glucose levels and prevention of microvascular and macrovascular complications.

Human insulin is recommended for newly diagnosed diabetic patients treated with insulin, to prevent allergies and local reactions such as lipoatrophy and the development of insulin antibodies.

Type 2 diabetes, with very high glucose levels, is more effectively managed initially with insulin to bring glucose into the range of 200-250 mg/mL; then oral agents are introduced.

Continued

PEARLS FOR THE PA—cont'd

Hemoglobin A_{1c} should be monitored every 3 months as an objective measure of control and compliance.

If the $HgbA_{1c}$ elevation does not correlate with patient reports of well-controlled glucose, the reason is probably postprandial hyperglycemia.

Metformin is a good first-line agent for the overweight diabetic. It may help the patient to achieve weight loss of a few pounds.

Obtain a glucose monitor for each patient with diabetes or the prediabetic state of impaired glucose tolerance/impaired fasting glucose.

The "white foods" (flour products: bread, tortillas, pastas, white potatoes, white rice) are the foods more likely to raise blood glucose concentrations.

Dyslipidemia

Edward Gaile, Sr., BA, BHS, PA-C, and
Nassoma King, PA-C

DEFINITION

Elevation in serum cholesterol, triglyceride (TG), very-low-density lipoprotein (VLDL), and/or low-density lipoprotein (LDL) levels. Classified as *hypercholesterolemia*, *hypertriglyceridemia*, and *mixed hyperlipidemia*.

HISTORY

Symptoms. Those related to vascular pathology including coronary atherosclerotic heart disease (CASHD), which may be manifested by angina, arrhythmias, dyspnea, cerebrovascular disease with transient or permanent neurologic deficit, or peripheral vascular disease with claudication. The patient may experience abdominal pain, nausea, and vomiting as a result of pancreatitis. With marked elevations in the serum triglyceride level, patients may experience memory defects, joint pain, or paresthesias.

General. A history of atherosclerotic risk factors should be obtained from the patient, such as family history of hypercholesterolemia, CASHD, ileal bypass surgery, hypothyroidism, acute or chronic liver disease, chronic renal failure, lupus, stress, sepsis, alcohol abuse, lipodystrophy, nephrotic syndrome, anorexia nervosa, diabetes mellitus, cigarette smoking, peripheral vascular disease, medication use, and obesity. A full medical history and review of systems should be obtained to evaluate for contributing disorders.

Age. Elevated cholesterol in the young and in infants is usually due to genetic factors, whereas elevated cholesterol due to lifestyle and dietary habits increases in frequency with advancing age. Persons with genetic factors have a mean age for occurrence of myocardial infarction between the fifth and sixth decades.

Onset. Slow and progressive, but many conditions secondary to elevated cholesterol, such as myocardial infarction and stroke, occur acutely.

Duration. Once diagnosis is confirmed, dietary and (possibly) medical management is lifelong. If dyslipidemia is corrected, surveillance may be adequate.

Intensity. Patients may be asymptomatic throughout life. Severe, life-threatening manifestations are related to the secondary effects of vascular disease.

Aggravating Factors. Dietary excess of saturated fatty acids and cholesterol. Obesity, stress, and alcohol contribute to overproduction of VLDL, whereas cigarette smoking, elevated serum triglycerides, physical inactivity, malnutrition, and certain drugs (e.g., beta blockers, anabolic steroids) decrease serum high-density lipoprotein (HDL).

Certain patients who are predisposed may experience a more marked hypertriglyceridemia in response to certain stressors, (e.g., obesity, alcohol, estrogen, isotretinoin, thiazide diuretics, bile acid sequestrants, beta blockers, protease inhibitors, glucocorticoids).

Alleviating Factors. Weight reduction, regular exercise, dietary modification, and control of coexisting disease (e.g., diabetes mellitus).

Associated Factors. Increased risk for CASHD especially in mixed hyperlipidemia. In young or middle-aged men, elevating the serum cholesterol from 200 to 250 mg/dL can double the risk of CASHD. Elevation from 250 to 300 again doubles the risk. Severe cases of dyslipidemia often have a genetic component. Pancreatitis is a risk in patients in whom the serum triglyceride levels exceed 1000 mg/dL.

Underlying medical disorders put patients at higher risk for dyslipidemias: diabetes mellitus, hypothyroidism, liver disease, pituitary dysfunction, steroid or estrogen use, anorexia nervosa, renal disease, and alcohol abuse.

PHYSICAL EXAMINATION

General. The patient generally appears normal. Blood samples appear lipemic (pale and creamy).

Cardiovascular. Vascular bruits and diminished pulses may be present due to atherosclerotic disease.

Extremities. Yellow-white or yellow-orange papules with erythemic halo called xanthomas may be present bilaterally and appear as nodular irregularities in the Achilles and patellar tendons or the extensor tendons of the hands.

Gastrointestinal.   Hepatomegaly and splenomegaly may be encountered. The abdomen may be somewhat distended, tender, or rigid, or rebound tenderness or absence of bowel sounds may be noted in the presence of pancreatitis.

Ophthalmologic.   Facial and lid xanthelasma and corneal arcus may be present. Pale white retinal vessels (lipemia retinalis) may be seen on funduscopy.

Skin.   Xanthomas (eruptive or planar) may be seen on the extensor surfaces such as elbows, knees, buttocks, and other pressure-sensitive areas, and on the palms and in the palmar creases.

PATHOPHYSIOLOGY

LDL is a major atherogenic lipoprotein and the most important cholesterol-carrying protein in the serum. LDL is derived from catabolism of VLDL, which is produced by the liver. It functions as a transport lipoprotein that carries cholesterol, which easily filters into the walls of arteries. Chylomicrons, the largest lipoproteins, carry triglycerides (which are byproducts of ingested dietary fat) from the intestinal mucosa. Both chylomicrons and VLDL undergo enzyme lipolysis to form remnant lipoproteins. Chylomicron remnants are removed by the liver, whereas VLDL remnants can be either removed by the liver or transformed into LDL. These remnants are cholesterol-rich and may play a role in atherogenesis. HDL, conversely, transfers cholesterol from peripheral tissues to the liver for excretion and is therefore antiatherogenic.

Hypertriglyceridemia alone is a risk factor for CASHD and is commonly associated with other lipid and nonlipid risk factors.

DIAGNOSTIC STUDIES

Laboratory

Cholesterol, Triglyceride, HDL, VLDL, and LDL Levels.   Obtained after a 10- to 15-hour fast (see Table 4-1).

Liver Function Tests.   Rule out hepatic disease as a cause for impaired metabolism.

Blood Urea Nitrogen (BUN)/Creatinine Levels.   Rule out nephrotic syndrome as a cause for elevated VLDL/LDL; renal failure can cause elevated TGs and low HDL.

Urinalysis and 24-Hour Urine for Protein.   Rule out nephrotic syndrome as a cause for elevated VLDL/LDL; renal failure can cause elevated TGs and low HDL.

Serum Glucose.   As a screen for diabetes mellitus causing elevated VLDL and TGs and low HDL.

Thyroid Function Test.   Rule out hypothyroidism as a cause for elevated serum LDL/TGs.

Table 4–1. ATP Classification of Lipids and Lipoproteins

Total Cholesterol (mg/dL)	
Desirable	<200
Borderline high	200-239
High	≥240
LDL Cholesterol (mg/dL)	
Optimal	<100
Near optimal/above optimal	100-129
Borderline high	130-159
High	160-189
Very high	≥190
HDL Cholesterol (mg/dL)	
High	≥160
Low	<40
Serum Triglycerides (mg/dL)	
Normal	<150
Borderline high	150-199
High	200-499
Very high	≥500

HDL, high-density lipoprotein; LDL, low-density lipoprotein.
Adapted from National Cholesterol Education Program, Adult Treatment Panel (ATP) III Report, 2001.

Radioimmunoassay and Gel Electrophoresis. May be performed when seeking a specific cause for hyperlipidemia, as it measures an abnormal lipoprotein pattern.

Radiology
Coronary Artery Catheterization/Site-Specific Angiography: Carotid, Cerebral, Aortic, Renal, or Femoral/Popliteal. Performed to evaluate the presence or extent of vascular involvement.

Other
ECG. May show evidence of myocardial ischemia in patients with significant CASHD.

DIFFERENTIAL DIAGNOSIS

Traumatic. Not applicable.
Infectious. Not applicable.

Metabolic
Diabetes mellitus (moderate or untreated) may cause hypertriglyceridemia. Diabetic treatment corrects the deficit.

Uremia and *dialysis* may cause an elevated VLDL and TG and decreased HDL levels.

Hypothyroidism may cause elevations in serum LDL and TGs. Thyroxine replacement reverses the defects.

Nephrotic syndrome/renal failure may increase VLDL, LDL, and TGs and cause low HDL.

Cushing syndrome is due to excess glucocorticoid levels. Associated with elevated VLDL and/or LDL levels.

Pituitary disease (hypopituitarism, acromegaly) may cause elevations in VLDL.

Neoplastic.   Not applicable.
Vascular.   Not applicable.

Congenital
Inborn errors of lipid metabolism may cause elevated lipid levels.

Acquired
Administration of *glucocorticoid* is associated with elevated VLDL and/or LDL levels.

Estrogen or *oral contraceptive therapy* may cause elevations in the VLDL.

Protease inhibitors for HIV infection may cause elevations in triglycerides.

TREATMENT

The goal of therapy is prevention of end-organ disease such as CASHD and atherosclerotic and peripheral vascular disease.

A total cholesterol of less than 200 mg/dL and a serum LDL of 100 mg/dL or lower is the objective. Aggressiveness of therapy depends on the patient's relative risk factors for CASHD. For those patients with multiple risk factors, or with an existing history of CASHD, drug therapy should be initiated with baseline LDL cholesterol of 130 mg/dL in concert with therapeutic lifestyle changes.

Consider deferring drug therapy in persons with high levels of HDL (e.g., pre- and postmenopausal women and young men).

Treat all identifiable underlying deficits such as hypothyroidism, diabetes mellitus, renal disease.

Dietary management varies with the degree of dyslipidemia:

Mild dyslipidemia: Most patients will respond to dietary changes such as reduced intake of saturated fatty acids and cholesterol (e.g., animal fats, egg yolks, whole milk, cream, ice cream, cheese, butter, processed meats). Weight reduction is important. Consider consultation of nutritional support service.

Moderate dyslipidemia: Dietary treatment should be tried for several months before instituting drug therapy. Drug therapy should be reserved for those patients with significant CASHD risk factors.

Severe dyslipidemia: Dietary modification and exercise constitute the first line of therapy. If this approach is unsuccessful, medications should be considered (see Table 4-2). Dietary changes include strict avoidance of cholesterol and saturated and *trans* fatty acids.

Table 4-2. Lipid Drug Therapy

Drug Class	Lipid Effect	Dose* Range: starting dose; maximum dose
HMG CoA reductase inhibitors	LDL cholesterol ↓ 18-55% HDL cholesterol ↑ 5-15% Triglycerides ↓ 7-30%	Lovastatin: 20 mg; 80 mg Pravastatin: 20 mg; 80 mg Simvastatin: 20 mg; 80 mg Fluvastatin: 20 mg; 80 mg Atorvastatin: 10 mg; 80 mg
Bile acid sequestrants	LDL cholesterol ↓ 15-30% HDL cholesterol ↑ 3-5% Triglycerides: No effect	Cholestyramine: 4-16 g; 24 g Colestipol: 5-20 g; 30 g Colesevelam: 2.6-3.8 g; 4.4 g
Nicotinic acid	LDL cholesterol ↓ 5-25% HDL cholesterol ↑ 15-35% Triglycerides ↓ 20-50%	Crystalline: 1.5-3 g; 4.5 g Sustained release: 1-2 g; 2 g Extended release: 1-2 g; 2 g
Fibric acid derivatives	LDL cholesterol ↓ 5-20% HDL cholesterol ↑ 10-35% Triglycerides ↓ 20-50%	Gemfibrozil: 600 mg bid; 1200 mg Fenofibrate: 54-160 mg qd; 160 mg

*Dose per day, unless otherwise specified.
HDL, high-density lipoprotein; HMG CoA, 3-hydroxy-3-methylglutaryl coenzyme A; LDL, low-density lipoprotein.
Adapted from National Cholesterol Education Program, Adult Treatment Panel III Report, 2001.

According to the National Cholesterol Education Program, the recommended caloric intake for hypercholesterolemia is as follows:
- Total fat less than 30%
- Carbohydrates 50% to 60%
- Protein 10% to 20%

Total cholesterol intake should be less than 200 mg daily; 10% to 15% of total caloric intake should be from monounsaturated fats, less than 10% polyunsaturated, and less than 7% saturated.

Bile acid sequestrants improve the action of LDL receptors, binding bile acids in the intestine, increasing the synthesis of new bile acids from cholesterol, and interrupting enterohepatic recycling of bile acid. Bile acid sequestrants can lower LDL 15% to 30%. Gastrointestinal side effects may be encountered with high doses including constipation, abdominal pain, and bloating. These agents may also increase triglycerides.

Nicotinic acid decreases synthesis of LDL and VLDL; the mechanism of action is not understood. Compliance may be reduced owing to the side effects of gastrointestinal distress, pruritus, flushing, and rash. Patients may also develop hepatotoxicity, hyperglycemia, or hyperuricemia.

3-Hydroxy-3-methylglutaryl coenzyme A (HMG CoA) reductase inhibitors are the most efficacious agents. They act by inhibiting cholesterol synthesis by the liver and increasing LDL receptors. Side effects may include liver function abnormalities, severe myopathies, elevated CPK, and lens opacities.

Fibric acids increase LDL and TG hydrolysis, decrease VLDL synthesis, and increase LDL catabolism. Side effects include gastrointestinal distress, myopathy, cardiac arrhythmias, and cholesterol cholelithiasis.

PEDIATRIC CONSIDERATIONS

Infants with certain inborn errors of triglyceride metabolism may manifest an intolerance to fatty foods. Lipid profile studies should be performed if there is a significant family history of significant hyperlipidemia, history of inborn errors of lipid metabolism, and/or complications occurring prior to the age of 50. Pancreatitis may be encountered. Diabetes or glucocorticoid therapy may cause an abdominal pain or "milky" plasma as the result of triglyceride abnormalities.

OBSTETRIC CONSIDERATIONS

Cholesterol levels are usually elevated during pregnancy. During the third trimester, triglycerides will normally be elevated. Dietary intake of fats and cholesterols should NOT be limited during pregnancy.

Most of the antilipidemic drugs are to be avoided during pregnancy unless the benefits of their use justify the risk to the fetus. Cholestryamine is considered relatively safe when used at the recommended dose. Lovastatin and pravastatin are *absolutely contraindicated* owing to findings of skeletal defects in animal safety studies.

GERIATRIC CONSIDERATIONS

Treatment of the geriatric patient with dyslipidemia should be based more on complications and symptoms of vascular disease rather than on laboratory data alone.

PREVENTIVE CONSIDERATIONS

Encourage lifestyle modifications such as weight reduction, exercise, decreased alcohol consumption, and smoking cessation. Aggressive treatment is generally warranted to reduce and prevent atherosclerotic vascular lesions and subsequent complications. Periodic screening should commence at age 35 in men and age 45 in women.

PEARLS FOR THE PA

The primary goal of therapy is prevention of vascular complications (CASHD, stroke).

Consider deferring drug therapy in patients with high levels of HDL.

Always rule out underlying medical conditions.

Aggressive therapy is warranted in patients with multiple risk factors or coexisting CASHD.

Treatment planning should always include therapeutic lifestyle changes regardless of the necessity for drug therapy.

Metabolic Bone Disorders

Daniel Wood, MPAS, PA-C

DEFINITION

Osteomalacia: Defined as excess organic bone matrix secondary to the inability to mineralize bone properly. The usual causes are a lack of vitamin D, calcium, or phosphorus.

Osteoporosis: A skeletal disorder characterized by a progressive decrease in the amount of normal bone mass and a disruption of skeletal microarchitecture, with an increase in bone fragility. High risk of fracture (especially back or hip fracture). Various types occur and may be due to advancing age, excess steroid use, lack of estrogen or androgen, inactivity, and low calcium intake.

Hyperparathyroidism: Hyperparathyroidism represents a loss of homeostasis leading to excessive parathyroid hormone secretion. Primary hyperparathyroidism is usually caused by an adenoma and may be seen in conjunction with multiple endocrine neoplasia. Secondary hyperparathyroidism can be seen with renal failure or four-gland hyperplasia. Both may cause osteitis fibrosa cystica.

Hypoparathyroidism: May be idiopathic or encountered after surgery involving removal of the parathyroid gland, resulting in a deficiency of parathyroid hormone, leading to neuromuscular symptoms secondary to hypocalcemia.

Pseudohypoparathyroidism: Due to peripheral resistance to the effects of parathyroid hormone.

Renal bone disease: May be due to hyperparathyroidism, low 1,25-dihydroxyvitamin D_3 (1,25-$(OH_2)D_3$), or aluminum bone disease from aluminum oral phosphate binders.

Paget disease: A metabolic imbalance, with osteolytic bone formation followed by disorganized excessive bone formation. Results in osteoblastic lesions with sclerosis. This bone structure is weak and prone to fractures.

HISTORY

Symptoms. Height loss, bone pain, proximal muscle weakness (seen with elevated parathyroid hormone) and symptoms of hypercalcemia (e.g., constipation, pancreatitis, or peptic ulcer disease, polyuria and, if the calcium level is high enough, central nervous system changes).

General

Osteoporosis. Multiple nonmodifiable and modifiable risk factors have been found to contribute to osteoporosis. Nonmodifiable risk factors include advanced age, female gender, white/Asian race, family history of osteoporosis, vitamin D resistance, dementia, and lactose intolerance. Modifiable risk factors include smoking, low calcium intake, sedentary lifestyle, low body weight, and low vitamin D intake or insufficient sunlight exposure.

Osteomalacia. May be encountered in patients with decreased sun exposure or decreased dietary intake of vitamin D, and in some malabsorption syndromes.

Paget Disease. The second most common bone disorder that causes abnormal bone growth, which can cause pain. Paget disease occurs in up to 3% of people over age 50. It is not common in people under age 40.

Age. Any, but more common in adults older than age 40.

Onset. Gradual.
Duration. Lifelong.
Intensity. Asymptomatic to severe pain.
Aggravating Factors. Fractures, advancing age, dietary lack of calcium or vitamin D, limited sunlight, renal failure, chronic acidosis, inactivity, and menopause.
Alleviating Factors. Exercise, administration of calcium or selective estrogen receptor modulator for osteoporosis, correction of hyperparathyroidism, correction of vitamin D deficiency in osteomalacia, and calcitonin or diphosphates for Paget disease.

Associated Factors
Osteoporosis. Hyperthyroidism, vitamin D deficiency, or lack of androgen may contribute to osteoporosis.
Osteomalacia. Phosphate-binding antacids, diphenylhydantoin (Dilantin), or gastrointestinal malabsorbtion may contribute to osteomalacia.
Pseudohypoparathyroidism. May cause skeletal abnormalities in children (neck, metacarpals, and metatarsals are short).

PHYSICAL EXAMINATION

General. Patients may appear quite normal unless bone deformity is present such as dowager's hump in osteoporosis.
Cardiovascular. Calcium abnormalities may cause abnormal ECG findings (see Diagnostic Studies).
Extremities. Pseudohypoparathyroidism may cause a short neck, metacarpals, and metatarsals.
Genitourinary. Kidney stones may cause flank pain (associated with hyperparathyroidism and vitamin D excess).
Head, Eyes, Ears, Nose, Throat. Pseudohypoparathyroidism may cause rounded facies.
Neurologic. Pseudohypoparathyroidism may cause mental retardation. Hypercalcemia can cause lethargy and, if the calcium is high enough, coma.
Skin. Dry skin and brittle hair may be seen with chronic hypocalcemia or hypoparathyroidism. Subcutaneous calcium phosphate accumulation with renal failure may cause pruritus, dry skin, secondary infections due to scratching, and subcutaneous nodules.

PATHOPHYSIOLOGY

The skeletal system is a dynamic specialized living organ with constant turnover of its constituents through a process of osteoclastic bone resorption and osteoblastic bone formation. The skeletal system undergoes constant remodeling and is affected by a variety of stimuli. Hormones such as parathyroid hormone, calcitriol ($1,25\text{-}(OH)D_3$), estrogens, and minerals such as calcium, phosphorus, and magnesium all are important in regulation and maintenance of normal bone turnover. Abnormalities in any of these systems may adversely affect bone and cause metabolic disease.

DIAGNOSTIC STUDIES

Laboratory

Calcium. Normal: 8.5-10.5 mg/dL. High to high-normal in hyperparathyroidism, low in hypoparathyroidism and pseudohypoparathyroidism and osteomalacia. Normal in Paget disease or elevated with an elevated alkaline phosphatase.

Phosphate. Normal: 2.3-4.8 mg/dL. Low to low-normal in hyperparathyroidism and osteomalacia. High in hypoparathyroidism and pseudohypoparathyroidism, and normal in Paget disease.

Albumin. Normal: 3.5-5.0 mg/dL. Used to monitor for correction of serum calcium (for every decrease of 1.0 mg/dL of albumin, calcium drops by 0.8 mg/dL).

Intact Parathyroid Hormone. Normal: 10-65 pg/mL. High in hyperparathyroidism and in pseudohypoparathyroidism, low in hypoparathyroidism. May be high in secondary hyperparathyroidism.

Serum 1,25-(OH_2)D_3. Normal: 20-76 pg/mL. Low in hypoparathyroidism and renal failure, elevated in hyperparathyroidism.

Serum Alkaline Phosphatase. Normal: 20-140 IU/L. May be high in osteomalacia, Paget disease, and hyperparathyroidism

24-Hour Urine for Calcium. Normal: 100-300 mg/24 hours. Used to document calcium intake; high in hyperparathyroidism and Paget disease and low in hypoparathyroidism.

Random Urine for Calcium. Normal: 1.0-11.5 mmol/L. Elevated in hyperparathyroidism.

Radiology

Bone Radiographs. Osteopenia may be seen with osteomalacia and osteoporosis. Looser fracture seen in osteomalacia (scapula and long bones). Increased bone resorption in fingers and clavicle ends with hyperparathyroidism. Aids in the diagnosis of pseudohypoparathyroidism if short metacarpal bones are present. Paget disease changes evident in the pelvis or skull.

Bone Densitometry. Quite helpful in determining bone density and fracture risk with osteoporosis.

Bone Scan. Will help in the diagnosis of Paget disease, as affected areas will demonstrate strong uptake of the isotope.

Other

ECG. Hypercalcemia causes a shortened ST segment on decreased corrected Q-T interval. With very high calcium (greater than 16 mg/dL), the T wave widens. With hypocalcemia, the ST segment is lengthened and the corrected Q-T interval may be prolonged.

Bone Biopsy. Helpful in the management of renal bone disease or osteomalacia.

DIFFERENTIAL DIAGNOSIS

Traumatic
Looser fractures may appear like tree fractures (e.g., osteomalacia).

Infectious
Chronic osteomyelitis, from infection of bone.

Metabolic
Hyperthyroidism may be a cause of osteoporosis.
Hypomagnesemia may affect parathyroid hormone release.

Neoplastic
Multiple myeloma may cause hypercalcemia, increased calcium loss, or renal failure.

Vascular
With *Looser fractures*, nutrient arteries going to bone may be severed, with resulting malnutrition of bone, if there is no secondary vascular supply due to osteomalacia.

Congenital
Hormone resistance patterns in pseudohypoparathyroidism.

Acquired
Alcoholism may be a cause for osteoporosis or it may occur in conjunction with hepatic failure or osteomalacia.

TREATMENT

Treatment of all forms of metabolic bone disease often requires calcium or vitamin D. Careful follow-up of serum calcium is essential to avoid hypercalcemia.

Osteomalacia
Correction of underlying cause if possible. Screen for and treat renal failure if present. Discontinue the use of aluminum hydroxide binders.
   Vitamin D Therapy.   With normal renal function give vitamin D 2000-4800 IU once a day; then reduce gradually. With renal failure give 1,25-$(OH_2)D_3$, 0.25-0.5 µg/day.

Osteoporosis
Lifestyle Changes. Increase the level of exercise if possible. Avoid prolonged bed rest. Reduce the risk of falls by providing ample room lighting and removing clutter from the floors

Pharmacologic Therapies
High-risk patients (thin, white females with a low calcium intake) should be apprised of the risks of osteoporosis and increase dietary intake of calcium. Recommendations for premenopausal women include daily calcium intake of at least 1200 mg elemental calcium. Postmenopausal women should maintain a calcium intake of of 1.5 g/day.

Estrogen therapy as menopause begins is currently under review.

Thiazide diuretics (25 mg/day) may help to prevent renal retention of calcium.

Calcitonin (Miacalcin) (50-100 IU/day) may aid in controlling bone pain and is indicated as second-line agent when patients may not be able to sit upright to take more effective medications. May be given as nasal spray (one spray is 200 IU/day).

Etidronate (Didronel) given cyclically at 400 mg/day for 2 weeks and repeated every 3 months has been used in Europe and in the United States to treat Paget disease.

Raloxifene (Evista) (60 mg/day), a selective estrogen receptor modulator, is approved for prevention and treatment of osteoporosis. It is particularly indicated in women at increased risk for breast cancer and osteoporosis.

Bisphosphonates such as alendronate (Fosamax) (for prevention, 5 mg/day; for treatment, 10 mg/day) and risedronate (Actonel) (5 mg once a day) act on osteoclasts to decrease cell resorption. They should be taken on an empty stomach.

Hyperparathyroidism
If adenoma is present, parathyroidectomy is indicated.

If the patient presents with renal failure, treatment consists of phosphate control (to achieve PO_4 level of less than 6.0 mg/dL), normalization of calcium, and administration of $1,25\text{-}(OH_2)D_3$ (oral dose 0.25-0.5 µg/day, pulse biweekly dose of 2-5.0 mEq, or intravenous dose 0.5-5 µg/day three times a week). This will often suppress parathyroid hyperplasia. This treatment is usually not effective in nodular hyperplasia, and parathyroidectomy may be necessary. Renal transplantation is often curative.

Hypoparathyroidism
Treatment with 25-hydroxyvitamin D_3 100,000 units/day or its analogue $1,25\text{-}(OH_2)D_3$ 0.25-0.5 µg/day. Calcium 1.0-2.0 g/day should be instituted.

Pseudohypoparathyroidism
Same as for hypoparathyroidism.

Paget Disease
Calcium 1.0 g/day.

Calcitonin (Miacalcin) is begun at 100 IU/day by subcutaneous injection. Dose may be decreased to 50 IU depending on response. Course is 1.5 to 3 years.

Bisphosphonates: alendronate (Fosamax) 40 mg/day, taken for 6 months, or risedronate (Actonel) 30 mg/day, taken for 2 months.

Nonsteroidal anti-inflammatory drugs (NSAIDs) or cyclooxygenase-2 (COX-2) inhibitors are used for secondary osteoarthritis.

PEDIATRIC CONSIDERATIONS

Osteopenia has been noted in premature infants, especially those with birth weights under 1000 g and those with chronic diseases of prematurity. In such infants, the rate of fetal bone mineralization is not always maintained by breastfeeding infants or those feeding on standard formulas. X-ray studies reveal bone demineralization and fractures. Serum alkaline phosphatase levels may be as high as two to three times normal. Sequelae may be prevented with formulas containing higher levels of calcium, phosphate, and vitamin D. Such dietary supplements are also used for treatment when indicated.

Patients with metabolic disorders may appear normal at birth and then begin to manifest signs of bone disease after or simultaneously with the manifestations produced by the underlying metabolic disorder. Treatment of inborn errors of metabolism must be aimed at correcting the specific disorder. Hypoparathyroidism may occur in premature infants

The key is to correct any vitamin D abnormalities rapidly, to prevent abnormal bone growth.

OBSTETRIC CONSIDERATIONS

Osteoporosis. Osteoporosis almost always occurs during the postmenopausal period or after oophorectomy. If a patient develops clinically significant osteoporosis during the perimenopausal years and becomes pregnant, she will need to pay very careful attention to maintaining adequate calcium and vitamin D levels. Ongoing follow-up is indicated because she is at high risk for developing fractures. If a patient is suffering from a form of secondary osteoporosis, control of the underlying condition, along with adequate maintenance of calcium and vitamin D levels, is appropriate.

Osteomalacia. Occurs secondary to nutritional vitamin D deficiency, renal failure, steatorrhea, or vitamin D–resistant rickets. Pregnant patients need careful attention to the underlying disease process and should take vitamin D in doses sufficient to maintain adequate levels for the fetus and to control the osteomalacia.

Paget Disease. Calcitonin (Miacalcin) and etidronate (Didronel), both used for treatment of Paget disease, should be used only when necessary. Etidronate is a pregnancy category B drug. Calcitonin (Miacalcin) and risedronate (Actonel) are pregnancy category C drugs. Bisphosphonates such as alendronate (Fosamax) should not be taken during pregnancy.

GERIATRIC CONSIDERATIONS

In the elderly, hypocalcemia is fairly common and may be due to any of various abnormalities.

PREVENTIVE CONSIDERATIONS

Encourage all patients, when indicated, to take proper amounts of calcium and vitamin D and to incorporate physical activity, including cardiovascular and resistance exercise, into the daily routine.

PEARLS FOR THE PA

Osteoporosis is a common problem in women as well as men and is treatable if identified early.

Osteoporosis is preventable if at-risk patients are identified and risk factors are corrected.

Paget disease may require surgical intervention for joint symptoms or neurologic complications.

Many patients presumed to have osteoporosis may also have osteomalacia.

Osteomalacia and hyperparathyroidism and hypoparathyroidism are uncommon problems in the general population. Persons at risk include those with vitamin D deficiency and renal failure. It is important to correct these conditions early.

Pituitary Adenoma

Roland G. Ottley, JD, PA-C

DEFINITION

Pituitary adenoma is a neoplasm arising from the anterior lobe (adenohypophysis) of the pituitary gland and accounts for 8% to 10% of all intracranial tumors. Pituitary adenomas are classified as prolactin-secreting (40%-50%), growth hormone (GH)-secreting (15%-20%), adrenocorticotropic hormone (ACTH)-secreting (10%-15%), follicle-stimulating hormone (FSH) and luteinizing hormone (LH)-secreting (5%-10%), thyroid-stimulating hormone (TSH)-secreting (less than 1%), and nonsecreting (10%-20%) tumors.

HISTORY

Symptoms

Symptoms are due to active endocrine secretion by the tumor, endocrine dysfunction, or compression of adjacent neural structures. Non–tumor-specific symptoms include headache, diplopia (with involvement of cranial nerves III, IV, and VI), visual field cut (with optic nerve or optic chiasm compression), hypothalamic syndrome (abnormalities of thirst, appetite, sleep, temperature regulation, and occasionally diabetes insipidus or syndrome of inappropriate antidiuretic hormone secretion [SIADH]), facial pain (with cranial nerve V involvement), and cerebrospinal fluid rhinorrhea. The patient may present with symptoms of hypopituitarism such as decreased energy level, muscle weakness, anorexia, and episodic confusion.

Endocrine Symptoms

Prolactin

With *hypersecretion*, women may present with breast growth, galactorrhea, and amenorrhea; men may be impotent.

With *hyposecretion*, women may have failure of postpartum lactation.

Growth Hormone

With *hypersecretion*, patients present with acromegaly, characterized by increased size of the hands and feet (after the growth plates have fused), mandibular prominence (prognathism), skin changes, hoarseness, new onset or worsening of snoring, heat intolerance, carbohydrate intolerance, and neuropathic and cardiac symptoms (e.g., congestive heart failure [CHF]). With onset before the growth plates fuse, patients may present as "pituitary giants."

Adrenocorticotropic Hormone

With *hypersecretion*, patients present with Cushing syndrome characterized by fat deposits in the face, trunk, and cervicothoracic area; skin changes; spontaneous bruising; new growth of facial hair; fatigue; and weakness.

With *hyposecretion*, hypoadrenocorticism (Addison disease) includes weakness, hyperpigmentation, nausea, vomiting, anorexia, loss of body hair, amenorrhea.

Thyroid-Stimulating Hormone

With *hypersecretion*, patients present with thyrotoxicosis characterized by toxic nodular goiter and/or Graves disease.

With *hyposecretion*, hypothyroidism includes cold intolerance, lethargy, periorbital edema, and decreased sweating.

Follicle-Stimulating Hormone/Luteinizing Hormone

Patients present with hypogonadism.

General. Nonsecreting tumors tend to grow to larger size owing to the relative endocrinologic silence; therefore, patients tend to present with symptoms of neural compression. FSH- and LH-secreting tumors were formerly categorized as nonsecreting tumors because of their previously undetectable levels of LH or FSH.

Patients may be reluctant to discuss certain symptoms or may have dismissed their symptoms as normal occurrences. Inquiry should be made about energy level, visual field disturbance (e.g., with driving or participating in sports activities), thirst, urinary habits, presence of double vision in certain visual fields, clear colorless drainage from the nose, galactorrhea, menstrual history, impotence, changes in ring or shoe size, increase in snoring, new weight gain, and/or additional facial hair. It may also be helpful to examine and compare previous photographs of the patient from the not too distant past.

Age. Adenomas may occur at any age, but GH-secreting tumors tend to occur in the third or fourth decade of life; prolactin-secreting tumors tend to manifest with symptoms in the child-bearing years with infertility.

Onset. Usually slow and insidious.

Duration. Progressive without treatment.

Intensity. Patients may be asymptomatic or present with severe endocrinologic disturbance. GH-secreting tumors may be life-threatening owing to nasopharyngeal closure or cardiac disturbance.

Aggravating Factors. None.

Alleviating Factors. Appropriate therapy.

Associated Factors. Are due to endocrine-dependent organs. Thyroid abnormalities, diabetes mellitus, and hypertension/hypotension.

PHYSICAL EXAMINATION

General. Observe the patient for appearance. Patients with ACTH-secreting tumors will have truncal obesity, moon facies, and a so-called buffalo hump. Patients with GH-screting tumors will have the appearance of acromegaly.

Vital signs should be evaluated for hypertension, postural hypotension, pulse rate, and rhythm. Patients with GH-secreting tumors and CHF may be dyspneic.

Cardiovascular. Evaluate GH-secreting tumor patients for CHF by inspecting neck veins for distention; auscultate for S_3 gallop (the hallmark finding).

Extremities. Test strength to evaluate for generalized weakness; inspect for wasting, especially in patients with ACTH-secreting tumors. Bilateral lower extremity edema in patients with CHF.

Head, Eyes, Ears, Nose, Throat. Palpate for thyroid enlargement or goiter. Test for cerebospinal fluid rhinorrhea by asking the patient (while sitting) to lean over. Observe for clear, colorless fluid coming from the nose. The fluid may test positive on glucose stick if it is cerebrospinal fluid (if any blood is present, the glucose test is void, as blood contains glucose).

Neurologic. A full neurologic examination needs to be performed in all patients with a suspected or known intracranial lesion. Test eye movements for paresis (cranial nerves III, IV, VI). Check the sensation of both sides of the face (cranial nerve V). Sensory examination should be performed in patients with GH-secreting tumors if there is any symptom of peripheral neuropathy.

Ophthalmologic. Funduscopic examination may show optic atrophy with long-standing optic nerve or chiasm compression. Papilledema may be present with increased intracranial pressure. Invasion of tumor into the cavernous sinus may result in proptosis or even sudden unilateral blindness from occlusion of the ipsilateral internal carotid artery. Visual fields are tested, initially to gross confrontation and then by formal means through ophthalmologic consultation. Suprasellar tumor extension with compression of the optic chiasm classically causes a bitemporal hemianopsia.

Pulmonary. Moist rales may be heard on auscultation or the chest may be dull to percussion in GH tumor patients with CHF.

Skin. Evaluate skin for turgor, acne, sweat production, and greasy appearance (with GH- and ACTH-secreting tumors). ACTH-secreting tumor patients may have purple striae and hirsutism.

PATHOPHYSIOLOGY

The pituitary is divided into two lobes:
- The anterior lobe—the adenohypophysis, from which tumors arise, develops from Rathke's pouch.
- The posterior lobe—the neurohypophysis—is formed from the infundibulum, which develops from the floor of the diencephalon.

The pituitary gland is under the control of the hypothalamus via hypothalamic releasing hormones. The anterior pituitary normally secretes GH, TSH, ACTH, prolactin, FSH, and LH, whereas the posterior pituitary secretes antidiuretic hormone (ADH) and oxytocin. When tumors develop, they may oversecrete certain hormones or, if a local mass effect is present, inhibit release of normal circulating hormones, eventually culminating in what is known as a panhypopituitary state.

Tumors are classified by size. Microadenomas are less than 10 mm in diameter. Macroadenomas can grow to a much larger size and extend superiorly, compressing the optic chiasm, hypothalamus, or third ventricle. The pituitary gland is connected to the hypothalamus via the pituitary stalk, which travels through the diaphragma sella (DS). In about 70% of cases the optic chiasm lies over the DS. In about 15% of cases the chiasm lies anterior and in 15% of cases it lies posterior to the DS. Lateral extension into the cavernous sinus occurs in 60% to 70% of cases, which may cause compression of cranial nerve III, IV, V, or VI. Inferior extension into the sphenoid sinus may potentially cause cerebrospinal fluid rhinorrhea. Macroadenomas tend to erode the sella. The sella then enlarges and remodels itself to accommodate the mass. This accounts for the large sella seen on plain radiographs or CT images. About 33% of pituitary tumors become invasive and permeate the pituitary capsule, bone, and dural sinuses. Most of these tumors are either prolactin-secreting or nonsecreting. Metastasis from pituitary carcinoma to distant extracranial sites or from seeding within the cerebrospinal fluid pathways occurs in less than 1% of cases.

DIAGNOSTIC STUDIES

Laboratory
Electrolytes.   May see hypokalemia with ACTH tumors.

Thyroid Function Studies.   If serum thyroxine is normal, then it is likely that the hypothalamic-pituitary-thyroid axis is intact. If the serum thyroxine is low, a thyrotropin-releasing hormone study is performed. A baseline TSH level is drawn, followed by an intravenous injection of thyrotropin-releasing hormone. TSH levels are obtained at 30 and 60 minutes after the injection. A normal test reveals an increase of twice the baseline level of TSH at 30 minutes. A low TSH response indicates a pituitary abnormality. A delayed TSH response (60 minutes) indicates a hypothalamic abnormality.

Hormone Assays by Radioimmunoassay
Prolactin.   Normal: women, 0-23 ng/mL; men, 0-20 ng/mL. Levels greater than 200 almost always indicate a tumor; a level greater than 1000 suggests an invasive tumor.

Growth Hormone.   Normal: women, less than 10 ng/mL; men, less than 5 ng/mL. Elevated with GH tumors. The two most sensitive confirmatory tests are the oral glucose tolerance test (OGTT) and determination of insulin-like growth factor-1 (IGF-1) [formerly somatomedin C] levels; these tests are helpful in patients suspected of having acromegaly, who do not have significantly elevated basal hormone levels. A normal OGTT result is a fall in serum GH to less than 2 ng/mL within 1 to 2 hours after 75-100 g of oral glucose. Sampling error from circadian variations can confuse actual GH levels. IGF-1 remains constant and therefore has more diagnostic reliability than OGTT.

Adrenocorticotropic Hormone (ACTH).   Using dexamethasone supression test, urine and plasma free cortisol are normally supressed with low-dose dexamethasone (0.5 mg every 6 hours). Levels are also supressed with high-dose dexamethasone (2 mg every 6 hours) in pituitary-dependent Cushing disease. There is no suppression of levels in nonpituitary Cushing disease.

Radiology
Plain Skull Radiographs.   True lateral views will show an enlarged sella with macroadenomas. May see erosion of bone.

High-Resolution CT Scan with Contrast.   This study, including coronal reconstruction views of the sella, will demonstrate micro- and macroadenomas. May see hydrocephalus with large tumor obstructing the third ventricle.

MRI Scan with Gadolinium.   The most sensitive test to identify micro- and macroadenomas. Should include coronal views of the sella. Suprasellar and lateral extension to the optic chiasm and cavernous sinuses, respectively, can be evaluated. May see hydrocephalus with a large tumor obstructing the third ventricle.

Cerebral Angiogram. Rule out giant aneurysm if the diagnosis of pituitary tumor is uncertain. Used less frequently since the advent of three-dimensional magnetic resonance angiography (3D-MR angiography), which does not require gadolinium and is therefore less invasive. However, a 3D-CT angiogram is more beneficial for evaluating any aneurysm and the surrounding bony structures.

Other

ECG. Rule out arrhythmia.

Echocardiography. Rule out cardiomegaly in GH-secreting tumor patients.

Sleep Studies. Rule out sleep apnea in GH-secreting tumor patients.

DIFFERENTIAL DIAGNOSIS

Traumatic

With *basilar skull fracture with avulsion of the pituitary stalk*, history of trauma. Raccoon eyes, Battle sign, or hemotympanum may be present. May have cerebrospinal fluid rhinorrhea. CT/MRI shows intracranial air in the acute stage.

Infectious

With *pituitary abscess*, presence of tissue destruction. Histologically differentiated by the presence of cell necrosis and polymorphonuclear lymphocytes.

Metabolic

Sarcoidosis may involve the hypothalamus or pituitary gland. Well-circumscribed mass seen on CT/MRI. Requires histologic confirmation.

Neoplastic

Adrenal adenoma/carcinoma may cause elevated ACTH production; secretion may be adrenal or from oat cell cancer of the lung or other ectopic sources. Ninety percent of patients with an elevated ACTH will have a pituitary source.

Craniopharyngioma is a cystic tumor, usually with flecks of calcium seen on CT/MRI. May enlarge the sella owing to pressure on the intrasellar contents.

Glioma may affect the hypothalamus or optic nerve. MRI may identify an intramedullary tumor or enlargement of the optic nerve.

Meningioma may occur in the suprasellar region. May see dural and homogenous enhancement of the tumor on MRI with gadolinium.

Granular cell tumors, chordomas, germinomas, teratomas all may affect the pituitary. Diagnosis requires histologic confirmation.

Vascular

Giant aneurysm may resemble an extrasellar pituitary tumor. A cerebral angiogram may be necessary to differentiate.

Pituitary apoplexy is a rare emergency resulting from an acute hemorrhage into the pituitary tumor, with resultant compression of the optic structures and destruction of the pituitary and hypothalamus. Patients may present with severe headaches, altered mental status, meningismus, and visual impairment.

Congenital

Rathke cleft cyst is probably a derivative of Rathke's pouch. May be confused with craniopharyngioma.

Acquired

Empty sella syndrome can be seen congenitally, postoperatively, with pseudotumor cerebri, or after radiation therapy. There is herniation of the arachnoid into the sella. This can occur with elevated intracranial pressure or hydrocephalus. Patients may be asymptomatic, have nonspecific symptoms, or present with cerebrospinal fluid rhinorrhea.

Postpartum women are at high risk for developing pituitary apoplexy (Sheehan's syndrome). They may also have transient increased size of hands, feet, or nose owing to circulating fetal GH.

TREATMENT

Treatment is dependent on the degree of endocrinologic or neural compromise. There are no medically curative measures, only therapies directed at reducing the excessive hormone levels or size of the tumors. Appropriate management of most pituitary adenomas will require a multispecialty team approach involving an internist, an endocrinologist, and a neurosurgeon.

Medical

Prolactin-secreting tumors can be effectively treated with the long acting dopamine agonist bromocriptine or pergolide, which inhibit prolactin synthesis and release. Although pergolide is approved only for treating Parkinson disease, it has been shown to be safe and effective in treating prolactin secreting tumors. A daily oral dose of bromocriptine may reduce or normalize the prolactin level, reduce tumor size, decrease galactorrhea, and allow for resumption of menses and fertility. Drug cessation because of pregnancy results in a resumption of the hyperprolactinemic state and regrowth of the tumor. Side effects include nausea, vomiting, and postural hypotension. The new very-long-acting dopamine agonist cabergoline is more effective and better tolerated than bromocriptine. However, women who wish to become pregnant should be treated with bromocriptine because of its long history of safety during pregnancy.

Tumors secreting GH, mixed GH, and prolactin may respond to bromocriptine. Bromocriptine can reduce GH levels up to 75%, but much larger doses are required to achieve this result. The dopamine agonist caber-goline is more effective and better tolerated than bromocriptine for acromegaly. However, the most effective medical therapy for acromegaly is the somatostatin analogue octreotide. The most common adverse effects of octreotide are abdominal discomfort, diarrhea, nausea, and mild malabsorption that subsides with continued use. In addition, new gallstones may develop in 26% of patients.

ACTH-secreting tumors may be treated with several inhibitors of steroidogenesis. These include ketoconazole (an imidazole derivative, liver function tests should be monitored), metyrapone, aminoglutethimide, and mitotane.

TSH-secreting tumors are best treated with octreotide.

Panhypopituitary patients require repletion of deficient hormones by treatment with hydrocortisone, estrogen/progestin, thyroxine, testosterone, GH, or 1-deamino-8-D-arginine-vasopressin (DDAVP) if diabetes insipidus is present. These patients are at increased risk of developing cardiac complications and therefore require close attentive medical management.

Surgical
Surgery to resect the tumor, performed through a transsphenoidal route or by frontotemporal craniotomy, is indicated with neural compression, acromegaly, ACTH-secreting tumors, and failure of medical treatment.

Radiation Therapy
There is a 20% 5-year and 44% 10-year relapse in patients with nonirradiated pituitary adenomas. Radiation therapy is indicated for patients who have undergone subtotal excision of the tumor, patients in whom general anesthesia and surgery are contraindicated, and those with intracavernous tumor, or if postoperative endocrine levels remain elevated.

PEDIATRIC CONSIDERATIONS

Pituitary tumors in children may result in retarded development of secondary sex characteristics or, in the case of GH-secreting tumors, result in "pituitary gigantism."

Stereotactic radiosurgery has been introduced in the management of certain pediatric pituitary adenomas. This therapy has been shown to be safe and effective in this age group, but long-term follow-up studies are still needed.

OBSTETRIC CONSIDERATIONS

Infertility is a symptom of prolactinoma. However, the patient may become pregnant during treatment with bromocriptine. After a positive pregnancy test, bromocriptine is stopped. Consider reintroducing bromocriptine if the patient has a macroadenoma and/or becomes symptomatic. Bromocriptine treatment can considered for growth hormone secreting tumors. The safety of pergolide or cabergoline treatment during pregnancy has not been established. It is rare for a woman with Cushing syndrome to become pregnant. Medical treatment is not recommended.

GERIATRIC CONSIDERATIONS

The age, endocrine symptoms, and medical condition of the patient should be considered in formulating the treatment plan.

PREVENTIVE CONSIDERATIONS

Close monitoring of endocrine status is imperative. Medical therapy is not curative, so continued follow-up is essential. After surgery, long-term hormone replacement may be required.

PEARLS FOR THE PA

Always consider pituitary adenoma in the differential diagnosis of endocrine abnormality or visual field deficit.

Always consider pituitary apoplexy in patients with a pituitary mass who experience acute clinical deterioration with worsening of symptoms.

There is no medical cure for pituitary adenomas, only interventions that inhibit hormone secretion and tumor size.

Thyroid Disorders

Michaela C. Gallagher-Gonzales, PA-C

DEFINITION

The thyroid is a butterfly-shaped gland in the anterior inferior neck. The lateral lobes are larger than the isthmus, which has a pyramidal lobe at the top. Conditions associated with the thyroid are underactivity, or *hypothyroidism*; overactivity, or *hyperthyroidism*; and *nodules*, which can occur with either condition.

HISTORY

Symptoms
Hypothyroidism. Fatigue, depression, abnormal weight gain or difficulty losing weight, dry skin and hair, hair loss (both diffuse scalp hair loss and loss of lateral eyebrows), brittle nails, joint aches, irregular menses (including oligomenorrhea and amenorrhea), cold intolerance, constipation, memory problems, paresthesias, carpal tunnel syndrome symptoms.

Hyperthyroidism. Fatigue, weight loss, palpitations, tremors, weakness, increased defecation, increased thyroid size, occasionally angina.

Thyroiditis. A temporary hyperthyroidism, thought to be caused by a virus and exhibiting the same symptoms as for hyperthyroidism in the acute phase. This is followed by hypothyroid symptoms, which may self-resolve or remain permanent. Resolution, if it occurs, usually does so within 3 months.

Thyroid Nodules. May be asymptomatic if nonfunctional. Symptoms of hyperthyroidism may be present if functional. Discovered during thyroid examination or by patient.

General
Symptoms depend on the degree of elevation or depression of thyroid-stimulating hormone (TSH). More women than men are affected.

With thyroid cancer, enlarging nodule, which may be solitary, hard.

Age
All increase with advancing age, although special populations exist (see Pediatric and Obstetric Considerations sections).

Onset
Hypothyroidism. Gradual unless due to thyroidectomy

Hyperthyroidism. Gradual, but can be acute with administration of iodine

Thyroiditis. Acute, if due to viral or bacterial cause.

Thyroid Nodule. Gradual or acute. Abrupt presentation can occur when a preexisting nodule experiences an interior capillary bleed.

Duration
Hypothyroidism. Months to years. If occurring as the recovery phase of thyroiditis, 2 to 3 months. May be permanent.

Hyperthyroidism. Months to years. There is a tendency for eventual burnout of Graves disease leading to a hypothyroid state.

Thyroiditis. Viral causes last from a few weeks to 3 months. Bacterial causes are acute. Hashimoto thyroiditis is lifelong.

Thyroid Nodule. Months to years.

Intensity. Symptoms may be mild, or severe enough to precipitate angina, depending on the amount of dysfunction of the gland.

Aggravating Factors

Hypothyroidism. Antithyroid medications, beta blockers, lithium, iodide, failure to routinely take thyroid supplementary medicine (levothyroxine).

Hyperthyroidism. Exogenous thyroid hormone (levothyroxine), iodine, stimulants.

Alleviating Factors

Hypothyroidism. Administration of thyroid replacement hormone.

Hyperthyroidism. Antithyroid medication, beta blockers (these alleviate symptoms only; they do not treat).

Thyroiditis. Beta blockers.

Associated Factors

Associated with a family history of thyroid problems.

Thyroid Nodules. Multiple endocrine neoplasia (MEN), history of neck irradiation. The condition known as multinodular goiter is thought to occur from long-standing mild hypothyroidism.

PHYSICAL EXAMINATION

General

Hypothyroidism. Overweight, puffy eyelids, sparse lateral eyebrows, slow movements.

Hyperthyroidism. Thin, may have "stare," nervous, jittery.

Cardiovascular

Hypothyroidism. Hypertension. May see distended neck veins.

Hyperthyroidism. Tachycardia, atrial fibrillation.

Extremities

Hypothyroidism. Nonpitting edema (myxedema) of legs, hands, feet.

Hyperthyroidism. Wasting of muscles, pretibial myxedema, fine resting tremor, onycholysis, achropachy (clubbing of fingertips).

Head, Eyes, Ears, Nose, Throat

Hypothyroidism. Enlarged thyroid (goiter), puffy facies, ptosis.

Hyperthyroidism. Enlarged thyroid (goiter), may hear bruit over gland, exopthalmos/proptosis, with stare, lid lag (can be unilateral).

Thyroiditis. Gland may be tender to palpation.

Thyroid Nodule. Palpable nodule(s). If palpable lymph nodes are appreciated, may signal metastasis.

Neurologic

Hypothyroidism. Hypoactive deep tendon reflexes.

Hyperthyroidism. Hyperreflexia.

Pulmonary
Hypothyroidism. Decreased lung sounds at bases suggesting pleural effusion (rare).

Skin
Hypothyroidism. Cool hands and feet. Dry, rough skin; coarse, dry hair; brittle nails; myxedema.
Hyperthyroidism. Warm moist palms. Fine hair.

PATHOPHYSIOLOGY

Hypothyroidism. Lymphocytic thyroiditis, Hashimoto disease, the autoimmune destruction of the thyroid gland, and status post iodine 131 (^{131}I) ablation for Graves disease are the most common causes for hypothyroidism. Hashimoto disease often manifests with thyromegaly. Iodine deficiency, thyroidectomy, iodinated drugs (lithium, amiodarone, interferon, antithyroid medications) are the next most common. Dietary-related hypothyroidism from turnips and cabbage is rare. Postpartum thyroiditis often has a hypothyroid phase. External irradiation to the neck can decrease thyroid function.

Hyperthyroidism. Graves disease, toxic multinodular goiter/autonomous nodule, and thyroiditis are the three most common causes. Graves disease is caused by continuous overproduction of hormone by thyroid-stimulating antibodies. It is frequently associated with thyromegaly/goiter. Toxic multinodular goiter or a single autonomous nodule produces hormone independently of the rest of the gland. Thyroiditis is a temporary condition caused by viral infection. Resolution of the hyperthyroid phase is followed by a temporary or permanent hypothyroidism. The gland may be tender or nontender (silent thyroiditis). Common in the postpartum period.

Thyroid Nodules. Functioning nodules are described as "warm" (demonstrate normal or increased isotope uptake) on an iodine scan. Hyperfunctioning nodules are "hot." Nonfunctioning nodules are "cold" and may be seen in multinodular goiter, follicular adenomas (benign), and malignancies of thyroid origin (papillary, follicular, medullary, Hurthle cell, or anaplastic carcinoma), as well as lymphomas metastatic to the thyroid.

DIAGNOSTIC STUDIES

Laboratory
Thyroid Function Tests
Thyroid-Stimulating Hormone. Normal range: 0.4-4.5 µU/mL. The best test to evaluate thyroid abnormality in dealing with primary thyroid disease (which is the most common cause). TSH assay is the first test indicating thyroid dysfunction, in advance of any other thyroid tests. Pituitary and hypothalamic disease can cause the TSH to be abnormal.

Thyroxine (T_4). Normal range: 4.5-12.0 µg/dL. Up to 99% bound to protein. May be elevated in estrogen use.

Triiodothyronine (T_3). Normal range: 60-90 ng/dL. Active thyroid hormone up to 98% bound to protein.

Free T_4, Free T_3. Unbound, physiologically active thyroid hormone in the blood stream. Less affected by protein binding. Gives a more accurate assessment than the total T_4 and T_3 assays. Free T_4 is also available by direct dialysis to remove protein interference.

Antibody Tests

Anti-Thyroid Peroxidase Antibody (TPO). Positive in Hashimoto disease.

Thyroid-Stimulating Immunoglobulins. Positive in Graves disease. Used to confirm diagnosis in the few cases in which the diagnosis is in question.

Thyroglobulin. Used in monitoring for recurrence of thyroid cancer after thyroidectomy. Less reliable when anti-thyroglobulin antibodies are present.

Calcitonin. Elevated in medullary thyroid cancer and C-cell hyperplasia, a familial precursor. Use to follow medullary thyroid cancer for recurrence.

Thyrotropin-Releasing Hormone Stimulation Test. Is the administration of an intravenous bolus of thyrotropin-releasing hormone, then measuring the TSH within a specified period of time. Hypothyroidism shows a brisk elevation of the TSH. Hyperthyroidism shows decreased or absent response. Used to elucidate occult hypothyroidism, in which there are symptoms of hypothyroidism but normal TSH.

Westergren Sedimentation Rate. Elevated in thyroiditis.

Complete Blood Count (CBC). Follow in patients using antithyroid medication (propylthiouracil or methimazole for control of Graves disease), which can cause agranulocytosis, leaving the patient prone to serious infection. A CBC sample is obtained immediately if the patient is feverish while using these medicines. If the white blood cell count is shown to be decreased, and differential indicates abnormally low granulocytes/segmented neutrophils, discontinue medication. Cessation of antithyroid medications usually results in normalization of the CBC.

Sodium. May be reduced in hypothyroidism.

Radiology

Iodine Radioisotope Uptake and Scan. Either iodine 123 (^{123}I) or ^{131}I may be used. Used to determine causes for hyperthyroidism, and if a thyroid nodule is functioning or cold. Increased uptake values in a diffuse pattern are typical of Graves disease. Very low uptake is seen in thyroiditis, with surreptitious thyroid hormone use, and in iodine-induced problems from other medications. Autonomous nodules may show normal or increased uptake percentages, but the hyperfunctioning nodule(s) show as darker areas on the scan. Markedly decreased uptake in the area of a known nodule shows that it is nonfunctioning and may indicate the necessity for fine needle aspiration biopsy. Twenty percent of cold nodules are at risk for malignancy. Hot or warm nodules rarely indicate cancer.

Other

Thyroid Ultrasound Examination. Used to determine if nodules are present, if they are cystic or solid, and interval change in size.

DIFFERENTIAL DIAGNOSIS

Trauma

Thyroid trauma can cause damage to the gland and subsequent endocrine effects.

Infectious

With *bacterial thyroiditis*, most cases are caused by gram-positive organisms, with symptoms of acute pain in the gland and fever. May require abscess drainage and antibiotics.

Metabolic

Thyroid Storm. Life-threatening condition of release of catecholamines and increased sensitivity of various tissues to catecholamines, in combination with thyrotoxicosis. Symptoms are fever, agitation, flushing, sweating, tachycardia, atrial fibrillation, jaundice, delirium, nausea, vomiting, diarrhea, and coma. May lead to heart failure and shock.

Sick Euthyroid Syndrome. Abnormally low T_3, normal to low T_4 during a nonthyroidal illness. TSH is slightly low at the onset of the illness; then may elevate minimally. Await resolution of the illness and recheck the thyroid function tests at a later date.

Neoplastic

TSH-secreting tumors are very rare causes of hyperthyroidism.

With *thyroid carcinoma*, risk factors are previous head or neck irradiation, family history of multiple endocrine neoplasia (MEN) or medullary cancer, young age, and male gender. A large, rapidly enlarging or rock-hard nodule, imaging cold on ^{123}I scan, is the main finding. Carcinoma is relatively less frequent in multinodular goiter. Papillary carcinoma is the most common variety. Follicular, medullary, and anaplastic are other types. The medullary variety shows elevated calcitonin levels and is not responsive to iodine for post-thyroidectomy ablation. Anaplastic type is extremely aggressive.

Vascular. Not applicable.
Congenital. See Pediatric Considerations.

TREATMENT

Hypothyroidism. Discontinue potential thyroid-harming medications such as amiodarone or lithium, if possible. Treat with synthetic levothyroxine (T_4). Avoid desiccated animal thyroid because of its variable bioavailability. Start levothyroxine at a low dose (generally 25-50 µg with an adult), and adjust at 6-week intervals to achieve a TSH of low normal levels of 1.0-2.0 IU/ml. Keep the TSH within the normal range, to avoid creating a risk for osteoporosis.

Hyperthyroidism
Medical Therapy

Antithyroid medication can cause chemical hepatitis and agranulocytosis. Monitor CBC and liver function tests prior to and at 6 to 8 hours after starting therapy. Adjust medication to maintain free T_4 and TSH in the normal range. May need to reduce dosage after several months. Treat for 9 to 12 months; then discontinue and observe thyroid function tests for recurrence. Medical therapy is less likely to be curative of Graves disease if the gland is very large or if the patient smokes. Not curative for hyperfunctioning nodules.

The following agents are used in the treatment of hyperthyroidism.

Propylthiouracil: The dose will depend on the degree of hyperthyroidism and gland size. Dose range: 100-600 mg/day, given two or three times daily in divided doses. Inhibits peripheral T_4 to T_3 conversion.

Methimazole (Tapazole): 5-60 mg/day, given four times a day for smaller doses, or twice daily for larger doses. Greater likelihood of compliance because of easier dosing schedule.

Iodine: Rarely used, to prepare patient for surgery, at 5-10 mg a day. Short-lived effects.

Beta blockers—atenolol, propranolol: Used to control tachycardia and other symptoms. Also helps to inhibit T_4 to T_3 conversion. Atenolol: 25-75 mg/day, in 2 or 3 divided doses. Propranolol: 10-360 mg/day, in 2 or 3 divided doses.

Corticosteroids: Inhibit T_4 to T_3 conversion. In thyroid storm may be given for several days to help achieve control.

Thyroiditis. Pain relief with aspirin or nonsteroidal anti-inflammatory medication. If thyrotoxic, use beta blockers. Steroids have been used for particularly difficult cases but are not generally recommended. In the hypothyroid phase of thyroiditis, levothyroxine may be needed temporarily (or permanently, as some thyroiditis results in permanent hypothyroidism).

Thyroid Nodules. Cold thyroid nodules necessitate fine needle aspiration biopsy. If carcinoma is found, treatment is thyroidectomy, followed by iodine ablation in most cases (except medullary, which is not sensitive to iodine). After ablation, the patient becomes permanently hypothyroid, requiring lifelong replacement therapy.

Warm nodules need no treatment unless patient is hyperthyroid. Levothyroxine is often administered to discourage the nodule's growth.

Hot nodules are treated with iodine I-131 ablation (which gives approximately a 50% chance that the thyroid will maintain sufficient function to remain euthyroid), or with surgical removal of the nodule (not generally recommended as more nodules can form later). Antithyroid medication will control an autonomous nodule while the medication is being taken, but the problem reemerges after the medication is discontinued.

PEDIATRIC CONSIDERATIONS

Rapid workup for evaluation of any nodules should be performed owing to the risk for malignancy.

Neonatal hypothyroidism can occur in children born to mothers with hypothyroidism in the first trimester. This may lead to impairment of psychomotor and intellectual development later in life. Neonates are checked for hypothyroidism at the time of PKU testing.

Hyperthyroidism in infants of women with Graves disease occurs from transplacental passage of thyroid-stimulating immunoglobulins. Fetal tachycardia, low birth weight, intrauterine growth restriction, and premature delivery can occur with inadequate treatment of Graves disease during pregnancy. After delivery, these infants may be irritable, hyperkinetic, or jaundiced, may be poor feeders, or may demonstrate thrombocytopenia, failure to thrive, craniosynostosis, and goiter. If the hyperthyroidism is severe, infants are given antithyroid medicines until antibody levels decrease, which may take up to 20 weeks.

OBSTETRIC CONSIDERATIONS

Hypothyroidism in pregnancy must be monitored in each trimester. Owing to the increased amount of thyroid-binding globulins, the dosage of levothyroxine may need to be raised up to 50 μg over the pre-pregnancy requirements, and reduced soon after delivery. Inadequately treated hypothyroidism during pregnancy is associated with anemia, congestive heart failure, abruptio placentae, preeclampsia, and postpartum hemorrhage. Pregnant patients should not take their prenatal vitamins closer than 2 hours to their thyroid replacement hormone.

Postpartum thyroiditis may be present after delivery.

Graves disease developing in pregnancy is treated medically, with propylthiouracil dosed three or four times a day. Methimazole is not used in pregnancy or nursing because it can cause aplasia cutis (scalp abnormalities). It also passes the placental barrier and can cause hypothyroidism and cretinism in the fetus. Surgery is an option in the second trimester. Iodine ablation is contraindicated because it can destroy fetal as well as maternal thyroid tissue. An exacerbation (or initial presentation) of Graves disease can occur post partum. Avoid treating to hypothyroidism with propylthiouracil, for this can adversely affect the fetal thyroid status. Monitor thyroid status carefully in pregnancy. Inadequately treated Graves disease can lead to maternal atrial fibrillation, congestive heart failure, left ventricular dysfunction and thyroid storm, and hyperthyroidism in the neonate.

GERIATRIC CONSIDERATIONS

The elderly and very sensitive hypothyroid patients may need decreased medication doses initially.

Elderly patients may be asymptomatic (apathetic hyperthyroidism). Apathetic hyperthyroidism in the elderly causes vague symptoms such as weakness or new-onset atrial fibrillation.

In this population, workup for weight loss, lethargy, or low sodium may show hypothyroidism.

PREVENTIVE CONSIDERATIONS

Prompt diagnosis and effective treatment. Regular monitoring should be scheduled with the treating provider. Compliance with the medication regimen.

PEARLS FOR THE PA

Thyroid replacement hormone should be taken on an empty stomach, at least 2 hours separated from any calcium, iron supplements, or vitamins.

Hashimoto thyroiditis, the autoimmune disorder, is not the same thyroiditis that produces hyperthyroidism.

Radioisotope imaging studies: [123]I is short-lived and can be given in a smaller dose to determine hyperthyroidism. It is also more expensive than ^{131}I, which is longer-lived, given in higher dose, and less expensive.

It takes about 6 weeks after changing a levothyroxine dose to be able to accurately measure the TSH response.

Levothyroxine is generally ordered as a brand name, because there can be too much variability between generics. It is a relatively inexpensive medicine, and a 3-month supply may be less expensive for the patient to buy out of pocket.

Further Reading
Beers MH, Berkow R (eds): Merck Manual, 17th ed. Whitehouse Station, NJ, Merck Research Laboratories, 1999.
Beers MH, Berkow R (eds): The Merck Manual of Geriatrics, 3rd ed. Whitehouse Station, NJ, Merck Research Laboratories, 2000.
Braunwald E, Fauci AS, Kasper DL, et al (eds): Harrison's Principles of Internal Medicine, 15th ed. McGraw-Hill, 2001.
Edelman S, Henry R: Diagnosis and Management of Type 2 Diabetes, 5th ed. Professional Communications, Inc., 2001.

Finberg L, Kleinman R (ed): Saunders Manual of Pediatric Practice, 2nd ed. Philadelphia, WB Saunders, 2002.

Greenspan F, Strewler G: Basics of Clinical Endocrinology. Norwalk, CT, Appleton & Lange, 1997.

Labus JB, Lauber AA: Patient Education and Preventive Medicine. Philadelphia, WB Saunders, 2001.

Leahy J, Clark N, Cefalu W (eds): Medical Management of Diabetes Mellitus. New York, Marcel Dekker, 2000.

LeRoith D, Olefsky J: Diabetes Mellitus: A Fundamental and Clinical Text, 2nd ed. New York, Lippincott Williams & Wilkins, 2000.

McDermott M: Endocrine Secrets, 3rd ed. Philadelphia, Hanley & Belfus, 2002.

Moser RL: Primary Care for Physician Assistants: Clinical Practice Guidelines, 2nd ed. Norwalk, CT, McGraw-Hill/Appleton & Lange, 2001.

Physician Assistants' Prescribing Reference, Fall 2003. New York, Prescribing Reference Inc., 2003.

Rakel R (ed): Saunders Manual of Medical Practice. Philadelphia, WB Saunders, 1996.

Web Sites

American Association of Clinical Endocrinologists: www.aace.com

American Association of Diabetes Educators: www.aadenet.org

American Diabetes Association: www.diabetes.org

National Diabetes Education Program of the National Institutes of Health: ndep.nih.gov/health/diabetes

GASTROENTEROLOGY

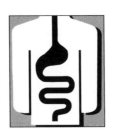

5

Appendicitis
James W. Becker, PA-C

DEFINITION

Acute inflammation of the appendix due to obstruction or infection.

HISTORY

Symptoms. Sequential onset of abdominal pain that usually becomes localized to the right lower quadrant. Frequently associated with anorexia and nausea.

General. Most common cause of acute abdominal pain in the young, otherwise healthy patient.

Age. Most common between 10 and 30 years of age.

Onset. May be rapid over a few hours or insidious over a few days.

Intensity. Usually mild to moderate epigastric pain progressing over 12 to 18 hours to moderately severe right lower quadrant pain.

Aggravating Factors. Sudden movements (e.g., going over bumps while riding in a car or stretcher).

Alleviating Factors. Fetal position, knees flexed.

Associated Factors. None.

PHYSICAL EXAMINATION

General. The patient may appear ill. Usually is in no distress when lying still. Temperature may be elevated (i.e., greater than 100° F), especially if the patient is dehydrated.

Gastrointestinal. Abdomen is nondistended. There may be guarding in the lower quadrants with point tenderness at McBurney's point (one-third of the distance between the iliac crest and the umbilicus). There is rebound tenderness with pain intensity of 5 to 7 (on a scale of 1-10) on percussion. Bowel sounds will be diminished. Peritoneal signs will be present with perforation (e.g., psoas sign: hyperextension of the right hip joint causing pain; obturator sign: pain on flexion and internal rotation of the right thigh). The patient may also demonstrate a Rovsing sign—tenderness in the right lower quadrant of the abdomen when pressure is applied in the left lower quadrant.

PATHOPHYSIOLOGY

The appendix is most commonly located in the right lower quadrant at the tip of the cecum. The appendix may flip into the retrocecal space, where tenderness is greater. Appendicitis is caused by obliteration of the appendiceal lumen by either a fecalith, a fibrous obliteration, or microorganisms (most commonly, enteric pathogens such as *Escherichia coli* and *Klebsiella*). Amebic organisms have also been implicated. Chronic appendicitis with smoldering symptoms has been reported.

DIAGNOSTIC STUDIES

Laboratory
Complete Blood Count. White blood cell (WBC) count is frequently but not always elevated (i.e., greater than 10,000/mm³). WBC differential may show a left shift.

Urinalysis. May reveal leukocytes (more than 10 cells/high-power field [hpf]).

Erythrocyte Sedimentation Rate (Westergren Method). May be elevated (to greater than 20 mm/hour).

Human Chorionic Gonadotropin. Should be assayed to rule out ectopic pregnancy.

Radiology
Flat and Upright Abdominal Films. Indicated to evaluate for fecalith and to rule out other abdominal pathology.

Pelvic Ultrasound Examination. Performed to rule out tubo-ovarian process or to look for free fluid or abscess.

Abdominal CT Scan. May show cecal inflammation, phlegmon, or abscess.

Other
Diagnostic Laparoscopy. For direct visualization of the appendix.

DIFFERENTIAL DIAGNOSIS

Traumatic. Not applicable.

Infectious
Colitis, especially with inflammation of the cecum, can mimic appendicitis. This can be caused by a viral or bacterial agent or may be due to a parasitic infection (e.g., giardiasis). The patient may have a history of exposure to contaminated water 1 to 2 weeks earlier.

Urinary tract infection usually manifests with elevated temperature and very high urinary leukocyte count.

With *tubo-ovarian infection*, tenderness on pelvic examination.

Metabolic
With *acute cholecystitis*, may have elevated liver enzymes, tender right upper quadrant; gallbladder ultrasound examination may show calculi or edema.

Crohn disease usually mainfests more insidiously. Previous episodes may have been less severe.

Renal calculi would show an elevated erythrocyte count on urinalysis. Calculi may be apparent on radiograph. Intravenous pyelogram is positive.

With *ectopic pregnancy*, a positive result on human chorionic gonadotropin assay.

Ruptured diverticulum may show as free air on radiograph.

Neoplastic
Ovarian cyst rupture is usually seen on ultrasound examination.

Carcinoid tumor, the most common neoplasm of the appendix, is found at approximately 0.3% of appendectomies. These tumors are considered incidental if they are small in size (less than 1.5 cm in diameter), but more aggressive surgical resection is indicated if the carcinoid is greater than 2 cm across.

Adenocarcinoma of the appendix is rare, but can occur.

Vascular
A *leaking abdominal aortic aneurysm*, especially if involving the right iliac artery, can mimic the presentation of appendicitis.

Congenital
Not applicable.

Acquired
With *perforated duodenal ulcer,* may have positive test for occult blood in stool and free air evident on radiograph.

TREATMENT

The following approach is recommended, if clinical findings warrant it:
   Hydration with lactated Ringer solution or 5% dextrose in half-normal saline ($D_5\frac{1}{2}NS$).
   Surgical consultation to consider appendectomy.
   Intravenous antibiotics with anaerobic and gram-negative coverage (e.g., timentin 3.1 g every 6 hours, OR a combination of cefoxitin [Mefoxin] 2 g every 6 hours and metronidazole [Flagyl] 500 mg every 8 hours), for 24 hours in the uncomplicated case and for 7 days with a ruptured appendix.

If an appendiceal abscess is noted on CT and the patient is not acutely ill, CT-guided drainage may be performed, followed initially by intravenous and then by oral antibiotics. A semielective appendectomy can be scheduled approximately 6 weeks later.

PEDIATRIC CONSIDERATIONS

Appendicitis is the most common cause of an acute abdomen in adolescents and older children. It is also the most common reason for abdominal surgery in childhood.

Clinical manifestations include a 1- or 2-day history of dull or crampy periumbilical pain that remains constant and localizes to McBurney's point. Anorexia and nausea (with or without vomiting), mild fever, and constipation also occur. Diarrhea may substitute for constipation. Atypical presentations are common among children. In children younger than 2 years of age, the pain of appendicitis is poorly localized. Serial examination of the abdomen over a period of several hours is recommended to interpret evolving signs and symptoms. Appendectomy is indicated whenever the diagnosis of appendicitis cannot be ruled out after a period of close observation. Despite the high incidence of perforation (40% in infants and children), the mortality rate is less than 1% during childhood.

OBSTETRIC CONSIDERATIONS

Pregnant women with appendicitis usually present with symptoms similar to those found in nonpregnant patients. The exception is that the classic right lower quadrant pain may be displaced superiorly owing to the enlarging uterus. Rebound tenderness also may not be as pronounced.

Obstetric patients are more prone to widespread peritonitis secondary to a perforated appendix because of appendiceal displacement by the gravid uterus. There is an approximately 20% perinatal mortality associated with a perforated appendix; the inflammation accompanying the peritonitis can lead to premature labor and fetal loss.

If appendicitis is diagnosed early with prompt surgical intervention, the outcome should be positive for both mother and baby. There may be an increased risk of premature delivery during only the first week after uncomplicated appendectomy.

Regional anesthesia is preferred for the appendectomy.

GERIATRIC CONSIDERATONS

Appendicitis can occur in any age group. The elderly patient may present in a critical situation and in shock, requiring rapid assessment and treatment.

PREVENTIVE CONSIDERATIONS

Incidental appendectomy, if performed with another surgical procedure, and after adequate bowel preparation, will prevent the onset of acute appendicitis later in life.

PEARLS FOR THE PA

In a majority of cases of appendicitis, the diagnosis is made by history.

Radiographic and laboratory data are frequently nondiagnostic.

The patient may be observed for 24 hours with serial white blood cell determinations if diagnosis is in doubt.

Cholecystitis

James W. Becker, PA-C, and Michelle Heinan, EdD, MS, PA-C

DEFINITION

Cholecystitis is inflammation of the gallbladder from any cause. *Cholelithiasis* is stones of the gallbladder. *Cholangitis* is inflammation of any bile duct due to stone, tumor, cyst, or stricture.

HISTORY

Symptoms

Symptoms are due to transient obstruction by stones (cholelithiasis), inflammation of the gallbladder secondary to the obstruction or infection (cholecystitis), or significant obstruction of the biliary tract causing significant damage and infection of the bile duct (cholangitis).

The predominant symptom is pain located in the right upper quadrant (RUQ) of the abdomen. Pain is described initially as dull, aching, and continuous and can radiate posteriorly to the scapula, parathoracic area, or shoulder. Symptoms may resolve over hours or can progress to generalized peritonitis. Nausea and vomiting may be present but are not consistent or specific findings. Other signs and symptoms may include fever, chills, anorexia, dyspepsia, and jaundice.

In cholangitis, *Charcot's triad* of fever/chills, RUQ pain, and jaundice may be present but is not a consistent sign. Shock and mental status changes suggest biliary sepsis.

Acalculous cholecystitis accounts for about 5% to10% of cases of cholecystitis. It has a more rapidly progressive clinical course. It is encountered with major trauma or significant illness (e.g., diabetes mellitus).

General. May have a history of prior attacks or known cholelithiasis. Cholangitis can occur without the gallbladder being present (bile duct inflammation).

Age.   Uncommon in children. Any age, but incidence increases with age.

Onset.   Subacute, with progression of symptoms within hours.

Duration.   Continuous pain lasting 30 minutes to 6 hours with cholelithiasis. Pain lasting over 6 hours suggests development of acute cholecystitis. If the obstruction (stone) clears, the symptoms may resolve and return after a week or longer, usually at about the same time of day.

Intensity.   May be relatively mild with spontaneous resolution of symptoms, or the patient may present with sepsis from severe obstruction and infection.

Aggravating Factors.   Recent ingestion of fatty foods. Persistent obstruction.

Alleviating Factors.   Passage of the stone.

Associated Factors.   Disease states such as diabetes mellitus, cystic fibrosis, intestinal malabsorbtion, chronic liver disease (alcoholism), hemolytic disease, hepatitis, HIV infection, herpesvirus infections. Also, other factors such as obesity, significant weight loss/fasting, oral contraceptive use, positive family history, Asian race, history of biliary infection, or biliary parasites.

PHYSICAL EXAMINATION

General.   Patients may be in mild, moderate, or severe distress depending on the degree of obstruction and inflammation/infection of the gallbladder. Vital signs may reveal tachycardia and fever.

Gastrointestinal.   Murphy's sign is worsened pain on inspiration with palpation of the RUQ. The inspiration may be halted owing to the pain. Percussion and rebound tenderness will be present with peritonitis. Bowel sounds may be hypoactive. Presence of generalized peritoneal signs suggests perforation.

Skin.   Observe for jaundice due to chronic hemolysis or hepatic involvement.

PATHOPHYSIOLOGY

Bile is manufactured in the liver and transported to the gallbladder for storage. Bile is released into the duodenum through the common bile duct at the ampulla of Vater. The pancreatic duct may merge with the common bile duct proximal to the ampulla of Vater. Bile is released in response to secretion of the hormone cholecystokinin from the mucosal cells of the small intestine. Cholecystokinin is released in response to ingestion of fats and amino acids that enter the duodenum.

Symptoms of cholelithiasis are due to stones causing obstruction that lead to bile stasis. Obstruction can occur in the gallbladder neck, cystic duct, or common bile duct. The stone may be extruded by pressure from the contracting gallbladder, leading to intermittent symptoms.

If the blockage does not clear, the result is acute cholecystitis. Retrograde pressure in the gallbladder leads to distention, inflammation and mucosal damage, ischemia, and infection. Ascending cholangitis is due to obstruction from any source of the common bile duct. This leads to increased pressure and bacterial overgrowth.

Acalculous cholecystitis is usually due to acute illness that leads to biliary stasis and mucosal ischemia. Gangrene of the gallbladder may occur with or without perforation (emphysematous cholecystitis) and leads to sepsis.

Gallstones may be composed of cholesterol (70% of stones), pigment (20%), or a combination (mixed, 10%). Cholesterol stones form when the bile is saturated with cholesterol. The other type of stone is composed of calcium bilirubinate (pigmented). Pigmented stones are associated with hemolytic anemias, Asian race, bacterial/parasitic infection, and liver disease. Owing to the presence of calcium, pigmented stones may be seen on radiographs.

Bacterial infections are most commonly due to members of the family Enterobacteriaceae (e.g., *Escherichia coli*, *Klebsiella*), which account for about 70% of infections; of these, enterococci account for approximately 15%, *Bacteroides* around 10%, *Clostridium* 10%, and group D streptococci and staphylococci the remainder.

DIAGNOSTIC STUDIES

Laboratory
Complete Blood Count.   Evaluate for elevated white blood cell (WBC) count in infection.

Liver Function Tests.   Elevation of direct bilirubin and alkaline phosphatase suggests obstruction or cholangitis. May increase over 1 or 2 days.

Electrolytes.   May be abnormal if the patient is dehydrated.

Amylase and Lipase.   Elevated with pancreatic involvement.

Urinalysis.   May have hematuria or proteinuria with urinary tract etiology. Bilirubinuria indicates common bile duct obstruction or hepatitis.

Human Chorionic Gonadotropin.   Should be assayed in appropriate patients to exclude pregnancy.

Cardiac Enzymes.   Determination of cardiac isoenzymes used to evaluate for a cardiac cause of symptoms.

Radiology
Ultrasound Examination.   Used as screening and for diagnosis.

Radionuclide Scanning with dimethyl iminodiacetic acid (HIDA).   Used for hepatobiliary imaging if clinical findings suggest cholecystitis even with negative result on ultrasonography. Can detect acalculous disease. Can diagnose common bile duct obstruction or cholecystitis, but not gallstones. HIDA scan is useful only if the serum bilirubin measurement is less than 5 mg/dL. With bilirubin levels 5 mg/dL or greater, the diisopropyl iminodiacetyl acid scan is used.

Abdominal Radiographs.   Rule out free air from intestinal perforation; gallstones may be seen in 20% of patients.

Abdominal CT Scan.   Used if other conditions need to be excluded.

Chest Film.   Can rule out a pulmonary cause of symptoms.

Endoscopic Retrograde Cholangiopancreatography (ERCP). To evaluate the biliary tree for tumors, congenital abnormalities, and stones.

Magnetic Resonance Cholangiopancreatography (MRCP). Another way to visualize the biliary tree, especially in those patients who cannot undergo ERCP (e.g., because of previous stomach surgery).

Other
ECG. As indicated to rule out a cardiac etiology for symptoms.

DIFFERENTIAL DIAGNOSIS

Traumatic. Not applicable.

Infectious
Fitz-Hugh–Curtis syndrome is caused by ascending infection due to *Chlamydia trachomatis* or *Neisseria gonorrhoeae* from pelvic inflammatory disease. It is accompanied by RUQ pain as a result of inflammation of the liver capsule or diaphragm.

With *hepatitis*, positive hepatitis profile; elevated liver enzymes.

In *pneumonia/pleurisy*, positive findings on chest film.

Appendicitis during pregnancy or with retrocecal involvement can manifest with RUQ pain.

Pyelonephritis can be differentiated on urinalysis with culture and sensitivity testing.

HIV infection can lead to AIDS-related sclerosing cholangitis. Positive HIV assay.

With *pelvic inflammatory disease*, positive findings on pelvic examination.

Metabolic
With *myocardial infarction*, positive ECG, cardiac enzymes.

Pancreatitis may be associated with cholelithiasis or exist alone. Negative findings on ultrasound examination and HIDA scan.

With *duodenal perforation*, free air evident on abdominal radiograph.

With *peptic ulcer disease*, may be *Helicobacter pylori* positive. Symptoms relieved by meals.

Gastritis causes more epigastric pain and may require endoscopy for diagnosis.

Kidney stone may cause hematuria detectable on urinalysis. Positive intravenous pyelogram (IVP).

Intestinal obstruction seen on plain film of abdomen with intestinal distention. If the obstruction is associated with air in the biliary tree, consider gallstone ileus with a cholecystoenteral fistula and a large gallstone obstructing the small bowel.

With *gastroesophageal reflux disease* (GERD), epigastric burning relieved by meals.

Neoplastic
Pancreatic tumor seen on CT study of abdomen.
Hepatic tumor seen on CT study of abdomen.

Vascular
Abdominal aortic aneurysm seen on CT study of abdomen. May have abdominal bruit.

Congenital
Not applicable.

Acquired
With ectopic pregnancy, positive human chorionic gonadotropin assay.

TREATMENT

Pharmacologic/Medical
For cholelithiasis, treat symptomatically for nausea and pain:
  Glycopyrrolate (Robinol) as an antispasmodic 1-2 mg orally two or three times a day; 0.1-0.2 mg IV or IM every 4 hours.
  Promethazine (Phenergan) 25 mg every 4-6 hours as needed.
  If symptoms continue beyond 6 hours, consider the possibility of acute cholecystitis.
  Support vital functions. Begin intravenous fluids if nausea, vomiting, and dehydration are present.
  Broad-spectrum antibiotics are begun. If there is no evidence of sepsis, begin a third-generation cephalosporin. If there is an obvious infection, begin parenteral ampicillin, gentamicin, and clindamycin (or piperacillin and metronidazole as alternatives for clindamycin).
  Keep the patient NPO. Consider placement of a nasogastric tube if there is ileus, if the patient is experiencing significant vomiting, or if complete bowel rest is indicated.
  Septic shock requires aggressive management (see "Shock" in Chapter 3, Emergency Medicine).
  Cholangitis can be fatal if left untreated.

Surgery
Surgery is indicated acutely for perforation or sepsis. It is also performed for acute cholecystitis, cholangitis, pancreatitis, obstruction, frequent attacks, congenital defect in the biliary system, and in patients with diabetes mellitus.
  Surgical techniques include the laparoscopic approach and open cholecystectomy.
  Endoscopic retrograde cholangiopacreatography (ERCP) may be used for endoscopic sphincterotomy and drainage.

PEDIATRIC CONSIDERATIONS

Gallstones are rare in children and if present are usually associated with hemolytic anemias (e.g., sickle cell disease, thalassemias). Acalculous cholecystis is more common and is associated with systemic illness such as sepsis.

Cholangitis is rare but can be found even after previous gallbladder surgery. Biliary atresia should be considered in an infant with jaundice, elevated liver enzymes, and decreased stool production.

OBSTETRIC CONSIDERATIONS

Prolonged labor may lead to acalculous cholecystitis. Cholelithiasis can develop in pregnancy but symptoms are usually delayed until after delivery. Preeclampsia and fatty liver can cause elevated liver enzymes on liver function testing. Cholecystectomy can be performed in pregnancy if necessary.

GERIATRIC CONSIDERATIONS

Murphy's sign may not be present in the elderly patient. Consider ultrasound examination to evaluate any abdominal pain or signs of sepsis.

Acalculous cholecystitis is more common in this age group.

PREVENTIVE CONSIDERATIONS

A high index of suspicion needs to be maintained to identify gallbladder disease in the early stages prior to progression to cholecystitis and ascending cholangitis.

PEARLS FOR THE PA

Symptoms of uncomplicated cholelithiasis should resolve within 6 hours.

Cholecystitis and ascending cholangitis can progress to peritonitis and sepsis.

Only about 20% of gallstones (pigmented type) can be seen on plain films.

Crohn's Disease

Michelle L. Heinan, EdD, MS, PA-C

DEFINITION

Crohn's disease is an inflammatory process that can affect any part of the gastrointestinal (GI) mucosa. It frequently involves the colon or small bowel, primarily the right colon and distal ileum. Crohn's disease is associated with human leukocyte antigen B27 (HLA-A2).

HISTORY

Symptoms. Low-grade fever, weight loss, malaise, fatigue, pain or mass in the right lower quadrant (RLQ) of the abdomen, cramping, postprandial lower abdominal pain, altered bowel habits (in the young), and watery diarrhea. Steatorrhea may accompany the other symptoms if there is small bowel involvement. Some patients with chronic disease will present with nausea and vomiting, which signals obstruction. Occult blood may be found in mild cases, with frank GI bleeding in severe cases.

General. The hallmark of the disease is a history of chronic and recurrent pain in the RLQ with associated diarrhea. Crohn's disease patients have a fivefold risk for developing cancer of the small bowel. Surveillance should start 10 years after the initial diagnosis of Crohn's disease, with routine colonoscopy every 1 to 2 years. A sudden change in the patient's bowel habits should prompt an evaluation.

Age. Crohn's disease can develop between 10 and 40 years of age and also 60 and 80 years. Peak age range is between 20 and 30 years.

Onset. Gradual.

Duration. Chronic.

Intensity. The pain is described as colicky.

Aggravating Factors. Consumption of food usually is the aggravating factor.

Alleviating Factors. Defecation.

Associated Factors. Extraintestinal manifestations may develop; these include uveitis, episcleritis, pyoderma gangrenosum, cholelithiasis, nephrolithasis, arthritis, sacroiliitis, erythema nodosum, aphthous ulcers, ankylosing spondylitis, clubbing, arthritis, folate deficiency, and vitamin B_{12} deficiency. With malabsorption of vitamin D and calcium or glucocorticosteroid use, osteoporosis and osteomalacia may be seen.

PHYSICAL EXAMINATION

General. The patient usually presents as thin and undernourished, with a history of weight loss and a low-grade temperature.

Head, Ears, Eyes, Nose, Throat
Eyes. Look for signs of uveitis and episcleritis.
Mouth. Aphthous ulcerations.

Gastrointestinal
Abdomen. Tenderness or mass in the right lower quadrant.
Rectal. Perianal disease including abscesses, skin tags, fissures, scarring, fistulas, and sinus tract.
Skin. Clubbing, erythema nodosum, and pyoderma gangrenosum.
Musculoskeletal. Signs of arthritis, sacroiliitis, and ankylosing spondylitis.

PATHOPHYSIOLOGY

Crohn's disease involves all layers of the intestinal mucosa. The disease is characterized by the ulcerations, fissures, and crypts filled with noncaseating granulomas. The bowel becomes inflamed, stenotic, and inflexible. "Skip areas" can be found between normal and diseased areas of the bowel. Patients can develop fistulas, fibrotic strictures, or perirectal fissures from the inflammation present in this transmural disease. Approximately half of the patients have lesions in the proximal colon and distal ileum; of these, a third of the lesions are found in the small bowel and/or colon, and a quarter are confined to the colon.

DIAGNOSTIC STUDIES

Laboratory
Complete Blood Count with Iron, Vitamin B$_{12}$, and Folate Levels. Will show a mixed anemia or iron and B$_{12}$ deficiency. The white blood cell (WBC) count will be increased. Sulfa drugs may lower the folate levels after the patient has been taking the medications chronically.
Erythrocyte Sedimentation Rate. Elevated.
Chemistry Profile. Decrease in albumin, calcium, and sodium. Alkaline phosphatase and gamma globulins will be increased.
C-Reactive Proteins. Should be used as a marker to determine the patient's progress in recovery.
Fat-Soluble Vitamin Deficiencies. Deficiencies of vitamins A, D, E, and K also can be found.

Radiology
Barium Enema. Should precede an upper GI series with small bowel follow-through. The studies may show flattening, thickening, straightening, or blunting of the normal bowel due to mucosal edema. Distortion of landmarks may be seen owing to fibrotic stenosis. May also show long longitudinal ulcerations, fistula, abscess, perforations, or rectal sparing.

CT Scan of the Abdomen. Can show fistulous tracts in the retroperitoneum, bladder, or skin. Transmural thickening will also be present.

Plain Abdominal Films. Can be used to demonstrate an intestinal obstruction, toxic megacolon, sacroiliitis, or arthritis.

Other

Endoscopy. Is used to complement the foregoing studies for evaluation.

DIFFERENTIAL DIAGNOSIS

Traumatic. Not applicable.

Infectious

In *tuberculosis*, positive findings on purified protein derivative (PPD) skin test, chest film, or culture for acid-fast bacilli.

In *gonorrheal/chlamydial pelvic inflammation*, positive genitourinary cultures.

Fungal infections such as those due to actinomycetes, *Histoplasma*, *Candida*, and *Aspergillus* can be differentiated on appropriate cultures.

With *clostridial toxin–induced diarrhea* (*Clostridium difficile* toxin), may have a history of antibiotic use. Positive cultures.

With *amebic colitis*, organisms may be seen on microscopic examination.

Infectious colitis (e.g., from *Yersinia* or *Campylobacter*) can be differentiated on culture.

Infectious diarrhea may be caused by bacteria (enterotoxigenic *Escherichia coli*, *Salmonella*, *Shigella*, *Aeromonas*, *Plesiomonas*, *Chlamydia trachomatis*,), parasites (*Entamoeba histolytica*, *Cryptosporidium*, *Isospora belli*), or viruses (herpes simplex virus, cytomegalovirus).

Pseudomembranous colitis can be caused by the use of antibiotics. The presentation may appear to be a toxic megacolon. The main pathogen is *C. difficile*.

Metabolic

With *diverticulitis*, diverticula are seen on barium enema or endoscopy.

Ulcerative colitis is differentiated on sigmoidoscopy or barium enema (See "Ulcerative Colitis" in this chapter).

Lymphogranuloma venereum is identified by positive serology/culture for *C. trachomatis*.

Neoplastic

Lymphoma/colon carcinoma can be identified on colonoscopy and/or CT.

Vascular

Ischemic colitis is a very common problem in the geriatric population, particularly after aortoiliac reconstructive surgery. Findings indicative of a necrotic colon necessitate immediate surgical intervention. Colonoscopy will demonstrate edema, petechiae, and ulcers. A sharp demarcation can be found just proximal to the splenic flexure.

Congenital.   Not applicable.

Acquired
With *drug-induced eosinophilic gastroenteritis* due to NSAIDs, history of NSAID use.

Antibiotic-associated/ischemic/radiation proctitis can be differentiated by the history.

Other
In *irritable bowel syndrome*, all studies negative.

Intestinal obstruction may be caused by Crohn's disease or another process. Acute condition.

Acute abdomen may be of traumatic, vascular, or structural etiology. May require immediate surgical intervention.

TREATMENT

Pharmacologic
Prednisone in combination with sulfasalazine and a delayed-release mesalamine, which is 5-aminosalicylic acid (5-ASA) (Asacol or Rowasa), can give improvement in up to three-quarters of patients with uncomplicated ileal disease.

- 5-ASA agents: for colon involvement
    Sulfasalazine 500 mg/dose, for a total dose of 3-6 g/day, in acute phase of mild to moderate disease; 2-4 g/day for maintenance.
    Patients not able to tolerate sulfasalazine can take:
    Olsalazine 250 mg/dose, up to a total of 1-3 g/day, which is found to be less toxic.
- Mesalamine agents
    Balsalazide 500-750 mg/dose, up to a total of 2-6 g/day, induces remission in patients.
    Delayed release for ileum/colon involvement:
    Asacol 400 mg/dose, up to a total of 1.6-4.8 g/day in acute phase; 0.8-4.8 g/day for maintenance therapy. Assists in treating ileocolitis, colitis, and ileitis to induce and maintain remission.
    Sustained release:
    Pentasa 250 mg/dose, up to a total of 1.5-4 g/day, or up to 4 g/day in the acute phase; 1.5-4 g/day for maintenance. Dissolves in the stomach.
    Topical mesalamine enemas are effective in relieving rectal symptoms.
- Glucocorticoids
    Prednisone 40-60 mg/day in active disease unresponsive to 5-ASA therapy. Once remission is achieved, taper dose by 20 mg every

7 to 14 days until the patient is on only 20 mg a day; then reduce by 5 mg every other day.

Adrenocorticotropic hormone (ACTH) is occasionally used, but a risk of adrenal hemorrhage is associated with its administration.

Topical glucocorticoids are beneficial for distal colitis (used for adjunctive therapy in patients who have rectal involvement and more proximal disease).

Hydrocortisone enemas or foam may control active disease; highly absorbed and may cause adrenal suppression. Use 7-14 days in active disease.

Glucocorticoids have no role in maintenance therapy for Crohn's disease.

- Antibiotics

   Metronidazole in a dose of 750-2000 mg/day is as effective as sulfasalazine. It is efficacious in active inflammation and in fistulous and perianal Crohn's and may prevent recurrence after ileal resection. Using metronidazole reduces the need for corticosteroid therapy.

- Azathioprine or 6-mercaptopurine (6-MP)

   Azathioprine 1.5-2.5 mg/kg/day.

   6-MP 1-1.5 mg/kg/day.

   Used in glucocorticoid-dependent disease, with efficacy seen in 3 to 4 weeks. Monitor 6-thioguanine levels for compliance.

- Methotrexate

   Methotrexate can be administered as follows:

   25 mg IM per week for 12 weeks: effective in inducing remission and reducing glucocorticoid dosage.

   15 mg IM per week after 12-week regimen: effective in maintaining remission in active Crohn's disease.

   Long-term methotrexate therapy can cause complications including pulmonary and hepatic fibrosis and pneumonitis.

- Nutritional therapy

   Patients with severe Crohn's disease respond well to bowel rest along with total enteral nutrition or total parenteral nutrition For maintenance, keep the patient on a high-protein diet with supplemental fat-soluble vitamins and B_{12}.

- Anti–tumor necrosis factor (TNF) antibody—infliximab

   TNF is found to be increased in inflammatory bowel disease. The monoclonal antibody infliximab is an effective agent in Crohn's disease, particularly in cases refractory to other treatment regimens. In such cases, use of infliximab 5 mg/kg IV has shown a 65% response rate. Infliximab can be repeated every 8 weeks. As long as the patient is responding, the treatment can continue for up to 14 weeks on the every-8-week regimen.

- Newer immunosuppressive agents

  Tacrolimus, an agent similar to cyclosporine in mechanism of action, has been efficacious in pediatric refractory inflammatory bowel disease and adult small bowel involvement (extensive).

  Mycophenolate mofetil 500 mg twice daily OR 15 mg/kg/day causes reduction in glucocorticoid requirement in Crohn's disease.

  Thalidomide inhibits TNF production. Effectiveness is found in those patients who have fistulas or whose disease is refractory to glucocorticoids. More randomized controlled trials are needed.

- Anti-inflammatory cytokines

  These newer agents need more controlled trials of use in Crohn's disease.

Surgical

Bowel resection is performed for abscess drainage, obstructions, perforations, intractable disease, and fistulas. Surgery is also done for ostomy function failure, toxic megacolon, and an inability to thrive. Recurrence of disease after surgery is common.

PEDIATRIC CONSIDERATIONS

About one-fifth of cases begin in childhood.

OBSTETRICAL CONSIDERATIONS

Medication must be used with *extreme* caution and in consultation with the obstetrician due to potential fetal harm.

GERIATRIC CONSIDERATIONS

Crohn's disease can develop in the elderly patient. A full evaluation is warranted because the geriatric patient is also more at risk for neoplastic and other diseases.

Crohn's disease occurs mainly in elderly women, and diagnosis is usually delayed. Crohn's disease involves the colon and has a distal distribution. The incidence of surgery is high, and it is often performed on an urgent basis. Morbidity rates for these patients are high.

PREVENTIVE CONSIDERATIONS

Smoking and use of oral contraceptives may be direct causes of or may increase risk for the disease.

PEARLS FOR THE PA

Crohn's disease affects all layers of the intestinal mucosa and is characterized by pain or mass in the right lower quadrant, cramping, postprandial lower abdominal pain, altered bowel habits (in the young), and watery diarrhea.

The disease causes fistulous tracts, perirectal disease with abscess formation, and perforations.

Patients are at risk for cancer of the small bowel.

Diverticulitis

James W. Becker, PA-C

DEFINITION

Acute inflammatory process occurring in outpouchings of the colonic mucosa called *diverticula*. Most commonly occurs in the sigmoid colon.

HISTORY

Symptoms. Rapid onset of abdominal pain, usually located in the left lower abdominal quadrant. Frequently associated with tenderness, fever, and chills.

General. Some patients may experience left lower quadrant discomfort with alternating constipation and diarrhea.

Age. Diverticular disease increases as age advances. Approximately 50% of patients older than 60 will have diverticula. Acute diverticulitis will develop in 25% of these patients.

Onset. Rapid. Acute onset with associated peritoneal signs (e.g., rebound tenderness) and shock, suggest acute perforation of an inflamed diverticulum.

Duration. Several hours to a few days.

Intensity. Moderate pain with diverticulitis. Severe pain with acute perforation.

Aggravating Factors. Consumption of food.

Alleviating Factors. None.

Associated Factors. Most commonly found in cultures that have less natural dietary fiber in the diet (United States and Western Europe).

PHYSICAL EXAMINATION

General. Patient appears generally uncomfortable or in severe pain. May be febrile (100.5° to 101° F).

Gastrointestinal. Abdomen may be slightly distended and nontympanic. Bowel sounds may be normal or diminished. There is usually guarding and/or tenderness to palpation over the left lower quadrant. An inflammatory mass or abscess may be palpable in a thin patient. Rectal examination may reveal gross blood. Guaiac testing may reveal occult blood. If a fistula has formed between the colon and the bladder, the patient may report passing air through the urethra while urinating (pneumaturia).

PATHOPHYSIOLOGY

Diverticula of the colonic wall form where blood vessels permeate the connective tissue to supply the mucosa. In patients with chronically high intraluminal colonic pressure (e.g., constipation), herniations develop at the blood vessel permeation site, forming small pouches that can entrap fecal debris. This allows for infection and microscopic abscess formation with possible perforation or fistula formation.

DIAGNOSTIC STUDIES

Laboratory
Complete Blood Count. White blood cell (WBC) count frequently elevated (more than 10,000/mm^3). Hemoglobin may be decreased (less than 10 g/dL) with lower GI bleed with diverticulitis.
Stool Guaiac Test. May be positive for occult blood.

Radiology
Flat and Upright Abdominal Films. May show free air if perforation is present.
Abdominal Ultrasound Examination. May reveal a mass from inflammatory response or abscess formation.
CT Scan of the Abdomen. Performed to visualize an abscess. May see inflammatory changes or diverticula.
Barium Enema. Not indicated in the acute setting of diverticulitis. May be performed no sooner than 2 weeks after the acute process has cleared.

Other
Colonoscopy. Performed after the acute process has cleared. Used to confirm the presence of diverticula.

DIFFERENTIAL DIAGNOSIS

Traumatic
Foreign body ingestion may cause intestinal perforation.

Infectious

With *pseudomembranous colitis*, positive test for *Clostridium difficile* in stool.

Metabolic

Peptic ulcer disease may cause intestinal perforation.

Crohn's disease may cause abscess or fistula formation and most commonly affects the terminal ileum (seen on CT scan).

Neoplastic

Colon cancer may cause intestinal perforation or obstruction.

Vascular

Intestinal ischemia due to either atherosclerotic disease, embolus, or hypotensive episode.

Congenital

Volvulus of the sigmoid colon will give counterclockwise appearance of sigmoid colon on flat plate film of the abdomen.

Acquired

With *acute colitis*, history of recent antibiotic use or exposure to contaminated food or water.

TREATMENT

Medical/Pharmacologic

For intravenous hydration, treat shock with volume expansion; give 5% dextrose in half-normal saline ($D_5\frac{1}{2}NS$) or 5% dextrose and lactated Ringer's solution.

Broad-spectrum antibiotics with both anaerobic and gram-negative coverage may be begun orally for initial episode, with close follow-up.

Keep the patient NPO during the severe attack; begin a low-residue diet as pain and fever resolve.

Surgical

CT-guided aspiration of abscess is indicated if patient is unresponsive to the medical regimen.

Surgery is indicated in those patients with evidence of perforation, large abscess, fistula, or severe hemorrhage.

The patient will frequently require a temporary colostomy, which can be closed after several months.

Patients with recurrent bouts of diverticulitis may benefit from elective resection of the affected colon. With adequate bowel preparation, colostomy may not be required.

PEDIATRIC CONSIDERATIONS

Meckel diverticulum is the most common anomaly of the GI tract. It represents the vestigial remnant of the omphalomesenteric duct. Although it rarely causes symptoms, complications most frequently appear within the first 2 years and more frequently in males than in females. The clinical signs include painless rectal bleeding and intestinal obstruction (from intussusception or volvulus). Diverticulitis occurs in 10% to 20% of symptomatic cases and clinically mimics appendicitis. Perforation and peritonitis may occur. Treatment is surgical resection.

OBSTETRIC CONSIDERATIONS

No specific indications.

GERIATRIC CONSIDERATIONS

Diverticulitis is a common ailment of the older population. Conservative management to avoid surgery may be the preferred course if comorbid factors significantly increase the risk associated with surgery.

PREVENTIVE CONSIDERATIONS

Increasing dietary fiber can prevent the formation of diverticula. However, once diverticula have been diagnosed, a low-residue diet is advised.

PEARLS FOR THE PA

Diverticula are most common in the sigmoid colon.

A diet low in fiber can lead to diverticulum formation.

Avoid barium enemas in the acute setting.

Dyspepsia
Michelle L. Heinan, EdD, MS, PA-C

DEFINITION

Dyspepsia occurs in approximately 25% of the population. There are several different causes of dyspepsia. *Nonulcer* and *functional dyspepsia* are terms used to describe the symptoms associated with peptic ulcer disease, malignancy, pancreatic pathology, and gastroesophageal reflux disease (GERD). In peptic ulcer disease, organic pathology cannot be detected in 15% to 25% of the population. *Helicobacter pylori* causes chronic gastritis or peptic ulcer disease in 30% to 60% of the patients, but in 50% to 60% of the patients, a specific etiology cannot be identified. Approximately 15% to 25% of the patients with dyspepsia have peptic ulcer disease, 5% to 15% have reflux esophagitis, and less than 2% have gastric and esophageal cancer. As noted, GERD also may cause dyspepsia. Sometimes patients have anxiety associated with dyspepsia. Dyspepsia causes substantial lost time from work and health care costs. Patients usually present after failing self-treatment with over-the-counter medications.

HISTORY

Symptoms. The patient presents with upper abdominal pain or discomfort that may be chronic or recurrent in nature. Pain can be worsened or relieved by meals. Associated symptoms are hypersalivation, bloating, belching, heartburn, nausea, sour taste, and vomiting. Patients who experience early satiety, nausea, or postprandial bloating may have a motility-related dyspepsia (e.g., delayed gastric emptying). Reflux may manifest with epigastric pain described as burning in nature. Depending on severity of symptoms, hematemesis, diarrhea, or melena may present. Other possible signs and symptoms that rarely may be noted are chest pain, hoarseness, pharyngitis, and cough. Occasionally odynophagia (pain on swallowing) develops. If odynophagia occurs, a workup needs to be done to evaluate for infectious esophagitis.

General. Obtain a thorough history from the patient to assist in determining cause of dyspepsia. Obtain information on smoking and alcohol ingestion as well as use of medications (prescribed, over-the-counter, and alternative).

Causes of Dyspepsia
Post-traumatic
  Head trauma
  Multiple trauma
Endocrine
  Diabetes mellitus
  Thyroid disease
  Hypercalcemia
  Parathyroidism
Respiratory
  Tuberculosis
Renal
  Renal cell carcinoma
Gastrointestinal
  GERD
Cholecystitis
Aerophagia
Pancreatic disease
Peptic ulcer disease
Gastric cancer
Pancreatic cancer
Ischemic bowel disease
Malabsorption syndromes
Esophageal spasms
Irritable bowel syndrome
Biliary tract disease
Celiac sprue
Pancreatitis
Gynecologic
Ovarian carcinoma

Infectious
Intestinal parasites (*Giardia*, *Strongyloides*)
Candida
Herpes simplex virus
Cytomegalovirus
Other

Connective tissue disorders
Use of nonsteroidal anti-inflammatory drugs (NSAIDs) and digitalis
Electrolyte disorders
Sarcoidosis
Hyperkalemia

Age. Dyspepsia can occur in persons younger than 25 years of age. With peptic ulcer, dyspepsia usually occurs between the ages of 45 and 54. Gastric ulcer disease occurs between the ages of 55 and 64 years. Past the age of 70, ulcers can be found in 60% of affected patients, and cancer in 33%.

Onset. Occasional flare-ups depending on cause of aggravation. Onset can be acute and vary with the extent of the problem (e.g., ulcer, perforation, hemorrhage).

Duration. Variable.

Intensity. Varies, ranging from mild dyspepsia to severe chest pain or epigastric pain.

Aggravating Factors. Tobacco, coffee, alcohol, and high-fat foods. Some medications such as NSAIDs, chemotherapy agents, theophylline, erythromycin, acarbose (Precose), alendronate (Fosamax), codeine, iron, metformin (Glucophage), orlistat (Xenical), potassium, progesterone, and corticosteroids. Herbal causes include garlic, gingko, saw palmetto, feverfew, chaste tree berry, and white willow. If a gastric ulcer is present, consumption of food will aggravate the ulcer.

Alleviating Factors. Milk, food, or antacids if the cause is peptic ulcer. Gastric ulcers are alleviated by fasting or sometimes by antacids.

Associated Factors

Smokers are at a higher risk of developing duodenal ulcer disease and experiencing delayed healing or symptom recurrence. A family history of dyspepsia is not uncommon. Weight gain may be experienced in uncomplicated peptic ulcer disease, whereas loss of appetite and weight may be experienced in gastric ulcer disease and gastric carcinoma.

Associated conditions include biliary tract disease, pancreatitis, carbohydrate malabsorption (lactose, sorbitol, fructose), metabolic disturbances (hypercalcemia, hyperkalemia), hepatoma, bowel ischemia, systemic disorders (diabetes mellitus, thyroid and parathyroid disorders, connective tissue disease), intestinal parasitic infections (e.g., with *Giardia*, *Strongyloides*), and abdominal cancer, especially pancreatic or gastric.

PHYSICAL EXAMINATION

General. Observe for jaundice, weight loss, and dehydration.

Mouth. Poor dentition can occur with reflux.

Gastrointestinal. Abdominal distention with tenderness in the epigastric region may be present. Gastric outlet obstruction can be determined by auscultating for a succussion splash. If perforation occurs, peritoneal signs, percussion changes, ascites, and guarding will be present. Palpate for masses. Rectal examination may show guaiac-positive stool.

PATHOPHYSIOLOGY

Dyspepsia can be caused by defects in the mucosa that penetrate into the submucosa but can go deeper than the muscularis propria. An exposure of the mucosa to gastric acid, pepsin, or medications as well as development of an *H. pylori* infection can cause symptoms. Erosion into the mucosa causes ulceration. The location of the ulcer will define whether it is peptic or gastric. In cases of erosive gastritis, edema of the mucosa develops with an infiltrate of neutrophils. With *H. pylori* infection, the organism is found within the layer overlying the superficial mucosal epithelium.

Pathogenesis of GERD includes factors such as those affecting the antireflux mechanism (e.g., lower esophageal sphincter tone, frequency of inappropriate lower esophageal sphincter relaxation, angle of esophagogastric junction, presence or absence of hiatal hernia), volume of gastric contents, composition and potency of refluxed material, efficiency of the esophageal clearance mechanism, and the esophageal mucosa's resistance to injury and its reparative abilities.

DIAGNOSTIC STUDIES

Laboratory
Complete Blood Count. Performed to evaluate for anemia.

Thyroid Function Studies. Performed to evaluate for hypothyroidism or hyperthyroidism.

Calcium. Hypercalcemia can cause dyspepsia.

Amylase, Lipase, and Liver Function Studies. Performed to check for pancreatic or obstructive biliary disease.

Stool Guaiac Test. For occult blood.

Lactase Deficiency. Can be detected by performing a hydrogen breath test after lactose ingestion.

Helicobacter pylori *Serum Titer or Breath Test:* For urease response using carbon radiolabeled urea.

Radiology
Upper Gastrointestinal Series. Will show strictures and rings as well as peptic ulcers.

Abdominal Utrasonography or CT. Used as indicated to identify lesions that may be responsible for symptoms.

Other
Endoscopy. Endoscopy should be performed in any patient who has new onset of dyspepsia or in whom medical treatment fails. Biopsy specimens should be obtained during the endoscopy, particularly of gastric ulcers. For

diagnosis of *H. pylori* infection, a rapid urease test or histologic examination is performed.

Esophageal Manometry. Indicated for patients who are undergoing surgery for GERD.

Esophageal pH Testing. Performed in patients who have unexplained chest pain that does not respond to medications.

DIFFERENTIAL DIAGNOSIS

Traumatic. Not otherwise applicable.
Infectious. Not otherwise applicable.
Metabolic. Not otherwise applicable.
Neoplastic. Not otherwise applicable.

Vascular
Ischemic heart disease/congestive heart failure may mainfest with symptoms attributable to dyspepsia. ECG and cardiac enzymes differentiate.

Congenital. Not otherwise applicable.
Acquired. Not otherwise applicable.

Other
In *psychiatric conditions* such as conversion disorder, the patient may exhibit dyspepsia as a prominent symptom.

TREATMENT

Pharmacologic
Sometimes patients will be treated empirically for the dyspepsia, but as soon as the treatment ceases, the discomfort returns. If over-the-counter medications have failed, a proton pump inhibitor (PPI) may be useful. PPIs should also be used for severe cases of GERD. Medications that can be used for treatment are:

Lansoprazole 30 mg daily

Omeprazole 20 mg daily

Histamine H_2 receptor antagonists such as ranitidine, cimetidine, famotidine, or nizatidine also may be beneficial. Treatment should be given for 4 weeks before considering endoscopy in mild to moderate cases of GERD.

Delayed gastric emptying will manifest as postprandial bloating, early satiety, or nausea. Use of a prokinetic agent (e.g., Reglan 5–15 mg) taken approximately 30 to 60 minutes before a meal is beneficial in the younger population. Reflux that occurs as burning epigastric pain can be treated with acid-reducing agents such as an H_2 receptor antagonist twice a day, a PPI daily, or a prokinetic agent before meals. If testing for *H. pylori* yields a positive result, dual, triple, or quadruple therapy needs to be instituted. (See regimen for eradicating *H. pylori* under Treatment in "Peptic/Gastric Ulcer Disease" later in this chapter.)

Endoscopy should be performed if the patient is older than 45, fails to respond to treatment, or experiences new-onset symptoms. Endoscopy along with other diagnostic procedures should be performed for unexplained weight loss, protracted vomiting, volume depletion, hematemesis, early satiety, dysphagia, evidence of bleeding or anemia, lymphadenopathy, abdominal mass, upper positive fecal occult blood test, melena, family history of upper gastrointestinal (GI) malignancies, or anorexia.

Surgical
Surgical intervention is needed in patients who fail to respond to medical management.

GERIATRIC CONSIDERATIONS

Geriatric patients tend to develop GERD. The most common symptom is heartburn (pyrosis). The severity of the heartburn does not correlate well with the amount of damage.

PREVENTIVE CONSIDERATIONS

Primary prevention includes maintaining ideal body weight, increasing physical exercise, and instituting dietary changes as needed. Avoid regular and decaffeinated coffee, tea, cocoa, alcohol, chocolate, foods high in fat, tobacco, and NSAIDs. Avoid foods, medications, and herbs that seem to cause symptoms to develop.

Secondary preventive measures include elevating the head of the bed, eating small frequent meals, and avoiding eating 2 to 3 hours before bedtime. Explore psychological issues and include a stress reduction program if needed. Make sure the patient does not take restrictions to extremes so that nutrition is impaired.

PEARLS FOR THE PA

There are multiple causes of dysphagia.

Endoscopy should be performed for new-onset dyspepsia and in patients in whom medical treatment has failed.

Prevention includes weight control, physical activity, and dietary changes.

Esophageal Disorders

James W. Becker, PA-C, and Michelle L. Heinan, EdD, MS, PA-C

DEFINITION

Disorders of the esophagus can range from mild to serious. Gastroesophageal reflux disease (GERD) and motility disorders are the most common esophageal disorders. Infection can also occur in patients who are immunocompromised, diabetic, or postoperative; have poor nutritional status; or are on antibiotics or steroids.

HISTORY

Symptoms

Some of the symptoms that occur are achalasia, heartburn, dysphagia, odynophagia, hematemesis, and noncardiac chest pain. Other potential symptoms include hoarseness, obstruction, and cough (with aspiration). The major symptom categories are as follows:

Achalasia: Manifests as chest pain, cough, respiratory problems, or progressive dysphagia. Patients may present with recurrent pneumonia or upper respiratory infections. As the disease progresses, patients have difficulty increasing introthoracic pressure to belch or vomit. Some will complain of a cough that is caused by regurgitated material.

Heartburn (pyrosis): Considered the most common symptom in esophageal disorders; described as a burning sensation that usually radiates upward. Symptoms can range from mild to severe and can be associated with complaints of dysphagia, regurgitation, water brash, belching, and odynophagia.

Dysphagia: Actual difficulty swallowing or the sensation of a blockage causing difficulty swallowing. Some patients will complain of food sticking in the throat or the need to swallow several times before the food will go down. Regurgitation can occur either orally or nasally, with associated coughing or choking. Dysarthria or nasal quality to the patient's voice can also be present.

Odynophagia: Pain on swallowing. The patient may refuse to eat because of the pain and present with weight loss and malnutrition.

Hematemesis: The vomiting of blood. The blood is usually bright red, but if the bleeding is not acute, the blood will have a darker color or "coffee grounds" appearance.

Noncardiac chest pain: Patients who present with chest pain require evaluation to rule out cardiac disease. GERD can cause chest pain with eating and is substernal in location.

Symptoms are specific to the disorder. Symptoms can be caused by the inability of the upper esophageal sphincter to prevent aspiration or the inability of the lower esophageal sphincter to prevent gastric contents from refluxing. Swallowing uses several muscle groups and five cranial nerves (V, VII, IX, X, and XII). Motility disorders can arise from a dysfunctional upper esophageal sphincter, a neurologic problem, or a structural lesion. It is important to ask what medications the patient is taking, as some medications can lead to esophagitis or esophageal injury, causing strictures.

General

It is important to get a thorough history to determine the origin of the problem. If bleeding has occurred, inquire about previous history of bleeding, use of NSAIDs, illnesses, medications, vitamin deficiencies, use of alcohol or tobacco, and family history of blood disorders.

If a patient has dysphagia, it is important to ask whether the difficulty is in initiating the swallowing or if the food gets "stuck" after being swallowed. If the patient feels the food is stuck at the xiphoid process, evaluate for a stricture, cancer, or ring in the lower esophageal area. Patients with neuromuscular disorders may have difficulty with both solids and liquids. Those with a mechanical obstruction complain of difficulty swallowing solids which then progresses to difficulty with liquids.

Age.   Achalasia usually appears in young adulthood but can develop as early as in infancy. Dysphagia can occur earlier in life but is mostly found in the geriatric population. Odynophagia can appear at any age depending on the etiology. Noncardiac chest pain usually occurs in the fourth decade or later, causing a suspicion of a cardiac etiology. Hematemesis can occur at any age.

Onset.   Problems associated with motility disorders can have either a gradual or rapid onset, depending on the cause. Heartburn can appear suddenly after ingesting particular foods, drinking alcohol, or using tobacco. Odynophagia will usually occur with a rapid onset following ingestion of a caustic substance. Odynophagia caused by a viral or fungal infection will be of slower onset. Dysphagia progresses rapidly to difficulty swallowing solids if cancer is present. In stroke, dysphagia can occur suddenly. Occasional bouts of dysphagia may be produced by Schatzki's ring.

Duration.   Acute or chronic. Depending on the cause of the esophageal disorder, the symptoms may be progressive.

Intensity.   Can be relatively mild or interfere with nutritional intake. Hematemesis due to rupture of esophageal varices can be fatal.

Aggravating Factors.   Aggravating factors for heartburn include spicy and fatty foods, chocolate, alcohol (red wines in particular), caffeine, nicotine, stress, and lying down or bending over. Hematemesis is aggravated by persistent vomiting, retching, or increased pressure from the portacaval system. Aggravation of noncardiac pain occurs with continued reflux of acids.

Alleviating Factors.   Heartburn is alleviated by milk, antacids, some foods, and baking soda unless the symptoms are severe. The remainder of the esophageal problems are more difficult to alleviate.

Associated Factors

Dysphagia
Neuromuscular disorders (e.g., stroke, Parkinson disease, amyotrophic lateral sclerosis [ALS], multiple sclerosis, poliomyelitis), peripheral neuropathy, motor myasthenia gravis, or skeletal muscle diseases (e.g., dermatomyositis, muscular dystrophy). Also, obstructive lesions such as cancer, strictures,

rings, web, foreign body, lymphadenopathy, substernal thyroid, anterior mediastinal mass, cervical osteophyte, or enlarged aorta or left atrium.

Odynophagia
Odynophagia is usually associated with an infection (e.g., due to *Candida*, cytomegalovirus, herpesvirus). Other causes are ingestions of medications or caustic substances. Patients with AIDS or who are otherwise immuno-compromised may develop Kaposi sarcoma or lymphoma.

Hematemesis
Hematemesis has been associated with rupture of esophageal varices occurring as a complication of cirrhosis or from a laceration associated with Mallory-Weiss syndrome. Hematemesis can also be caused by prolonged vomiting, retching, or ingestion of caustic substances.

Noncardiac Chest Pain
Noncardiac chest pain may be secondary to GERD.

PHYSICAL EXAMINATION

General.   Possible weight loss due to malignancy or lack of eating due to progressive symptoms. Evaluate vital signs. Hypotension may be found in those with hematemesis. Dehydration can be found in severe cases.

Cardiovascular.   A cardiovascular examination should be performed when the patient presents with chest pain.

Gastrointestinal.   Findings on examination usually are normal. Abdominal distention with tenderness in the epigastric region may be present. Gastric outlet obstruction can be determined by auscultating for a succussion splash. If perforation occurs, peritoneal signs, percussion changes, ascites, and guarding will be found. Rectal examination may show guaiac-positive stool. Hepatomegaly may be present in patients with cirrhosis.

Head, Eyes, Ears, Nose, Throat.   Halitosis and hoarseness may be present. Look for oral ulcers that may suggest GERD. Observe for swallowing ability and palpate the thyroid for enlargement or nodules. Occasionally patients will have hiccups depending on where the lesion is located. Evidence of pseudobulbar or bulbar palsy including ptosis, tongue atrophy, dysphonia, or hyperactive jaw jerk can be found in neuromuscular disease.

Pulmonary.   Auscultation of the lungs to check for rales, wheezes, and rhonchi. Percuss for consolidation. Observe for respiratory difficulty and use of accessory muscles. Look for deformities that may cause esophageal problems.

Neck.   If the presentation is acute, cervical subcutaneous emphysema suggests esophageal rupture.

Skin.   Observe for skin and hair changes consistent with hypothyroidism. Hyperkeratosis of the palms or soles may be present. Telangiectasis may be present in scleroderma. Spider angiomas and jaundice may be seen in patients with cirrhosis.

Lymph Nodes.   Palpate for lymph node enlargement related to possible lymphoma or cancer.

Musculoskeletal/Neurologic. Look for muscle atrophy particularly of the extremities. A full neurologic exam should be done to evaluate for central or peripheral nerve involvement. Observe and examine for neurologic deficits such as tremor, paresis, or ptosis. Evaluate gait and posture.

PATHOPHYSIOLOGY

Dysphagia
Dysphagia can be caused by upper esophageal dysfunction, neurologic or musculoskeletal disorders, or local structural lesions. The cause can be in the oropharynx or in the esophagus. Most neurologic disorders mainfest with oropharyngeal dysphagia.

Achalasia
Achalasia is a motor disorder of unknown etiology. A degenerative lesion of the vagus nerve is suspected. Patients with achalasia have little or no peristalsis, with the inability of the lower esophageal sphincter to relax.

Heartburn
Heartburn is caused by recurrent or prolonged reflux. The reflux materials produce inflammation. Healing occurs by reepithelialization. Pathogenesis of GERD includes factors affecting the antireflux mechanism (e.g., lower esophageal sphincter tone, frequency of inappropriate lower esophageal sphincter relaxation, angle of esophagogastric junction, and presence or absence of hiatal hernia), volume of gastric content, composition and potency of refluxed material, efficiency of the esophageal clearance mechanism, and esophageal mucosal resistance to injury and its reparative abilities. Prolonged reflux can lead to a Barrett's esophagus.

Odynophagia
Odynophagia is caused by an infection in immunocompromised patients. The offending organisms can be *Candida*, herpes simplex virus, or cytomegalovirus. Other causes are ingestions of caustic substances or medications that cause an inflammatory response.

Hematemesis
Associated with Mallory-Weiss tear, a longitudinal tear of the esophagus. The tear(s) may penetrate the wall of the esophagus or extend just into the mucosa. Infection is possible, leading to inflammation, ulceration, or mediastinitis. Varices develop from cirrhosis, which causes the blood flow through the portal vein to be impeded. This problem causes collateral bypass channels for the systemic and portal system to meet. When the varices rupture, there is an effusion of blood into the lumen and esophageal wall.

Noncardiac Chest Pain
Noncardiac chest pain is usually esophageal in nature caused by the pathogenesis related to GERD.

DIAGNOSTIC STUDIES

Laboratory
Complete Blood Count.   Indicated to rule out anemia if bleeding is present.
Serum Electrolytes.   Used to evaluate for dehydration.
Liver Function Studies.   Performed to rule out hepatic disease.

Radiology
Chest Film.   Indicated to rule out a primary chest abnormality causing symptoms. May also identify aspiration pneumonia.
Esophagogram.   Esophagography employing barium-coated marshmallows, soaked bagels, or other symptom-provoking foodstuffs together with fluoroscopic video recording is often helpful. The diagnosis of achalasia is often based on the classic esophagram depicting dilatation and "bird's beak" distal esophagus. An air-filled esophagus on the esophagram indicates an incompetent lower esophageal sphincter. Heartburn can be studied using reflux-producing maneuvers.
CT/MRI of the Brain.   Indicated if neurologic etiology of symptoms is suspected.
Cervical X-Ray Studies.   Indicated to evaluate esophageal position and evidence of neck edema.
Nuclear Medicine Scan.   With tagged red blood cells, used to detect obscure upper gastrointestinal bleeding.
Barium Swallow.   Can view anomalies, also used to assess function of the esophagus.

Other
ECG.   Indicated to rule out myocardial infarction, especially in persons with chest pain.
Holter Monitoring.   Used if a cardiac source of symptoms is suspected.
Upper Gastrointestinal Endoscopy.   Used for direct visualization and to obtain biopsy specimens to rule out neoplasms and for culture (bacterial, viral, tissue).
Esophageal Manometry.   Used to evaluate esophageal motility.

DIFFERENTIAL DIAGNOSIS

Traumatic
Foreign body must be ruled out in children with new-onset dysphagia. May be seen on radiograph.
   With *costochondritis/rib fractures*, history of trauma to the chest wall. May cause respiratory splinting and noncardiac chest pain. Chest wall is tender to palpation.
   With *bowel perforation/peritonitis*, free air will be seen on kidney-ureter-bladder (KUB) films. Patient may have a history of trauma, recent surgery, or diverticular disease.

Infectious

In *pneumonitis/pneumonia*, chest film will usually show an infiltrate. Patient may be febrile or have concurrent upper respiratory infection or a history of such infection.

Pericarditis may manifest as chest pain. ECG, chest film, or echocardiogram may be required.

Metabolic

Neurologic disease such as amyotrophic lateral sclerosis, multiple sclerosis, myasthenia gravis, or Parkinson disease may cause dysphagia.

With *Zenker's diverticulum*, the patient may notice a "gurgling" noise when swallowing. This lesion tends to occur after the age 50 and is thought to be secondary to increased pressure with swallowing.

With *thyromegaly*, goiter may be palpable or visible on examination.

Esophageal stricture may be due to chronic inflammation (e.g., in GERD). Seen on barium studies or endoscopy.

Schatzki's ring may be associated with GERD. Seen on endoscopy or barium studies.

Esophageal web may be congenital or acquired. Associated with Plummer-Vinson syndrome. Composed of thin structures of mucosa or submucosa in the mid or proximal esophagus.

Gastric or *duodenal ulcer* may cause hematemesis. Will be differentiated on endoscopy or barium studies.

Pleuritis may cause noncardiac chest pain. Chest film and esophageal workup negative. Pain on inspiration.

In *degenerative disease* of the cervical spine, spurs abutting the esophagus may be evident on cervical spine radiographs.

In *biliary colic/cholecystitis*, pain may radiate to the shoulder or back and may be associated with the intake of fatty foods. Ultrasound examination will identify cholecystitis.

In *pancreatitis*, patient may have a history of alcohol abuse. Amylase is elevated.

Neoplastic

Neoplasm of adjacent structures (squamous cell carcinoma and adenocarcinoma) may impinge on the esophagus, causing dysphagia. Will be differentiated on imaging studies or intraoperatively.

Brain stem lesion with cranial nerve involvement may cause swallowing difficulty.

Vascular

Stroke may cause motor paralysis with anterior circulation involvement or cranial nerve involvement with posterior circulation involvement.

Pharyngeal hemorrhage may cause hematemesis. Will be differentiated on endoscopy.

Pulmonary artery or *aortic aneurysm* may cause noncardiac chest pain. May be seen on chest film or chest CT scan.

Coronary atherosclerotic heart disease (CASHD) may manifest as chest pain in a typical or an atypical fashion. ECG and cardiac isoenzymes will be abnormal with ischemia. Cardiac catheterization may be required in patients at high risk for cardiac events.

Congenital
Not otherwise applicable. See Pediatric Considerations section.

Acquired
In *psychiatric disease*, the patient may present with chest pain or dysphagia. All studies will be normal. Patient may exhibit signs of psychiatric illness.

TREATMENT

In the acute setting, airway must be maintained. A nasogastric tube is placed if hemorrhage is suspected and/or an upper gastrointestinal bleed needs to be ruled out.

The blood-free bilious material in the gastric aspirate excludes upper gastrointestinal bleeding in most cases.

Intravenous fluids are provided if the patient is dehydrated or is unable to take food or fluids.

Speech therapists can provide valuable treatment for primary and secondary esophageal disorders.

Dysphagia
Treatment varies depending on the etiology. In many cases, only palliative therapy may be available. Dilation procedures may clear nonmalignant obstructive lesions. Malignant lesions may be surgically resected or vaporized using an endoscopic laser followed by a stent placement. Motility disorders may be treated with agents to enhance motility such as bethanechol, metoclopramide (Reglan), or domperidone.

Heartburn and Associated Gastrointestinal Reflux
Elevate the head of the bed; avoid chocolate, caffeine, high-fat meals, acidic foods, peppermint oils, and nicotine. Antacids may offer temporary relief from symptoms, but aggressive treatment of esophagitis usually requires one of the following medications.
- Proton Pump Inhibitors (PPI)
    Omeprazole 20 mg/day
    Lansoprazole 30 mg/day
    Rabeprazole 20 mg/day
    Pantoprazole 40 mg/day
- Histamine H_2 receptor antagonists
    Cimetidine 800 mg at bedtime
    Ranitidine 300 mg at bedtime
    Famotidine 40 mg at bedtime

Nizatidine 300 mg at bedtime

In severe cases, incompetence of the lower esophageal sphincter may be treated surgically with fundoplication and selective parietal cell vagotomy.

Odynophagia

With infectious etiology, responds to appropriate antimicrobial therapy. Viscous lidocaine swish/swallow preparations may offer temporary relief during meals but carry a high risk for cardiac side effects with frequent use.

Hematemesis

If esophageal in origin, usually spontaneously resolves if the lesion is minor. Hemodynamic fluid status and hematocrit should be monitored and deficiencies treated accordingly. With loss of larger amounts of blood due to an esophageal lesion, aggressive treatment with therapeutic-endoscopic procedures is necessary.

Noncardiac Chest Pain

Pain related to esophageal spasm may be treated with nitrates and calcium channel blockers after careful evaluation and after other potentially serious conditions have been ruled out. Treat the underlying process if esophageal symptoms are caused by a primary neurologic disorder.

PEDIATRIC CONSIDERATIONS

Most infants tend to manifest poor esophageal tone, especially in the lower esophagus, which results in achalasia and reflux. In infants, GERD may mainfest as coughing, wheezing, or choking, especially after nursing, which may lead to failure to thrive. Most symptoms of GERD in infancy spontaneously resolve by age 9 to 13 months. This condition should not be confused with pathologic acid reflux occurring after infancy, which usually manifests with marked symptoms such as recurrent pneumonia, nocturnal apnea, paroxysmal nocturnal asthma, night cough, and possibly sudden infant death syndrome.

Persistent drooling, coughing, and gagging with nursing from birth suggests congenital esophageal atresia. Diagnosis may be made when attempts to insert a nasogastric tube are unsuccessful and/or aspiration pneumonitis occurs. Esophageal atresia is a surgical emergency and requires meticulous preoperative airway management and constant suction of secretions.

With foreign body aspiration, obtain a consultation with a gastrointestinal specialist if the ingested item is likely to cause additional damage (sharp).

OBSTETRIC CONSIDERATIONS

Heartburn is a particularly prominent problem during pregnancy, occurring in approximately 25% of patients.

GERD, which can lead to esophagitis, is often due to decreased lower esophageal sphincter pressure during pregnancy as a result of elevated estrogen and progesterone levels.

H_2 blockers have proved to be safe for use in pregnancy. Sucralfate and metoclopramide also have a similar safety profile. Omeprazole should be used with caution, and misoprostol (Cytotec) is *absolutely contraindicated,* as it is an abortifacient.

GERIATRIC CONSIDERATIONS

Approximately 30% to 40% of nursing home patients have dysphagia. About 80% of the oral and pharyngeal dysphagia cases are related to neuromuscular causes, and 10% are related to cancer. Symptoms of dysphagia should not be considered psychogenic.

Geriatric patients with esophageal hemorrhage may present with constipation, diarrhea, loss of appetite, or change in mentation. Oropharyngeal disorders have a poorer prognosis in the geriatric population owing to a high incidence of aspiration pneumonia.

PREVENTIVE CONSIDERATIONS

Primary prevention of GERD includes avoidance of nicotine, caffeine, high-fat meals, and acidic foods. Secondary prevention involves aggressive treatment of GERD to prevent potential complications such as Barrett's esophagus or Schatzki's ring.

PEARLS FOR THE PA

Disorders of the esophagus can be divided into five diagnostic categories: dysphagia, heartburn (reflux), odynophagia, hematemesis, and noncardiac pain based on the anatomic site involved.

Heartburn (pyrosis) is the most common of all organic gastrointestinal symptoms and is the most prominent symptom of GERD.

Aggressive treatment of GERD is indicated to prevent later complications (e.g., Barrett's esophagus).

Weight loss of variable degree may suggest malignant or complicated disease.

Gastrointestinal Bleeding: Lower Tract

James W. Becker, PA-C

DEFINITION

Bleeding from any site in the lower gastrointestinal (LGI) tract including the colon or rectum.

HISTORY

Symptoms. May be insidious with a mild anemia or obvious in the case of bright red blood from the rectum or melena.

General. LGI bleeding is usually painless. If the patient complains of crampy abdominal pain, it is usually due to other causes (e.g., colitis, diverticulitis).

Age. Young (second decade) to the elderly.

Onset. Insidious to severe with obvious hemorrhage.

Duration. Variable, depending on the degree of hemodynamic compromise.

Intensity. The patient may be asymptomatic or may present in shock due to blood loss.

Aggravating Factors. Bleeding dyscrasias (e.g., thrombocytopenia).

Alleviating Factors. Dependent on the etiology of the bleed.

Associated Factors. Recent anticoagulant or aspirin therapy.

PHYSICAL EXAMINATION

General. The patient may present in very little distress or in hypovolemic shock. Assess heart rate and blood pressure (including orthostatic). The supine position should be avoided if it results in hypotension, and it may be hazardous for the patient to sit or stand for orthostatic measurement.

Gastrointestinal. Left lower quadrant tenderness suggests diverticular disease or colitis, although neither is generally associated with massive GI bleeding. A silent abdomen with rebound tenderness may indicate perforation or ischemic colitis. Check the stool for occult blood. Inspect for jaundice, ascites, spider angiomas, hepatomegaly, and dilated superficial abdominal veins to rule out chronic liver disease.

PATHOPHYSIOLOGY

The most common cause of LGI blood is upper gastrointestinal (UGI) bleeding. Melena usually indicates bleeding from the small intestine to the transverse colon. Bright red blood usually indicates bleeding from a site in the left colon, sigmoid colon, or rectum.

The most common sources of LGI bleeding are tumors, diverticula, and arteriovenous malformations.

With diverticulitis, dietary changes and perforations may cause a flare-up.

With arteriovenous malformation, spontaneous bleeding may be triggered by anticoagulants. This cause is the most difficult to detect on routine studies.

With GI neoplasm, the tumor is visualized by endoscopic procedures and contrast studies.

In colitis, the source of the bleeding can be viewed on proctoscopy.

With perianal disease, the bleeding source can be viewed on anoscopy.

DIAGNOSTIC STUDIES

Laboratory

Complete Blood Count.   Elevated white blood cell (WBC) count may be seen with infections. Decreased hemoglobin and hematocrit with acute blood loss (may see a microcytic anemia consistent with chronic blood loss).

Prothrombin Time (PT)/Partial Thromboplastin Time (PTT)/ Platelets/ Bleeding Time.   Indicated to rule out bleeding dyscrasias or used in evaluating patients taking warfarin, heparin, or aspirin. Rule out idiopathic thrombocytopenic purpura (ITP).

Serum Chemistry.   May show electrolyte imbalance with dehydration or elevated values on liver function tests with hepatic disease.

Typing and Cross-Matching Blood.   For transfusions as indicated. Fresh frozen plasma should be available to correct coagulation deficits.

Radiology

Obstruction Series.   Including flat and upright films of the abdomen.

Chest Film.   Used to look for signs of obstruction or intra-abdominal or mediastinal air.

Technetium Bleeding Scan.   Patient must be actively bleeding for the test to be positive.

Arteriography.   Performed if findings on endoscopy are negative. Patient must be actively bleeding for the test to localize the site of the hemorrhage.

Barium Enema.   Performed if a neoplastic source of LGI bleeding is suspected. Should be performed *only* if the decision is made not to proceed with angiography, as residual barium may obscure the angiogram.

Other

Nasogastric Tube.   Placed to rule out UGI source of the bleeding.

Proctosigmoidoscopy.   Mandatory (after UGI source of the bleeding is excluded) to rule out a tumor as the cause of the bleeding or colitis.

Colonoscopy. May be attempted if the bleeding is not vigorous. Visualization may be poor.

DIFFERENTIAL DIAGNOSIS

Traumatic
With *rectal trauma*, may have a history of recent GI or abdominal surgery.

Infectious
In *pseudomembranous colitis*, positive culture for *Clostridium difficile*.

Metabolic
Gastric or *esophageal varices* may be a UGI source of bleeding. May be viewed on esophagogastroscopy.

Neoplastic
GI neoplasms can arise at any site from the esophagus to the rectum.
   Benign intestinal lipomas may be friable and bleed.

Vascular
Hemorrhoids may be apparent on inspection of the anus. Visualization may require anoscopy.

Congenital
Not applicable.

Acquired
Aortoduodenal fistula may be seen following aortic bypass surgery.
   Anal fissures usually are associated with a recent bout of constipation.

TREATMENT

Immediately recognize and treat shock with intravenous hydration, maintenance of blood pressure (with pressors if necessary), and monitoring of urine output.
   Correct coagulation deficits if present.
   Transfuse as necessary.
   Rule out a UGI site of the bleed.

Medical
Indicated for any form of colitis (see "Ulcerative Colitis" later in this chapter).
   Perianal diseases are usually self-limited and will resolve with conservative therapy.

Close follow-up is required for any case of LGI bleeding to evaluate for recurrence.

Surgical
Indicated for tumors, arteriovenous malformations, and diverticula or any source of LGI bleeding that fails to respond to the medical regimen.

PEDIATRIC CONSIDERATIONS

The clinical manifestations of blood loss are far more dramatic than those seen in an adult. For this reason, monitoring hemoglobin and hematocrit is crucial in the developing child.

OBSTETRIC CONSIDERATIONS

No specific indications. In bleeding causing hypotension, restoration of an adequate fluid volume is crucial to avoid fetal damage (see "Shock" in Chapter 3, Emergency Medicine).

GERIATRIC CONSIDERATIONS

The clinical manifestations of blood loss are far more dramatic than those seen in the younger patient. Conditions that cause and contribute to LGI bleeding are more common in the elderly (e.g., diverticulitis, neoplastic disease, anticoagulation).

PREVENTIVE CONSIDERATIONS

Prevention of underlying conditions that cause LGI bleeding involves a high-fiber diet, avoidance of caffeine and nicotine, and a regular exercise program. Periodic sigmoidoscopy or colonoscopy and routine stool guaiac examinations should be considered as a screening measure in patients older than 40 years of age.

PEARLS FOR THE PA

The most common sources for lower gastrointestinal bleeding are tumors, diverticula, and arteriovenous malformations.

Patients' symptoms may be insidious with a mild anemia or obvious in the case of bright red blood from the rectum or melena.

Gastrointestinal Bleeding: Upper Tract

James W. Becker, PA-C

DEFINITION

Bleeding from any site in the upper gastrointestinal tract (UGI) tract including the esophagus, stomach, or small intestine. It is a symptom of underlying gastrointestinal (GI) pathology.

HISTORY

Symptoms

Hematemesis. With hematemesis (vomiting of blood), the vomitus may have the appearance of "coffee grounds" or may be grossly bloody. A thorough history of the hematemesis is important. Was blood present on the initial vomitus or only on subsequent episodes? Was the hematemesis associated with recent ingestion of food or alcohol, or a recent choking episode? Was the emesis grossly bloody or blood-streaked or did it have a coffee grounds appearance? What was the approximate amount? (Dilution with stomach contents or toilet bowl water may make accurate estimate difficult.)

Abdominal Pain. Determine whether the pain was present before the emesis, relation of the pain to meals, and any radiation of the pain to the shoulder or back.

General. Presentations may range from insidious with a mild anemia to obvious loss of blood via hematemesis or melena. Obtain a history of recent systemic illness; current use of medications (over-the-counter and prescription), especially aspirin, NSAIDs or anticoagulants; recent epistaxis; or history of ulcer disease, liver disease, pancreatitis, bleeding disorders, alcohol abuse, or previous surgery, either ulcer or vascular reconstruction using an aortic graft (aortoduodenal fistula).

Age. Young (teens) to the elderly.
Onset. Can be sudden or insidious.
Duration. Days to months.
Intensity. Severe (with hematemesis) or minimal (with chronic anemia).
Aggravating Factors. Dependent on etiology.
Alleviating Factors. Dependent on etiology.
Associated Factors. Recent anticoagulation therapy.

PHYSICAL EXAMINATION

General. The patient may present in very little distress or in hypovolemic shock. Assess heart rate and blood pressure (including orthostatic). The supine position should be avoided if it results in hypotension, and it may be hazardous for the patient to sit or stand for orthostatic blood pressure measurement.

Gastrointestinal. Abdominal tenderness on examination is of little use in the acute setting. A rigid, silent abdomen suggests perforation or ischemic bowel that may require immediate surgical intervention (after hemodynamic stabilization). Inspect for jaundice, ascites, spider angiomas, hepatomegaly, and dilated superficial abdominal veins to rule out chronic liver disease.

PATHOPHYSIOLOGY

Esophageal Etiology
Varices are seen in patients with chronic liver disease.

With *ulceration*, the patient may have a history of chronic reflux esophagitis.

Laceration from a foreign body is more common in younger age groups. Usually of acute onset with a readily identifiable object. The object may be present in the esophagus or stomach.

Ingestion of corrosives usually is associated with an acute onset. It is important to determine the type of agent so that appropriate treatment can be started immediately.

Malignancy has a higher incidence in the black population. Male predominance, with a sex ratio of 4:1. Increased incidence in smokers.

With *Mallory-Weiss tear*, acute hemorrhage common in persons with a history of heavy alcohol use.

Gastric Etiology
Gastric varices are associated with chronic liver disease, splenic vein thrombosis secondary to trauma.

With *ulceration*, increased incidence with NSAID, aspirin, and steroid and tobacco use. Associated with infection with *H. pylori* (see "Peptic/Gastric Ulcer Disease" later in this chapter).

Malignancy occurs with increased incidence in patients with previous (remote) history of subtotal gastrectomy and in patients with a positive family history of gastric cancer.

Foreign body laceration is more common in younger age groups. Usually has an acute onset with a readily identifiable object.

Small Intestine Etiology
Duodenal ulceration is associated with hyperacidity of the stomach and infections with *H. pylori.*

Association with *Crohn's disease* is unknown (see "Crohn's Disease" earlier in this chapter).

Tumors—both benign (adenomas) and malignant (carcinoma)—may be associated with bleeding.

With *aortoduodenal fistula*, the patient will have a history of a previous surgical aortic graft.

DIAGNOSTIC STUDIES

Laboratory
Complete Blood Count with Red Blood Cell Indices (MCV, MCH, MCHC). Elevated white blood cell (WBC) count may be seen with infections. Decreased hemoglobin and hematocrit with acute blood loss (may see a microcytic anemia consistent with chronic blood loss).

Prothrombin Time (PT)/Partial Thromboplastin Time (PTT)/Platelets/ Bleeding Time. Indicated to rule out bleeding dyscrasias or used in evaluating patients taking warfarin, heparin, or aspirin.

Serum Chemistry. May show electrolyte imbalance with dehydration or elevated values on liver function tests with hepatic disease.

Typing and Cross-Matching Blood. For transfusions as indicated.

Radiology
Obstruction Series. Including flat and upright films of the abdomen.

Chest Film. Indicated to look for signs of obstruction or intra-abdominal or mediastinal air.

Barium Swallow Studies. Used to examine additional lengths of small bowel inaccessible to endoscopy.

Technetium Bleeding Scan. Patient must be actively bleeding for the test to be positive.

Arteriography. Performed if findings on endoscopy are negative. Patient must be actively bleeding for the test to be positive.

Other
Upper Endoscopy. Performed to attempt to determine the origin of the bleeding. Diagnostic in the majority of cases. Therapeutic intervention may be applied.

Nasogastric Tube. Placed to rule out UGI source of the bleeding.

DIFFERENTIAL DIAGNOSIS

Traumatic. Not applicable.
Infectious. Not applicable.

Metabolic
Pancreatitis may produce hemobilia. Differentiated on endoscopy.

Neoplastic. Not applicable.
Vascular. Not applicable.
Congenital. Not applicable.

Acquired
Epistaxis, whether traumatic, spontaneous, or due to blood dyscrasias, may cause symptoms of UGI bleeding. History may be positive for anterior epistaxis, and physical examination will reveal a posterior epistaxis.

TREATMENT

Immediately recognize and treat shock with intravenous hydration, maintenance of blood pressure (with pressors if necessary), and urine output. Correct coagulation deficits if present.

Esophageal Varices
Upper endoscopy is performed to control bleeding by one of the following:
1. Sclerotherapy: Injection of 2% sodium tetradecyl sulfate. Successful in 80% to 90% of cases, but rebleeding rate can occur in 3% to 66% of patients. If a shunt procedure is performed, rebleeding rates will decrease. Complications of sclerotherapy occur in up to 40% of patients and include esophageal ulceration, altered esophageal motility, esophageal stricture, perforation, and pleural effusion.
2. Endoscopic band ligation: Application of rubber bands directly onto varices. Up to a 60% rate of success. Complications include recurrent bleeding, postbanding ulcers, esophageal stricture, and esophageal perforation. Results are improved if a shunt procedure is performed.
3. Blakemore tube placement: Balloon catheter is applied with traction at the gastroesophageal junction to tamponade bleeding varices. This allows for stabilization of the patient until definitive treatment can be instituted.

Ulcer
Place nasogastric tube. Gastric lavage can be performed to assess the severity of any gastric bleeding and to lavage stomach to assist endoscopic examination.

Upper endoscopy is performed to diagnose and treat bleeding ulcers by use of a thermal probe (bipolar circumactive probe), laser, or heater probe or by injection of epinephrine.

Surgery is performed to control bleeding, close perforations, and perform antrectomy and/or vagotomy.

Medical therapy with:
Histamine H_2 receptor blockers (e.g., ranitidine 150 mg orally twice a day; 50 mg intravenously three times a day; cimetidine 300 mg four times a day, 400 mg two times a day, or 800 mg at bedtime; famotidine 40 mg at bedtime; nizatidine 150 mg twice a day), OR
Treatment with proton pump inhibition with lansoprazole 30 mg/day, esomeprazole magnesium 20–40 mg/day, or omeprazole 20–40 mg/day, OR
Treatment with carafate 1 g four times a day, OR
Antacids.
Embolization of visible bleeding sites through angiographic catheter can also be performed.

PEDIATRIC CONSIDERATIONS

The clinical manifestations of blood loss are far more dramatic than those seen in an adult. For this reason, monitoring hemoglobin and hematocrit is crucial in the developing child.

OBSTETRIC CONSIDERATIONS

No specific indications. In bleeds causing hypotension, restoration of an adequate fluid volume is crucial to avoid fetal damage (see "Shock" in Chapter 3, Emergency Medicine).

GERIATRIC CONSIDERATIONS

The clinical manifestations of blood loss are far more dramatic than those seen in the younger patient. Conditions that cause and contribute to upper gastrointestinal bleeding are more common in the elderly (e.g., neoplastic disease, anticoagulation).

PREVENTIVE CONSIDERATIONS

Prevention of underlying conditions that cause upper gastrointestinal bleeding involves a high-fiber diet, avoidance of caffeine and nicotine, and a regular exercise program. Periodic sigmoidoscopy or colonoscopy and routine stool guaiac examinations should be considered as a screening measure in patients older than 40 years of age.

PEARLS FOR THE PA

Do not perform barium studies until the need for an arteriogram has been ruled out.

HEMORRHOIDS

James W. Becker, PA-C, and Michelle L. Heinan, EdD, MS, PA-C

DEFINITION

A common malady that results from enlargement, inflammation, prolapse, or thrombosis of the hemorrhoidal veins.

HISTORY

Symptoms.   Small amounts of transient, spotty rectal blood seen with bowel movements. Generally painless. Reduceable or irreduceable prolapse of the hemorrhoid may occur with bowel movements. Mucous discharge and pruritus may be present with prolapse. Irreduceable prolapse leads to painful strangulation and thrombosis.

General.   It is important to determine the amount of blood produced. A "coffee grounds" appearance suggests upper gastrointestinal (GI) bleed. Large volumes of bright red blood suggest lower GI bleed.

Age.   Uncommon in children. Any, but incidence increases with age.

Onset.   Chronic; may have acute symptoms with thrombosis.

Intensity.   Generally mild; may be irritating. Pain can be severe with thrombosis.

Aggravating Factors.   Chronic constipation, straining with bowel movements, anal intercourse, requirement for long periods of sitting on the job; prominent with pregnancy, with resolution afterwards.

Alleviating Factors.   Appropriate treatments, increased fiber in diet, stool softeners.

Associated Factors.   Increased portal venous pressure can cause internal hemorrhoid enlargement. Rectal and sigmoid colon tumors; hypertension.

PHYSICAL EXAMINATION

General.   The patient should be in no acute distress.

Gastrointestinal.   Inspection for external hemorrhoids. Digital rectal examination to evaluate for mass (internal hemorrhoids are nonpalpable); stool guaiac test.

PATHOPHYSIOLOGY

Hemorrhoids can occur from the internal or external hemorrhoidal venous system. The superior system empties into the superior rectal veins, and the external system drains into the pudendal and iliac veins. There is communication between the internal and external hemorroidal veins.

Internal and external hemorrhoidal venous system drains the anorectal area. Proximal to the dentate line are the internal hemorrhoidal veins. External veins are distal to the dentate line and can be viewed externally.

Association with straining and constipation. Prevalent during pregnancy. Possibly due to sustained increased pressure on the venous drainage of the rectum. Increased portal system pressure (that drains the internal hemorrhoids) may lead to venous dilatation.

DIAGNOSTIC STUDIES

Laboratory
Complete Blood Count. Indicated in cases with hemorrhage to rule out anemia.
Radiology. Not applicable unless other conditions need to be ruled out.

Other
Anoscopy. For direct visualization of the extent of the hemorrhoids.

DIFFERENTIAL DIAGNOSIS

Traumatic
With *anal trauma*, history of injury or abuse.

Infectious
Perirectal abscess seen on inspection.

Metabolic
Anal fissure seen on inspection.

Neoplastic
Tumors of the rectum and sigmoid colon can be viewed on anoscopy. May be the cause of the hemorrhoid.

Vascular. Not otherwise applicable.
Congenital. Not applicable.

Acquired
Rectal prolapse seen on inspection.

TREATMENT

Pressure control of active bleeding if present. Symptomatic relief using hot sitz baths three times a day and after each bowel movement.

Bulk-forming laxative or stool softener may be given to reduce straining.

Topical over-the-counter medications (Preparation H, Anusol) or steroid-containing ointments for pain or pruritus.

NSAID may be used if there is pain.

Prolapse can be manually reduced if possible.

Surgery may be necessary for nonreduceable prolapse, inflammatory bowel disease, or strangulated hemorrhoid. Other indications may include coagulopathy (to prevent subsequent hemorrhage), immunocompromised status (to prevent infection), and severe pain or pruritus attributable to the lesion.

Surgical intervention may consist of:
Surgical referral for inpatient procedures
Sclerosing injections, rubber band ligation.

PEDIATRIC CONSIDERATIONS

Rare.

OBSTETRIC CONSIDERATIONS

Hemorrhoids are common in pregnancy.

GERIATRIC CONSIDERATONS

Any rectal bleeding in the elderly patient should be fully investigated to rule out a malignant process.

PREVENTIVE CONSIDERATIONS

Increase fiber intake and fluid intake and reduce dietary fats to prevent the onset of hemorrhoids. Avoid long periods of sitting.

PEARLS FOR THE PA

Hemorrhoids classically manifest as small amounts of spotty blood with bowel movements.

Internal hemorrhoids are nonpalpable.

Rectal or sigmoid colon tumors may cause hemorrhoid.

Pancreatitis (Acute)

James W. Becker, PA-C

DEFINITION

Inflammation of the pancreas due to obstruction, alcohol abuse, trauma, or underlying metabolic disorder.

HISTORY

Symptoms. Mild ache to severe, constant, boring abdominal pain. Usually located in the epigastric and midabdominal regions but may alternate between right and left upper quadrants. Frequently radiates to the back. Intractable vomiting, uncontrolled by nasogastric suctioning. Vomiting does *not* relieve the symptoms.

General. The patient may have a history of alcohol abuse, biliary disease, or previous episodes of pancreatitis.

Age. Usually occurs in the adult, but can occur in children.

Onset. Usually rapid over several (4 to 8) hours.

Duration. Several days, possibly several weeks in severe cases.

Intensity. Varies, ranging from mild tenderness to intense pain.

Aggravating Factors. Food intake, supine position.

Alleviating Factors. Food avoidance, sitting position (usually leaning forward), lying on side.

Associated Factors. Hypertriglyceridemia, abdominal trauma, alcohol abuse, cholelithiasis, prescription medications, and hypercalcemia.

PHYSICAL EXAMINATION

General. The patient appears generally ill, frequently in shock. The breath may smell of alcohol.

Pulmonary. Decreased breath sounds in bases bilaterally due to pain on inspiration.

Gastrointestinal. Abdomen may be somewhat distended or rigid, or there may be rebound tenderness or absence of bowel sounds. Presence of Grey Turner sign (erythema along the flank, bluish discoloration) or Cullen sign (discoloration and bruising at the umbilicus) indicates hemorrhagic pancreatitis.

Ophthalmologic. Sclerae may be icteric.

PATHOPHYSIOLOGY

Depending on the population, 40% to 50% of patients with pancreatitis will have concomitant cholelithiasis, which is associated with transient obstruction of the ampulla of Vater.

Approximately 25% of patients will have a history of alcohol abuse for at least 6 years.

Ten percent of patients will have suffered blunt trauma (e.g., motor vehicle accident, fall, or surgery) that injures the pancreas.

Hyperlipidemia (types I, IV, V) and hypercalcemia (secondary to renal disease or hyperparathyroidism) are metabolic causes.

Suspected drugs that may cause pancreatitis include corticosteroids, estrogen, oral contraceptives, and thiazide diuretics.

DIAGNOSTIC STUDIES

Laboratory
Complete Blood Count.   Leukocytosis with cell counts of up to 20,000/mm^3.

Hematocrit.   Elevated with dehydration, depressed with hemorrhage.

Chemistry Profile.   Plasma amylase and lipase elevation can be seen. These tests, although not unequivocally diagnostic of the disease, are usually elevated for the first several days of the acute illness.

Urinalysis.   Amylase elevated (greater than 5000 IU/dL) in the first week of illness.

Hyperlipidemia Profile.   May show elevated triglycerides, cholesterol, and low-density liproprotein (LDL), depressed high-density liproprotein (HDL). Obtained during the acute phase and repeated at 4- to 6-week intervals.

Radiology
Flat and Upright Abdominal Films.   May reveal calcified gallstones or a sentinel loop (dilated duodenum).

Abdominal CT.   May show dilated biliary and/or pancreatic ducts. Surveillance CT scan 10 to 14 days after the acute onset may show pseudocyst or abscess.

Ultrasound Examination.   Used initially to rule out cholelithiasis/cholecystitis. May be repeated after 4 to 6 weeks if the initial study is negative and no other explanation for pancreatitis is found.

Chest Film.   Used to rule out pneumonia from aspiration of emesis or from splinting. Rule out acute respiratory distress syndrome (ARDS) in severe pancreatitis.

Endoscopic Retrograde Cholangiopancreatography (ERCP).   May be indicated during the acute episode to remove common bile duct stone or may be performed after the pancreatitis resolves.

Magnetic Resonance Cholangiopancreatography (MRCP).   A relatively new form of imaging the biliary and pancreatic duct system for common bile duct stone or other abnormalities. Most beneficial in patients with previous gastrointestinal surgery that would make ERCP not feasible.

DIFFERENTIAL DIAGNOSIS

Traumatic
Abdominal trauma, especially deceleration injuries such as from motor vehicle accidents.

Infectious.   Not applicable.

Metabolic
With *perforated duodenal* or *gastric ulcer*, serum amylase may be slightly elevated (greater than 250 IU/dL). Free air may be apparent on plain

abdominal films; peripancreatic inflammation secondary to perforation may be seen on CT scan.

With *acute cholecystitis*, amylase is usually normal, pancreas appears normal on CT and ultrasound examinations.

Neoplastic. Not applicable. Pancreatic cancer rarely causes acute pancreatitis.

Vascular

With *ruptured* or *leaking abdominal aortic aneurysm*, decreased to absent pulses in the lower extremities, rapid drop in hematocrit. CT will show retroperitoneal blood.

With *ischemic intestinal injury/obstruction*, amylase may be slightly elevated; physical presentation can be identical. CT scan may reveal ischemic or thrombosed vessels. Colonoscopy may be helpful if the large intestine is thought to be compromised.

Congenital. Not applicable.
Acquired. Not applicable.

TREATMENT

The patient should be kept NPO. In severe cases of pancreatitis, especially with emesis, a nasogastric tube may be indicated.

Intravenous fluids (e.g., lactated Ringer's) to prevent hypovolemic shock. May require 4 to 5 L/24 hours.

Maintain urine output at greater than 60 mL/2 hours.

Central venous pressure or Swan-Ganz catheter monitoring to evaluate fluid status.

Plasma expanders (e.g., albumin, hetastarch [Hespan]) to maintain serum albumin of greater than 3 g/dL.

Replenish serum calcium as needed.

Consider empiric broad-spectrum antibiotic coverage (somewhat controversial).

Analgesics such as meperidine (Demerol) 75 mg intramuscularly every 3 to 4 hours for pain control or 25 mg intravenously every 2 hours.

Maintain a gastric pH greater than 4 with antacids by nasogastric tube or with histamine H_2 receptor blockers (e.g., ranitidine [Zantac] 50 mg IV every 8 hours; cimetidine [Tagamet] 300 mg IV every 6 hours).

Begin total parenteral nutrition once fluid status is stabilized.

Treat hyperlipidemia if lipids remain elevated 8 weeks after the acute episode.

After the acute episode is resolved, a thorough search for the underlying causative disorder is indicated.

PEDIATRIC CONSIDERATIONS

Acute pancreatitis in children is most often the result of drugs (e.g., corticosteroids, thiazides, valproic acid, sulfonamides, acetaminophen,

L-asparaginase), infections (e.g., mumps, coxsackievirus infection, hepatitis, influenza, *Mycoplasma* infection), systemic disease (e.g., cystic fibrosis, systemic lupus erythematosus, α_1-antitrypsin deficiency, chronic renal failure), or abdominal trauma. Alcohol-induced pancreatitis should also be considered.

The typical presentation includes severe epigastric pain occasionally radiating to the back, nausea, vomiting, and fever. The abdomen is tender and may or may not be rigid. Abdominal distention is common in infants and young children. A mass may be palpable if a pseudocyst has formed. Leukocytosis and elevated levels of serum amylase and lipase are expected. Infants younger than 6 months of age may have hypoamylasemia. With conservative management (rest, fluids, electrolyte replacement, and other supportive measures), the prognosis is good for the pediatric patient.

OBSTETRIC CONSIDERATIONS

Acute pancreatitis should be considered in any pregnant patient with severe epigastric pain, persistent nausea and vomiting, and jaundice. Sixty-five percent of these cases are secondary to gallstones. The overall management is the same as in the nonpregnant patient. Pancreatitis poses an increased risk of fetal and maternal death if not managed properly.

GERIATRIC CONSIDERATIONS

Elderly patients with severe pancreatitis have a much higher mortality rate and should be monitored in a critical care setting.

PREVENTIVE CONSIDERATIONS

Enthusiastic alcohol usage should be discouraged. Patients with symptomatic cholelithiasis should be considered for cholecystectomy. Patients with documented hypertriglyceridemia should undergo pharmaceutical intervention.

PEARLS FOR THE PA

Aggressive treatment of hypovolemia is essential in the management of pancreatitis.

Treat the underlying cause after the acute phase has passed.

Remember pancreatitis in the differential diagnosis for abdominal pain.

Peptic/Gastric Ulcer Disease

Michelle L. Heinan, EdD, MS, PA-C

DEFINITION

Peptic ulcer disease (PUD) is four times more prevalent than gastric ulcer. The causative factor in over 80% of patients is infection with *Helicobacter pylori*. Areas affected by peptic ulcer disease are areas vulnerable to acid, bile, pepsin, and pancreatic enzyme effects. These effects occur around the area of the mucosal transition zones.

HISTORY

Symptoms. The prominent symptom of a peptic ulcer is described as a deep, gnawing, dull, or burning pain located in the epigastric region of the abdomen. The pain occurs 1 to 3 hours after meals and causes the patient to awaken at night. Nausea with possible vomiting occurs in patients who have severe pain. Sometimes patients complain of accompanying thirst, melenic stools, syncope, and/or dizziness. Pain radiating to the back suggests a posterior ulcer. The pain is relieved by food intake and/or antacids. Weight loss is common.

General. The most common complication of an ulcer is bleeding. Bleeding can be a life-threatening problem in very young and geriatric patients owing to dehydration and inadequate organ perfusion. Perforation occurs in 5% of the patients presenting with acute abdominal pain and peritoneal signs. Patients can be predisposed to gastric carcinoma with chronic gastric irritation. The irritation leads to atrophic changes. There is a possible link between *H. pylori* and gastric cancer. There is also a possibility of a link between *H. pylori* and gastric lymphoma as a result of chronic *H. pylori* infection.

Age. Peptic ulcer disease occurs in 2% of the U.S. population between the ages of 45 and 54 years. Males have a slightly higher prevalence. Gastric ulcer disease occurs most frequently between the ages of 55 and 64 years, with a gender ratio of about 1:1. The equivalent incidence in men and in women is attributed to the increased use of NSAIDs in women.

Onset. Acute.

Duration. Peptic ulcer symptoms may be intermittent, with several episodes of pain over a short period followed by long periods of remission. Gastric ulcers must be followed closely to ensure that the lesion heals.

Intensity. Some patients are asymptomatic, whereas others have mild, moderate, or severe epigastric pain. In some cases, patients present with perforation and/or change in sensorium due hemorrhage. Gastric ulcer pain is less severe than that of peptic ulcer.

Aggravating Factors. Peptic ulcers can be aggravated by alcohol, tobacco, coffee, aspirin, NSAIDs, tolazoline, and corticosteroids. Stress can also aggravate symptoms. The pain of gastric ulcer is usually worsened with meals.

Alleviating Factors.   Peptic ulcer pain is relieved by food and sometimes by vomiting. Gastric ulcer pain is relieved by fasting or (sometimes) by antacids.

Associated Factors.   Peptic ulcers can be a secondary effect of significant trauma or illness, such as burn injuries, intracranial trauma, shock, hypoglycemia, dehydration, renal failure, vasculitis, cystic fibrosis, nephrolithasis, gastrinoma, hyperparathyroidism, coronary artery disease, chronic pancreatitis, systemic mastocytosis, α_1-antitrypsin deficiency, type I multiple endocrine neoplasia (MEN I), chronic obstructive pulmonary disease (COPD), chronic liver disease, and polycythemia. Development of malignancy correlates highly with gastric ulcer disease.

PHYSICAL EXAMINATION

General.   Signs of dehydration, tachycardia, stupor, loss of consciousness, or orthostatic problems may be present if significant bleeding has occurred.

Gastrointestinal.   Epigastric tenderness can be present in adults. Hyperactive bowel sounds may occur. Children may have generalized pain or tenderness localized to the periumbilical region. If perforation occurs, peritoneal signs, percussion changes, ascites, and guarding will be found. Rectal examination may show guaiac-positive stool.

PATHOPHYSIOLOGY

Peptic ulcers are more commonly found in the first portion of the duodenum. The ulcers have sharp demarcation and can go as deep as the muscularis propria. NSAID-induced ulcers, acid secretion problems, and *H. pylori* infection commonly cause peptic ulcers. Gastric ulcers can become malignant. Damage can be caused by NSAIDs and *H. pylori* infection. Patients with gastric ulcers usually have normal or low acid secretion with an impaired mucosal defense. Gastric ulcers are usually found distal from the junction in the area between the antrum and the acid secretory mucosa.

DIAGNOSTIC STUDIES

Laboratory

Complete Blood Count.   Performed to evaluate for anemia due to blood loss.

Serum Chemistry.   Used as a baseline and to rule out other conditions.

Stool Guaiac Test.   Reveals presence of blood. Will be positive with upper or lower GI bleed.

Helicobacter pylori *Serum Titer or Breath Test.* For urease response using carbon radiolabeled urea.

Serum Gastrin Level and Secretin Stimulation Tests. Performed if Zollinger-Ellison syndrome is suspected. If the ulcer has not healed after 8 weeks of full therapy or if the patient has recurrence, serum gastrin (usually greater than over 500 pg/mL) along with serum calcium should be measured. These levels are measured to check for a gastrinoma or MEN.

Gastric Acid Analysis. Should be performed to determine if there is gastric acid hypersecretion or an impairment in mucosal protection.

Radiology
Upper Gastrointestinal Series with Small Bowel Follow-Through. Features such as strictures, incompetent sphincter, hiatal hernia, contour changes, masses, and ulcers can be visualized. May diagnose PUD. Barium studies are not sufficient to determine whether a gastric ulcer is malignant. Ulcer shrinkage with therapy makes it difficult to make determinations based on the study.

Other
Endoscopy. The gold standard for diagnosing *H. pylori* infection is histologic examination of endoscopic biopsy specimens of the gastric antrum. Will definitively diagnose PUD. Should be performed if there is a concern about gastric carcinoma, bleeding, or obstruction.

DIFFERENTIAL DIAGNOSIS

Traumatic
Corrosive ingestion may occur accidentally in children or with suicide attempt.

Infectious
With *acute gastroenteritis*, acute onset after ingestion of contaminated food. Other persons may be affected.

Metabolic
With *depression*, negative results on GI studies. May be elicited on comprehensive history.

In *pancreatitis*, pain can radiate to the back. Elevated amylase/lipase.

In *gallbladder disease*, pain radiates to the right upper quadrant.

In *liver disease*, elevated liver function studies. Positive hepatitis profile.

In Zollinger-Ellison syndrome, abnormal serum gastrin level.

Nonulcer dyspepsia is differentiated on diagnostic studies.

Gastroesophageal reflux disease (GERD) is differentiated on endoscopy.

In *Crohn's disease*, may have associated dyspepsia alone with lower abdominal symptoms (see "Crohn's Disease" earlier in this chapter).

Atrophic gastritis is differentiated on endoscopy.

Neoplastic
With *gastric carcinoma*, tumor is seen on endoscopy. May have symptoms of weight loss, anorexia, early satiety, nausea, and vomiting or regurgitation.

Vascular

With *variant angina pectoris/myocardial infarction*, positive ECG and/or cardiac enzymes.

Abdominal angina (mesenteric insufficiency) may require angiography for diagnosis.

Congenital. Not applicable.

Acquired

With *drug addiction* or *withdrawal*, history of use. Differentiated on toxicology screen.

TREATMENT

Pharmacologic

Eradication of *H. pylori* is indicated if infection is present and symptomatic. Use NSAIDs cautiously.

- Antacids: rarely used except in patients who have dyspepsia.

  Mylanta or Maalox, as directed, at 1 hour before and 3 hours after meals is recommended for dyspepsia. Patients with chronic renal failure should not use aluminum owing to possible neurotoxicity, and the magnesium can cause hypermagnesia. Long-term use of calcium carbonate and sodium bicarbonate can lead to milk alkali syndrome, and sodium can induce systemic alkalosis. Tums or Gaviscon also can be used before meals and at bedtime.

Other agents:

- Mucosal-protective agents: These replace aluminum hydroxide and sulfate.

  Sucralfate 1 g twice a day

  Avoid aluminum hydroxide agents in patients with chronic renal insufficiency, as these agents can cause aluminum-induced neurotoxicity.

- Histamine H_2 receptor antagonists: For treatment of active ulcers for 4 to 6 weeks; use with antibiotics to eradicate *H. pylori.*

  Cimetidine 800 mg at bedtime

  Ranitidine 300 mg at bedtime

  Famotidine 40 mg at bedtime

  Nizatidine 300 mg at bedtime

- Proton pump inhibitors (PPIs): Inhibit effect at 2 to 6 hours after administration; lasts 72 to 96 hours with daily dosing.

Omeprazole	20 mg/day
Lansoprazole	30 mg/day
Rabeprazole	20 mg/day
Pantoprazole	40 mg/day

- Bismuth-containing preparations also are effective against *H. pylori* infection.

  Colloidal bismuth subcitrate and bismuth subsalicylate (BSS, Pepto-Bismol) are used.

- Prostaglandin analogues: Used in the treatment of peptic ulcer disease and for prevention of NSAID-induced ulcers.
  Misoprostol 200 μg four times a day

Eradication of Helicobacter pylori

For eradication of *H. pylori*, treat the patient for 14 days with one of the following:

Amoxicillin, metronidazole, tetracycline, clarithromycin, and bismuth compounds are used in various combinations.

Dual Therapy

Dual therapy for 14 days works well and is tolerated well by patients:

Omeprazole 20 mg twice a day plus clarithromycin 500 mg three times a day

Triple Therapy

Approximately 20% to 30% of the patients have side effects with triple therapy.

Bismuth 2 tablets four times a day, metronidazole 250 mg three times a day, and tetracycline OR amoxicillin 500 mg three times a day

Ranitidine bismuth citrate 400 mg twice a day, tetracycline 500 mg twice a day, and clarithromycin OR metronidazole 500 mg twice a day

Quadruple Therapy

Omeprazole 20 mg daily, bismuth subsalicylate 2 tablets daily, metronidazole 250 mg four times a day, and tetracycline 500 mg four times a day

Anti-*H. pylori* prepackaged preparations include:

Prevpac (lansoprazole, clarithromycin, amoxicillin) for 14 days

Helidac (bismuth subsalicylate, tetracycline, metronidazole) for 14 days

NSAID-Induced Disease

If the ulcer is NSAID-induced, discontinue NSAID and administer an H_2 receptor antagonist or PPI. If continued NSAID use is absolutely necessary, treat with a PPI. To treat NSAID-induced ulcers:

Prophylactic misoprostol 200 μg PO two or three times a day

For adjunctive PPI therapy:

Omeprazole 20 mg OR

Lansoprazole 30 mg PO daily

Selected cyclooxygenase-2 (COX-2) inhibitors

Surgery

Surgery is usually performed for ulcer-related complications (hemorrhage, peritoneal perforations, inflammatory pyloric channel ulcers, or scarring from a gastric outlet obstruction). Hemorrhage occurs in 15% to 25% of the

patients, usually in those age 60 and older. Some GI bleeds cease spontaneously, whereas others require endoscopic control of the hemorrhage.

Surgery will decrease the secretion of gastric acid. Some of the procedures
used to correct this problem are vagotomy and drainage by pyloroplasty,
antrectomy with a Billroth I anastomosis for antral ulcer, vagotomy (only
for duodenal ulcer), gastroduodenostomy or gastrojejunostomy, vagotomy
with antrectomy, or a subtotal gastrectomy with Roux-en-Y esophagogas-
trojejunostomy

Monitoring

Peptic ulcer.   Patients with peptic ulcers should have a follow-up radiologic or endoscopic evaluation only if there is a persistence or recurrence of
pain, presenting symptoms of a gastric outlet obstruction, or any evidence
of bleeding. Stool guaiac tests and a complete blood count assist in detecting bleeding. Monitor the patient's symptoms.

Gastric Ulcer.   Patients with gastric ulcers do not generally need follow-up
evaluation if the symptoms resolve completely and there are no clinical findings
that suggest cancer or complications of the disease. Symptoms should dissipate
in 4 to 6 weeks and not recur. If the patient has continued pain after 8 weeks
on a full medical regimen, endoscopy and biopsy are required, especially in
patients older than 40 years of age, to evaluate for gastric cancer.

PEDIATRIC CONSIDERATIONS

Children may have pain localized to the periumbilical region, or the pain can
be generalized. Symptoms of concern include weight loss, anorexia, early
satiety, nausea, and vomiting or regurgitation. These symptoms suggest an
obstruction caused by stricture, gastric outlet syndrome, or carcinoma.
Further workup is required.

GERIATRIC CONSIDERATIONS

Geriatric patients can present with frank shock, angina, cardiac failure,
orthostatic changes, or a change in sensorium due to hemorrhage from peptic or gastric ulcer. Many patients will be taking over-the-counter and prescription NSAIDs for underlying medical conditions. Approximately 50% of
the patients older than 70 years of age have complications, the most common of which is bleeding. Geriatric patients have a higher mortality rate.

An H_2 receptor antagonist can be given at bedtime for prophylaxis in
high-risk patients.

Theophylline, phenytoin, and warfarin levels are increased by cimetidine.
Most of the H_2 receptor antagonists cause central nervous system effects
(e.g., lethargy, disorientation) in the geriatric population.

PREVENTIVE CONSIDERATIONS

The patients should be instructed to avoid smoking (especially over {½}
pack per day), alcohol, coffee, stress, and medications that can cause gastric

distress such as NSAIDs and steroids. The patient should also follow a low-fat diet.

PEARLS FOR THE PA

Geriatric patients may present with frank shock or a change in sensorium when they have a peptic or gastric ulcer.

Patients with gastric ulcers are prone to develop gastric carcinoma.

H. pylori infection is a very common cause of peptic and gastric ulcers.

Peptic ulcers can be aggravated by alcohol, tobacco, coffee, aspirin, NSAIDs, tolazoline, corticosteroids, and stress.

With gastric ulcer, pain is usually worsened with meals.

Ulcerative Colitis

Michelle L. Heinan, EdD, MS, PA-C

DEFINITION

Only the mucosa and submucosa are affected in ulcerative colitis unless the disease is in the fulminant stage. The crypts are distorted. The mucosa will be erythematous and have a sandpaper quality in the mild stages. In the fulminant stage, the intestine will be edematous, ulcerated, and hemorrhagic. Eventually it will become atrophic and shortened.

There is rectal involvement in 95% of the cases, with extension to the left colon or possibly the entire colon. Full extension of the colonic involvement is called pancolitis. Nonsmokers and former smokers are at greater risk.

HISTORY

Symptoms. Usually will be localized to the left lower quadrant. The characteristic feature is diarrheal stools containing blood or mucus. Other associated symptoms are fever, fatigue, anorexia, and weight loss.

General. Diagnosis can be made on the basis of the patient's history and symptoms; sigmoid colon appearance; negative stool examination for bacteria, *Clostridium difficile*, and ova and parasites; and absence of abnormalities on rectal or colonic biopsy specimens.

Approximately one-third of patients with ulcerative colitis will develop colon cancer. Cancer workups are required with disease exacerbation or at 10 years after diagnosis (with or without remission). Colonoscopy with biopsy is recommended annually. Other complications include liver disease, hemorrhage, toxic megacolon, obstruction, extracolonic disease, intractable disease, and perforation.

Age.   Ulcerative colitis usually develops between 10 and 40 years of age and again in the seventh decade of life. Males and females are affected equally.

Onset.   Symptoms can be slow in onset, can increase over a 24- to 48-hour period, or can be abrupt.

Duration.   Ulcerative colitis is a chronic disease. The disease may be intermittent with periods of remission.

Intensity.   The patient can experience symptoms that are virtually undetectable and may not seek medical treatment. The patient can also experience symptoms of abdominal pain, hemorrhage, and dehydration.

Aggravating Factors.   None.

Alleviating Factors.   Defecation.

Associated Factors.   Associated factors include erythema nodosum, pyoderma gangrenosum, jaundice, skin lesions, cataracts, keratopathy, episcleritis, uveitis, central serous retinopathy, and corneal ulceration. Approximately 20% of the patients have arthritis (inflammatory, migratory, or peripheral in the elbows, wrists, ankles, and hips). Ankylosing spondylitis is a complication. Anemia and iron deficiency may occur. Cirrhosis can be found in 1% to 5% of the patients. Rare associated conditions include bile duct carcinoma, thromboembolic disease, hepatomegaly, primary sclerosing cholangitis, and pericarditis amyloidosis.

PHYSICAL EXAMINATION

General.   Patients may appear ill and pale. Jaundice is possible. Skin turgor may be increased. Temperature may be greater than 103° F. Patients are frequently hypotensive, hypovolemic, and tachycardic.

Eyes.   Look for signs of cataracts, episcleritis, keratopathy, uveitis, central serous retinopathy, and corneal ulceration.

Gastrointestinal.   The abdomen appears distended. Bowel sounds are decreased to absent. There is tenderness to palpation in the left lower quadrant on light and deep palpation. The bowel wall is tender and bleeds easily on rectal examination. Tenesmus may be a feature. Stool is Hemoccult-positive. Occasionally hemorrhoids, perianal abscess, and anal fissures are found.

PATHOPHYSIOLOGY

The etiology of ulcerative colitis is unknown. Theories include psychologic, immune, and infectious causes. There is possible genetic involvement with presence of human leukocyte antigen B27 (HLA-B27). Ulcerative colitis is common in the Jewish population of Eastern European descent. Caucasians are affected more often than African Americans. There is a tenfold increased risk for the development of ulcerative colitis if a first-degree relative has the disease.

DIAGNOSTIC STUDIES

Laboratory
Complete Blood Count.   May show anemia. Leukocytosis will also be present.

Iron Level.   May be decreased.

Platelet Count.   Increased.

Liver Function Tests.   Values will be elevated.

C-Reactive Protein and Orosomucoid Levels (Acute Phase Reactants). Increased.

Fecal Leukocytes and Cultures/Stool Examination for Ova and Parasites. May be positive.

Electrolytes.   Used to evaluate the degree of dehydration.

Amylase.   May be elevated.

Erythrocyte Sedimentation Rate.   Elevated.

Serum Albumin.   Hypoalbuminemia and hypoproteinemia may be present. In severe cases, the serum albumin will fall quickly.

Radiology
Plain Abdominal Film.   Thickening and dilatation can be visualized.

Barium Enema.   Used to reveal the extent and severity of disease. Haustral markings may be normal early in the disease process. As the disease progresses, haustral markings can disappear. Early in the disease, a fine mucosal granularity can be seen until later when the mucosa develops ulcerations and narrowing of the intestinal lumen.

Abdominal CT.   Not as useful as barium enema and sigmoidoscopy in making the diagnosis.

Other
Sigmoidoscopy.   Should be done to determine disease activity and before instituting treatment. The examination will reveal ulcerations and an irregular mucosal surface.

DIFFERENTIAL DIAGNOSIS

Traumatic.   Not applicable.

Infectious
Bacterial infections including those due to *Shigella*, *Salmonella*, *Campylobacter*, *Yersinia*, *C. difficile*, *Neisseria gonorrhoeae*, and *Chlamydia trachomatis*. Differentiated on culture.

Parasitic infections including those due to *Isospora*, hookworm, *Stronglyoides*, amebae, and *Trichuris trichura*. Seen on ova and parasite culture.

Viral infections including those due to cytomegalovirus, herpes simplex virus, and HIV. May require special cultures if suspected. HIV positive.

Fungal infections including those due to *Histoplasma*, *Candida*, and *Aspergillus*. Differentiated on fungal cultures.

Mycobacterial infections including tuberculosis and *Mycobacterium avium* infection. Differentiated on serologic or special cultures.

Metabolic

Diverticulitis is differentiated on barium enema, CT, or colonoscopy.

Crohn's disease is differentiated on sigmoidoscopy/colonoscopy, barium enema.

Hemorrhoids are differentiated on sigmoidoscopy.

Neoplastic

Neoplasms including colon cancer, lymphoma, carcinoid, and familial polyposis. May be seen on CT, or sigmoidoscopy/colonoscopy, or suspected on barium enema. Differentiated on biopsy.

Vascular

Ischemic proctitis is differentiated on sigmoidoscopy.

Arteriovenous malformation is diagnosed with angiogram.

Congenital. Not applicable.

Acquired

With *radiation proctitis*, history of a condition requiring treatment with radiation.

Drugs and chemicals including NSAIDs, gold, oral contraceptives, cocaine, chemotherapeutic agents, oral sodium phosphate solution (Phospho-Soda), and cathartics. History of use or found on drug screen.

With *pseudomembranous colitis*, history of antibiotic use. *Clostridium difficile*–positive.

Other

Intestinal obstruction from any cause is differentiated on diagnostic studies.

With *irritable bowel syndrome*, all studies negative

TREATMENT

Pharmacologic

- Sulfasalazine: Used in mild to moderate disease.
  Sulfasalazine 500 mg, for a total of 2-6 g/day in acute phase;
  2-4 g/day for maintenance
  Olsalazine is less toxic and can be used in place of sulfasalazine:

Olsalazine 500 mg twice a day, for a total of 1-3 g/day, OR

Balsalazide 500-750 mg, for a total of 2-6 g/day for 8-12 weeks

- Mesalamine agents: For ileum-colon involvement.

    To induce and maintain remission:

    Asacol 2.4-4.8 g/day in acute phase; 0.8-4.8 g/day for maintenance

    Topical-mesalamine enemas are effective in mild to moderate distal ulcerative colitis: 4 g/60 mL suspension or 500 mg suppositories twice a day.

- Glucocorticoids

    For management of moderate to severe ulcerative colitis:

    Prednisone 40-60 mg/day in active disease unresponsive to 5-acetylsalicylic acid therapy (e.g., sulfasalazine, olsalazine, mesalamine, balsalazide)

    Intravenous hydrocortisone 300 mg/day OR methylprednisone 48-60 mg/day

    Topical glucocorticoids are beneficial in distal colitis (useful for adjunctive therapy in patients who have rectal involvement and more proximal disease).

    Hydrocortisone enemas (90 mg per rectum per day) or foam may control active disease.

    Glucocorticoids have no role in maintenance of ulcerative colitis after the acute phase.

- Antibiotics: No role in the treatment of active or quiescent disease.

    If a patient develops pouchitis (post colectomy or ileal pouch anal anastomosis), ciprofloxacin or metronidazole can be effective.

- Azathioprine and 6-mercaptopurine (6-MP): Purine analogues commonly employed in the management of glucocorticoid-dependent irritable bowel syndrome. Inhibit immune response; efficacy in 3 to 4 weeks; monitor compliance by measurement of level of 6-thioguanine, an end product of 6-MP metabolism.

    Azathioprine 50 mg orally daily up to 2.5 mg/kg/day

    6-MP 1-1.5 mg/kg/day

- Cyclosporine

    In cases that are refractory to intravenous glucocorticoids:

    Cyclosporine 4 mg/kg/day IV in severe cases

    Oral cyclosporine is not helpful except in a higher dose (7.5 mg/kg/day) and will not maintain remission.

- Nutritional therapy: Ulcerative colitis patients do not benefit from total parenteral nutrition or total enteral nutrition in active disease.

Surgery

Some patients will require a colectomy, protocolectomy, protocolectomy with continent ileostomy, or an ileoanal anastomosis for management of complications. Most ulcerative colitis patients will require surgery in the first 10 years after diagnosis.

OBSTETRIC CONSIDERATIONS

If sulfasalazine is given to the pregnant patient, folic acid supplementation is imperative. Patients with ulcerative colitis may have a flare of symptoms in the first trimester. Spontaneous abortion rates are higher in this population. Patients may wish to consider deferring pregnancy until there have been no flares for 1 year.

PEDIATRIC CONSIDERATIONS

Inflammatory bowel disease usually does not appear until adolescence.

GERIATRIC CONSIDERATIONS

The second peak of inflammatory bowel disease occurs after the age of 60 years. Presenting symptoms are usually diarrhea, abdominal pain, and weight loss. Geriatric patients who have colitis-type symptoms need to be evaluated for other conditions.

Patients usually have a more distal distribution than is seen in their younger counterparts. Patients do well on medical therapy, especially with immunosuppressants and 5-ASA, with low doses of glucocorticoids. Cyclosporine is used frequently, but dosage has to be calculated carefully to compensate for age-related decrease in renal clearance. The use of glucocorticoids can cause osteoporosis and hyperglycemia.

Sulfasalazine is to be used at the lowest dose possible for mild or moderate active colitis. Folic acid should be given as a supplement. For patients allergic to sulfa drugs or those who cannot tolerate the side effects, 5-ASA compounds can be used. Distal colitis or proctitis may respond initially to treatment with enemas containing corticosteroids or a 5-ASA compound.

Moderate to severe colitis may require oral corticosteroid therapy for 2 to 3 months. Long-term high-dose corticosteroid therapy is associated with significant complications. Antibiotic therapy appears to be more effective in patients with Crohn's disease, especially for fistulous disease or perianal involvement. 6-MP does not appear to be effective as a single agent but can diminish the corticosteroid dose needed. Both cyclosporine and methotrexate are toxic medications and should probably be reserved for treatment of Crohn's disease.

Long-term maintenance therapy for inflammatory bowel disease includes use of sulfasalazine, 5-ASA, metronidazole, or 6-MP (in combination with low-dose corticosteroid therapy).

PREVENTIVE CONSIDERATIONS

Colonoscopy will need to be done annually after the disease has been present for 8 to 10 years, as colon cancer will occur in approximately one-third of patients. A biopsy should accompany the colonoscopy. Liver function tests should be monitored closely, especially in patients who have pancolitis. Cholangiography should also be done to evaluate for cholestasis.

PEARLS FOR THE PA

A barium enema study should be avoided in acute cases of ulcerative colitis.

Pain is usually located in the left lower quadrant.

Cancer workups are required with disease exacerbation or at 10 years after diagnosis (with or without remission).

Colonoscopy with biopsy is recommended annually.

Further Reading

American Gastroenterological Association medical position statement: Evaluation of dyspepsia. Gastroenterology 114:579-581, 1998.

Andreoli TE (ed): Cecil Essentials of Medicine, 5th ed. Philadelphia, WB Saunders, 2001.

Bazaldua OV, Schneider FD: Evaluation and management of dyspepsia. Am Fam Physician 60:1773-1784, 1999.

Bonapace ES, Parkman HP: Dysphagia and esophageal obstruction. In Rakel RE (ed): Conn's Current Therapy 2000. Philadelphia, WB Saunders, 2000.

Braunwald E, Fauci AS, Kasper DL, et al (eds): Harrison's Principles of Internal Medicine, 15th ed. New York, McGraw-Hill Medical Publishing Division, 2001.

Dambro MR (ed): Griffith's 5-Minute Clinical Consult. Philadelphia, Lippincott Williams & Wilkins, 2000.

Goff JS: Bleeding esophageal varices. In Rakel RE (ed): Conn's Current Therapy 2000. Philadelphia, WB Saunders, 2000.

Goldstein J, Oshin P: Peptic ulcer disease. In Rakel RE (ed): Conn's Current Therapy 2000. Philadelphia, WB Saunders, 2000, pp 496-501.

Goroll AH, Mulley AG: Primary Care Medicine: Office Evaluation and Management of the Adult Patient, 4th ed. Philadelphia, Lippincott Williams & Wilkins, 2000.

Koop E: Wellness and prevention of dyspepsia. Available at http://www.drkoop.com/dyncon/article.asp?id=6153

Kumar V, Cotran RS, Robbins SL: Basic Pathology, 6th ed. Philadelphia, WB Saunders, 1997.

Kutty K, Sebastian JL, Mewis BA, et al: Kochar's Concise Textbook of Medicine. Baltimore, Williams & Wilkins, 1998.

Labus JB, Lauber, AA: Patient Education and Preventive Medicine. Philadelphia, WB Saunders, 2001.

Moser RL: Primary Care for Physician Assistants: Clinical Practice Guidelines, 2nd ed. New York, McGraw-Hill Medical Publishing Division, 2001.

Rosen P, Barkin RM, Hayden SR, et al (eds): The 5 Minute Emergency Medicine Consult. Philadelphia, Lippincott Williams & Wilkins, 1999.

Shaker R, Dua SK, Koch TR: Gastroenterologic disorders. In Duthie EH Jr, Katz PR (eds): Practice in Geriatrics, 3rd ed. Philadelphia, WB Saunders, 1998, pp 505-523.

Stobo JD, Hellmann DB, Ladenson PW, et al (eds): The Principles and Practice of Medicine, 23rd ed. Stamford, CT, Appleton & Lange, 1996.
Tintinalli JE, Kelen GD, Stapczynski JS (eds): Emergency Medicine: A Comprehensive Study Guide, 5th ed. New York, McGraw-Hill, 2000.

GYNECOLOGY

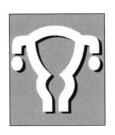

6

Cervicitis

Jodi L. Cahalan, MPH, MS, PA-C

DEFINITION

An inflammation of the cervix, usually infectious in etiology.

HISTORY

Symptoms. The majority of cases are asymptomatic, but patients may have a vaginal discharge, deep dyspareunia, and/or postcoital bleeding.

General. Symptoms are generally mild when present. Asymptomatic cases may be detected on speculum examination.

Age. Generally adolescent and adult women who are sexually active.

Onset. Variable; may be difficult to ascertain because many cases are asymptomatic.

Duration. Variable.

Intensity. Usually mild discomfort unless an ascending infection occurs, causing pelvic inflammatory disease.

Aggravating Factors. None.

Alleviating Factors. None.

Associated Factors. Unprotected intercourse, multiple sexual partners, history of sexually transmitted diseases.

PHYSICAL EXAMINATION

General. The patient appears to be in no acute distress.

Gastrointestinal. Abdomen should be soft and nontender, with no palpable masses or organomegaly.

Gynecologic. Inspect external genitalia for signs of inflammation, and look for discharge in the vaginal vault. Inspect cervix for signs of a mucopurulent discharge from the os, inflammation, and any lesions; palpate for cervical motion, uterine or adnexal tenderness, enlargement, or masses. Positive findings include an erythematous cervix with a mucopurulent, often yellow discharge from the os. The cervix may be edematous and hypertrophic. Nabothian cysts may be present. Cervix may be seen to be friable when endocervical smear is obtained, and cervix may be mildly tender to palpation.

PATHOPHYSIOLOGY

An inflammatory process involving the columnar epithelium and subepithelium of the endocervix, generally occurring as a result of an infectious agent.

DIAGNOSTIC STUDIES

Laboratory
Wet Preparation.   Look for white blood cells (WBCs) or trichomonads.
Culture.   Indicated to rule out gonorrhea.
DNA Probe or Polymerase Chain Reaction (PCR) Assay.   Performed to rule out *Chlamydia* infection.

Radiology.   Not applicable.
Other.   Not applicable.

DIFFERENTIAL DIAGNOSIS

Traumatic
With *irritation from cervical cap/diaphragm*, history of use, negative results on testing for infectious causes, normal Papanicolaou (Pap) smear.
  With *inflammation due to cryosurgery*, history of cryosurgery.

Infectious
Chlamydial infection, the most common cause, can be present without any signs or symptoms. DNA probe or antigen testing required for diagnosis.
  In *gonorrhea*, profuse, purulent cervical discharge usually present. Requires culture for diagnosis.
  Trichomoniasis causes petechiae on cervix. Involves the ectocervix rather than the endocervix.
  Herpes simplex virus (HSV) *infection* causes vesicular lesions that may involve the cervix. Often associated with vulvar pain and tenderness.
  Human papillomavirus (HPV) *infection* is often asymptomatic but may be identified on Pap smear.

Neoplastic
With *cervical cancer*, any visible lesions should be biopsied. Pap smear should be done if lesions are persistent without identifiable cause.

Acquired
Columnar eversion is protrusion of endocervical glandular tissue, which mimics cervicitis. This is a physiologic process caused by pregnancy and oral contraceptives that does not require treatment.

Metabolic.   Not applicable.
Vascular.   Not applicable.
Congenital.   Not applicable.

TREATMENT

Chlamydial Infection
  A single dose of Azithromycin 1 g PO (especially for patients in whom follow-up may not occur or when poor compliance is suspected) OR

Doxycycline 100 mg PO twice a day for 7 days
Alternative regimens:
Erythromycin base 500 mg PO four times a day for 7 days OR
Erythromycin ethylsuccinate 800 mg PO four times a day for 7 days OR
Ofloxacin 300 mg twice a day for 7 days OR
Levofloxacin 500 mg PO once a day for 7 days

Gonorrhea
A single dose of cefixime 400 mg PO OR
A single IM injection of ceftriaxone 250 mg 1 dose IM OR
A single dose of ciprofloxacin 500 mg PO OR
A single dose of ofloxacin 400 mg PO OR
A single dose of levofloxacin 250 mg PO
PLUS, if chlamydial infection has not been ruled out,
A single dose of azithromycin 1 g PO OR
Doxycycline 100 mg twice a day for 7 days

PEDIATRIC CONSIDERATIONS

Presence of gonococci or *Chlamydia* in a child requires evaluation for sexual abuse.

OBSTETRIC CONSIDERATIONS

Neisseria gonorrhoeae *Infection*
Women with gonococcal cervicitis are at increased risk for disseminated gonoccocal infection during pregnancy, which has been associated with premature labor. Infants born to mothers with cervicovaginal gonorrhea may develop gonoccocal conjunctivitis, pharyngeal, respiratory, or rectal infections, or sepsis during the neonatal period.

Chlamydia trachomatis *Infection*
Chlamydial infection is usually asymptomatic during pregnancy. *Chlamydia* can cause preterm delivery, low birth weight in the infant, chorioamnionitis, stillbirth, postpartum endometritis, and neonatal conjunctivitis and pneumonia. This infection also has been implicated in causing habitual spontaneous abortions.

Human Papillomavirus Infection
Podofilox should not be used in the treatment of HPV infection in pregnant women.

Herpes Simplex Virus Infection
HSV infection complicates 1% to 2% of all pregnancies. The risk of infection to the fetus occurs during delivery. If the mother is experiencing a pri-

mary active outbreak (attack), a vaginal delivery creates a 50% chance of HSV transmission to the infant. Delivery by cesarean section is recommended if the woman has genital herpetic lesions. Up to 60% of women who deliver infected infants may be asymptomatic at the time of delivery. In addition, approximately 1% to 2% of all people (pregnant women and nonpregnant) chronically shed the virus in saliva and genital excretions. Women who carry an active herpes infection of the cervix have no symptoms. Infants born to mothers who acquired the infection late in the pregnancy are at much greater risk of serious neonatal sequelae.

HSV infection in the neonate is often catastrophic, with an approximate 50% mortality rate. Serologic testing may be considered. Primary HSV infection in the mother increases the risk of prematurity and intrauterine growth retardation (IUGR).

Acyclovir use in pregnancy has yet to be defined as being safe for the fetus. Its use should be limited to severe, life-threatening maternal primary HSV infections. Disseminated maternal infection is more likely in a woman who is pregnant.

GERIATRIC CONSIDERATIONS

A higher index of suspicion should be maintained for cervical cancer.

PREVENTIVE CONSIDERATIONS

Barrier method for contraception is recommended to help prevent sexually transmitted disease. Having multiple sexual partners is also a risk factor.

PEARLS FOR THE PA

History is important in the diagnosis of cervicitis.

Infectious agents, especially Chlamydia, *may be present without signs or symptoms; consider screening high-risk patients.*

Dysmenorrhea

Jodi L. Cahalan, MPH, MS, PA-C

DEFINITION

Painful menstruation classified as either primary (from excess prostaglandin production in an ovulatory cycle) or secondary (associated with other disorders such as endometriosis, adenomyosis, leiomyomas, or pelvic inflammatory disease [PID] or with an intrauterine device [IUD]).

HISTORY

Symptoms.   Discomfort may range from a dull ache to severe and painful cramping felt in the lower abdomen. Pain may radiate to hips, lower back, and inner thighs. May be described as constant, intermittent, and wave-like.

Patient may also report having headaches, nausea, vomiting, diarrhea, fatigue, and lightheadedness as well as tachycardia and tremulousness in severe cases.

Age.   Primary dysmenorrhea typically begins in the mid- to late teens. It generally does not begin at menarche, but generally appears within 1 to 2 years of menarche.

Secondary dysmenorrhea most commonly affects women older than 20 years of age.

Onset.   The pain usually begins with the onset of menstrual flow but may start soon before or soon after the onset of flow.

Duration.   The discomfort typically lasts 2 to 3 days.

Intensity.   Varies, ranging from mild to severe in intensity.

Aggravating Factors.   Menorrhagic cycles, smoking.

Alleviating Factors.   Palliative measures may include rest, heat, and elevation of the legs. Symptoms generally lessen in severity after pregnancy and delivery.

Associated Factors.   Increased production of prostaglandins associated with the ovulatory cycle.

PHYSICAL EXAMINATION

General.   The patient may appear normal or be in significant discomfort if symptoms are present.

Gynecologic.   There may be generalized tenderness if the examination is performed during a symptomatic episode. Otherwise, the physical examination is generally unremarkable in patients with primary dysmenorrhea.

Signs of infection, IUD, or fibroids may be evident in patients with secondary dysmenorrhea.

PATHOPHYSIOLOGY

The pain of primary dysmenorrhea is thought to arise from an increased production of prostaglandins by the endometrium, which may lead to increased uterine contractility and uterine ischemia.

The pain of secondary dysmenorrhea is not physiologic but rather is caused by other disorders such as endometriosis, adenomyosis, leiomyomas, or PID or is associated with the presence of an IUD. A thorough search for the etiologic factor is necessary.

DIAGNOSTIC STUDIES

Laboratory
Complete Blood Count.   Elevated white blood cell (WBC) count with infection as a cause for secondary dysmenorrhea.

Cervical Culture and Sensitivity Testing for Pathogens Including Agents of Sexually Transmitted Diseases.   Indicated to rule out or identify an infectious agent.

Radiology.   Not generally applicable for primary dysmenorrhea, but pelvic/uterine ultrasound examination may be used to seek structural cause of the pain.

Other.   On occasion, laparoscopy may be necessary to differentiate between primary and secondary dysmenorrhea.

DIFFERENTIAL DIAGNOSIS

Infectious
PID differs in the timing of pain and manifests with signs of infection.

Neoplastic
Leiomyoma uteri is a benign uterine tumor usually palpable on bimanual examination. Usually associated with pelvic pressure and/or bloating throughout cycle, not just accompanying menstruation. Usually associated with older age group than typical for primary dysmenorrhea.

Congenital
Malformations such as imperforate hymen are present with regular monthly discomfort but without menstruation. Prompt recognition and surgery are indicated.

Other
With *endometriosis*, pain usually begins premenstrually, is associated with symptoms of dyspareunia, and may be accompanied by abnormal pelvic examination findings.

Foreign body, typically an IUD, may exacerbate menstrual cramping.

Traumatic.   Not applicable.
Metabolic.   Not applicable.
Vascular.   Not applicable.
Acquired.   Not applicable.

TREATMENT

Prostaglandin synthase inhibitors such as nonsteroidal anti-inflammatory drugs (NSAIDs) are often the agents of choice for initial treatment.

Ibuprofen 400-600 mg four times a day OR
Naproxen 500 mg twice a day OR
Ketoprofen 50 mg three times a day OR
Vioxx 50 mg PO once a day for a minimum of 5 days

Other NSAIDs may also be tried, but the patient be instructed to take the medication regularly, rather than on an as-needed basis, to achieve improved pain control. The patient should begin the NSAID approximately 3 days before the expected onset of menstruation and should take it with food or milk to decrease gastrointestinal irritation.

Oral contraceptives constitute the second line of therapy if the prostaglandin synthase inhibitors fail to relieve symptoms. Should be used as primary treatment if patient also is seeking a contraceptive method.

In rare cases, no medication will relieve the pain. Cervical dilatation is of little use. Uterosacral ligament division and presacral neurectomy are infrequently performed but may be helpful.

PEDIATRIC CONSIDERATIONS

Dysmenorrhea is the most common gynecologic complaint of adolescent girls and is the leading cause of short-term school absenteeism among female students. Most cases of dysmenorrhea in adolescents is primary spasmodic dysmenorrhea. Secondary dysmenorrhea is uncommon in adolescents and, when present, is usually secondary to infection or endometriosis.

OBSTETRIC CONSIDERATIONS

No specific indications.

GERIATRIC CONSIDERATIONS

Not a consideration in the postmenopausal female. Pelvic pain must be fully evaluated to rule out pathology.

PREVENTIVE CONSIDERATIONS

Smoking cessation and regular exercise may help. Regular rather than as-needed NSAID use may prevent or lessen the symptoms.

PEARLS FOR THE PA

If an adequate trial of prostaglandins and oral contraceptives has failed to reduce dysmenorrhea sufficiently, laparoscopy should be considered to rule out a secondary cause.

Endometriosis

Pam Harrison Chambers, MPH, PA-C

DEFINITION

A disorder in which abnormal growth of tissue, histologically resembling the endometrium (uterine lining), is present in locations other than the uterine lining.

HISTORY

Symptoms.   The cardinal symptoms are pelvic pain and infertility. Pain can be constant, premenstrual, or menstrual. Deep dyspareunia and intermenstrual spotting are common. Less common are painful defecation, dysuria, and hematuria.

General.   Infertility is the only symptom in many women.

Age.   Women of reproductive age (15 to 44 years). From 5% to 10% of women have endometriosis.

Onset.   Gradual; however, patients may present with acute pain. The disorder tends to be progressive until menopause.

Duration.   Can be present from menarche to menopause. Symptoms tend to be cyclic.

Intensity.   Some patients are asymptomatic. If pain is present, it can be severe. May be asymptomatic at times during the cycle.

Aggravating Factors.   Pain is usually worse premenstrually, during menses, and with intercourse and defecation.

Alleviating Factors.   Menopause, either natural, surgical, or medical.

Associated Factors.   May cause infertility. If implants form over bowel or ureters, obstruction may occur. Endometriomas may rupture and cause peritonitis or ovarian torsion.

PHYSICAL EXAMINATION

General.   The patient may appear normal or be in significant discomfort if symptoms are present.

Gynecologic.   Classically, the pelvic examination reveals tender nodules in the cul-de-sac and pain on uterine motion. The uterus may be fixed and retroverted as a result of adhesions. Tender adnexal masses may indicate endometriomas.

PATHOPHYSIOLOGY

Endometrial implants vary in size, color, and location. Multiple lesions are typical and are usually found in the ovary, cul-de-sac, uterosacral ligaments, and pelvic peritoneum. Ovarian cysts (endometriomas or chocolate cysts) caused by endometriosis can enlarge to several centimeters in diameter.

DIAGNOSTIC STUDIES

Laboratory.   Not applicable.

Radiology.   Pelvic ultrasound examination may be helpful if endometriomas are present. Endometriosis is not ruled out by a negative ultrasound examination.

Other.   Definitive diagnosis can be made only by laparoscopy or laparotomy.

DIFFERENTIAL DIAGNOSIS

Traumatic

Physical or *emotional abuse* should be considered, as pelvic pain is a more common complaint in abused women.

Infectious

In *PID*, symptoms do not vary with menses.

Neoplastic

Endometriomas must be differentiated from *other pelvic neoplasms*. Ultrasound examination can be helpful, but surgery is often required for definitive diagnosis.

Metabolic.   Not applicable.

Vascular.   Not applicable.

Congenital.   Not applicable.

Acquired.   Not applicable.

TREATMENT

The patient's age, desire for fertility, severity of symptoms, and stage of the disease dictate treatment. Analgesia with NSAIDs can be helpful for control of symptoms. For mild cases, pseudopregnancy can be induced by hormone regimens such as oral contraceptives or medroxyprogesterone acetate. Induction of pseudomenopause using danazol or a gonadotropin-releasing hormone agonist (leuprolide acetate or nafarelin acetate) is an effective therapy for 6 to 9 months. These agents offer better suppression than that obtained using female steroids such as oral contraceptives.

Laporascopic surgery may be used to ablate implants and adhesions by means of electrocautery, sharp dissection, or laser.

Total abdominal hysterectomy (TAH) with bilateral salpingo-oophorectomy (BSO) with excision of all implants and adhesions provides definitive therapy.

Hormone replacement therapy may be advised after TAH-BSO, depending on the patient's age, health, and family history.

PEDIATRIC CONSIDERATIONS

Endometriosis can be present in teenagers.

OBSTETRIC CONSIDERATIONS

Pregnancy decreases the incidence and severity of endometriosis. Danazol, used for symptomatic treatment, can cause masculinization of a female fetus if a patient becomes pregnant while taking the medication.

GERIATRIC CONSIDERATIONS

Menopause alleviates the symptoms.

PREVENTIVE CONSIDERATIONS

Appropriate treatment to relieve symptoms. Age and desire for fertility are significant considerations in treatment of endometriosis. Definitive therapy by TAH-BSO obviously prevents conclusively any future pregnancy and should not be entered into lightly in the young, fertile patient.

PEARLS FOR THE PA

Ultrasound examination should not be used to screen for endometriosis. The only way to diagnose endometriosis definitively is through laparoscopy or laparotomy.

The clinician should maintain a high index of suspicion and not be afraid to treat endometriosis aggressively to preserve fertility and to decrease patient discomfort.

Fibrocystic Breast Disease

Pam Harrison Chambers, MPH, PA-C

DEFINITION

Fibrocystic breast disease, also known as mammary dysplasia or chronic cystic mastitis, is the most common benign breast condition. It is characterized by the presence of multiple tender nodules in one or both breasts. It probably represents a variant of normal rather than a true disease.

HISTORY

Symptoms. The patient usually presents with multiple, often bilateral painful breast masses that fluctuate in size. Pain is usually cyclic, occurring late in the cycle, but may be constant. Occasional clear nipple discharge may be present.

General. The history should include relation of menses to symptoms, caffeine intake, family history of breast cancer, and mammogram history.

Age. Most commonly affects women 30 to 50 years of age.

Onset. Symptoms may be constant but worsen during the premenstrual phase.

Duration. Symptoms tend to abate after menses.

Intensity. Varies, ranging from mild to severe.

Aggravating Factors. Caffeine intake, trauma, lack of supportive bra.

Alleviating Factors. Wearing a good support bra, eliminating dietary caffeine.

Associated Factors. Breast cancer and fibroadenoma may be difficult to differentiate from fibrocystic breast lesions.

PHYSICAL EXAMINATION

General. The patient usually appears to be in no acute distress.

Breasts. Single or multiple, usually tender, soft, rubbery nodules. Often bilateral involvement. The upper outer quadrant is affected most often. There should be no dimpling or skin retraction. Mass size may vary with cycle. Twenty percent of affected women may have palpable axillary lymph nodes.

PATHOPHYSIOLOGY

Fibrocystic breast disease is probably due to ovarian activity, as symptoms are rare in postmenopausal women. Symptoms occur as the result of an imbalance between estrogen and progestin that causes ductal stimulation and proliferation. Microscopic findings include cysts, papillomatosis, adenosis, fibrosis, and ductal hyperplasia.

DIAGNOSTIC STUDIES

Laboratory. Pathologic examination of mass aspirate or nipple discharge is warranted.

Radiology. Mammography may be helpful; however, young women have dense breasts, which may preclude an adequate mammogram.

Other. Ultrasonography can differentiate a solid (possibly malignant) from a cystic lesion (probably benign). Biopsy of suspicious lesions is advised, as it is often difficult to differentiate fibrocystic breast lesions from carcinoma.

DIFFERENTIAL DIAGNOSIS

Traumatic
Breast trauma is easily distinguishable from chronic fibrocystic changes by history and physical findings.

Infectious
Mastitis/breast abscess manifests as acute-onset discomfort, erythema, induration, and warmth. Usually occurs in nursing mothers.

Neoplastic
Carcinoma usually presents as a single, painless and firm nodule that may be fixed to underlying structures. Nipple retraction and skin retraction may be present. It is often difficult to differentiate fibrocystic breast lesions from carcinoma, so biopsy of suspicious lesions is advised.

Fibroadenoma is a benign, round, firm, discrete nodule that is relatively movable and nontender. Excision is required for diagnosis.

Metabolic. Not applicable.
Vascular. Not applicable.
Congenital. Not applicable.
Acquired. Not applicable.

TREATMENT

The first step is accurate diagnosis of the fibrocystic condition by aspiration of lesions. Pain may be temporarily decreased if fluid is removed from the mass.

Treatment of fibrocystic breast disease is often based on reassuring the patient that it is unlikely she has cancer. Recommend avoidance of caffeine, and advise the patient that there may be no improvement for 1 to 2 months.

Instruct patient on wearing supportive bra.

PEDIATRIC CONSIDERATIONS

Sometimes seen in older adolescents. Consider the value of reassurance and emphasizing the importance of breast self-examination.

OBSTETRIC CONSIDERATIONS

Patients with fibrocystic condition have dramatic improvement in symptoms when pregnant or lactating due to hormonal changes occurring at that time.

GERIATRIC CONSIDERATIONS

No specific considerations other than continued breast self-examination and biopsy/removal of suspicious lesions.

PREVENTIVE CONSIDERATIONS

Avoidance of aggravating factors such as caffeine and trauma, and wearing a good supportive bra can help alleviate symptoms.

PEARLS FOR THE PA

Patients may be trained in breast self-examination as early as the time of menarche. Technique must be reviewed annually.

Functional Ovarian Cysts

Pam Harrison Chambers, MPH, PA-C

DEFINITION

Enlargement of the ovary due to the presence of fluid-filled sacs, caused by a transient abnormality of a normal physiologic process, usually ovulation.

Two types of cysts fall into this category: follicular cysts and corpus luteum cysts.

HISTORY

Symptoms

Frequently asymptomatic. Pelvic pain, menstrual irregularities, and dyspareunia are relatively common symptoms.

General.   Inquire about the possibility of pregnancy.

Age.   Affects menstruating women.

Onset.   Variable, depending on cyst type.

Duration.   Variable, depending on cyst type. Most follicular cysts resolve within 60 days if not treated.

Intensity.   Usually mild, but a ruptured cyst or ovarian torsion can cause severe pain.

Aggravating Factors.   None.

Alleviating Factors.   None.

Associated Factors.   None.

PHYSICAL EXAMINATION

General.   The patient usually appears well but may be in acute distress.

Gastrointestinal.   Abdomen should be soft and nontender. Rupture of a cyst can cause acute pain and mimic an acute abdomen.

Gynecologic.   On bimanual examination, a cystic mass 4 to 8 cm in diameter may be palpable in the adnexal region. The mass is mobile, unilateral, and tender and should regress following the next menstrual cycle.

PATHOPHYSIOLOGY

Follicular cysts result from the failure of a mature follicle to rupture or from incomplete absorption of the fluid in an immature follicle.

Excessive bleeding in the central cavity of the corpus luteum causes corpus luteum cysts.

DIAGNOSTIC STUDIES

Laboratory

Human Chorionic Gonadotropin.   Should be assayed to rule out pregnancy.

Radiology

Pelvic Ultrasound Examination.   Indicated to exclude extrauterine pregnancy or solid mass and to measure the cyst.

Other

Not applicable.

DIFFERENTIAL DIAGNOSIS

Infectious

With *tubo-ovarian abscess*, history of PID, complex mass; patient appears generally ill.

Neoplastic
Benign and *malignant tumors* arising in the ovaries are solid or nonchanging masses on repeat ultrasound examination; require surgical exploration.

Acquired
Ectopic pregnancy is a possibility, so always rule out pregnancy.

Other
With *endometrioma*, history usually consistent with endometriosis.

With *ovarian torsion*, patient is usually in acute pain. Urgent surgical intervention is indicated.

Traumatic. Not applicable.
Metabolic. Not applicable.
Vascular. Not applicable.
Congenital. Not applicable.

TREATMENT

In menstruating women with cysts less than 8 cm in diameter, observation for 6 to 8 weeks is appropriate. Oral contraceptives are frequently prescribed during the observation period. A solid ovarian mass in any woman and any ovarian mass in a premenarchal girl or postmenopausal woman require immediate surgical exploration. Surgical management is also indicated for a mass greater than 8 cm in diameter or a mass 5 to 8 cm in size that has persisted for more than 8 weeks.

PEDIATRIC CONSIDERATIONS

At puberty, and in girls with true isosexual precocious puberty, larger follicular cysts are seen. Any adnexal mass in a prepubescent girl requires surgical exploration.

OBSTETRIC CONSIDERATIONS

This is a disorder of menstruating women.

GERIATRIC CONSIDERATIONS

This is a disorder of menstruating women.

PREVENTIVE CONSIDERATIONS

No specific preventive measures.

Pelvic Inflammatory Disease

Nina Multak, MPAS, PA-C

DEFINITION

Pelvic inflammatory disease (PID) is an inflammation, usually infectious, of the upper female genital tract. Involvement of the uterus is termed *endometritis*; of the fallopian tubes, *salpingitis*; of the ovaries, *oophoritis*; and of the pelvioperitoneum, *peritonitis*.

HISTORY

Symptoms. Symptoms are related to the causative organism and extent of the infection. Lower abdominal pain, which is present in 90% of patients with acute PID, increases with movement and sexual intercourse. Abnormal vaginal bleeding, increased vaginal discharge, or vaginal odor can be present. Nonspecific symptoms that may be present include fever, malaise, gastrointestinal symptoms, dysuria, and headache.

General. Greatest risk factor is multiple sex partners. Other risk factors involve situations in which mucosal injury occurs (i.e., endometrial biopsy, curettage, IUD insertion, hysterosalpingogram).

Age. Generally occurs in women 15 to 44 years of age.

Onset. When *Neisseria gonorrhoeae* is the primary pathogen, onset is typically acute. The onset of *Chlamydia trachomatis* infection is variable, and the infection can be asymptomatic.

Duration. Related to timing of patient evaluation and onset of treatment.

Intensity. Variable.

Aggravating Factors. Pregnancy, human immunodeficiency virus (HIV) infection.

Alleviating Factors. None.

Associated Factors. Multiple sexual partners, intrauterine procedure, transperitoneal spread of upper genital tract organisms from appendicitis, diverticulitis, or traumatic viscus rupture.

PHYSICAL EXAMINATION

General.   Usually acute onset of lower abdominal pain and pelvic pain (usually bilateral). Back pain may be present and radiate down the legs. Purulent vaginal discharge, headache, malaise, and nausea and vomiting are common.

Gastrointestinal.   Tenderness of lower abdominal quadrants. Rebound tenderness is evident when peritonitis occurs.

Gynecologic.   Examine external genitalia for signs of inflammation; look for discharge in the vaginal vault; examine the cervix for signs of inflammation and abnormal lesions; palpate for cervical motion and for uterine or adnexal tenderness. Positive findings include an erythematous cervix with a purulent discharge from the os; enlarged and edematous cervix; exquisite cervical motion tenderness; and uterine and adnexal tenderness. Tubo-ovarian enlargement may be palpable. The examination may be limited owing to guarding.

PATHOPHYSIOLOGY

Pathogens ascend from the lower to the upper genital tract, potentially affecting the vagina, cervix, uterus, tubes, ovaries, and peritoneum. *N. gonorrhoeae* is a causative organism in one-third of acute PID cases. *N. gonorrheae* has been identified with mixed aerobic and anaerobic flora. *C. trachomatis* has been found in up to 30% of cases in conjunction with other organisms. Anaerobes such as *Bacteroides*, *Peptostreptococcus*, and *Peptococcus* are identified when abscesses are noted. Aerobes commonly involved in PID include *Escherichia coli*, group B streptococci, *Streptococcus faecalis*, and coagulase-negative staphylococci.

DIAGNOSTIC STUDIES

Laboratory
Wet Preparation.   Look for white blood cells (WBCs), trichomonads.
Complete Blood Count.   WBC count cannot be relied on.
Serum Pregnancy Test.   If positive, consider ectopic pregnancy.
Electrolytes.   Used to evaluate for dehydration.
Liver Function Studies.   Indicated for evaluation of perihepatic inflammation.
Culture.   Cervical cultures for *N. gonorrhoeae*.
DNA Probe   Used to rule out *C. trachomatis*.
Urinalysis.   Urinalysis of specimen obtained by catheterization is useful to rule out urinary tract infection.

Radiology
Kidney-Ureter-Bladder (KUB) Films and Upright Film of Abdomen. Identify obstruction, ileus, or free peritoneal gas.
Abdominal Ultrasound Examination/CT.   Indicated to evaluate masses, rule out abscess.

Transvaginal Ultrasound Examination. Reveals peritoneal fluid, thickened edematous structures, hydrosalpinx.

Other
Laparoscopy. "Gold standard" for definitive diagnosis.

DIFFERENTIAL DIAGNOSIS

Traumatic
With *hematoperitoneum*, history of abdominal trauma.

Infectious
In *urinary tract infection*, positive urine culture.

In *pyelonephritis*, positive costovertebral angle tenderness; urine may show casts. Blood urea nitrogen (BUN)/creatinine levels may be elevated.

In *gastroenteritis*, presence of nausea and vomiting, prominent diarrhea, no cervical motion tenderness.

Neoplastic
Mass effect from neoplasms will be evident on CT or ultrasound examination of the abdomen/pelvis.

Acquired
In *ectopic pregnancy*, positive pregnancy test.

With *septic abortion*, enlarged uterus, open cervical os, positive pregnancy test, and elevated WBC count.

Other
Appendicitis can be differentiated by history, unilateral tenderness. Right rectal wall tenderness is difficult to differentiate.

Ruptured corpus luteum cyst can be differentiated by history. Laboratory studies are normal; pain tends to subside quickly after onset.

With *ovarian torsion*, no evidence of infectious process; unilateral mass.

Ulcerative colitis can be differentiated by history. Scarring and adhesions on examination.

Metabolic.   Not applicable.
Vascular.   Not applicable.
Congenital.   Not applicable.

TREATMENT

Hospitalization is indicated with uncertain diagnosis; for pregnant patients and those with sepsis, tubo-ovarian abscess, or immunodeficiency state; and for patients who are unable to tolerate oral medications or in whom outpatient treatment has failed. Patients requiring hospitalization should have bed rest, NPO status initially, intravenous fluids, and nasogastric suction when indicated.

Inpatient Treatment

Regimen A
Cefoxitin 2 g IV every 6 hours OR
Cefotan 2 g IV every 12 hours
PLUS
Doxycycline 100 mg IV every 12 hours continued until 48 hours after
   clinical improvement; then 100 mg PO twice a day for 10 to 14 days

Regimen B
Clindamycin 900 mg IV every 8 hours
PLUS
Gentamicin IV, loading dose 2 mg/kg, followed by 1.5 mg/kg every 8
   hours, continued until 48 hours after clinical improvement
THEN
DOXYCYCLINE 100 mg twice a day for 10 to 14 days

Outpatient Treatment

Regimen A
Ceftriaxone 250 mg IM once OR
Cefoxitin 2 g IM
PLUS
Probenecid 1 g PO OR
Other parenteral third generation cephalosporins PLUS
Doxycycline 100 mg PO twice a day WITH OR WITHOUT
Metronidazole 500 mg PO twice a day for 14 days. Is advocated to
   cover anaerobes associated with bacterial vaginosis.

Regimen B
Oflaxicin 400 mg PO twice a day for 14 days
PLUS
Metronidazole 500 mg PO twice a day for 14 days
The outpatient should be reevaluated in 48 to 72 hours after starting therapy. If no improvement is noted, hospitalization is indicated. Cervical cultures should be performed 2 weeks after therapy to verify cure.

PEDIATRIC CONSIDERATIONS

Young women aged 13 to 19 years have the highest rate of PID. The younger the sexually active teenager, the greater the risk of developing PID.

OBSTETRIC CONSIDERATIONS

Chlamydia trachomatis *Infection*

Chlamydial infection in the obstetric patient is associated with grave risk to the mother and fetus. *Chlamydia* can cause preterm delivery, low birth weight, chorioamnionitis, stillbirth, and postpartum endometritis; it also causes neonatal conjunctivitis and pneumonia in the infant. This infection also has been implicated in causing habitual spontaneous abortions. Treatment should consist of erythromycin base 500 mg PO four times a day for 7 days or amoxycillin 500 mg three times a day for 7 days.

Neisseria gonorrhoeae *Infection*

Women with gonococcal cervicitis are at increased risk for disseminated gonoccoccal infection during pregnancy. Gonococcal infection has been associated with premature labor. Infants born to mothers with gonorrhea may develop gonococcal conjunctivitis. The infant may also develop pharyngeal, respiratory, or rectal infections or sepsis during the neonatal period. Treatment of gonorrheal cervicitis in the pregnant patient consists of administration of erythromycin base, 500 mg PO four times a day for 7 days, or amoxycillin 50 mg PO three times a day for 7 days, or erythromycin ethylsuccinate 800 mg PO four times a day for 7 days, or azithromycin 1 g orally in a single dose.

GERIATRIC CONSIDERATIONS

No specific considerations. PID generally occurs in the young to middle-aged female.

PREVENTIVE CONSIDERATIONS

Risk factors include multiple sexual partners, sexually transmitted diseases, and HIV infection. Measures to reduce risk such as barrier contraception should be used.

PEARLS FOR THE PA

The "gold standard" for the diagnosis of PID is laparoscopy.

The most common organisms implicated with PID are Neisseria gonorrhoeae *and* Chlamydia trachomatis.

Uterine Prolapse

Nina Multak, MPAS, PA-C

DEFINITION

Prolapse of the uterus into the vagina, with possible protrusion from the vagina.

HISTORY

Symptoms. Patient complains of a pelvic heaviness. Additional complaints may include low back pain, a mass protruding from the vagina, and a sensation that something is "falling out" of the vagina.

General. Multiparous Caucasian women most commonly develop uterine prolapse.

Age. Uterine prolapse occurs most commonly in postmenopausal women.

Onset. Variable onset.

Duration. Duration dependent on timing of diagnosis and surgical intervention.

Intensity. Usually mild.

Aggravating Factors. Prolonged standing, increased intra-abdominal pressure.

Alleviating Factors. Lying down.

Associated Factors. Multiparity, menopause.

PHYSICAL EXAMINATION

General. The patient appears well.

Gastrointestinal. Abdomen should be soft and nontender.

Gynecologic. Vaginal examination can be performed with the patient in a recumbent or a standing position. The extent of prolapse identified on physical examination parallels the degree of separation of the supporting structures. A *first degree prolapse* exists when the uterus is located in the lower part of the vagina. When the uterus protrudes beyond the introitus, a *second degree prolapse* exists. A *third degree prolapse* occurs when the entire uterus is outside the introitus.

PATHOPHYSIOLOGY

The pelvic musculature is weakened from stretching and trauma during vaginal delivery. Postmenopausal atrophy of vaginal tissues is a contributing factor. Chronic increased intra-abdominal pressure can increase the stress on the muscle providing pelvic support.

DIAGNOSTIC STUDIES

Laboratory.   Not applicable.
Radiology.   Pelvic ultrasound examination is indicated if a mass is suspected.

DIFFERENTIAL DIAGNOSIS

Neoplastic
Cervical or *uterine tumor* (rare) can be differentiated with pelvic ultrasound examination or CT scan.

Congenital
Congenital abnormalities of the pelvic musculature can cause uterine prolapse.

Acquired
With *cystocele*, a protrusion of the bladder from its normal position into the vagina, the usual symptoms include a sensation of fullness or pressure. On examination, a soft reducible mass is present in the anterior vagina.

With *rectocele*, a protrusion of the rectum into the vagina due to loss of support from the rectovaginal septum and posterior vaginal wall, symptoms include sensation of incomplete emptying of rectum with bowel movement, bearing-down sensation, vaginal heaviness, and constipation.

Enterocele, a herniation of the pouch of Douglas, usually contains small bowel. Herniation into the vagina occurs. Symptoms are minimal and usually include sensation of internal weakness or heaviness.

Traumatic.   Not applicable.
Infectious.   Not applicable.
Metabolic.   Not applicable.
Vascular.   Not applicable.

TREATMENT

Mild, asymptomatic prolapse does not require treatment. Kegel exercises to help strengthen the pelvic musculature can help in mild first degree prolapse. Pessaries, prosthetic devices inserted into the vagina, can support the uterus and provide symptomatic relief. Surgery is the most definitive treament. The most common surgical repair is vaginal hysterectomy with restoration of vaginal support using the cardinal and uterosacral ligaments.

PEDIATRIC CONSIDERATIONS

Not applicable.

OBSTETRIC CONSIDERATIONS

The uterus should be supported with a pessary to prevent entrapment within the vagina.

GERIATRIC CONSIDERATIONS

Uterine prolapse is primarily a disorder of multiparous geriatric women.

PREVENTIVE CONSIDERATIONS

Kegel exercises to help strengthen the pelvic musculature can help prevent prolapse and may help in mild first degree prolapse.

PEARLS FOR THE PA

Uterine prolapse occurs in mutiparous older women as a result of weakening of the pelvic musculature from stretching and trauma during delivery of a child.

Definitive treatment is surgical.

VAGINITIS

Nina Multak, MPAS, PA-C

DEFINITION

An inflammation of the vagina. Usually caused by *Candida albicans*, *Trichomonas vaginalis*, *Candida glabrata*, *Gardnerella vaginalis*, *Mobiluncus* species, *Mycoplasma hominis*, and atrophic factors.

HISTORY

Symptoms

Candidal Infection
Thick white vaginal discharge, moderate to severe pruritus, vulvar burning pain, vulvar dysuria due to urine contact with inflamed mucosa and labia; odor not typical with discharge.

Bacterial Vaginosis
Malodorous vaginal discharge, often described as "fishy"; odor frequently more obvious following intercourse.

Trichomoniasis
Increased vaginal discharge (frothy), staining of underwear, occasional odor present with discharge, occasional vulvar pruritus.

Atrophic Vaginitis
Intense itching of vagina and vulva.

General. Vulvovaginitis is one of the most common reasons for women to seek health care.
Age. All ages susceptible; most frequently identified in sexually active women.
Onset. Variable; symptoms can manifest from a few days to 4 weeks following contact with an infected sex partner.
Duration. Generally resolves with 7 days following onset of treatment.
Intensity. Variable.
Aggravating Factors. Diabetes, antibiotic therapy, human immunodeficiency virus (HIV) infection, pregnancy, oral contraceptives.
Alleviating Factors. None.
Associated Factors. Multiple sexual partners.

PHYSICAL EXAMINATION

General. The patient is moderately comfortable.
Gastrointestinal. Abdomen should be soft and nontender.

Gynecologic

Vulvovaginal Candidiasis
Vulvar erythema with occasional edma or fissures; discharge is usually scant, white, curd-like, adherent to vaginal mucosa.

Bacterial Vaginosis
Scant to moderate discharge, usually white, homogeneous; appears to be coating vaginal walls or labia. No erythema.

Trichomoniasis
Vast amount of homogeneous, purulent discharge usually present; occasional petechiae on the cervix; bubbles may be present in vaginal secretions.

Atrophic Vaginitis
Friable mucosa; symmetrically reddened, smooth and shiny appearance to mucosa.

PATHOPHYSIOLOGY

A transudate is normally present in the vagina consisting of vaginal epithelial cells, cervical mucus, and secretions from Bartholin's and Skene's glands. Infectious organisms cause white blood cell (WBC) infiltration. *Candida* infection is identified by the presence of hyphae and spores. *Trichomonas* infection is identified by motile trichomonads. Bacterial vaginosis alters the normal vaginal flora. Atrophic changes are reflected by reduced estrogen levels.

DIAGNOSTIC STUDIES

Laboratory
Wet Preparations. In bacterial vaginosis, WBCs, clue cells (epithelial cells stippled with bacteria), and a fishy odor will be apparent when potassium hydroxide (KOH) is applied. Motile trichomonads are identified in trichomoniasis. Hyphae and spores are evident in candidiasis.
Culture. Occasionally used in difficult cases.

Radiology
Not applicable.

DIFFERENTIAL DIAGNOSIS

Traumatic
Foreign body such as a retained tampon may be seen on pelvic examination.

Infectious
Herpes simplex virus infection causes exudate, presence of vesicular or ulcerative lesions.

Metabolic
Increased mucus production may be due to *hormonal stimulation*.

Neoplastic
Cancer may appear in a similar fashion, so it is imperative to biopsy any lesions.

Acquired
Chemical reaction to products such as douche or spermicide may occur.

Vascular. Not applicable.
Congenital. Not applicable.

TREATMENT

Candidal Infection
For acute infection:
   Fluconazole 150-200 mg PO (single dose)
   An imidazole cream or suppository used intravaginally for 3 to 7 days:
      butoconazole, clotrimazole, tioconazole, econazole, miconazole,
      terconazole
For prevention of recurrent infection:
   Fluconazole 100 mg PO once weekly
   Clotrimazole 500 mg intravaginally once weekly

Bacterial Vaginosis
   Metronidazole 500 mg PO twice a day for 7 days OR
   Metronidazole 2 g PO, single dose
   Metronidazole 0.75% gel, 5 g intravaginally daily or twice daily for 5
      days OR
   Clindamyacin in 2% cream, 5 g intravaginally daily for 7 days

Trichomoniasis
   Metronidazole 2 g PO, single dose, for patient and sexual partner
If single-dose treatment fails:
   Metronidazole 500 mg PO twice daily for 7 days

Atrophic Vaginitis
   Estrogen cream
   Hormone replacement therapy if appropriate

PEDIATRIC CONSIDERATIONS

Vaginitis
A physiologic milky-white vaginal discharge associated with maternal hormone
withdrawal is common in the female newborn. The leukorrhea gradually
resolves within the first 2 to 3 weeks. The discharge may appear blood-tinged.

The prepubertal child is susceptible to vulvovaginitis. Vulvar irritation
and inflammation may be the result of poor hygiene (contamination of the
vagina with bowel flora), chronic irritation from masturbation, and contact
with play equipment and sand from sand boxes. Pinworm infestation causing perianal pruritus may lead to perineal irritation and vulvitis. Pinworms
may migrate to the vagina and cause a discharge. A vaginal discharge may
also result from a foreign body.

Group A streptococci are a common cause of vaginitis in prepubertal
girls. On physical examination, erythema, serous discharge, and irritation of
the vulvar area may be seen. Discomfort in walking and dysuria are associated complaints.

Candida albicans may frequently cause vaginitis in young infants or in children following antibiotic therapy. Sexual abuse is highly likely if infection due to *Neisseria gonorrhoeae, Chlamydia trachomatis,* herpes simplex virus, or human papillomavirus is diagnosed in a child.

OBSTETRIC CONSIDERATIONS

Bacterial Vaginosis
Bacterial vaginosis may be a causative factor in preterm labor, premature rupture of membranes, and chorioamnionitis. It has been associated with postpartum endometritis. Bacterial vaginosis is often diagnosed concurrently with other sexually transmitted infections that can increase the possibility of adverse effects on a pregnancy. Oral metronidazole, the usual treatment in a nonpregnant patient, is contraindicated during the first trimester of pregnancy. Clindamycin can be safely used in pregnancy when indicated.

Trichomonas Vaginalis
Infection with *T. vaginalis* may be associated with premature delivery, low birth weight, and postpartum endometritis. Metronidazole should be avoided during the first trimester of pregnancy. Infection also has been shown to worsen with pregnancy.

Candida Vaginitis
Candidiasis is more prevalent in pregnant women. This is the most commonly seen infection of the perineum and the vagina. Pregnancy increases the glycogen content of the vaginal epithelium and promotes a greater degree of acidity. This can lead to an overgrowth of yeast. Terconazole is safe to use during pregnancy.

GERIATRIC CONSIDERATIONS

Most frequently occurs in sexually active women and can affect women of any age.

PREVENTIVE CONSIDERATIONS

Barrier contraception is recommended to help prevent partner-to-partner infection. Associated with multiple sexual partners.

PEARLS FOR THE PA

Vulvovaginitis is one of the most common reasons for women to seek health care.

May be caused by bacterial agents, Trichomonas, *or atrophic factors.*

Further Reading

Beckmann C, Ling F, Herbert W, et al: Obstetrics and Gynecology, 3rd ed. Baltimore, Williams & Wilkins, 1998.

Bickley LS, Szilagyi PG: Bates' Guide to Physical Examination and History Taking, 8th ed. Philadelphia, Lippincott Williams & Wilkins, 2002.

Bland K, Copeland E: The Breast: Comprehensive Management of Benign and Malignant Diseases, vol 1, 2nd ed. Philadelphia, WB Saunders, 1998.

Chan, PD, Winkle CR: Gynecology and Obstetrics, 2002 Edition. Current Clinical Strategies Publishing, 2002.

Hacker NF: Essentials of Obstetrics and Gynecology, 2nd ed. Philadelphia, WB Saunders, 1998.

Handsfield H: Color Atlas and Synopsis of Sexually Transmitted Diseases, 2nd ed. New York, McGraw-Hill, 2001.

Pernoll ML: Benson and Pernoll's Handbook of Obstetrics and Gynecology, 10th ed. New York, McGraw-Hill, 2001.

Speroff L, Glass RH, Kase NG: Clinical Gynecologic Endocrinology and Infertility, 6th ed. Baltimore, Williams & Wilkins, 1999.

Stenchever MA, Droegenmueller W, Herbst AL, Mishell DR: Comprehensive Gynecology, 4th ed. St. Louis, Mosby, 2001.

Stovall TG, Ling FW: Gynecology for the Primary Care Physician. Philadelphia, Current Medicine, 1999.

Youngkin, E, Davis, M: Women's Health: A Primary Care Clinical Guide, 2nd ed. Stamford, CT, Appleton & Lange, 1998.

HEMATOLOGY

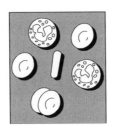

7

Anemia

Charles W. Reed, MEd, MPAS, PA-C

DEFINITION

A reduction in the oxygen-carrying capacity of the blood, frequently associated with a decrease in red blood cell (RBC) mass. Clinically, anemia usually is defined by a hemoglobin less than 14 g/dL in males and less than 12 g/dL in females.

HISTORY

Symptoms. Fatigue, weakness, lightheadedness, dyspnea, palpitations, sore tongue, ataxia, dysesthesias, fever, anorexia, weight loss. Pallor may be noted by the patient or family. Mild jaundice may occur with hemolytic anemias. Unusual bleeding such as hematemesis, hematochezia, melena, hemoptysis, epistaxis, hematuria, or excessive bleeding with menstruation.

General. Most patients with anemia are relatively asymptomatic. The symptoms of anemia tend to be nonspecific and usually occur late or only when the anemia is severe. Symptoms also are more likely to occur with rapidly developing anemias. Except in patients with preexisting respiratory or cardiac disease, slow-developing anemias tend to be well tolerated until the hemoglobin approaches approximately 8 g/dL. More specific symptoms may relate to the underlying cause or specific type of anemia. With anemia in blacks, Asians, and persons of Mediterranean descent, consider hemoglobinopathy, G6PD deficiency, and thalassemias.

Age. Children or adults.

Onset. Most anemias have an insidious onset. Anemia associated with hemorrhage or hemolysis may occur acutely.

Duration. Variable. Depends on underlying cause.

Aggravating Factors. See Pathophysiology section.

Alleviating Factors. Appropriate treatment.

Associated Factors. History of previous anemias or blood transfusion. Several pregnancies in rapid succession. Peptic ulcer disease or inflammatory bowel disease. Alcohol use. Drug and medication history, especially use of aspirin or nonsteroidal anti-inflammatory drugs (NSAIDs). Previous gastrointestinal surgery. Chronic renal, infectious, inflammatory, or endocrine disease. Diet deficient in protein, iron, vitamin B_{12}, or folate. Pica—compulsive eating of clay, earth, ice, or other nonfood substances. Positive family history for anemia or need for frequent blood transfusions.

PHYSICAL EXAMINATION

General. Postural hypotension if there has been rapid blood loss. Peripheral lymphadenopathy.

Cardiovascular.   Tachycardia, systolic "flow" murmur. Signs of heart failure may occur if the cardiovascular system can no longer compensate for anemia.

Gastrointestinal.   Ascites or abdominal mass. Splenomegaly or hepatomegaly. Rectal mass. Hemorrhoids. Prostate enlargement and induration. Frank or occult blood in stool.

Genitourinary.   Uterine bleeding or cervical lesion.

Head, Eyes, Ears, Nose, Throat.   Icterus. Glossitis or angular stomatitis (iron deficiency or megaloblastic anemias). Pallor of conjunctivae or oral mucosa. Retinal hemorrhages may be seen in severe anemias.

Neurologic.   Distal muscle weakness, ataxia, decreased proprioception, or mental status changes may be noted with pernicious anemia.

Pulmonary.   Increased respiratory rate. Signs of pulmonary edema may occur if respiratory system can no longer compensate for anemia.

Skin.   Pallor, jaundice, koilonychia (spoon-like concavity in nails occasionally seen with iron deficiency), petechiae, purpura, spider angiomata. Pallor of palmar skin creases usually indicates severe anemia.

PATHOPHYSIOLOGY

Anemia results from one or more of the following mechanisms:
- Decreased RBC production by the bone marrow (inadequate erythropoiesis)
- Loss of RBCs from the circulation (hemorrhage)
- Shortened RBC lifespan within the circulation (hemolysis)

Common causes of inadequate erythropoiesis are lack of some nutrient essential for RBC production or hemoglobin synthesis (iron, vitamin B_{12}, folate, protein); injury to bone marrow (immune, toxic, radiation); marrow replacement by neoplasm or fibrosis; chronic inflammatory collagen disease (systemic lupus erythematosus [SLE], rheumatoid arthritis); and endocrine deficiency (chronic renal failure, hypothyroidism).

Hemorrhage may be occult, and the bleeding frequently originates from the gastrointestinal or genitourinary tract.

Hemolysis can result from an intrinsic RBC defect or an extracorpuscular injury to the RBCs. Intrinsic hemolytic anemias include conditions associated with abnormal hemoglobin (sickle cell anemia), defective globin synthesis (thalassemia), defective heme synthesis (porphyria), defective RBC membrane (hereditary spherocytosis), defective or deficient enzymes necessary for glucose metabolism (glucose-6-phosphate dehydrogenase [G6PD], pyruvate kinase), and defective RBC stem cell (paroxysmal nocturnal hemoglobinuria). Extrinsic causes of hemolysis include autoimmune or connective tissue diseases (SLE), isoimmunization (transfusion reaction, hemolytic disease of newborn), splenomegaly, drug reaction, disseminated intravascular coagulation (DIC), and infection (malaria, clostridial infection, gram-negative sepsis).

DIAGNOSTIC STUDIES

Laboratory

Complete Blood Count. With RBC indices: mean corpuscular volume (MCV), mean corpuscular hemoglobin (MCH), MCH concentration (MCHC), and reticulocyte count. The MCV is useful in identifying the underlying cause of the anemia; specifics on this aspect of diagnosis are given at the end of this section.

Wright-Stained Smear of Blood. Used to evaluate RBC morphology. Abnormal RBC morphology may be seen with some hemolytic anemias. The combination of nucleated RBCs and immature white blood cells (WBCs) is suggestive of bone marrow infiltration by malignancy. Hypersegmented neutrophils may be seen with vitamin B_{12} and folate deficiency.

Reticulocyte Count. If MCV is normal, used to rule out hemolysis versus bone marrow failure, anemia, or chronic disease.

Serum Ferritin, Serum Iron, and Total Iron-Binding Capacity (TIBC). If anemia is microcytic (MCV of less than 80 fL).

Serum Vitamin B_{12} and Folate Levels. If anemia is macrocytic (MCV of greater than 100 fL).

Erythrocyte Sedimentation Rate (ESR), Rheumatoid Factor, and Antinuclear Antibody (ANA). If anemia of chronic disease is suspected.

Thyroid Function Tests. If hypothyroidism is suspected.

Total and Direct Serum Bilirubin, Lactate Dehydrogenase (LDH), Serum Haptoglobin, Sickle Cell Preparation, G6PD Screen, Hemoglobin Electrophoresis, and Coombs Test. May be useful in the diagnosis and differentiation of hemolytic anemias.

Chemistry Profile. Used to assess renal and hepatic function if indicated.

Radiology

Chest Film, Bone Scans, Barium Enema, CT Scans of Chest, Abdomen, and Pelvis. If malignancy is suspected as a cause for anemia.

Other

Bone Marrow Aspiration and Biopsy. May be indicated to diagnose aplastic anemia, leukemia, myelodysplasia, sideroblastic anemia, or neoplastic infiltration of bone marrow. Useful when there is difficulty diagnosing iron deficiency anemias, anemia of chronic disease, or the macrocytic anemias.

Schilling Test. May help differentiate among the various causes of vitamin B_{12} deficiency.

Sigmoidoscopy. May be indicated to evaluate possible colonic malignancy in the setting of iron deficiency anemia in a middle-aged adult.

Diagnosing the Cause of the Anemia

The usual approach to differentiating among the various causes of anemia is to first classify the patient by MCV.

Microcytic Anemias: MCV Less than 80 fL

Iron Deficiency Anemia. Diagnosed by decreased ferritin, decreased serum iron, increased TIBC. Rule out chronic bleeding (especially from occult gastrointestinal or genitourinary malignancy). Dietary iron deficiency is rare in the United States; however, increased fetal demands for iron make iron deficiency common in pregnancy. Iron deficiency may also occur after subtotal gastric resection.

Thalassemic Traits. Diagnosed by abnormal hemoglobin electrophoresis (increased hemoglobin A_2, increased hemoglobin F, presence of hemoglobin H). Iron studies normal. May have family history of anemia. Thalassemias most common among persons of Asian ancestry, blacks, and people of Mediterranean descent.

Anemia of Chronic Disease. Evidence of renal failure, malignancy, chronic infection, or inflammatory collagen diseases. ESR may be elevated. Serum iron and TIBC often decreased. Serum ferritin usually normal or increased.

Lead Poisoning. Usually in children. History of environmental lead exposure (e.g., old paint). RBCs may show basophilic stippling on smear. Elevated serum lead levels are diagnostic.

Macrocytic Anemias: MCV Greater than 100 fL

Vitamin B_{12} deficiency. Consider pernicious anemia (presence of circulating antibodies to intrinsic factor; Schilling test demonstrates reduced B_{12} absorption corrected with oral intrinsic factor). Other causes include ileal surgery or total gastrectomy, malabsorption, blind loop syndrome, infestation with *Diphyllobothrium latum* (tapeworm). Dietary B_{12} deficiency is rare in the United States. Neurologic signs and symptoms may occur with B_{12} deficiency.

Folate deficiency. Consider nutritional deficiency (pregnancy, elderly, alcoholism) or malabsorption (celiac and tropical sprue, partial gastrectomy, Crohn's disease). Unlike B_{12} deficiency, folate deficiency is not associated with neurologic manifestations.

Normal vitamin B_{12} and folate. Consider alcoholism, chronic liver disease, or hypothyroidism. Refer for bone marrow aspiration and biopsy to rule out myelodysplastic and preleukemic syndromes.

Normal MCV with Increased Reticulocytes

Hemolytic Anemias. Reticulocytosis is an important hallmark of hemolysis but may be present in any anemic state with appropriate erythropoiesis. Increased unconjugated (indirect) serum bilirubin, increased LDH, and decreased haptoglobin levels are also seen with hemolysis. Examination of Wright-stained blood smear may reveal abnormal RBC morphology (e.g., target cells, sickle cells, spherocytes, elliptocytes, fragmented RBCs). Intravascular hemolysis may be associated with hemoglobinuria. A positive direct Coombs test is useful for distinguishing immune from nonimmune causes of hemolysis. A clinically significant cold agglutinin titer may indicate malignancy (rare).

Normal MCV with Decreased Reticulocytes

Anemia of Chronic Disease. Evidence of renal failure, malignancy, chronic infection, or inflammatory disease. ESR may be elevated. Serum iron and TIBC often decreased. Serum ferritin usually is normal or increased.

Aplastic Anemia. Anemia is accompanied by decreased WBC and platelet counts. May have a history of drug or radiation exposure. Bone marrow studies are required to confirm the diagnosis.

Leukemia, Neoplastic Infiltration of Bone Marrow, Myelodysplasia. Bone marrow studies are required to confirm the diagnosis.

DIFFERENTIAL DIAGNOSIS

Because anemia is a laboratory diagnosis, the underlying cause must be determined. The concept of differential diagnosis does not apply.

TREATMENT

Iron Deficiency. Identify and eliminate underlying cause (especially gastrointestinal or genitourinary bleeding or occult malignancy). Iron replacement therapy with plain ferrous salts. The optimal dosage is approximately 65 mg of elemental iron (equivalent to 325 mg of ferrous sulfate) three times a day.

Pernicious Anemia. Lifetime monthly intramuscular injections of 1000 mg of vitamin B_{12}. If there are neurologic manifestations, 1000 mg is administered intramuscularly every 2 weeks for the first 6 months.

Folate Deficiency. Correct underlying cause if possible. Oral folic acid 1 mg/day is recommended. Patients with hemolytic anemias, hemoglobinopathies, symptomatic thalassemia, anemia of chronic disease, bone marrow failure, or suspected malignancy should be referred to a hematologist for further workup and management.

PEDIATRIC CONSIDERATIONS

With anemia in children, consider hemoglobinopathy or aplastic anemia.

OBSTETRIC CONSIDERATIONS

Seventy-five percent of all cases of anemia noted during pregnancy are due to iron deficiency. The consequences of uncompensated anemia include postpartum hemorrhage, infection, and failure of the patient to recuperate rapidly from childbirth. Anemia has also been linked to an increased risk of spontaneous births during the second trimester, prematurity, low birth weight of the infant, fetal distress, and death.

The average normal hemoglobin is 11.5 to 12.5 g/dL. The hemoglobin values uniformly will decrease in early pregnancy owing to expansion of the plasma volume.

GERIATRIC CONSIDERATIONS

The geriatric patient with anemia, particularly acute or progressive, should be thoroughly evaluated for common geriatric causes such as gastrointestinal/genitourinary bleeding from carcinoma, anemia of chronic disease, myelodysplastic syndrome, leukemia, or NSAID overuse secondary to arthritis and its treatment. Malabsorption may be the cause of pernicious anemia in the elderly.

PREVENTIVE CONSIDERATIONS

A diet containing adequate amounts of iron, B vitamins, and folate is important, particularly in teens. An adequate diet is always preferable, but for those who cannot or will not engage in healthy dietary practices, a daily multivitamin supplement will usually meet requirements for hematopoiesis.

Avoidance of alcohol abuse is also an important consideration.

PEARLS FOR THE PA

Iron deficiency, thalassemia, and vitamin B_{12} and folate deficiencies may produce changes in MCV before the hemoglobin and hematocrit decrease.

Although reticulocytosis is most commonly associated with hemolysis, it can also occur after acute hemorrhage and in response to therapy for iron, vitamin B_{12}, or folate deficiency.

Common medications associated with hemolysis, megaloblastic anemia, or bone marrow depression are as follows: hemolysis: *penicillin, cephalosporins, L-dopa, sulfonamides, phenothiazines, aldomet, quinidine, antimalarials, aspirin;* megaloblastic anemia: *anticonvulsants, antineoplastics, trimethoprim-sulfamethoxazole;* bone marrow depression: *chloramphenicol, phenylbutazone, phenytoin, trimethadione.*

Bleeding Disorders

Charles W. Reed, MEd, MPAS, PA-C

DEFINITION

Abnormal bleeding or impaired coagulation caused by a breakdown in normal hemostatic mechanisms.

HISTORY

Symptoms. Localize bleeding: multiple versus single sites, joints, deep muscle, superficial cut, skin or mucous membrane, epistaxis, gingivae, urine, gastrointestinal tract, menstrual. Identify precipitating cause (spontaneous or after trauma). Determine temporal relationship between trauma and bleeding (immediate or delayed). Ascertain whether or not bleeding is easily controlled with direct pressure.

General. Previous history of bruising or bleeding (recent onset of symptoms suggests acquired disorder versus congenital problem). Excessive bleeding following dental extraction, surgery, or obstetric delivery. The need for blood transfusions due to past bleeding.

Types of bleeding disorders include:

- Idiopathic thrombocytic purpura (ITP)

  Predominantly a disease of childhood that frequently begins abruptly 2 to 21 days after a viral infection. Spontaneous recovery usually occurs after 1 to 2 months. Chronic ITP is primarily a disease of adults and rarely resolves spontaneously. Both acute and chronic forms of ITP are mediated by antiplatelet autoantibodies. Clinically, ITP is manifested by petechiae, epistaxis, and bleeding from gums and gastrointestinal and urinary tracts. The spleen is enlarged in only about 10% of cases. Decreased platelet counts and prolongation of the bleeding time are typical laboratory features. Medication history, examination of platelets on a Wright-stained blood smear, and bone marrow aspiration and biopsy are important for ruling out other causes of thrombocytopenia.

- Hemophilia A

  A hereditary, X-linked recessive bleeding disorder caused by deficient or defective factor VIII. Its estimated incidence is about 1 in every 10,000 male births. Clinically, hemophilia A is classically characterized by deep hematomas and hemarthrosis either occurring spontaneously or after trauma. Intracranial hemorrhage and severe bleeding after surgery may also occur. Mildly affected hemophiliacs may have infrequent bleeding episodes. Laboratory features of the disease include a prolonged PTT, normal PT, and normal bleeding time. Diagnosis is confirmed by demonstrating decreased factor VIII levels.

- Hemophilia B
  Sex-linked bleeding disorder caused by deficiency of factor IX. Less common than hemophilia A. Clinical and laboratory features are similar to those of hemophilia A. Diagnosis is confirmed by demonstrating decreased factor IX levels.
- Von Willebrand disease (vWD)
  An inherited bleeding disorder occurring in both genders. Characterized by variable degrees of dysfunction in Von Willebrand factor and, occasionally, factor VIII abnormalities. Several subtypes of the disease exist, and there is a great deal of variability in bleeding tendency. Epistaxis, menorrhagia, gingival bleeding, and easy bruising are the most common symptoms. Abnormal bleeding after dental extraction, trauma, and surgery is also common. Gastrointestinal bleeding is rare. Typical laboratory features include prolonged bleeding time with a normal platelet count. The PTT may occasionally be prolonged. Confirmation of diagnosis may require specialized hemostatic testing.
- Acute disseminated intravascular coagulation
  An acquired hemostatic disorder that complicates a number of conditions including obstetric emergencies (abruptio placentae, septic abortion, toxemia, amniotic fluid embolism), sepsis, neoplastic disease, trauma, burns, hemolysis, and snake bites. Shock and widespread, fulminant bleeding (intracerebral, skin, mucous membrane, gastrointestinal, or renal) are common clinical features of acute DIC. Organ damage by microthrombi is also part of the clinical picture. Common thrombotic manifestations include skin necrosis, central nervous system dysfunction (delirium, coma), and renal failure. The laboratory abnormalities reflect the multiple hemostatic defects that are associated with this condition. Typically, there is thrombocytopenia and prolongation of the PT, PTT, and thrombin time. Fibrin degradation products will be present in the serum.

Age. Infancy, childhood, or adulthood.

Onset. Usually acute.

Duration. Variable. Depends on specific diagnosis.

Intensity. Variable. Wide spectrum of clinical expression.

Aggravating Factors. Trauma or surgical procedures.

Alleviating Factors. Appropriate treatment.

Associated Factors. Medications (especially aspirin, NSAIDS, warfarin and heparin, and antineoplastic agents). Alcoholism, liver disease, uremia, malignancy, systemic lupus erythematosus (SLE). Family history of bleeding problems suggests congenital disorder. However, a negative family history does not rule out a congenital hemostatic defect. Recessive diseases may not produce disease in every generation of a family.

PHYSICAL EXAMINATION

Extremities. Joint swelling (especially involving knees, ankles, and elbows) may represent hemarthrosis.

Gastrointestinal. Hepatomegaly, splenomegaly, or ascites may suggest liver disease, lymphoma, or other malignancy.

Lymphatics. Lymphadenopathy may suggest lymphoma or other malignancy.

Neurologic. Focal neurologic deficits and fever may indicate disseminated intravascular coagulation (DIC) or an intracranial bleed.

Skin. Petechiae, ecchymoses (note number and size), telangiectasia, jaundice, spider angiomata.

DIAGNOSTIC STUDIES

Laboratory

Bleeding Time. Screening test for disorders of primary hemostasis and vWD. When interpreting the bleeding time, it is important to obtain a medication history to ascertain use of aspirin or other drugs that affect platelet function.

Platelet Count. Screening test for quantitative platelet disorders (thrombocytopenia, thrombocytosis). Spontaneous bleeding and bleeding after surgery is unlikely to occur until the platelet count drops below 50,000/mm^3.

Prothrombin Time (PT). Screens for deficiencies in the concentration or function of fibrinogen, prothrombin, and coagulation factors V, VII, and X. Also used to monitor oral anticoagulant (coumadin) therapy.

Partial Thromboplastin Time (PTT). Screens for deficiencies in the concentration or function of coagulation factors V, VIII, IX, X, XI, and XII, and prothrombin. Also used to monitor heparin therapy and to screen for pathologic coagulation inhibitors. The PTT also may be prolonged if fibrinogen levels are greatly decreased or if high concentrations of fibrin degradation products are present (e.g., with DIC).

Thrombin Time. Screens for marked reduction in concentration of plasma fibrinogen. Also prolonged in the presence of fibrin degradation products.

Fibrin Degradation Products. The presence of fibrin degradation products in serum is an indicator of DIC.

Special Studies. Other studies, usually available only in specialized referral laboratories, include platelet function studies and assays for specific coagulation factors, von Willebrand factor, and the various components of the fibrinolytic system.

Radiology. Not applicable.
Other. Not applicable.

PATHOPHYSIOLOGY

Problems with abnormal bleeding can be traced to defects in either or both of two basic mechanisms:

- Primary hemostasis—the formation of a hemostatic plug by means of the adherence and aggregation of platelets to injured vascular endothelium or subendothelial collagen
- Secondary hemostasis—the formation of an adequate fibrin clot from fibrinogen and plasma coagulation factors (see Table 7-1)

Primary Hemostasis

Common disorders of primary hemostasis include thrombocytopenia resulting from immune-mediated destruction of platelets (e.g., idiopathic thrombocytopenic purpura [ITP]); suppression of bone marrow platelet production by drugs, infection, or neoplastic infiltration; and platelet sequestration by an enlarged spleen. Defective platelet function without a reduction in platelet numbers is another common cause of primary hemostatic problems (e.g., with aspirin or NSAID use, uremia). Congenital platelet disorders and vessel wall abnormalities are rare causes of primary hemostatic defects.

Secondary Hemostasis

Common disorders of secondary hemostasis include congenital deficiencies in plasma coagulation factors (hemophilia A and B) and acquired coagulation factor disorders (vitamin K deficiency, anticoagulation therapy, liver disease, nephrotic syndrome). Congenital afibrinogenemia, disorders of fibrinolysis, and the development of pathologic coagulation inhibitors are rare causes of coagulation defects.

Multiple Hemostatic Defects

Von Willebrand disease involves abnormalities in both platelet function and fibrin formation. Acute DIC is a syndrome caused by the abnormal activation of the coagulation and fibrinolytic systems and is associated with the consumption of both platelets and plasma coagulation factors.

DIFFERENTIAL DIAGNOSIS

The strict concept of differential diagnosis does not apply. It is instead imperative to determine the cause of the bleeding disorder.

TREATMENT

Idiopathic Thrombocytopenic Purpura. Mild acute ITP may not require any treatment other than protecting the patient from trauma and avoiding aspirin. More severe thrombocytopenia is managed initially with drug therapy to include intravenous immunoglobulin (IVIG), $Rh_0(D)$ immune globulin (i.e., intravenous anti-D antibodies), and oral steroids. $Rh_0(D)$ immune globulin has gained more popularity as studies continue to show improvement in many cases of ITP refractory to other therapies. Splenectomy is generally reserved for patients in whom drug therapies have proved ineffective.

Table 7–1. Clinical Differentiation of Bleeding Disorders

History	Disorders of Primary Hemostasis	Disorders of Secondary Hemostasis
Sex distribution	Female > male	Male > female
Family history of bleeding problems	Rarely positive	Usually positive
Time relationship between trauma and bleeding	Immediate	Delayed (2-3 days)
Prolonged bleeding from a superficial cut	Yes	No
Control of bleeding by local pressure	Effective	Not effective
Petechiae	Very common	Not common
Ecchymosis	Small, multiple	Large, solitary
Hemarthrosis	No	Yes
Screening test	Prolonged bleeding time	Prolonged PT and /or PTT

PT, prothrombin time; PTT, partial thromboplastin time.

Failure of one treatment modality does not necessarily predict the failure of any other treatment. Platelet transfusions are not routinely used; however, they may provide transient benefit when there is life-threatening hemorrhage. Overuse of platelet transfusions may result in the development of autoantibodies, negating their effectiveness during future episodes of serious bleeding.

Hemophilia A.　Therapy depends on the degree of factor VIII deficiency and the type of hemorrhage. Factor VIII concentrate or cryoprecipitate are effective in controlling hemorrhage. Mild hemophilia may be treated with desmopressin (desamino-D-arginine vasopressin [DDAVP]) (Stimate) to release factor VIII from endothelial cell stores.

Hemophilia B.　Factor IX concentrate (also called prothrombin complex concentrate) and fresh frozen plasma can correct the hemostatic defects in hemophilia B. A purified factor IX concentrate is now available.

Von Willebrand Disease

Mild vWD may be treated with DDAVP. Von Willebrand factor also is present in cryoprecipitate and fresh frozen plasma.

Disseminated Intravascular Coagulation

Life support measures such as oxygenation and fluid therapy to maintain adequate cardiac output and blood pressure. Treat underlying disorder. Specific treatment of DIC is controversial, and no standard therapy is recommended. However, some combination of an antithrombotic agent (heparin) and transfusion of platelets and coagulation factors is often used.

PEDIATRIC CONSIDERATIONS

In the neonate, post-circumcision or umbilical stump bleeding is an important clue to congenital coagulation factor deficiency. Umbilical stump bleeding is classically associated with factor XIII deficiency. Approximately half of the children born to mothers with chronic ITP will be thrombocytopenic at birth.

OBSTETRIC CONSIDERATIONS

In immune ITP, the cause is an antibody that is formed against platelets. These antibodies are capable of crossing the placenta, affecting the fetus. Corticosteroid therapy is indicated in pregnant patients with ITP.

In contrast, the disease of thrombotic thrombocytic purpura (TTP) does not involve the fetus. This disease has been associated with pregnancy-induced hypertension.

Approximately one-third of patients with vWD will have excessive bleeding associated with abortion or during the puerperium. Patients with type III disease may have fetal involvement with the bleeding diathesis.

GERIATRIC CONSIDERATIONS

Potential causes of acute bleeding in the geriatric patient are numerous, and the differential diagnosis most commonly includes NSAID or heparin use, cirrhosis due to chronic alcohol consumption or viral hepatitis, various carcinomas, vitamin K deficiency, myelodysplastic syndrome, renal failure, DIC, and leukemia.

PREVENTIVE CONSIDERATIONS

Important considerations in the prevention of coagulopathies include avoidance of NSAID and alcohol overuse, sufficient dietary vitamin intake, and vaccination against viral hepatitis. Early genetic screening of children with a family history of inborn coagulopathies could identify some at-risk children at an early age.

PEARLS FOR THE PA

Common drugs that may interfere with platelet production or function are alcohol, aspirin, NSAIDS, thiazide diuretics, heparin, quinidine, phenothiazines, penicillins, cephalosporins, calcium channel blockers, beta blockers, sulfonamides, and antineoplastic drugs.

An abnormal PT or PTT that fails to correct to within 4 to 5 seconds of normal by mixing the patient's plasma with an equal amount of normal plasma suggests the presence of an anticoagulant or of a pathologic coagulation inhibitor, rather than a coagulation factor deficiency. The most common pathologic coagulation inhibitor is the lupus anticoagulant. Lupus anticoagulant is rarely associated with abnormal clinical bleeding and, interestingly, may cause thrombosis.

A chronic form of DIC can occur in patients with malignancies or autoimmune diseases. The clinical picture usually involves some combination of bleeding, venous thrombosis, or nonbacterial endocarditis with systemic embolization. Occasionally some patients will have a subclinical course manifested only by laboratory abnormalities such as thrombocytopenia, hypofibrinogenemia, and positive assay for serum fibrin degradation products.

Deep Venous Thrombosis

Charles W. Reed, MEd, MPAS, PA-C

DEFINITION

Deep venous thrombosis (DVT) is a pathologic condition in which a clot is embedded in one of the deep veins of the lower legs, thighs, or pelvis, potentially resulting in blockage of return blood flow to the heart distal to the obstruction. The most commonly affected site is the calf.

HISTORY

Symptoms. Although this condition can be asymptomatic and most symptoms are nonspecific, the most common manifestations are pain, swelling, and erythema/warmth of the affected leg. These signs of irritation in a vein are termed *thrombophlebitis*. Onset of pain is usually gradual, and the pain often worsens with dorsiflexion of the foot. Nocturnal leg cramps may be another nonspecific sign. More serious symptoms of acute shortness of breath or chest pain may indicate pulmonary embolism (PE).

Age. Age at onset is variable but most patients are 40 years or older.

Onset. Variable.

Duration. May spontaneously resolve or require ongoing treatment.

Intensity. Can range from subacute to serious embolic events.

Aggravating Factors. See Associated Factors.

Alleviating Factors. Symptomatic relief of more superficial thromboses may be obtained with supportive measures including local heat, elevation of the limb, and aspirin.

Associated Factors. Predisposing factors leading to the development of DVT include vessel damage, changes to normal blood flow, and hypercoagulable states.

Risk factors include bed rest or prolonged sitting, often during extended travel; air travel at heights greater than 14,000 feet; recent surgery or trauma; obesity; myocardial infarction or congestive heart failure; recent childbirth; and use of estrogen or hormonal contraceptive therapy, particularly in smokers older than 35 years of age.

PHYSICAL EXAMINATION

General. Signs and symptoms are often nonspecific and unreliable for confirming the diagnosis. In cases of PE, 63% of the patients will appear apprehensive. Examination findings must be combined with other tests to make the diagnosis.

Skin. Characteristic findings of lower extremity pain, swelling, and erythema may or may not be present. Skin surrounding the area may be blue, white, or normal in color.

Extremities. Symptoms may be limited to an increase in calf circumference in the affected extremity. Palpable nodule or cord-like mass may or may not be present. Calf pain with rapid dorsiflexion of the toes (Homan sign) may be present or absent.

Pelvic. Extension of thrombosis into the pelvis may be palpable on examination.

Pulmonary (in Pulmonary Embolism). Chest pain (pleuritic and/or nonpleuritic) may be present in 85% of cases. Dyspnea or tachypnea is present in 85% and cough in 50%. Rales, particularly in lower lobes, are present in slightly more than half of all patients.

Cardiac (in Pulmonary Embolism). Tachycardia is found in almost 60% of patients.

PATHOPHYSIOLOGY

The Virchow triad of vessel wall injury, venous stasis, and presence of a hypercoagulable state is the primary mechanism for the development of DVT. However, this process is best understood as the activation of the coagulation pathway in an area of decreased venous flow.

In most cases, DVT resolves spontaneously without treatment. In approximately 20% of the cases, the condition will progress proximally. Thrombotic lesions with proximal progression are most likely to result in embolic complications. This is due to the innate instability of a progressing thrombus. A thrombus will begin to organize and adhere to the vessel wall about 5 to 10 days after formation. Although these thrombi are much less likely to propagate or embolize, they are also less likely to spontaneously lyse, so that there is an increased risk for the development of chronic venous insufficiency.

DIAGNOSTIC STUDIES

Although signs and symptoms of DVT/PE are not specific, a reliable diagnosis is possible when examination findings are combined with appropriate diagnostic studies. Diagnostic studies are most useful in patients with a high likelihood of having DVT/PE as evidenced by the preponderance of findings.

Laboratory

Arterial Blood Gas Analysis. Findings consistent with PE include PaO_2 below 80 mm Hg, usually accompanied by hypocapnia.

D-Dimer Test. A negative result may be used to rule out venous thrombosis in a patient in whom clinical suspicion for DVT is low. However, a negative D-dimer assay does not rule out DVT in a patient in whom clinical suspicion is moderate or high. Positive D-dimer assay results are common, have no diagnostic significance, and always require objective confirmatory testing.

Radiology

Chest Film. The chest radiograph is often unremarkable, or it may demonstrate evidence of subsegmental atelectasis (wedge defect). Pleural effusion is present in 30% to 50% of cases but is often small.

Ultrasonography. Real-time (duplex) ultrasonography is probably the most accurate of the noninvasive procedures in the diagnosis of proximal DVT but is less accurate in the diagnosis of isolated distal DVT.

Contrast Venography. Probably the most reliable test for DVT, but complicated by postvenography phlebitis in 5% to 10% of patients who undergo the procedure. Indicated for confirmation of negative findings on noninvasive procedures when clinical suspicion for DVT is moderate or high (or at least the procedures should be performed serially over the 10 to 14 days after presentation).

Other

ECG. The ECG will often indicate sinus tachycardia and may show evidence of right heart strain.

Impedance Plethysmography. A noninvasive procedure measuring changes in tissue volumes based on electrical impedance at the body surface. When combined with a thorough physical examination, it is both sensitive and specific for the diagnosis of proximal vein obstruction.

DIFFERENTIAL DIAGNOSIS

Traumatic

Lower extremity *trauma* usually can be differentiated by the history. Patients may develop DVT as a result of inactivity after trauma.

Infectious

Cellulitis is arguably the most common cause for misdiagnosis of DVT. Because cellulitis can also manifest with erythema, edema, and warmth, it is often difficult to make the distinction on the basis of physical findings alone. A confirmatory test may be required.

Metabolic

Lymphatic obstruction will generally demonstrate edema only and may be due to pelvic mass or lymph node enlargement.

Congestive heart failure results in bilateral pitting edema. DVT will exhibit unilateral edema, which is usually nonpitting.

Neoplastic. Not applicable.

Vascular

Thrombophlebitis is a common condition in patients who have diabetes and in others with poor peripheral venous return. It is superficial, with very low likelihood of clinically significant embolism. The superficial nature is readily apparent on physical examination. Warmth, rest, and elevation of the limb will usually suffice for treatment.

Congenital. Not applicable.
Acquired. Not applicable.

TREATMENT

Treatment goals of DVT include prevention of clot extension, prevention of PE, and prevention of recurrent DVT. To avoid these sequelae, treatment is begun as soon as there is clinical suspicion of disease.

Thrombosis confined to the calf veins carries a low risk of embolization and generally requires only supportive treatment. However, 20% of these thrombi will extend proximally. Thus, even calf-confined thrombi need to be monitored if anticoagulation is withheld. In these cases, noninvasive testing should be repeated 2 to 3 days after diagnosis and several more times during the following 2 weeks.

Anticoagulation

Heparin is the most commonly used agent in the acute treatment of DVT. Heparin prevents further thrombus growth, which allows the body's intrinsic thrombolytic system to dissolve the clot. Heparin is best administered through continuous intravenous infusion on an inpatient basis. A common dosing schedule for patients without contraindications to heparin therapy is a bolus of 80 U/kg of actual body weight followed by a maintenance infusion of 18 U/kg/hour for 5 to 7 days. The target for heparin therapy is a partial thromboplastin time (PTT) of 46 to 70 seconds, which corresponds to an PTT ratio (patient PTT/control PTT) of 1.5:2.3.

Oral warfarin also is started on day 1. The usual dosage is 5 mg PO daily, which is adjusted on the basis of the INR (international normalized ratio). An INR of 2.0 to 3.0 is considered adequate.

When the patient has received intravenous heparin therapy for at least 5 days and the INR has been therapeutic for 2 consecutive days, the heparin may be discontinued. Warfarin therapy is generally continued for 3 to 6 months depending on the risk of recurrent thrombosis.

The disadvantages of this standard treatment modality include the need for hospitalization, dosing adjustments, frequent monitoring of PTT, CBC, and INR, and significant bleeding risk.

A less complex treatment option is obtained through the use of low molecular weight heparin (LMWH). LMWHs have the same risk-benefit profile as for standard heparin. However, they offer an outpatient management option not found with heparin. The most commonly used LMWH is enoxaparin. LMWH is used only as a subcutaneous injection with a 12-hour dosing schedule. Dosing for DVT treatment is 1 mg/kg SC every 12 hours. This regimen allows patients with uncomplicated DVT to obtain treatment on an outpatient basis. If the diagnosis of DVT is not confirmed at onset of treatment, a loading dose of 5000 U of intravenous heparin should be given before instituting outpatient therapy with enoxaparin. As with heparin, enoxaparin should be continued for at least 5 days and until the INR is in therapeutic range with oral warfarin.

Selection of agents for anticoagulation/thrombolysis in patients with thromboembolic pathology such as PE depends largely on the location and severity of the embolism. Anticoagulants (such as heparin, LMWH, and warfarin) and thrombolytics (such as streptokinase, urokinase, and recombinant tissue plasminogen activator [t-PA]) often are used.

For recurrent DVT or large DVT, a Greenfield filter may be placed in the inferior vena cava to prevent clot extension and PE.

PEDIATRIC CONSIDERATIONS

DVT is less common in the pediatric patient, except during the peripartum period, and treatment is much the same as for adults. Thrombosis of the central venous system and embolic events generally are not the result of a single DVT episode in this population. Congenital and acquired factors must be considered.

OBSTETRIC CONSIDERATIONS

Pregnancy is itself a hypercoagulable state. DVT with PE is the most common cause of maternal death. The incidence during pregnancy is 1 to 5 cases/1000 pregnancies (including postpartum). Women with a history of previous DVT have a 12% to 35% risk of thrombosis. Etiologic factors include decreased levels of protein S and "free" protein S, decreased levels of antithrombin, and venous stasis. Increased levels of factors VII and VIII and fibrinogen also are seen.

GERIATRIC CONSIDERATIONS

Thromboembolic events are more common in geriatric patients. This is particularly true for the geriatric inpatient. Although prophylactic anticoagulation decreases the risk, thromboembolism may be the culprit causing the sudden system failure in the hospitalized patient.

PREVENTIVE CONSIDERATIONS

Important considerations are as follows:

Smoking cessation, particularly in women older than 35 years of age who use estrogen or hormonal contraceptives, is paramount.

Patients should be counseled to avoid prolonged sitting during long trips. Recommend standing and moving around every hour or two and to avoid crossing the legs.

Encourage weight loss in obese patients.

PEARLS FOR THE PA

Vigilance is the key. Mental status changes are common in hospitalized patients of any age, and many are due to medication-related issues. Wise is the PA who considers a thromboembolic event as the responsible etiologic factor.

Polycythemia Vera

Charles W. Reed, MEd, MPAS, PA-C

DEFINITION

A myeloproliferative disorder characterized by autonomous proliferation of red blood cells (RBCs) and an increased RBC mass, or erythrocytosis. Clinically, erythrocytosis is usually defined by a hematocrit greater than 55% to 60%.

HISTORY

Symptoms. Pruritus (in 40% of cases), headaches, dizziness, vertigo, tinnitus, visual disturbances, abdominal fullness, and early satiety.

Age. Middle and late adulthood. Peak incidence between 50 and 60 years of age.

Onset. Insidious. Often discovered after a routine blood count discloses an elevated hematocrit.

Duration. Median survival is approximately 10 years. The major causes of death in polycythemia vera are thromboembolism, acute leukemia, and hemorrhage.

Aggravating Factors. The pruritus associated with polycythemia may be aggravated by hot showers.

Alleviating Factors. None.

Associated Factors. Peptic ulcer disease occurs 3 to 5 times more frequently among patients with polycythemia vera than in the normal population. Complications of polycythemia may manifest as angina, intermittent claudication, epistaxis, ecchymoses, and gingival and gastrointestinal bleeding.

PHYSICAL EXAMINATION

General. Facial plethora. Increased blood pressure is common.

Gastrointestinal. Splenomegaly is present in about 75% of patients. Thirty percent of patients may have hepatomegaly.

Head, Eyes, Ears, Nose, Throat. Conjunctival injection. Funduscopic examination may reveal venous engorgement.

PATHOPHYSIOLOGY

Polycythemia vera results from a neoplastic transformation of hematopoietic stem cells in the bone marrow, which produces a clonal proliferation of RBCs. RBC production is autonomous and independent of erythropoietin, as erythropoietin levels are typically decreased in polycythemia vera. Although RBC proliferation dominates the clinical picture, there is usually an absolute increase in granulocytic cells and platelets as well. Increased RBC mass produces hypervolemia and hyperviscosity, which may impair blood flow to brain, heart, gastrointestinal mucosa, and other tissues. Associated platelet abnormalities contribute to an increased risk of thromboembolism or hemorrhage. Patients with polycythemia vera are at an increased risk for development of acute leukemia.

DIAGNOSTIC STUDIES

Laboratory
Complete Blood Count and Platelet Count. Hematocrit greater than 55% to 60%. Decreased platelets and granulocytes.

Arterial Blood Gas Analysis. May show hypoxia.

Leukocyte Alkaline Phosphatase (LAP). An enzyme found in the cytoplasmic granules of white blood cells (WBCs). When the number of WBCs is increased, the total concentration of this enzyme is increased. Secondary and relative forms of erythrocytosis are not associated with an increase in LAP.

Serum B_{12} or Unbound Vitamin B_{12}–Binding Capacity (UBBC). WBCs synthesize transcobalamin III, a serum transport protein for vitamin B_{12}. In polycythemia vera, the associated increase in WBCs also increases the availability of transcobalamin III and raises the levels of B_{12} in the serum. Secondary and relative forms of erythrocytosis are not associated with an increase.

Radiology
Head/Abdominal CT or MRI With and Without Contrast. Indicated to rule out tumors of the kidney, liver, ovaries, or brain.

Other
^{51}Cr-Labeled RBC Mass, Measurement of Plasma Volume, Bone Marrow Aspiration and Biopsy, Hemoglobin P_{50} (to Assess Hemoglobin-Oxygen Dissociation Curve), Hemoglobin Electrophoresis, Erythropoietin Level, Carboxyhemoglobin Concentration. Indicated in selected cases to distinguish polycythemia vera from other causes of erythrocytosis.

DIFFERENTIAL DIAGNOSIS

Traumatic. Not applicable.
Infectious. Not applicable.
Metabolic. Not applicable.

Vascular

Polycythemia vera must be distinguished from other causes of erythrocytosis such as *secondary* and *relative polycythemia* (see Table 7-2).

In secondary polycythemia, the increase in RBC mass results from a physiologic response to increased levels of erythropoietin, which can be induced by tissue hypoxia, as in pulmonary disease, congenital heart disease, exposure to high altitudes, smoking, or hemoglobinopathies. Or it may be inappropriately secreted owing to a tumor of the kidney, liver, ovaries, or brain; renal disease; adrenocortical hyperfunction; or drugs (e.g., corticosteroids, androgens).

Relative polycythemia is characterized by a normal RBC mass but an increased hematocrit due to a contracted plasma volume (e.g., with dehydration, diuretics, burns) or "stress polycythemia" (Gaisbock syndrome).

Neoplastic. Not applicable.
Congenital. Not applicable.
Acquired. Not applicable

TREATMENT

Phlebotomy. Periodic removal of 200 to 450 mL of blood relieves symptoms of hypervolemia and hyperviscosity. Volume and frequency of phlebotomy are dependent on age and cardiovascular status. The goal of phlebotomy is to maintain hematocrit between 42% and 46%. Remissions last less than 2 weeks. Patients treated with phlebotomy alone remain at risk for thromboembolism.

Intravenous Radioactive Phosphorus (^{32}P). Suppresses proliferation of RBC progenitors. Normalization of hematocrit and reduction of splenomegaly occur in about 10 weeks. Remissions may last as long as 6 to 24 months. Because ^{32}P is associated with an increased risk for acute leukemia, this therapy is usually avoided in younger patients and used mainly in patients older than 70 years of age.

Hydroxyurea. A myelosuppressive drug that does not appear to increase the risk for acute leukemia. Especially useful when there are thrombotic complications. Continuous therapy is required because unmaintained remissions last only about 2 weeks.

Histamine H$_1$ Receptor Blockers and H$_2$ Receptor Blockers. H$_1$ blockers such as diphenhydramine and hydroxyzine and H$_2$ blockers such as cimetidine are effective for symptomatic management of pruritus and may be useful in prevention of associated peptic ulcer disease.

Table 7-2. Differential Diagnosis of Increased Hematocrit

	Polycythemia Vera*	Secondary Polycythemia†	Relative Polycythemia‡
⁵¹Cr-radiolabeled RBC mass	Increased	Increased	Normal
Serum erythropoietin	Decreased	Increased	Normal
Po₂	Normal	Usually decreased	Normal
Splenomegaly	Usually present	Absent	Absent
Increased WBCs (>12,000/mL)	Yes	No	No
Increased platelets (>400,000/mL)	Yes	No	No
LAP score (>100)	Increased	Normal	Normal
B₁₂ level (>900 pg/mL)	Yes (30%)	No	No
UBBC (>2200 pg/mL)	Yes (75%)	No	No

*Uncontrolled proliferation of RBCs—"primary" erythrocytosis.

†Diagnosis of secondary polycythemia: chronic hypoxia (e.g., in pulmonary disease, congenital heart disease; with exposure to high altitudes); defective oxygen transport (e.g., with heavy smoking, some hemoglobinopathies); drugs (e.g., corticosteroids, androgens); inappropriate secretion of erythropoietin (e.g., with renal cysts; carcinoma of kidney, liver, ovaries; cerebellar hemangioblastoma).

‡Diagnosis of relative polycythemia: decreased plasma volume (e.g., with dehydration, diuretics, burns). "Stress" polycythemia (Gaisbock syndrome).

§With secondary polycythemia with normal Po₂ (greater than 92% O₂ saturation), consider heavy smoking associated with increased carboxyhemoglobin levels; renal disease or tumors of kidney, liver, ovaries, or cerebellum, diagnosed by appropriate CT or MRI studies; hemoglobinopathy—inheritance of abnormal hemoglobin with high affinity for oxygen (low hemoglobin P₅₀) and/or abnormal hemoglobin electrophoresis.

LAP, leukocyte alkaline phosphates; RBC, red blood cell; UBBC, unsaturated vitamin B₁₂–binding capacity; WBC, white blood cell.

PEDIATRIC CONSIDERATIONS

Polycythemia vera has been reported in only a few children.

OBSTETRIC CONSIDERATIONS

It is suggested that all patients of childbearing age who have polycythemia vera be managed with repeat phlebotomies alone. Hydroxyurea is a pregnancy category D drug and is teratogenic, although the carcinogenic potential is not known.

A massive uterine fibromyoma has been implicated in secondary polycythemia due to increased erythropoietin production.

GERIATRIC CONSIDERATIONS

Because the average age at onset is in this group, vigilance is necessary. In evaluation of a geriatric patient presenting with peptic ulcer disease, the complete blood count should be checked. This will be helpful in discovering a concomitant anemia or polycythemia.

PREVENTIVE CONSIDERATIONS

There are no preventive measures for primary polycythemia; however, smoking cessation is the top preventive consideration for secondary polycythemia.

PEARLS FOR THE PA

Polycythemia vera is an uncommon disorder. Secondary erythrocytosis and relative erythrocytosis are more likely causes of an increased hematocrit.

Gaisbock syndrome is a poorly understood condition associated with an increased hematocrit due to a reduction in plasma volume (e.g., relative erythrocytosis). Typically, it occurs in overweight, middle-aged men who smoke, use alcohol, and have hypertension. Controlling weight and blood pressure while reducing smoking and alcohol intake frequently corrects the increased hematocrit.

In about 10% of the patients, polycythemia vera progresses to a "spent" phase, characterized by marrow fibrosis, anemia, leukocytosis, and massive splenomegaly.

Sickle Cell Disease

Charles W. Reed, MEd, MPAS, PA-C

DEFINITION

A genetic disorder that produces a defect in the β-globin components of the hemoglobin molecule. The resulting structurally abnormal hemoglobin (hemoglobin S) alters the shape and stiffness of RBCs, leading to hemolysis and vascular occlusion. The abnormal β-globin gene is inherited in an autosomal recessive fashion. The homozygous state produces sickle cell anemia. Sickle cell trait is associated with the heterozygous state. Under normal conditions, sickle cell trait does not produce anemia or symptoms.

HISTORY

Symptoms. Pain (bone, abdomen, chest, hands, feet), jaundice, hematuria, dyspnea, painful erection. Central nervous system complications may be manifested by visual disturbances, drowsiness, convulsion, headache.

General. The patient has periodic attacks associated with physiologic stressors.

Age. Usually first diagnosed in early childhood.

Duration. Lifelong. Pattern of periods of well-being interrupted by symptomatic crises. Many adults live well into middle age.

Intensity. Variable. Broad spectrum of clinical expression.

Aggravating Factors. Fever, infection, dehydration, pregnancy, surgery.

Alleviating Factors. Adequate hydration and prompt recognition and treatment of infections.

Associated Factors. Family history of sickle cell anemia or sickle cell trait. Sickle cell anemia occurs in 1 out of every 650 American blacks. The prevalence of sickle cell trait in this population is approximately 8%. Because α-thalassemia is also common in the black population, concomitant inheritance of hemoglobin S and α-thalassemia genes can occur.

PHYSICAL EXAMINATION

General. Fever, tachycardia.

Extremities. Joint swelling or deformity. Bone tenderness.

Gastrointestinal. Hepatomegaly. Splenomegaly (prominent in early childhood, rare in adults).

Genitourinary. Priapism, testicular atrophy.

Head, Eyes, Ears, Nose, Throat. Retinal hemorrhages (usually at periphery and difficult to visualize).

Neurologic. Central nervous system complications may be associated with altered level of consciousness, cranial nerve dysfunction, or focal sensory/motor deficits.

Pulmonary. Splinting of respirations, crackles.
Skin. Jaundice, leg ulcers.

PATHOPHYSIOLOGY

Hemoglobin S functions normally in the oxygenated state. However, in the deoxygenated form, the abnormal hemoglobin polymerizes into long strands that distort the RBC into a characteristic "sickle" shape. Other common factors that precipitate sickling include dehydration, infection, low temperatures, and acidosis. The two major consequences of sickling are premature destruction of the fragile abnormal RBCs in the circulation (hemolysis) and occlusion of the microvascular circulation, causing ischemia or infarction of tissues (vaso-occlusive crisis). Painful vaso-occlusive crises involving bone, abdomen, or chest are the most common clinical manifestation of sickle cell disease. Other complications of sickle cell anemia include stroke, proliferative retinopathy with retinal detachment and blindness, priapism, renal insufficiency, infections (osteomyelitis, sepsis, pneumonia, meningitis), stasis ulcers of leg and ankle, and extrahepatic biliary obstruction by bilirubin stones. Sickle cells may become sequestered in the lung, producing fever, chest pain, and a pneumonia-like clinical picture with life-threatening hypoxia (acute chest syndrome).

DIAGNOSTIC STUDIES

Laboratory
Complete Blood Count. Hematocrits in the range of 18% to 30% are not unusual. Sickle cells may be seen on Wright-stained blood smears.
Reticulocyte Count. Increased during episodes of hemolysis.
Hemoglobin Electrophoresis. Demonstrates abnormal hemoglobin S.
Screening Sickle Tests. Demonstrates transformation of abnormal RBCs into sickle cells when exposed to solution of metabisulfite. Other tests produce turbidity when solutions containing hemoglobin S are exposed to high concentrations of salt.
Serum Bilirubin, Lactate Dehydrogenase (LDH), and Haptoglobin. May be abnormal during hemolytic episodes.

DIFFERENTIAL DIAGNOSIS

The diagnosis of sickle cell anemia is usually apparent when a patient from an ethnic group with a high prevalence of the sickle cell gene presents in painful crisis, with severe infections, and with sickle cells on Wright-stained blood smears. Patients presenting with hemolysis require evaluation to rule out other causes of hemolytic anemia. The strict concept of differential diagnosis does not apply, as this condition is essentially a laboratory diagnosis.

TREATMENT

No specific treatment is available. Therapy is largely supportive and geared to the management of complications.

Painful Vaso-occlusive Crisis.   Fluid therapy to maintain adequate hydration, analgesia, oxygen by nasal cannula. Evaluate for occult infection (e.g., osteomyelitis).

Infection.   Prompt diagnosis and vigorous antibiotic therapy are indicated.

Acute Chest Syndrome.   Rule out pulmonary infection. Oxygen therapy is indicated to maintain adequate oxygen saturation.

PEDIATRIC CONSIDERATIONS

Painful swelling of the hands and feet (hand-foot syndrome) is seen primarily in children. Infants and children with sickle cell anemia may experience a sudden, life-threatening fall in hematocrit and hemoglobin due to sequestration of RBCs in the spleen (splenic sequestration crisis) or suppression of bone marrow by viral infection (aplastic crisis); both normally require immediate RBC transfusion.

Almost all patients with sickle cell anemia lose splenic function because of repeated infarctions by the age of 6 to 8 years. This makes them particularly susceptible to infection by encapsulated microorganisms (e.g., pneumococci, *Haemophilus influenzae*). Immunization against these organisms should be part of the routine management of sickle cell patients.

OBSTETRIC CONSIDERATIONS

There is an increased incidence of fetal and maternal mortality among pregnant sickle cell patients. Oral contraceptives in female patients are associated with a significantly higher incidence of thromboembolism.

The frequency of severe sickle cell crisis is greatly increased during pregnancy. Maternal morbidity may involve severe anemia, megaloblastic crisis, acute sequestration of sickled erythrocytes, pneumonia, pulmonary embolism, antepartum hemorrhage, pyelonephritis, toxemia, and crises involving the bones, abdomen, or brain. Leukocyte-poor washed red cell transfusions or erythrocytopoiesis can be used starting at 24 to 28 weeks of gestation to maintain hematocrit and decrease the chances of a crisis. Simple transfusions have not been proved to reduce the likelihood of the development of a crisis during pregnancy.

The likelihood of spontaneous abortion is increased by 20% to 35%. Intrauterine growth retardation and premature labor are also more likely in sickle cell disease. Asymptomatic bacteriuria is more common in persons with sickle cell disease and trait. Therefore, urine cultures should be carefully checked during pregnancy.

Women with sickle cell disease should be maintained on routine doses of folic acid and iron supplementation during their pregnancy.

GERIATRIC CONSIDERATIONS

None.

PREVENTIVE CONSIDERATIONS

Avoiding known triggers of sickle cell crisis such as high altitudes and pressurized environments may prevent some occurrences.

PEARLS FOR THE PA

Drug addiction is a significant problem among adult patients requiring narcotic analgesics for frequent painful vaso-occlusive crises. However, pain is also undertreated in this patient group. Because of chronic narcotic use, these patients may require higher-than-normal doses of narcotics during crisis to adequately manage their pain. Inadequate control of pain in any patient is unacceptable.

Patients with sickle cell anemia who require surgery must be adequately hydrated and oxygenated preoperatively to reduce the risk of sickling. Some clinicians advocate the use of exchange transfusions prior to surgery.

Heparin-Induced Thrombocytopenia

Charles W. Reed, MEd, MPAS, PA-C

DEFINITION

Heparin-induced thrombocytopenia (HIT): Although a form of thrombocytopenia, this is a thromboembolic event due to an immune reaction to heparin therapy.

HISTORY

Symptoms.   Symptoms may range from a subclinical thrombocytopenia to an acute venous or arterial thrombosis with embolic complications.

General.   History of previous heparin treatment with or without complications increases the likelihood for development of HIT. The dosage of heparin and the route of administration do not appear to play a role in the frequency of HIT. Approximately 35% of patients with clinically diagnosed HIT will develop a clinically significant thrombosis.

Age.   Although most patients are adults, persons of any age may be affected.

Onset.   At 5 to 14 days after initiation of heparin. HIT may occur in just a few hours after heparin administration if the patient had been previously sensitized.

Duration.   Variable.

Intensity.   Dependent on the type of manifestations.

Aggravating Factors.   Continued heparin therapy.

Alleviating Factors.   See Treatment section.

Associated Factors.   Prior heparin use.

PHYSICAL EXAMINATION

General.   Rapid changes in level of consciousness, personality, or orientation may indicate an intracranial infarct. Rapid onset of pulmonary distress may indicate a pulmonary embolism even in the absence of deep venous thrombosis (DVT). Acute onset of hypotension may be another general indication of infarction. HIT may result in a worsening of the initial condition that prompted the heparin therapy.

Cardiac.   Thrombi developing in the cardiac arteries may result in myocardial infarction.

Pulmonary.   Rapid pulmonary collapse, shortness of breath, or poor oxygenation may indicate a pulmonary thrombus.

Gastrointestinal.   Acute development of abdominal pain or distention with or without fever may indicate bowel infarction.

Skin.   Digital pallor or necrosis resembling gangrenous changes may indicate superficial or deep arterial infarct. DVT may also develop.

PATHOPHYSIOLOGY

HIT is an immune-mediated, drug-induced thrombocytopenia. HIT occurs in about 1% to 3% of patients receiving unfractionated heparin for 7 to 14 days. The incidence of HIT resulting from small subcutaneous doses is small.

Endogenous (patient-produced) IgG antibodies bind to heparin and platelet factor 4 (PF_4), resulting in platelet clumping and strong platelet activation. Platelet-derived procoagulant microparticles are generated that accelerate thrombin generation. HIT antibodies also bind to the PF_4 receptors on the endothelial surface, leading to injury and activation. The damaged endothelium produces still more thrombin and acts as starting point for thrombosis.

DIAGNOSTIC STUDIES

Laboratory.   Currently there are no highly specific or sensitive laboratory analyses for the detection of HIT. Some of the assays used are the platelet aggregation assay (PAA) and the serotonin release assay (SRA). Both tests are inadequately sensitive and require large laboratories with highly skilled technicians.

A rapid decline in platelet count of 50,000/mm³ or more, or 50% or more from baseline if platelet count is low, that follows administration of heparin is generally considered adequate for a diagnosis of HIT in the absence of a thrombotic event. Other laboratory studies such as assay for fibrin degradation products or D-dimer and prothrombin time (PT) and partial thromboplastin time (PTT) are not affected.

Essentially, if HIT is suspected, then the patient has HIT.

Radiology.   Radiologic examinations, especially ultrasonography or impedance plethysmography, are useful only in the evaluation of a suspected thrombotic event.

DIFFERENTIAL DIAGNOSIS

Traumatic.   Not applicable.
Infectious.   Not applicable.
Metabolic.   Not applicable.

Vascular
Idiopathic thrombocytopenic purpura (ITP), *thrombotic thrombocytopenic purpura* (TTP), and *hemolytic-uremic syndrome* and other causes of thrombocytopenia are generally bleeding disorders accompanied by anemia.

Unrelated DVT is easily ruled out by absence of thrombocytopenia. Unlikely to develop while patient is on heparin.

Disseminated intravascular coagulation (DIC), while also unlikely to develop during heparin therapy, will result in prolonged PT and hypofibrinogenemia. Fibrin degradation products and D-dimer will be elevated. These tests are not affected by HIT.

Polycythemia vera will also demonstrate elevated hematocrit and red cell mass, which are normal in HIT.

Neoplastic.   Not applicable.
Congenital.   Not applicable.
Acquired.   Not applicable.

TREATMENT

First discontinue *all* heparin. Although low molecular weight heparin (LMWH) is less immunogenic, it will react with anti-heparin antibodies and is not an acceptable substitute. LMWH should also be avoided in patients with a history of HIT.

Reestablish anticoagulation if the underlying requirement for heparin therapy still exists or if a thrombotic event is suspected or confirmed. Some authorities suggest establishing anticoagulation even in the absence of thrombi owing to the high risk of thrombotic complications associated with HIT (30% to 50%). Alternative anticoagulants include argatroban, danaparoid, and lepirudin. Required duration of treatment is controversial; however, it has been shown that patients with HIT have up to a 50% chance of experiencing a thromoembolic event up to 30 days after heparin is discontinued.

Owing to a potential for warfarin-induced thrombotic complications, it should be avoided in acute HIT unless used in conjunction with therapeutic doses of argatroban, danaparoid, or lepirudin. Warfarin is acceptable for single-agent long-term anticoagulation in patients with HIT complicated by thrombotic events. Optimally, warfarin should be withheld until resolution of the thrombocytopenia.

Surgical thromboembolectomy or thrombolysis should be considered for patients with large-artery thrombi or significant pulmonary embolism.

Platelet transfusion is usually unnecessary in the absence of active bleeding.

PEDIATRIC CONSIDERATIONS

HIT is possible in any age group. Incidence is the same, but morbidity is less in the pediatric age group. Diagnosis of any platelet disorder in utero is much more difficult owing to the problem of obtaining an adequate sample and to the high likelihood of false results.

OBSTETRIC CONSIDERATIONS

The incidence of other forms of thrombocytopenia and hypercoagulable states is increased in this population. There is no greater incidence of HIT.

GERIATRIC CONSIDERATIONS

Geriatric patients are most likely to receive heparin therapy for other conditions, and treatment must be monitored closely. This presents a particular problem when the geriatric patient has a preexisting disorder of mentation. Confusion and change in mental status are particularly common in geriatric inpatients but could be the first signs of thromboembolic complications of

HIT. HIT should be considered in the differential diagnosis for any geriatric patient on heparin therapy who develops mental status changes.

PREVENTIVE CONSIDERATIONS

The potential for HIT in heparinized patients should not prevent the use of heparin when indicated. However, a thorough history and maintenance of a high index of clinical suspicion are the best preventive mechanisms. Any patient with a history of HIT should not receive heparin if anticoagulation is required. Heparin trials are dangerous and should not be used in these patients. Use of LMWH decreases the incidence of HIT but is unsafe in patients with a history of HIT. Porcine heparin is more immunogenic than bovine.

PEARLS FOR THE PA

Although HIT is more common at therapeutic heparin doses, any source of heparin may cause HIT. Such sources include heparin-coated catheters and stents and heparin lock intravenous lines.

Further Reading

Bussel J, Freiberg A, Tarantino M, et al: Current perspectives in treating immune thrombocytopenic purpura. Continuing Medical Education (CME) Monograph. Somerset, NJ, Dannemiller Memorial Education Foundation and Alpha & Omega Worldwide, 2000.

Chu E, DeVita V: Physician's Cancer Chemotherapy Drug Manual 2001. Sudbury, MA, Jones and Bartlett, 2001, pp 264-267.

Goldman L, Ausiello D (eds): Cecil Textbook of Medicine, 22nd ed. Philadelphia, WB Saunders, 2003.

Lichtman M, Beutler E, Kipps T (eds): Williams W: Manual of Hematology, 6th ed. New York, McGraw-Hill, 2003.

INFECTIOUS DISEASE

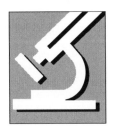

8

Endocarditis (Infectious)

Mary Beth Kvanli, MPAS, PA-C

DEFINITION

A microbial infection of a heart valve or of the endocardial surface of the heart produced by either bacterial, fungal, rickettsial, or chlamydial organisms.

HISTORY

Symptoms. Acute onset is usually associated with high fever, systemic toxicity, and leukocytosis. Subacute forms are associated with low-grade fever, night sweats, weight loss, and vague systemic complaints.

General. Because a variety of organisms can be involved, and also because septic emboli can travel to distant sites, patients can present with manifestations of remote organ involvement. These manifestations may include stroke, monocular blindness (from retinal artery occlusion), pulmonary embolism, and/or kidney failure.

Age. Over 50% of the cases occur in adults older than 50 years of age; 26% occur in those younger than 30.

Onset. May be acute, with rapid progression to death if the infection goes untreated, or subacute, with a slow indolent course leading to death after weeks to months in untreated endocarditis.

Duration. Course of progression to death in untreated endocarditis varies according to causative organism and mode of onset. In acute onset, death occurs in several days to less than 6 weeks. In subacute onset, death occurs after 6 weeks to 3 months.

Aggravating Factors. Immunocompromised status.

Alleviating Factors. Identification of the offending agent and appropriate treatment.

Associated Factors. A recent history of dental work, urethral instrumentation, surgery (particularly rectal or ear-nose-throat procedures), intravenous drug administration (therapeutic or related to illicit drug use), or recent skin or lower respiratory tract infection is found in two-thirds of patients with infective endocarditis. These factors are usually associated with acute onset.

Congenital heart abnormalities, prosthetic valves, indwelling transvenous pacemakers, and a history of rheumatic heart disease or other structural heart disease that results in turbulence of blood flow all can be etiologic factors in infective endocarditis. These factors are usually associated with subacute onset.

PHYSICAL EXAMINATION

General. Fever is usually present, but may be absent in the elderly. Acute onset may manifest with high fever (102° to 105° F; 38.9 to 40.6° C). Fever is classically low grade (99° to 100° F; 37.2 to 37.8° C) and not associated with rigors in subacute onset of disease.

Cardiovascular. Audible heart murmur occurs in over 85% of the cases. Murmurs can represent the underlying (predisposing) cardiac abnormality or may arise as a result of infection of the valve leaflet. A changing murmur and the development of a new regurgitant murmur are uncommon. When present, they are significant findings, often indicating a complicated course. In more than 90% of patients in whom new regurgitant murmur develops, congestive heart failure (CHF) also eventually develops. Most murmurs arise from left heart involvement; however, in the case of intravenous drug abusers, the right heart (particularly the tricuspid valve) is involved. Accordingly, there may be a distinct increase in the intensity of the murmur with deep inspiration (Carvallo sign). If pericarditis develops as a complication, a pericardial friction rub may be heard.

Gastrointestinal. Palpable splenomegaly is common, with occasional spontaneous splenic rupture.

Head, Eyes, Ears, Nose, Throat. Approximately 5% of patients will exhibit flame-shaped hemorrhages, petechial lesions, nerve fiber layer infarcts (cotton-wool patches), and Roth spots (oval white areas surrounded by hemorrhage) on funduscopic examination. Petechiae may be found on the conjunctivae, buccal mucosa, and palate.

Musculoskeletal. A monarticular or polyarticular arthritis may manifest as a warm, red, and tender joint with a rare effusion. Low back pain, which may be severe, and diffuse myalgias may accompany the arthritis.

Neurologic. A cerebral embolism is the most frequent event leading to abnormal findings. Hemiplegia, sensory loss, ataxia, aphasia, or an alteration in mental status can be the presenting complaint or can occur later in the course of the illness as a complication. A persistent focal headache may be produced by a cerebral aneurysm (always mycotic) with invasion of the arterial wall by the causative microbe. Brain abcesses occur rarely. Seizures may occur as a result of irritation by the emboli.

Skin. Pallor, produced by anemia, is commonly present, as are petechiae on the extremities. Pustular petechiae may be present, suggesting *Staphylococcus aureus* as the infecting bacterial agent. Subungual splinter hemorrhages of the nail bed can also be present. Osler nodes (subcutaneous nodules of the fingers that can be tender and often have a purplish hue) and Janeway lesions (which are small nonpainful hemorrhagic patches on the soles of the feet and palms) have been described but uncommon.

PATHOPHYSIOLOGY

Subacute bacterial endocarditis (SBE) is primarily a left-sided abnormality of the heart resulting in valvular insufficiency, with the mitral valve more commonly involved than the aortic valve. A valvular defect or an abnormal communication (ventricular septal defect) can produce a Venturi effect (fluid is driven from a high-pressure area through an orifice into a low-pressure reservoir). The low-pressure side is most often the site of microbial implantation (vegetation). Platelets can adhere to the abnormalities, forming a fibrin clot to which the organisms attach. Some organisms are capable of producing extracellular dextrans that aid their adherence to tissue.

Many bacterial species have been implicated in the cause of endocarditis. In SBE, the causative organisms are of a less virulent disposition and often indigenous. Because they are less invasive, they usually do not affect normal cardiac structures but will propagate on sites of congenital or acquired valvular disease or on other cardiac abnormalities. The most prominent bacteria are members of the normal flora of the gastrointestinal tract, genitourinary system, or oral cavity.

Pathogenic streptococcal species are as follows: viridans streptococci (gingival), *Streptococcus mutans, Streptococcus mitis,* and group D (*Streptococcus bovus*), group H (*Streptococcus sanguis*), and groups B, C, G, and K streptococci. Other pathogens are enterococci (lower gastrointestinal tract, female genitourinary tract, and perineum), *Enterococcus faecalis, Enterococcus faecium,* nonhemolytic streptococcus, beta-hemolytic streptococci, microaerophilic streptococci, and anaerobic streptococci.

Other, less common causative bacterial species include *Haemophilis aphrophilis, Actinobacillus actinomycetemcomitans, Haemophilus influenzae, Haemophilus parainfluenzae, Cardiobacterium hominis, Erysipelothrix insidiosa, Legionella* species, and diphtheroid organisms.

Nonbacterial causes include fungal agents such as *Candida albicans* and *Aspergillus* (seen in patients after cardiac surgery or on intravenous fluids), *Candida parapsilosis* (seen in intravenous drug users), *Histoplasma, Blastomyces, Cryptococcus, Coccidioides, Hansuela,* and *Mucor.*

Other causative microorganisms are *Rickettsia, Coxiella burnetii* (agent of Q fever) (usually seen in the face of preexisting valvular disease and thought to cause the most indolent form of infectious endocarditis), and *Chlamydia* species including *C. psittaci.*

Predisposing cardiac lesions include ventricular septal defect, bicuspid aortic valve, aortic stenosis, pulmonary stenosis, tetralogy of Fallot, complex cyanotic congenital heart disease, systemic to pulmonary artery shunts, patent ductus arteriosus, coarctation of the aorta, hypertrophic cardiomyopathy, and mitral valve prolapse.

Acute bacterial endocarditis (ABE) is caused by organisms that are more invasive than those seen in SBE. The organisms can affect normal heart valves and mural endocardium as well as hearts with congenital or acquired defects. *S. aureus* (cutaneous portal of entry) is the most common cause of ABE. Other causative organisms include *Streptococcus pneumoniae,* group A streptococci, *Neisseria gonorrhoeae,* and *Pseudomonas aeruginosa* (in intravenous drug abusers).

Complications.   CHF is the most common complication due to destruction of the affected heart valves. Leaflet perforation or scarring and fusion of the commissures can result in severe dysfunction. Conduction disturbances can also result from deeper invasion of the infection into cardiac tissue (particularly with involvement of the aortic valve). Extension of the infection into the pericardium from a valve ring abcess can result in pericarditis. Stroke, kidney infarct or abscess, glomerulonephritis, pulmonary embolism, splenic infarct, and mycotic aneurym can all be complications.

DIAGNOSTIC STUDIES

Laboratory

Complete Blood Count.   Usually demonstrates a normochromic, normocytic anemia. White blood cell (WBC) counts are usually normal in SBE and commonly elevated in ABE.

Erythrocyte Sedimentation Rate (ESR).   Almost always elevated.

Rheumatoid Factor.   Positive in 50% of patients affected for longer than 6 weeks.

Circulating Immune Complexes.   Present in 90% of patients.

Blood Cultures.   Positive in most cases for the causative microbe (less than 10% of patients are culture negative). Obtaining three sets of culture specimens in the first 24 hours is recommended.

Serologic Testing.   Necessary for suspected infections with *Legionella, C. psittaci,* and *C. burnetii.*

Urinalysis.   Often demonstrates proteinuria and microscopic hematuria.

Gram Stain/Cultures.   Staining or culture of pustular or petechial skin lesions (as seen in ABE with *S. aureus*) can be diagnostic.

Radiology

CT Scan of the Brain.   May show a stroke or abscess, if indicated.

Cerebral Angiography.   May show a mycotic aneurysm, if indicated.

Intravenous Pyelography.   May show evidence of renal involvement, if indicated.

Chest Film.   May demonstrate a pneumonia as a causative disorder or as a result of the endocarditis. Findings may be consistent with pericardial effusion (e.g., large cardiac silhouette with normal pulmonary vasculature).

Other

ECG.   ECG routinely done in all suspected cases. New changes demonstrating conduction disturbances during the course of the illness suggest extension of the infection into the valve ring or into deeper cardiac tissues (e.g., intraventricular septum).

Transesophageal Doppler Echocardiography.   Can be helpful in identifying vegetations on the valve leaflets.

M-Mode or Transthoracic Two-Dimensional Echocardiography.   Can be useful with prosthetic valves, as the valves produce echos that obscure the vegetations in regular echocardiographic studies.

DIFFERENTIAL DIAGNOSIS

Traumatic
Not applicable.

Infectious
In *meningococcemia*, infection may be due to bacteremia or cerebral emboli. Positive findings on cerebrospinal fluid examination, signs of meningeal irritation (Kernig/Brudzinski signs).

In *pneumonia*, septic emboli can infarct lung tissue. Positive findings on chest radiography, productive cough.

Metabolic
Renal calculi may be confused with renal emboli. Manifestations are flank pain and hematuria.

Acute rheumatic fever can cause fever, cardiac murmurs, and CHF; however, blood cultures and antistreptolysin O antibody titers are negative.

Neoplastic
Atrial myxoma can mimic infective endocarditis by giving rise to a cardiac murmur, cerebral emboli, elevated ESR, and anemia. A change in the murmur with position would favor myxoma. Echocardiography will confirm the lesion.

Hypernephroma (richly vascular) can be associated with anemia, cardiomegaly, murmur, and fever.

Vascular
Stroke may be the result of septic emboli or can be an isolated event. Positive focal neurologic signs and positive CT/MRI scan.

Congenital
Heart murmur may be asymptomatic. Echocardiography may be required for diagnosis.

Acquired
Not otherwise applicable.

TREATMENT

Medical
Antibiotics. Choice of antibiotic therapy depends on positive identification of the causative agent. Empiric antibiotic therapy can (and should) be initiated in rapidly progressing ABE and fulminant infection after blood cultures have been obtained. Generally, bactericidal antibiotics are used parenterally for 4 to 6 weeks.

Antithrombotic Therapy. Should be individualized and based on whether the patient has cardiac or extracardiac disease that would warrant such therapy in the absence of endocarditis. Therapy is not indicated to prevent systemic emboli in patients with normal sinus rhythm who have uncomplicated disease.

In patients with prosthetic heart valves who have cardiac disease that requires long-term warfarin therapy, warfarin therapy should be continued during an episode of infective endocarditis unless there are other contraindications. There is lack of evidence that antithrombotic therapy will prevent embolization from vegetations.

Surgical

Indications for valve replacement include valve destruction, vegetative valves, perivalvular extension of the infection (abscess), *Pseudomonas aeruginosa* (or other gram-negative organism) infections that fail to clear after 10 days of antibiotic therapy, relapsing disease in patients with prosthetic valves, and presence of systemic emboli. Persistent fever, ECG changes demonstrating heart block (particularly with aortic valve disease), and echocardiographic abnormalities can raise suspicion of such disease.

PEDIATRIC CONSIDERATIONS

Infective endocarditis in the pediatric age group is most commonly caused by viridans streptococci and *S. aureus*. Fungal infections make up the remainder of the cases. Although pediatric infective endocarditis is rare, its incidence appears to be increasing owing to increased survival rate for children with congenital heart disease and use of more aggressive techniques in treating critically ill newborns.

Prophylaxis is recommended for children with congenital or acquired heart disease when there is a known increased risk for bacteremia (dental or surgical procedures). Children with valve dysfunction who are on penicillin prophylaxis to protect against rheumatic fever may require an alternative prophylactic antibiotic. Prophylaxis is not necessary for children with functional murmurs.

OBSTETRIC CONSIDERATIONS

Pregnancy has been implicated as a factor in the development of endocarditis in patients with native heart valves who do not abuse drugs.

GERIATRIC CONSIDERATIONS

Elderly patients with infective endocarditis may not present with or complain of fever as readily as do younger patients. An early systolic ejection murmur may be dismissed as a normal finding consistent with calcific aortic stenosis common to older persons.

PREVENTIVE CONSIDERATIONS

Certain patients should receive prophylactic antibiotics to prevent bacterial endocarditis. These include patients with prosthetic heart valves; those with a previous history of bacterial endocarditis or previous rheumatic fever or other acquired valvular heart disease; and those with congenital or acquired cardiac abnormalities. Procedures that require antibiotic coverage include dental procedures (including routine cleaning), upper respiratory tract surgery (including bronchoscopy), intestinal surgery, genitourinary tract surgery or instrumentation, obstetric infections and surgery through or on the vagina, and surgery involving infected tissue.

PEARLS FOR THE PA

Infectious endocarditis should be suspected in any patient with an unexplained illness in whom a recent dental procedure has been performed.

Common organisms implicated include bacteria, fungi, rickettsiae, and Chlamydia.

The presenting symptom may be due to septic emboli traveling to distant organs.

Human Immunodeficiency Virus Infection

Diana Turner, PA-C

DEFINITION

An immune system disorder caused by a retrovirus known as human immunodeficiency virus (HIV).

HISTORY

Symptoms. Seroconversion illness may cause early symptoms of a viral or flu-like illness. Later in the course of the infection, systemic complaints such as recurrent fever, adenopathy, persistent diarrhea, night sweats, chronic fatigue, neurologic symptoms, and weight loss can occur. Opportunistic infections, malignancies, and HIV-related conditions cause symptoms specific to those processes, and may involve any organ system.

General. Risk factors include intravenous drug abuse, receiving blood products before March 1985, occupational exposure to blood or blood products, having multiple sexual partners, homosexual or bisexual experiences, or having unprotected sex with anyone who has the any of the foregoing risk factors. HIV infection can also be congenitally acquired.

Age. Can affect any age, newborn to elderly. Most commonly affects persons 25 to 44 years of age. Incidence is rising in the 45 to 64 age group.

Onset. During the early stages of the disease when the patient is only HIV seropositive, the patient may be totally asymptomatic. There is a gradual progression to acquired immunodeficiency syndrome (AIDS) over months or years. Without treatment, life expectancy following the diagnosis of AIDS (fewer than 200 CD4$^+$ cells/mm^3 or onset of opportunistic infection) is 2 to 4 years.

Duration. Without treatment, average of 8 to 10 years from initial exposure to HIV until death.

Intensity. Initially mild but may be incapacitating in the later stages of AIDS.

Aggravating Factors. Nonadherence to antiretroviral regimens leads to development of drug-resistant virus. Antiretroviral medications can cause adverse effects, many of them long term. Other chronic infections (hepatitis C, hepatitis B) can accelerate the course of HIV infection. Older age is associated with a less favorable course.

Alleviating Factors. Early detection by testing and early intervention may prolong life and improve the quality of life. Antiretroviral and prophylactic medications can halt or reverse disease progression.

Associated Factors. Some patients deny they have HIV infection and continue to expose themselves and others to the virus. Substance abuse, lack of access to care, lack of knowledge, and economic issues are barriers to diagnosis and treatment.

PHYSICAL EXAMINATION

General. Patients may appear completely healthy in early stage of infection, or may present acutely or terminally ill as a result of malignancies or opportunistic infections associated with AIDS. A complete physical examination to include vital signs is required to assess all organ systems.

Cardiovascular. Evaluate rate, rhythm, and presence of any new murmurs. Neck veins, carotid arteries should be examined.

Head, Eyes, Ears, Nose, Throat. Funduscopic examination evaluating for lesions such as the perivascular hemorrhages or fluffy exudates of cytomegalovirus (CMV) infection. Examine the oral mucosa, evaluating for the white plaques of thrush, apthous or viral ulcers, hairy leukoplakia, or purplish lesions of Kaposi sarcoma. Also note any bleeding or inflamed gums.

Lymphatic. Cervical, pre-and postauricular, occipital, supra-and infra-clavicular, axillary, epitrochlear, and inguinal nodes should be evaluated for enlargement.

Genital/Rectal. Ulcers of active herpes simplex or CMV infection may be present. Patient may also have multiple human papillomavirus (HPV) lesions. Fissures, fistulas, abcesses, and hemorrhoids are common. Digital or visual examination may reveal anal cancer or discharges of various types. Female patients should have vaginal examination for thrush, signs of sexually transmitted diseases (STDs), and Papanicolaou smear.

Neurologic. Cranial nerves II to XII should be evaluated, along with deep tendon reflexes and muscle strength. Examine dermatomes for sensory loss, which can occur secondary to a peripheral neuropathy. Neurologic examination may reveal focal deficits. Cognitive defects are common.

Pulmonary. Signs of consolidation, effusion, and pneumothorax and shortness of breath can be found in opportunistic infection. Auscultation, observation of accessory muscle use, and percussion are essential.

Skin. Examine for new rashes or lesions such as psoriasis, molluscum contagiosum, Kaposi sarcoma, or fungal infections. Seborrheic dermatitis, eosinophilic folliculitis, and furunculosis are common.

Abdominal. Hepatic or splenic enlargement may occur. Ascites or masses may be present, and presence of Murphy sign can indicate gallbladder disease.

PATHOPHYSIOLOGY

The human immunodeficiency virus is a retrovirus. After introduction of the virus into the blood, the virus is incorporated into the host's cellular DNA. This invasion occurs after the virus, composed of RNA, transforms into a proviral DNA particle via the reverse transcriptase enzyme. Once integrated, the DNA viral particles are copied with each division of the host cell. The infection results in reproducible virus in the resting memory of the $CD4^+$ T lymphocytes (also called T helper cells).

HIV infection causes deterioration of cellular immunity by decreasing the numbers of T helper cells. This deficit allows the patient to acquire potentially deadly infections. Autoimmunity may occur as a result of disordered cellular immune function or B lymphocyte dysfunction (e.g., idiopathic thrombocytic purpura [ITP]).

DIAGNOSTIC STUDIES

Asymptomatic Patients

Laboratory
HIV Enzyme-Linked Immunosorbent Assay (ELISA). Tests for HIV seropositivity.

Western Blot Test. Confirms positive ELISA result.

HIV Polymerase Chain Reaction (PCR) Assay. Can establish diagnosis before ELISA is positive.

Complete Blood Count with Differential. May reveal anemia, neutropenia, lymphopenia, or thrombocytopenia.

Chemistry Profile. May reveal increased values on liver function tests, increased creatine kinase (CK), lipid or glucose abnormalities, or electrolyte abnormalities.

Hepatitis A, B, C Serologic Testing. Indicated to evaluate for possible coinfections with the hepatitis virus and to establish need for immunizations.

CD4⁺ T Lymphocyte Count. Used to evaluate patients' cellular immunity status as follows:

- More than 350 cells/mm^3: Defer therapy and follow closely, unless patient is symptomatic or has HIV viral load greater than 55,000 copies.
- 200 to 350 cells: Treatment with antiretroviral medication should be offered, although controversy exists. Definitely treat if patient is symptomatic or has HIV viral load greater than 55,000.
- 200 cells and below: Diagnosis of AIDS can be made without history of opportunistic infections. *Pneumocystis carinii* pneumonia (PCP) prophylaxis should be given. Antiretroviral therapy is clearly indicated in this group.
- 50 cells and below: Start *Mycobacterium avium* complex infection prophylaxis with azithromycin, rifabutin.

HIV Genotype. Used to determine resistance profile of patient's viral strain to guide choice of antiretroviral regimen.

Rapid Plasma Reagin (RPR) and Venereal Disease Research Laboratory (VDRL) Tests. Used to evaluate for coinfection with syphilis.

Toxoplasma Immunoglobulin G (IgG). Used to establish need for prophylaxis.

Glucose-6-Phosphate Dehydrogenase (G6PD). In African American patients or those of Mediterranean descent, should be performed in patients prescribed dapsone for PCP prophylaxis.

Purified Protein Derivative (PPD). Indicated to evaluate for tuberculosis exposure or active disease. Controls are sometimes used to evaluate if patient is anergic.

Radiology

Chest Film. Indicated to evaluate for tuberculosis (TB) or possible infiltrates (e.g., in PCP).

Symptomatic Patients

Laboratory

Stool Cultures. For enteric pathogens, *Cryptosporidium*, microsporidia, *Clostridium difficile*, ova, and parasites.

Stool Smears. For white blood cell (WBC) count and acid-fast bacilli (AFB).

Fungal and M. avium Complex Blood Cultures. Evaluate for possible infection with *M. avium* complex or for histoplasmosis or cryptococcosis.

Cytomegalovirus (CMV) PCR Assay. Evaluate for possible infection with CMV.

Culture or Biopsy of Lesions Noted on Physical Examination. For herpes simplex virus (HSV), CMV, methicillin-resistant *Staphylococcus aureus* (MRSA), atypical mycobacteria, and fungi.

Radiology
MRI, CT, or ultrasonography as indicated to search for nervous system, abdominal, or pulmonary pathology.

Other
Colonoscopy. Indicated to obtain biopsy specimens to evaluate for infection due to CMV, *M. avium* complex, herpes simplex virus (HSV), *Histoplasma*, or other pathogens that could contribute to weight loss, such as diarrhea or rectal bleeding.

Patients Presenting with Neurologic Manifestations

Laboratory
Cerebrospinal Fluid (CSF). Including VDRL (for neurosyphilis), India ink preparation and cryptococcal antigen (cryptococcal meningitis), cell count, protein, glucose, and culture for bacteria, AFB (tuberculoma), PCR assay for HSV, AFB, or CMV if indicated.

Cryptococcal Antigen. Positive assay result may support the diagnosis of cryptococcal meningitis.

Toxoplasma Antibodies. Indicated to evaluate for positive serology to support diagnosis of toxoplasmosis.

Radiology
MRI or CT of Brain. Used to evaluate for cerebral lesions of toxoplasmosis, cryptococcosis, nocardiosis, tuberculosis, or CMV infection, or AIDS dementia complex.

Other
Not applicable.

DIFFERENTIAL DIAGNOSIS

HIV infection/AIDS, once considered as a possible diagnosis, is easily differentiated from other disease processes by HIV ELISA and Western blot testing, and HIV PCR assay.

Traumatic. Not applicable.

Infectious
With *tuberculosis*, weight loss, fatigue, night sweats, fever, chills, and abnormal chest radiograph. May coexist with HIV infection.

In *mononucleosis*, fatigue, acute viral syndrome, fever, chills, and weight loss. Patient may have CMV-positive serology.

Other viral syndromes may mimic early HIV disease with constitutional symptoms.

Metabolic
In *systemic lupus erythematosus* (SLE), fever, weight loss, skin and oral lesions, multiple organ system involvement. Patient may have a positive antinuclear antibody assay, and a further workup with anti-DNA and anti–extractable nuclear antigens may be diagnostic.

Neoplastic
With *lymphoma*, fever, chills, weight loss, adenopathy, fatigue, and possible diarrhea. Patient will have abnormal lymph node biopsy.

Testicular cancer/ovarian cancer/colon cancer, weight loss, fatigue, and other constitutional symptoms. Abnormal tissue on biopsy.

Vascular.   Not applicable.
Congenital.   Not applicable.
Acquired.   Not applicable.

TREATMENT

No current cure exists for HIV infection/AIDS. Treatment of opportunistic infections will prolong life and improve the quality of life. Highly active antiretroviral therapy (HAART), available since 1995, has prolonged life expectancy in HIV infection and AIDS.

Antiretroviral Medications
There are four categories of approved antiretroviral medications. Antiretroviral regimens should include at least three of these medications, preferably from two categories.

1. Nucleoside reverse transcriptase inhibitors (NRTIs)
   - Zidovudine
   - Didanosine
   - Zalcitabine
   - Stavudine
   - Lamivudine
   - Abacavir
2. Nucleotide reverse transcriptase inhibitor
   - Tenofovir
3. Non-nucleoside reverse transcriptase inhibitors
   - Nevirapine
   - Delavirdine
   - Efavirenz

4. Protease inhibitors
    Saquinavir   Nelfinavir
    Ritonavir   Amprenavir
    Indinavir   Lopinavir/ritonavir
5. Fusion inhibitor
    Enfuvirtide

These agents are used to decrease viral replication (see Diagnostic Studies for timing of therapy).

Treatment should include regular follow-up visits to monitor response to therapy and development of adverse effects.

PEDIATRIC CONSIDERATIONS

Children born to HIV-positive mothers should be undergo regular follow-up evaluation by infectious disease specialists until serologic HIV status can be confirmed. HIV DNA PCR assay is the preferred virologic method for diagnosing HIV infection during infancy. Testing should be performed on the infant at 48 hours, at age 1 to 2 months, and at age 3 to 6 months. Can be diagnosed in most infected infants by 1 month of age and in virtually all by 6 months of age. Newborns of HIV-positive mothers should receive antiretroviral chemoprophylaxis, and receive chemoprophylaxis against PCP at 4 to 6 weeks of age. Breastfeeding should be discouraged owing to possibility of infecting the infant.

OBSTETRIC CONSIDERATIONS

HIV-positive women should be counseled about the possibility of transmission of infection to their infant. Administration of standard antiretroviral therapy during pregnancy in accordance with current guidelines substantially reduces the risk of perinatal transmission, as does a three-part zidovudine chemoprophylaxis regimen. Zidovudine should be included in combination antiretroviral regimens, and efavirenz should be avoided during the first trimester. Ongoing studies are attempting to establish whether HIV treatments are teratogenic. Certain adverse effects of antiretroviral treatment may be increased in pregnancy (e.g., metabolic acidosis). Invasive procedures, such as use of scalp electrodes, should be avoided during labor, and cesarean section is generally the preferred method of delivery.

GERIATRIC CONSIDERATIONS

The number of elderly HIV-infected persons is growing. HIV infection therapies lead to multiple metabolic abnormalities, including lipodystrophy, hyperlipidemia, diabetes, and lactic acidosis, which are common in the geriatric population. Medications should be chosen with care to avoid as many adverse effects as possible. It may be necessary to differentiate other forms of age-related dementia in the elderly from HIV-related neurologic conditions. Elderly patients do not have as robust a reconstitution of CD4$^+$ counts as seen in younger patients when given HIV infection treatment.

PREVENTIVE CONSIDERATIONS

There is no preexposure prophylaxis (vaccine) for HIV infection other than modification of risky behaviors.

Postexposure prophylaxis (PEP) for health care workers depends on quality and volume of exposure, as well as patient factors (HIV-infected, noninfected, risk factors, and unknown). The risk of HIV infection from a percutaneous exposure is about 0.3%, and from mucous membrane exposure, approximately 0.09%. PEP should begin as soon as possible after the exposure.

PEP following sexual exposure is currently not an established recommendation and is dependent on physician decision. Universal safe sex practices are recommended, as the virus can be transmitted by people who are asymptomatic and unaware of their own infection.

PEARLS FOR THE PA

The history is the key to identifying patients at risk for HIV infection; if there is any question, HIV testing is indicated.

Findings on the physical examination in the early stages of the illness may be unremarkable.

HIV infection/AIDS allows opportunistic infections to involve every organ system of the body.

HIV infection/AIDS can affect anyone and can manifest in many ways.

If a patient is tested early, the ELISA may come back negative— for the high-risk patient, HIV PCR assay is indicated.

HIV patients treated by HIV specialists have better outcomes than those patients treated by other health care providers.

The definition of AIDS changes. PAs should consult the current Centers for Disease Control and Prevention (CDC) guidelines or the guidelines used by their employer.

Gastroenteritis

Mary Beth Kvanli, MPAS, PA-C

DEFINITION

Inflammation of the intestinal tract caused by viral, parasitic, or bacterial pathogens or toxins. Also known as *food poisoning*.

HISTORY

Symptoms. Symptoms may be relatively nonspecific such as general malaise, back pain, headache, fever, abdominal pain or cramping, nausea, and vomiting. Diarrhea is the most consistent sign of intestinal infection. Viral causes of gastroenteritis frequently cause upper gastrointestinal symptoms such as nausea, vomiting, anorexia, and bloating.

General. Small bowel involvement is manifested by few voluminous stools, and large bowel involvement is characterized by the presence of blood, pus, or mucus.

Inquire about the ingestion of improperly cooked or unrefrigerated foods. Food-borne disease can be essentially confirmed if two or more people ingesting the same food develop symptoms, if there is epidemiologic evidence of a specific food type causing illness, or if cultures confirm a source (e.g., food handler, food preparation area, food source, patient cultures). A history of travel, especially to developing areas of the world, or hiking and drinking water from wells or streams, should be ascertained. Risk for developing traveler's diarrhea persists for approximately 1 month after the trip. Sepsis or peritonitis can develop after infection with certain agents.

Age. Any.

Onset. May be acute (within 12 hours) or may occur 1 month after exposure to an infectious agent.

Duration. Dependent on the infectious agent and the incubation period. Symptoms usually last hours to 2 to 5 days, but symptoms due to certain agents, such as ciguatoxin, *Entamoeba histolytica*, *Giardia lamblia*, and *Clostridium botulinum*, may last for months.

Intensity. May be mild and self-limited or cause severe dehydration with profuse nausea and vomiting, or may be fatal owing to the presence of neurotoxins (e.g., from *C. botulinum*).

Aggravating Factors. Immunocompromised status, systemic disorders (e.g., diabetes mellitus), and low stomach acid concentration (e.g., in older people, in patients on antacids, H_2 blockers, or cyclooxygenase inhibitors) are risk factors for certain infections.

Alleviating Factors. Time and hydration in most cases.

Associated Factors. Improper food preparation, infection in food handler, incorrect handwashing, improperly sanitized water, and group centers (e.g., daycare centers, nursing homes).

PHYSICAL EXAMINATION

General. The patient may appear in significant distress due to the symptoms. Test for postural hypotension due to dehydration or the presence of neurotoxins. If sepsis is suspected, evaluate all organ systems for secondary effects (e.g., meningeal signs, heart murmur).

Gastrointestinal. Usually normal, or the patient experiences nonspecific discomfort. Certain organisms (e.g., *Yersinia*) may produce significant abdominal discomfort and features similar to those encountered with appendicitis. Rectal examination may reveal blood. Hepatomegaly and splenomegaly may be palpated in infections due to *Salmonella typhi.*

Head, Eyes, Ears, Nose, Throat.   Pharyngitis is present with infection due to certain organisms. Dry mucous membranes may be present, with dehydration secondary to diarrhea and vomiting.

Neurologic.   If ingestion of *C. botulinum* or other toxins is suspected, evaluate the extraocular muscles for ophthalmoplegia, check speech for dysarthria, test swallowing for dysphagia, and assess extremity strength for weakness.

Skin.   Poor skin turgor may be present with dehydration. The trunk may exhibit "rose spots" in typhoid fever.

PATHOPHYSIOLOGY

Diarrhea occurs as a result of either abnormal secretion or improper absorption of electrolytes and water. Abnormal secretion may occur in the presence of bacterial exotoxins produced by organisms such as *Vibrio cholerae, Escherichia coli,* strains of *Shigella, Yersinia enterocolitica,* or *Aeromonas.*

The most common pathogens in food-borne bacterial gastroenteritis in the United States are *Salmonella, S. aureus,* and *Clostridium perfringens.* Other bacterial organisms include *C. botulinum, Bacillus cereus, Shigella* species, *Vibrio parahaemolyticus, E. coli, Y. enterocolitica, V. cholerae, Campylobacter jejuni, Cyclospora* species, and *Campylobacter fetus. E. coli* is the organism primarily responsible for traveler's diarrhea.

The most common viral causes include Norwalk virus and hepatitis A virus. Other viral agents include rotavirus, enteric adenoviruses, and caliciviruses.

The most common chemical etiologic factors are ciguatoxin, scombrotoxin, poisonous mushrooms, heavy metals, monosodium-L-glutamate, and shellfish.

Amebiasis may be caused by *Entamoeba histolytica.*

The most common water-borne organism is *Giardia lamblia.* Other pathogens include *Campylobacter fetus, S. typhi, Shigella,* and viruses such as Norwalk virus and rotavirus.

Neurologic abnormalities can occur as a result of ingested toxins. *C. botulinum* produces a neurotoxin that blocks acetylcholine, impairing neuromuscular transmission. Ingestion of improperly prepared puffer fish, paralytic shellfish, and snapper/grouper (agents of ciguatera), which contain toxins, can lead to impairment of sodium conductance in the nerves. Mushroom and heavy metal poisoning will also cause neurologic abnormalities. The symptoms of scambroid fish poisoning are due to histamines produced in spoiled fish. Recent antibiotic use can lead to pseudomembranous colitis—infection with *C. difficile. C. difficile* also is transmitted as a result of improper handwashing by health care workers.

DIAGNOSTIC STUDIES

Diagnosis is obtained primarily by history and symptoms, but the following studies may be beneficial.

Laboratory

Complete Blood Count.   May reveal a leukocytosis, especially marked in the presence of secondary sepsis. Hemoglobin and hematocrit may be elevated owing to dehydration. Leukopenia and thrombocytopenia may be encountered in infections with *S. typhi* (typhoid fever).

Electrolytes.   Indicated to evaluate for dehydration (e.g., metabolic acidosis, hyponatremia, hypokalemia, elevated blood urea nitrogen, elevated creatinine).

Stool Cultures.   For the causative organism, virus toxin. Some potentially infectious agents are found in the stool of normal patients, and negative cultures do not rule out an infectious etiology. The first stool in the morning is often the most reliable, but samples should be fresh when examined. Laboratory experience in recognizing certain abnormal organisms may be a factor. Laboratory diagnosis of parasitic pathogens usually depends on visualization of characteristic forms in the feces.

Duodenal Aspirate.   Obtained if the index of suspicion is high for giardiasis, and stool cultures are negative.

Examination of Stool/Vomitus for Occult Blood.   Blood may be seen with infectious gastroenteritis. Serial specimens can be obtained to further guide therapy and to evaluate for other causes of diarrhea and vomiting.

Cultures of Suspected Sources.   Food cultures, if available, should be obtained. In certain instances, culture specimens from the skin and nasopharynx should be obtained from food handlers.

Blood Cultures.   Should be obtained if sepsis suspected.

Reverse Passive Latex Agglutination Test.   Specific for *C. perfringens.*

Serologic Testing.   For *E. coli, Yersinia,* or *Salmonella.* If index of suspicion for amebiasis is high and results on three consecutive stool cultures are negative, serologic testing with indirect hemagglutination should be performed.

Immune Electron Microscopy/Radioimmunoassay/ELISA.   Used as indicated to diagnose viral infection and microsporidia and *Isospora* infection in AIDS.

Enzyme Immunoassay (EIA).   Performed to detect *C. difficile* enterotoxin. Specimen must be fresh. The test is not valid if the patient has been administered oral contrast (e.g., barium, diatrizoate meglumine/sodium [Gastrografin]).

Specialized Concentration and Staining Methods.   Used to identify *Cyclospora* and *Cryptosporidium.*

Radiology

CT Scan/Ultrasound Examination of the Abdomen.   Used as indicated to rule out abscess, intestinal perforation, or other pathologic process that may mimic the symptoms of gastroenteritis.

Other
Endoscopic Procedures.   Can be used in refractory cases (duration longer than 5 days) for culture and biopsy and to differentiate other causes for the symptoms.

DIFFERENTIAL DIAGNOSIS

Diarrhea, nausea, and vomiting are nonspecific complaints associated with a multitude of disorders. Therefore, it is imperative to obtain a detailed history regarding the potential transmission of intestinal pathogens to aid in the diagnosis and to prevent expensive or invasive procedures from being performed unnecessarily.

Traumatic
Not applicable.

Infectious
Appendicitis may be difficult to distinguish, as symptoms may be similar and WBC count may be elevated with both conditions. Usually associated with nausea and vomiting as a principal complaint. Examination characteristically reveals guarding in the lower quadrants, right lower quadrant tenderness, rebound tenderness and pain on percussion, diminished bowel sounds, and point tenderness at McBurney's point.

Peritonitis, although rare, may be secondary to infection of the intestinal tract from cirrhosis or in peritoneal dialysis patients, or it may occur spontaneously. Commonly associated with nausea, vomiting, diarrhea, ascites, and abdominal tenderness. Differentiated on paracentesis. A high mortality rate necessitates early detection and treatment.

Metabolic
Eosinophilic gastroenteritis is due to infiltration of the gastrointestinal tract with eosinophils. May involve the entire alimentary tract (including the esophagus and stomach to the anus). Symptoms include diarrhea, abdominal pain, nausea, vomiting, and anorexia. Etiology is unknown, but allergies (especially to foods) have been implicated. Treatment is with steroids.

Lactose intolerance usually is a chronic condition associated with ingestion of lactose (e.g., cow's milk). Symptoms include distention, bloating, flatulence, abdominal pain, and diarrhea. Infection due to contaminated milk should be explored if there is no history to suggest lactose intolerance. Stool pH is usually acidic. More common in blacks.

With *gastritis,* nausea and vomiting are the primary symptoms. Gastric inflammation is not characteristic of gastroenteritis.

In *Guillain-Barré syndrome/myasthenia gravis,* symptoms may be similar to those produced by neurotoxins (e.g., from *C. botulinum*). Differentiated by history and electromyography.

Neoplastic

Gastrointestinal tumors can manifest with symptoms similar to those of gastroenteritis. The symptoms are usually progressive, and diagnostic studies (e.g., CT, endoscopy, barium studies) will reveal a neoplastic etiology.

Vascular

With *acute mesenteric ischemia*, nonbloody diarrhea that progresses to bloody diarrhea due to mucosal sloughing. Severe, continuous abdominal pain and nausea and vomiting. May lead to peritonitis. Obtain a history of atherosclerotic vascular disease. Diagnosed on angiogram.

Nonoccluding mesenteric ischemia (abdominal angina) is associated with severe abdominal pain after eating. Nonbloody diarrhea is common. Obtain a history of atherosclerotic vascular disease. Diagnosed on angiogram.

Congenital

Not applicable.

Acquired

Antibiotic use may cause diarrhea, and possibly colitis, as the result of destruction of normal intestinal flora. *C. difficile* is implicated in 15% to 25% of cases of diarrhea and in 70% to 95% of cases of colitis associated with antibiotics. The antibiotics likely to produce this effect are clindamycin, ampicillin, and the cephalosporins.

Gastroenteritis may be related to presence of a *nasogastric tube* or may have a *nosocomial* etiology. Enteral feedings can provide an ideal medium for the growth of bacteria whether the bacteria are introduced by contaminated feedings, as opportunistic organisms, or with overgrowth of normal flora. Gastroenteritis also may occur in the hospitalized patient via transmission from another patient or staff member, through procedures such as endoscopy, or through a common contaminated food source.

With *medication use/abuse*, similar symptoms may occur. Commonly implicated are laxatives, digoxin, and colchicine.

With *alcohol abuse*, similar symptoms may occur and may be associated with chronic or acute alcohol ingestion.

TREATMENT

As infectious gastroenteritis may be self-limited, supportive therapy with oral and intravenous fluids (e.g., Ringer lactated solution), and time may be all that is required. Recurrent infectious diarrhea resulting in colitis may be treated with metronidazole 500 mg three times a day for 7 to 10 days.

The following are specific infections requiring definitive therapy.

Salmonella Infection

Antibiotics should not be used unless there is sepsis, infection with a strain of *Salmonella* likely to produce sepsis, or focal infection, or unless the patient is a chronic typhoid carrier. DT104 *Salmonella* infection can become severe salmonellosis if the pathogen is exposed to an antimicrobial agent to which it is resistant.

C. difficile Infection
Oral vancomycin 500 mg PO every 6 hours for 10 days is the mainstay of treatment. Flagyl 500 mg PO three times a day for 2 weeks may also be given, although it is only 50% to 60% effective. Recheck stool cultures/EIA after treatment.

E. coli Infection
Use of antibiotics is controversial, as the disorder may be self-limited and, with certain strains, such agents may liberate toxins within the bowel. Antibiotic use depends on the strain of *E. coli* identified.

Listeria monocytogenes Infection
At-risk patients include pregnant patients and those who are immunocompromised. The patient may present with or progress to the development of severe sequelae such as sepsis. Ampicillin is the first-line therapeutic agent. Other effective agents include trimethoprim-sulfamethoxazole, tetracycline, chloramphenicol, erythromycin, and penicillin G.

C. botulinum Infection
Support vital functions. Intubation may be necessary if respiratory muscles are affected. Fatality rates continue to decrease as critical care improves, especially ventilatory support. Administer antitoxin early in the course of the illness. Hypersensitivity rates are between 9% and 20%, as the preparation is derived from horse serum. Skin testing is performed before administration of the antitoxin.

Salmonella typhi Infection
Immunization for prevention.

V. cholerae Infection (Cholera)
Uncommon in the United States but can be fatal owing to the volume of diarrhea. Begin treatment with oral and intravenous Ringer lactated solution. Antibiotic therapy should commence with tetracycline 250-500 mg every 6 hours for 3 to 5 days. Other antibiotics that may be used include streptomycin, chloramphenicol, trimethoprim-sulfamethoxazole, and ampicillin.

C. jejuni Infection
Erythromycin eradicates carriage of the organism and can shorten duration of illness if given early.

Cyclospora Infection
Can be treated with high-dose trimethoprim-sulfamethoxazole.

PEDIATRIC CONSIDERATIONS

Acute gastroenteritis is one of the most common pediatric illnesses. Viruses (primarily rotavirus) cause most infections. Bacteria and parasites are responsible for the remainder. Winter epidemics of rotavirus infection occur in daycare centers and hospitals. Transmission is by fecal-oral route. Proper handwashing in these situations will prevent spread of infection.

The differential diagnosis is extensive and, especially in the child younger than 2 years of age, should include more significant gastrointestinal problems (e.g., intussusception, volvulus, pancreatitis) and infection outside the gastrointestinal tract (e.g., pneumonia, otitis media, sepsis, urinary tract infection, meningitis).

Dehydration and electrolyte abnormalities are the most important acute complications, especially if diarrhea is accompanied by vomiting. Infants, especially those younger than 6 months of age, are most at risk. Infants and young children will often reduce their intake when they are ill, putting them at greater risk for dehydration and secondary sequelae. History should include duration, frequency, and description of stools; frequency of vomiting; frequency of urination (dehydration will decrease volume and frequency); and exposure to others with similar symptoms of vomiting or diarrhea.

Treatment requires the replacement of the fluid deficit. Oral solutions are most suitable for fluid replacement. Replacement volume should be administered by mouth over 12 to 24 hours.

Secondary lactase deficiency is common but is not a contraindication to breastfeeding in most infants. In uncomplicated viral gastroenteritis, a return to normal caloric intake should be fairly rapid. Continuation of clear liquid diet may lead to "starvation" stools and further weight loss. In formula-fed infants, when the number of stools decreases, a return to half-strength formula for 24 hours, and then to full-strength formula, may be initiated. Intestinal lactase levels will remain depressed for 7 to 14 days. Therefore, it may be advisable to use a lactose-free formula. Constipating solids (e.g., rice cereal, apple sauce, bananas, carrots) may be given to older infants and children when feeding is resumed. Antidiarrheal agents are rarely necessary and may be contraindicated. If vomiting or weakness prevents oral hydration, or in the presence of severe dehydration, shock, or acidosis, or with impending surgery, hospitalization and parenteral fluid therapy are indicated.

Raw honey may contain *C. botulinum* spores, and its ingestion been associated with a form of botulism. Therefore, it should not be given to infants younger than 1 year.

OBSTETRIC CONSIDERATIONS

In maternal cases of gastroenteritis caused by *Campylobacter*, bacteremic infections have been known to cause abortion or neonatal infection.

GERIATRIC CONSIDERATIONS

Older patients may present without fever and with indistinct abdominal complaints. Older persons seem less susceptible to traveler's diarrhea but are more susceptible to illness caused by other agents of gastroenteritis.

PREVENTIVE CONSIDERATIONS

Prevention remains the cornerstone of management. Handwashing by persons involved with food preparation, avoidance of improperly canned foods, proper food storage, and appropriate cooking are imperative to prevent outbreaks of food poisoning. Handwashing among child care workers, health care personnel, and nursing home attendants can reduce person-to-person spread.

PEARLS FOR THE PA

Diarrhea is the most consistent sign of intestinal infection.

A history of a common source for the symptoms (e.g., food handler, two or more affected individuals) needs to be obtained.

Most intestinal infections are self-limited and respond to oral or intravenous fluids.

Prevention remains the cornerstone of management (proper food preparation, handwashing).

Gonorrhea

Mary Beth Kvanli, MPAS, PA-C

DEFINITION

An infectious disease caused by *Neisseria gonorrhoeae* that primarily affects the genitourinary tract. Other sites that may be affected are the pharynx, rectum, eye, and joints.

HISTORY

Symptoms. Males may complain of urethritis, with white or creamy yellow, sometimes blood-tinged, purulent profuse discharge appearing 2 to 8 days following exposure; may have rectal discharge. A few males may be asymptomatic.

Females may have increased vaginal discharge, dysuria, urinary frequency and urgency, pelvic pain, purulent urethral discharge, or rectal discharge or itching, or may be asymptomatic.

Conjunctivitis may be present, with copious purulent discharge, often caused by (direct) inoculation from the genitalia. Disseminated conditions may manifest with intermittent fever; arthralgia; maculopapular, pustular, or hemorrhagic skin lesions; or arthritis/tenosynovitis of one or more joints such as knee, ankle, or wrist. Rare presentations include endocarditis and meningitis.

General. Determine the type of potential exposure (heterosexual, homosexual, bisexual/vaginal, oral, anal), history of sexually transmitted diseases (STDs), whether the encounter was unprotected.

Age. Greatest incidence in 15- to 29-year-old age group, but persons of any age can be infected, including infants during birth.

Onset. Usually 2 to 8 days after infection for urethritis or cervicitis.

Duration. Variable; patient may have asymptomatic infection in genitourinary gonorrhea.

Aggravating Factors. May have other STDs in conjunction with gonorrhea.

Alleviating Factors. Antibiotic therapy. However, even without therapy, patient may be asymptomatic.

Associated Factors. May have other STDs. Risk for concurrent HIV infection; multiple sex partners; illicit drug use.

PHYSICAL EXAMINATION

General. A complete physical examination should be performed in all patients to look for signs of other STDs. The patient may be febrile.

Genitalia/Rectum. Examination of discharge from penis/rectum is necessary in males. Specimens for Gram stain and culture should be collected. In the female, pelvic examination should be done to assess the external genitalia and Bartholin's glands. Speculum examination of the cervix may reveal an inflamed cervix with purulent discharge from the os. Rectum and urethra should be observed for discharge.

Cardiac. Endocarditis may produce valvular heart disease and murmur (see "Endocarditis (Infective)" earlier in this chapter).

Musculoskeletal. Evaluate for arthritis or tenosynovitis, especially in the knees, ankles, or wrists.

Neurologic. Meningeal signs such as nuchal rigidity (extreme discomfort on passive flexion of the neck), flexion of the hip and knee on flexion of the neck (Brudzinski sign), or inability to extend the legs fully (Kernig sign) may be present with meningitis.

Ophthalmologic. As indicated to evaluate for conjunctivitis with copious purulent discharge.

Skin. Observe for pustular or hemorrhagic skin lesions.

PATHOPHYSIOLOGY

N. gonorrhoeae attaches to epithelial cells, multiplies, and is internalized by endocytosis into the cell. The gonococci cause a nonspecific neutrophilic inflammatory reaction, producing large amounts of yellowish purulent discharge. Some strains of gonococci can escape the normal host defense mechanisms and are more prone to dissemination.

DIAGNOSTIC STUDIES

Laboratory
Gram stain. Will reveal gram-negative intracellular diplococci and increased leukocytes; smears in males are usually positive. Diagnosis by smear in women is more difficult because smears are often falsely negative.

Culture. Organism is grown on Thayer-Martin type medium. Organism is sensitive to cold temperatures, so medium should be warm prior to plating of specimen. All discharge specimens from patients in whom gonorrhea is suspected should be cultured. A positive culture for *N. gonorrhoeae* is diagnostic. Cultures of specimens from the urethra, cervical os, pharynx, conjunctiva, joints, and rectum should be performed as indicated by signs and symptoms noted during physical examination.

Cerebrospinal Fluid (CSF). As indicated by symptoms. Elevated white blood cell count, elevated CSF protein and low CSF glucose, positive CSF cultures.

DNA Probe. Can be done from a simple culture swab. Compared with culture, more rapid results and more effective when transport problems may make culture difficult; sensitivity equal to or better than that of culture.

HIV Assay. May be indicated to rule out coinfection.

Radiology
Not applicable.

Other
ECG. If cardiac disease is suspected.

DIFFERENTIAL DIAGNOSIS

Traumatic. Not applicable

Infectious. In *nongonococcal urethritis* or *cervicitis/vaginitis*, discharge may not be characteristic of gonorrhea. Wet preparation/mount, cultures, rapid plasma reagin (RPR) test are indicated to rule out other or coexistent infection.

Metabolic. In *Reiter syndrome*, patient may present with urethritis, conjunctivitis, mucocutaneous lesions, and arthritis. May follow infection with *Chlamydia, Campylobacter fetus, Salmonella*, or *Yersinia*. Arthritis is asymmetrical, involving weight-bearing joints (knees, ankles); initial attack is self-limiting and may resolve spontaneously. May have positive HLA-B27 titer. Treated with nonsteroidal anti-inflammatory drugs (NSAIDs).

Neoplastic. Not applicable.

Vascular. Not applicable.

Congenital. Not applicable.

TREATMENT

Definitive drug therapy is as follows:

Ceftriaxone 125 mg IM × one dose
PLUS
Doxycycline 100 mg PO twice daily for 7 days
Can give 125 mg ceftriaxone intramuscularly alone if cost or amount of medication is a factor, but it may not delay development of resistant strains.
Alternative treatment:
Ciprofloxacin 500 mg PO OR
Cefixime 400 mg PO OR
Ofloxacin 400 mg PO
PLUS
Azithromycin 1.0 g PO in a single dose OR
Doxycycline 100 mg PO twice daily for 7 days

PEDIATRIC CONSIDERATIONS

Ophthalmic infection of the newborn can occur with passage through the birth canal. Prophylaxis by instillation of 1% aqueous solution of silver nitrate into the conjunctivae soon after delivery is highly effective. Topical application of 0.5% erythromycin ointment or 1% tetracycline ointment is somewhat less effective. Gonorrhea in children is usually transmitted by sexual abuse. Infection is treated with ceftriaxone 25-50 mg/kg body weight daily for 7 to 10 days, IM or IV.

OBSTETRIC CONSIDERATIONS

Women with gonoccocal cervicitis are at increased risk for disseminated gonococcal infection during pregnancy. Gonococcal infection has been associated with premature labor. Infants born to mothers with cervicovaginal gonorrhea may develop gonococcal conjunctivitis. Infants may also develop pharyngeal, respiratory, or rectal infection or sepsis during the neonatal period.

Treatment of gonorrhea cervicitis in the pregnant patient consists of the following regimen:

Ceftriaxone 125 mg IM, FOLLOWED BY
Erythromycin base or stearate 500 mg PO four times a day for 7 days OR
erythromycin ethylsuccinate 800 mg PO four times a day for 7 days

Doxycycline 100 mg PO twice a day OR azithromycin 1 g PO in a single dose is an acceptable substitute for erythromycin.

Spectinomycin 2.0 g IM may be used in patients with penicillin and/or cephalosporin allergies to substitute for ceftriaxone.

GERIATRIC CONSIDERATIONS

No different than the normal adult population. Never assume that elderly patients are not having intercourse. Always inquire.

PREVENTIVE CONSIDERATIONS

Preventive measures are as follows:

Condoms are highly effective if properly used.

Use of female condoms, diaphragm, or cervical cap is probably protective.

Screening and treatment of sexual contacts of infected persons are required.

Screening of all sexually active persons is indicated.

Public education and personal counseling promoting these measures are recommended.

PEARLS FOR THE PA

All patients with gonorrhea should be evaluated for other STDs such as Chlamydia infection, a common coexistent infection.

All patients with gonorrhea should be counseled about their increased risk for HIV disease and tested if possible.

All cases of gonorrhea should be reported to the local health department. Sexual contacts should be evaluated and treated.

Hepatitis (Viral)

Diana Turner, PA-C

DEFINITION

Hepatitis is defined as an injury to hepatic cells and infiltration of inflammatory cells into the liver. It can be caused by viral infection, drugs, or toxic agents, with similar clinical manifestations for all three groups of etiologic agents. *Acute viral hepatitis* is caused by five distinct agents: hepatitis A virus (HAV); hepatitis B virus (HBV); hepatitis C virus (HCV), which is non-A, non-B virus; hepatitis D virus (HDV); and hepatitis E virus (HEV). *Chronic hepatitis* refers to three specific disorders: chronic persistent hepatitis, chronic lobular hepatitis, and chronic active hepatitis.

HISTORY

Symptoms.   Most patients with *acute* viral hepatitis present with similar clinical manifestations despite the etiologic agent. The most common early symptoms are fatigue, lassitude, anorexia, and nausea. Dark urine and clay-colored stools may be noticed. Low-grade fever, dull aching pain in the right upper quadrant exacerbated by movement, and pruritus are complaints in some patients. Typical viral symptoms such as myalgias and arthralgias also may be present. With the onset of jaundice (icterus), most constitutional symptoms diminish. Most patients with *chronic* hepatitis are asymptomatic, but some may complain of anorexia, fatigue, and nausea.

General.   Inquiry should be made about blood or blood product transfusion or intravenous drug use; presence of similar symptoms in others within the same household; travel history; and sexual history (oral/anal practices).

Age.   Any.

Onset.   The incubation period of HAV infection is about 30 days; of HBV infection, 60 to 90 days, infrequently up to 180 days; and of HCV infection, 2 to 20 weeks, with most cases becoming apparent between 6 and 10 weeks of exposure.

Duration.   Jaundice is usually maximal by the second week after onset and then decreases, disappearing within 6 to 8 weeks or earlier in most cases. Stool color may again darken. Full clinical recovery may be expected by the end of week 16 in 80% of patients and by the end of 6 months in 90% to 95% of patients.

Intensity.   Varies depending on the age at onset and the type of virus. Mild to severe symptoms with organ failure or dehydration are associated with nausea and vomiting.

Aggravating Factors.   Debility, malignancy, alcohol overuse/abuse, coinfections, and advancing age diminish the survival rate of affected patients.

Alleviating Factors.   None

Associated Factors.   Mild steatorrhea may occur during the icteric phase owing to deficiency of bile salts. Glomerulonephritis, pancreatitis, myocarditis, pericarditis, acute myelitis, aseptic meningitis, and peripheral neuropathy all have been reported to occur, although rarely, with viral hepatitis. If HBV and HCV infections are left untreated, they may cause chronic hepatitis, cirrhosis, and hepatocellular cancer.

PHYSICAL EXAMINATION

General.   Patient may appear mildly ill or significantly debilitated. In chronic hepatitis, findings on examination are usually normal.

Skin.   May be icteric, as can the sclera. Porphyria cutanea tarda is seen with HCV infection.

Gastrointestinal.   With acute hepatitis, the liver is often enlarged and tender to palpation. Punch tenderness may be elicited over the right rib cage. Transient splenomegaly is found in approximately 10% of patients. In chronic hepatitis, the liver may be slightly tender or enlarged, and ascites or splenomegaly may be present.

PATHOPHYSIOLOGY

HAV is a small, RNA-containing picornavirus first identified in 1973. It is transmitted primarily through the fecal-oral route. HAV infection occurs in small epidemics traced to fecal contamination of food or drinking water. There is an increased incidence of HAV infection among homosexual men who have multiple sexual partners or in those who have oral-anal sexual exposure.

HBV is a DNA-containing hepadnavirus. The virus is transmitted primarily by parenteral exposure (e.g., with needlesticks or blood transfusions) or by inapparent skin or mucosal exposure (e.g., sexual contact). All major body fluids (blood, saliva, semen) have been shown to harbor the virus. HBV is transmitted at least eight times as efficiently as human immunodeficiency virus (HIV) owing to its greater concentration in body fluids.

HCV is a small, enveloped, cytopathic RNA virus, similar to members of the flavovirus group. It is a major cause of transfusion-associated non-A, non-B hepatitis. Persons at highest risk for acquiring HCV infection are intravenous drug users and patients requiring multiple transfusions of blood or blood products (e.g., hemophiliacs, persons undergoing major surgery).

HDV, or delta agent, is a more recently discovered defective virus that requires coinfection with HBV in order to replicate. HDV infection has a worldwide distribution, but the areas of highest occurrence are in the Mediterranean basin, Middle East, and certain parts of South America. It occurs most commonly among intravenous drug users and patients requiring multiple transfusions.

HEV infection is an enterically transmitted non-A, non-B form of acute viral hepatitis. HEV is serologically distinct from the other viruses causing hepatitis and has been identified in stool. A viral antigen has been identified in infected liver cells in acute cases. Blood-borne transmission and a carrier state have not been demonstrated. Epidemics in some countries appear to be related to fecal contamination of water supplies.

Chronic persistent hepatitis and *chronic lobular hepatitis* result from infections with HBV and non-A, non-B hepatitis viruses. They are nonprogressive disorders that do not lead to liver failure or cirrhosis. *Chronic active hepatitis* is associated with multiple etiologic factors (although the primary cause is HBV and non-A, non-B viruses) and is characterized by continuing hepatic necrosis, active inflammation, and fibrosis. It may lead to liver failure, cirrhosis, and death. Approximately 85% of persons infected with HCV and 5% to 10% of persons infected with HBV develop chronic hepatitis. Approximately 20% of persons with chronic HCV infection and 10% of persons with chronic HBV infection will develop cirrhosis. *Hepatocellular carcinoma* is associated with HBV infection in 89% of cases and also is associated with HCV infection. Enveloped viruses can cause both acute and chronic disease. Nonenveloped viruses cause only acute disease. See Table 8-1.

DIAGNOSTIC STUDIES

Laboratory

Serologic Testing. Indicated to establish the diagnosis of hepatitis A, B, C, and D.

Tests for fecal or serum HAV are not readily available, so a diagnosis of type A hepatitis is based on detection of IgM anti-HAV during the acute illness ("anti" refers to "antibody").

The diagnosis of HBV can be made by detection of hepatitis B surface antigen (HBsAg) ("Ag" refers to "antigen"). Sometimes, the levels of HBsAg are too low during the acute phase to be detected. In these cases, the diagnosis can be established by the presence of IgM for anti-HBc. In chronic active hepatitis in HBV infection, HbsAg, HbeAg, and anti-HBc are present.

Diagnosis of acute infection with HCV is one of exclusion in the absence of HBsAg, IgM anti-HBc, and IgM anti-HAV, although HCV RNA titer is diagnostic. Diagnosis of chronic infection in HCV is made by finding persistent positive HCV RNA in persons who are HCV Ab positive.

The presence of HDV infection can be made by demonstrating antidelta seroconversion (a rise in titer of anti-HDV or de novo appearance of IgM anti-HDV) or positive HDV RNA titer.

Acute HEV infection can be diagnosed by the presence of IgM anti-HEV and, later in the course, finding of IgG anti-HEV. See Table 8-2.

Complete Blood Count with Differential. Most patients have a relative lymphocytosis.

Serum Glucose. May be decreased owing to vomiting or poor hepatic glycogen stores.

Alkaline Phosphatase. May be normal to mildly elevated.

Albumin. Low levels may be seen, but uncommon.

Bilirubin. Generally does not exceed 15 to 20 mg/dL.

Aspartate Transaminase (AST) and Alanine Transaminase (ALT) Levels. In acute hepatitis, these rise 1 to 2 weeks before the onset of symptoms and begin to fall shortly after symptoms appear. Peak levels generally exceed 500 IU/L, but the degree of elevation does not necessarily correlate with the severity of disease.

Gammaglobulin Fraction. Mildly elevated during acute viral hepatitis.

Serum ImmnoglobulinMG (IgM) and Immunoglobulin G (IgG). Are elevated in one-third of patients. IgM increase is seen mostly during acute HAV infection.

Antibodies to Smooth Muscle and Other Cell Constituents. May be present.

Table 8-1. Characteristics of the Hepatitis Virus Types

	Hepatitis A Virus	Hepatitis B Virus	Hepatitis C Virus	Hepatitis D Virus	Hepatitis E Virus	Hepatitis G Virus
Molecular structure	RNA	DNA	RNA	RNA	RNA	RNA
Incubation	15-45 days	30-180 days	15-160 days	20-140 days	15-60 days	15-160 days
Transmission route						
Fecal-oral	+++	–	–	?	+++	–
Percutaneous	–	+++	+++	+++	?	+++
Other nonpercutaneous	–	++	++	++	?	?
Progression to chronicity						
Chronic carrier	No	10%	50-60%	Yes	No	?
Chronic active hepatitis	No	Approximately 5%	50-60%	Up to 70%	No	?
Fulminant hepatitis	Approximately 0.1%	<1%	<1%	Up to 17%	10-20% in pregnant women	?

From Rakel RE, Bope ET: Conn's Current Therapy 2003. Philadelphia, Saunders, 2003, p. 568.

Table 8–2. Diagnostic Tests for Acute and Chronic Viral Hepatitis

Virus	Status	Diagnostic Test
HAV	Acute	IgM Ab (+)
	Resolved	IgG Ab (+)
	Vaccinated	IgG Ab (+)
HBV	Acute	Surface Ag (+), core IgM Ab (+)
		Surface Ab (−), core IgG Ab (−)
	Chronic active	Surface Ag (+), core IgG Ab (+), E Ag (+)
		HBV DNA (+)
		Surface Ab (−), E Ab (−)
	Chronic persistent	Surface Ag (+), core IgG Ab (+), E Ab (+)
		Surface Ab (−), E Ag (−), HBV DNA (−)
	Resolved	Surface Ab (+), core IgM/IgG Ab (+), E Ab (+)
		Surface Ag (−), E Ag (−), HBV DNA (−)
	Vaccination	Surface Ab (+)
		Core IgM/IgG Ab (−), surface Ag (−), E Ag/Ab (−)
HCV	Active	Ab (EIA) (+), RIBA (+), HCV RNA* (+)
	Resolved	Ab (+), RIBA (+), HCV RNA (−)
HDV	Acute	IgM Antibody (+)
	Chronic	IgG Antibody (+)
HEV	Acute	Antibody (+)
	Resolved	Antibody (+)

* By polymerase chain reaction or branched-chain DNA assay.

Ab, antibody; Ag, antigen; EIA, enzyme immunoassay; HAV, hepatitis A virus; HBV, hepatitis B virus; HCV, hepatitis C virus; HDV, hepatitis D virus; HEV, hepatitis E virus; RIBA, recombinant immunoblot assay.

From Rakel RE, Bope ET: Conn's Current Therapy 2001. Philadelphia, WB Saunders, 2001, p. 531.

Rheumatoid Factor, Antinuclear Antibody, and Heterophil Antibody. May be positive during the acute phase of viral hepatitis.
Prothrombin Time (PT). Prolonged value may reflect a severe defect of synthesis or significant hepatocellular necrosis.
Urinalysis. May reveal mild hematuria or proteinuria.

Radiology
CT Scan of the Abdomen. Performed to rule out mass lesions or other pathology as indicated.

Other
Liver Biopsy. Rarely necessary or indicated in acute viral hepatitis, except when there is a question regarding acute versus chronic disease. Liver biopsy is required to diagnose chronic hepatitis.

DIFFERENTIAL DIAGNOSIS

Traumatic
Not applicable.

Infectious
Mononucleosis, cytomegalovirus (CMV) *infection, herpes simplex virus* (HSV) *infection, coxsackievirus infection, adenovirus infection,* and *toxoplasmosis* can be differentiated on serologic testing.

Metabolic
Wilson disease and α_1-*antitrypsin deficiency* can be differentiated on serologic testing.

Neoplastic
Hepatic malignancies and *metastases* can be differentiated on serologic testing and imaging studies of the liver.

Vascular
Right ventricular failure may cause passive hepatic congestion or hypoperfusion syndromes such as those associated with shock, severe hypotension, and severe left ventricular failure.

Congenital
Not applicable.

Acquired
With *alcoholic hepatitis,* history of alcohol abuse. Differentiated on serologic testing.
Use of medications that are metabolized by the liver may cause symptoms similar to those of hepatitis (acute and chronic hepatitis) and elevated values on liver function studies. A full medication history must be obtained and these medications referenced to determine if hepatic toxicity is a side effect.

TREATMENT

There is no specific treatment for typical acute viral hepatitis once symptoms begin. Sometimes hospitalization is required for an uncertain diagnosis, clinically severe illness with failure to maintain nutrition, progressive worsening of coagulation status, or emerging encephalopathy, or for unusually high-risk patients such as those who are pregnant, are elderly, or have an underlying illness.

Some patients feel better with restricted physical activity, but complete bed rest is not necessary.

An increase in caloric intake is desirable, preferably in the early morning when it is more easily tolerated.

Parenteral nutrition may be necessary in patients with persistent vomiting. Alcohol and drugs that are metabolized by the liver should be avoided.

The use of bile acid–sequestering resin (cholestyramine) may help relieve pruritus.

Physical isolation of patients is not necessary except for those experiencing fecal incontinence infected with HAV or HEV, or in those infected with HBV or HCV with uncontrolled, voluminous bleeding.

Universal precautions should be observed in caring for any patient to prevent spread of infection.

Hepatitis A Virus Infection
Postexposure prophylaxis with early administration of immunoglobulin can prevent the symptoms of HAV infection in 80% to 90% of persons. Owing to the short incubation period, vaccinations should be given within 2 weeks of exposure. Recommended dose is 0.02 mL/kg. Preexposure prophylaxis with hepatitis A vaccine is recommended for routine childhood immunization, injecting drug users, travelers to developing countries, men who have sex with men, and persons coinfected with HCV and HBV.

Hepatitis B Virus Infection
Both immunoglobulin and hepatitis B immunoglobulin (HBIG) contain anti-HB. HBIG is preferred for postexposure prophylaxis owing to its high anti-HB titers (1:100,000). Administration of hepatitis B vaccine is the preferred method of preexposure prophylaxis. It is recommended as routine childhood immunization, for persons engaging in high-risk behavior, for persons exposed to blood and blood products occupationally, and for those infected with HCV.

Hepatitis C Virus Infection
There is no vaccine available for prevention of HCV infection. Postexposure prophylaxis is not recommended.

Hepatitis D Virus Infection
There are no specific means of preventing infection, but successful immunization against HBV will also prevent infection with HDV.

Chronic Persistent and Lobular Hepatitis
Once the diagnosis is made on liver biopsy, no specific therapy is required. Follow-up examination is recommended every 6 to 12 months until laboratory abnormalities have returned to normal.

Chronic Active Hepatitis
Chronic active hepatitis can lead to cirrhosis and liver failure, as well as hepatocellular carcinoma in HBV and HCV infection. Liver biopsy should be performed in persons with chronic active hepatitis to determine whether they are candidates for therapy. Lamivudine and adefovir dipivoxil are both oral medications approved for treatment of chronic HBV infection, and are

generally well tolerated. The preferred treatment for chronic HCV is combination therapy with peginterferon alpha-2b and ribavirin, for up to 1 year. The therapy is associated with significant adverse affects, and success in reaching sustained virologic response depends on the HCV genotype. Genotype 1, the most common in the United States, is associated with lower response to therapy than has been obtained with genotypes 2 and 3.

PEDIATRIC CONSIDERATIONS

Hepatitis in children is transmitted and acquired in the same manner as in adults. In children, however, viruses that do not affect adults (owing to exposure and immunity) may also cause hepatitis. Viral diseases that may be associated with hepatitis in children include CMV infection, herpesvirus infection, encephalomyocarditis due to coxackievirus (newborns), congenital rubella, AIDS, infectious mononucleosis, and complications of varicella, mumps, measles, and herpes virus infection and echovirus 2 infection in infants.

Children younger than 5 years of age frequently have anicteric disease. In adolescents and older children, hepatitis tends to resemble the more severe disease seen in adults. Hepatitis A is usually more acute, whereas hepatitis B is more insidious.

The presentation associated with hepatitis in children is different from that in adults. Hepatitis A manifests at its onset as systemic complaints of fever, malaise, digestive complaints of nausea, vomiting, anorexia, intolerance of food and tobacco, and abdominal pain and cramping. This prodrome may be mild and go unnoticed. Dull right upper quadrant pain or epigastric fullness may be exacerbated with exercise or vigorous movements. Jaundice and dark urine usually appear after the onset of systemic symptoms. Diarrhea, rather than constipation, is more common in children. Infants may fail to gain weight. As a whole, children tend to have less disability from hepatitis A than is experienced by adults.

Hepatitis B symptoms may be heralded by arthralgias or skin eruptions such as urticaria, purpura, or macular or maculopapular rashes. Papular acrodermatitis (Gianotti-Crosti syndrome) may also occur. The physical findings are usually the same as in adults: enlarged tender liver, splenomegaly, and lymphadenopathy.

Hepatitis C is more insidious in onset in the pediatric population. Transaminase elevations may be prolonged.

Hepatitis E is rare in children younger than 15 years of age.

Diagnosis is made the same as in adults. Prolongation of PT and partial thromboplastin time (PTT) is a serious sign, requiring immediate hospitalization. Although most children recover rapidly and uneventfully from hepatitis, some may suffer serious acute or chronic complications.

Infants born to women with evidence of active or chronic HBV infection should be given HBIG, and hepatitis B vaccination initiated. Breastfeeding is discouraged. Treatment of uncomplicated hepatitis is supportive. The presence of anorexia or vomiting may require intravenous hydration, as dehydration in children can be devastating. Generally, acute problems such as encephalopathy, bleeding, fluid retention, and electrolyte disturbances need to be managed while awaiting restoration of hepatic function.

OBSTETRIC CONSIDERATIONS

Pregnant women who have received no prenatal care should be routinely screened for hepatitis B at the time of delivery. Vertical transmission of HBV and HCV is common, especially during the third trimester in both the chronic carrier and the patient with active disease. Ninety percent of infants infected perinatally with HBV develop a chronic carrier status. In the obstetric patient with hepatitis B, the risk of premature delivery is increased. Pregnancy is *not* a contraindication to receiving the hepatitis B vaccination.

In hepatitis A, vertical transmission to the fetus rarely occurs.

GERIATRIC CONSIDERATIONS

No specific recommendations.

PREVENTIVE CONSIDERATIONS

General primary prevention includes strict attention to handwashing, especially in the food industry; avoidance of oral-anal contact; following recommendations for immunizations prior to travel; and use of barrier methods of contraception. Universal precautions should always be maintained in the health care setting.

Hepatitis A Virus Infection
Postexposure prophylaxis with early administration of immunoglobulin can prevent the symptoms of HAV in 80% to 90% of persons. Owing to the short incubation period, vaccinations should be given within 2 weeks of exposure. Recommended dose is 0.02 mL/kg. Preexposure prophylaxis with hepatitis A vaccine is recommended for routine childhood immunization, injection drug users, travelers to developing countries, men who have sex with men, and persons coinfected with HBV and HCV.

Hepatitis B Virus Infection
Hepatitis B is usually transmitted via the percutaneous route, but HBV can survive in dried blood for up to 1 week, making universal precautions an absolute necessity. Both immunoglobulin and hepatitis B immunoglobulin (HBIG) contain anti-HB. HBIG is preferred for postexposure prophylaxis owing to its high anti-HB titers (1:100,000). Administration of hepatitis B vaccine is the preferred method of preexposure prophylaxis. It is recommended as routine childhood immunization, for persons engaging in high-risk behavior, for persons exposed to blood and blood products occupationally, and for those infected with HCV.

Hepatitis C Virus Infection
There is no vaccine available for prevention of HCV infection. Postexposure prophylaxis is not recommended.

Hepatitis D Virus
There is no specific means of preventing infection, but successful immunization against HBV will also prevent infection with HDV.

PEARLS FOR THE PA

Transmission of hepatitis viruses occurs through the fecal-oral route, contaminated drinking water and food, blood transfusions, vertical transmission from mother to fetus, contaminated needles, mucosal exposure, or exposure to other body fluids (saliva or semen).

HBV is transmitted at least eight times more efficiently than HIV owing to its greater concentration in body fluids.

Chronic active hepatitis can lead to hepatic necrosis, liver failure, cirrhosis, and death.

Acute viral hepatitis is diagnosed by serologic testing, and chronic hepatitis is diagnosed by liver biopsy.

Mononucleosis
Diana Turner, PA-C

DEFINITION

An acute infectious disease caused by the Epstein-Barr virus (EBV), characterized by fever, malaise, sore throat, lymphadenopathy, and hepatosplenomegaly.

HISTORY

Symptoms. Patients usually present with nonspecific complaints including malaise, tender lymph nodes, fever, sore throat, anorexia, and headache. Less common complaints are cough, myalgia, jaundice, and skin rash.

General. The patient will usually present for evaluation after a 1-week history of symptoms. There may also be a history of sore throat or other viral-type illness approximately 1 to 2 months before the onset of symptoms.

Age. Young adults, especially in the 15 to 25 age group.

Onset. Incubation period lasts 4 to 6 weeks. Mild symptoms during the prodromal phase lasting 3 to 5 days. More specific symptoms, which vary in severity, occur over the succeeding 7 to 10 days.

Duration. Symptoms usually last 2 to 4 weeks. Most patients will clinically improve within 4 weeks. Some patients may experience mild to moderate symptoms for 2 to 3 months.

Intensity. Variable. Most intense during the second and third weeks of the clinical course.

Aggravating Factors. None.

Alleviating Factors. Aggressive symptomatic treatment.

Associated Factors. Approximately 20% of patients will have concurrent exudative pharyngitis. Complications may include central nervous system involvement, airway obstruction, and bacterial superinfections.

PHYSICAL EXAMINATION

General. Patients may be febrile with peaks of 101° to 104° F (38.3° to 40° C) and appear acutely ill. Due to the nonspecificity of symptoms, a complete physical examination is essential with special attention to the head-eyes-ears-nose-throat (HEENT), gastrointestinal, and lymphatic systems.

Head, Eyes, Ears, Nose, Throat. Most often will reveal inflammation and edema of the pharyngeal tissue. There may also be petechiae-like lesions near the border of the hard and soft palates.

Gastrointestinal. Splenomegaly is generally noted in 50% of patients. Less frequently, the liver may be palpable.

Lymphatic. Lymphatic enlargement is seen in almost all cases, primarily in the cervical region. Axillary and inguinal nodes may also be palpable. There is no correlation between the size of the lymph nodes and the severity of the illness.

Neurologic. Focal neurologic signs occur rarely.

Skin. Maculopapular rash occurs in about 10% of cases.

PATHOPHYSIOLOGY

Mononucleosis is caused by the Epstein-Barr virus, a lymphotrophic herpesvirus transmitted through intimate contact with saliva of an infected person. Commonly known as the "kissing disease."

DIAGNOSTIC STUDIES

Laboratory

Complete Blood Count with Differential. Will reveal a mild increase in the white blood cell (WBC) count (10,000 to 15,000/mm³) with a lymphocytosis. Approximately 10% to 20% of lymphocytes are noted to be atypical.

Monospot Test.   Will be positive in 40% of cases in first week of illness and in 80% to 90% in last 3 to 4 weeks of illness.

Liver Function Tests.   May reveal an increase in aspartate transaminase (AST) (formerly serum glutamate-pyruvate transaminase [SGPT]), alanine transaminase (ALT) (formerly serum glutamic-oxaloacetic transaminase [SGOT]), and alkaline phosphatase levels.

Radiology.   Not applicable.
Other.   Not applicable.

DIFFERENTIAL DIAGNOSIS

Traumatic.   Not applicable.
Infectious.   *Streptococcal infections, viral upper respiratory infections, rubella, hepatitis, tonsillitis, cytomegalovirus* (CMV) *infection,* and *toxoplasmosis* all may cause similar constitutional symptoms. Differentiated by laboratory tests, Monospot test.
Metabolic.   Not applicable.
Neoplastic.   *Leukemia, Hodgkin's disease, lymphoma* can be differentiated by laboratory tests and Monospot test. Any patient presenting with nonclassic symptoms should undergo a full evaluation to rule out these conditions.
Vascular.   Not applicable.
Congenital.   Not applicable.
Acquired.   Not applicable.

TREATMENT

Treatment is directed at providing symptomatic relief. Strenuous activity should be avoided while splenomegaly is present, usually for 1 month. Bed rest is recommended as dictated by severity of symptoms. Some experts prescribe a 5-day course of steroids. It is important to stress that supportive care combined with patient education is usually all that is required. In patients given ampicillin for concomitant bacterial infection, development of a rash has been reported.

Antibiotic therapy is needed only if a secondary bacterial infection is present and identified.

PEDIATRIC CONSIDERATIONS

The Monospot test result is frequently negative in a child younger than 5 years of age, regardless of immune status. In a child, the spleen is palpable far more frequently than in adults. Splenic rupture due to mononucleosis is more common in the pediatric population. Infants and young children are often asymptomatic or have only a mild pharyngitis.

OBSTETRIC CONSIDERATIONS

No specific indications.

GERATRIC CONSIDERATIONS

No specific issues—extremely unlikely to affect the elderly population, as 75% of cases occur in adolescents.

PREVENTIVE CONSIDERATIONS

Prevention involves not sharing drinking glasses or utensils with infected persons, as well as avoiding other intimate contact with their saliva.

PEARLS FOR THE PA

Patients with mononucleosis usually present with a triad of irregular fever, pharyngotonsillitis, and cervical lymphadenopathy.

This triad, along with splenomegaly and an atypical lymphocytosis, points to the diagnosis.

Sepsis

Mary Beth Kvanli, MPAS, PA-C

DEFINITION

Sepsis refers to the clinical effect of the presence of pathologic microorganisms or toxins in the blood stream. *Bacteremia* is defined as the presence of bacteria in the blood stream that can occur after any exposure of the blood supply to the environment (e.g., brushing teeth) and may be transient or may lead to sepsis.

HISTORY

Symptoms. Fever, tachycardia, tachypnea, mental status changes, hypotension, or symptoms related to the causative factor (e.g., flank pain with ascending urinary tract infection).

General. A thorough history of potential causative factors needs to be elicited. Possible modes of bacterial entry into the bloodstream include surgery, invasive procedures, dental procedures, skin lesions, urinary tract infections, gastrointestinal and respiratory infections, and meningitis.

Age. Any.

Onset. Hours to days after the organisms gain entry into the blood stream.

Duration. Once sepsis begins, it may be rapidly progressive.

Intensity. The patient may present with only modest complaints or be seriously ill.

Aggravating Factors. Immunocompromised patients (e.g., those with AIDS; those taking immunosuppressive medications, chemotherapeutic agents, or steroids), burn-injured patients, chronic alcoholics, and persons with conditions requiring invasive monitoring.

Alleviating Factors. The host response is usually adequate to manage simple bacteremias. Immediate empirical therapy after cultures have been obtained is essential to prevent clinical deterioration. Fluid resuscitation and maintenance of vital functions are important aspects of management.

Associated Factors. Recent infections or invasive procedures (including dental procedures).

PHYSICAL EXAMINATION

General. Vital signs should be documented. Blood pressure (if systolic measurement is less than 90 mm Hg or falls 40 mm Hg below the baseline level, septic shock should be suspected). Heart rate (tachycardia greater than 90 beats/minute may be present).

Respiratory rate (tachypnea) (greater than 20 breaths/minute) may be present. Temperature should be measured rectally; if it is greater than 101° F (38.3° C), sepsis should be suspected.

Cardiovascular. Auscultate for murmurs that may signify infected valve leaflets, which may lead to septic emboli.

Genitourinary. Examination should include percussion for flank tenderness, which may indicate renal infection.

Head, Eyes, Ears, Nose, Throat. Perform a full examination of the nose, throat, and ears to evaluate for infections and dental caries.

Neurologic. Evaluate for meningitis by testing signs of meningeal irritation. Nuchal rigidity (extreme discomfort on passive flexion of the neck), flexion of the hip and knee with flexion of the neck (Brudzinski sign), and the inability to extend the legs fully (Kernig sign) may be present with primary or secondary meningitis. These meningeal signs may not be present in infants, small children, the elderly, or persons in a coma.

Pulmonary. Auscultate for rales or rhonchi to evaluate for pneumonia or pulmonary infection as a cause for sepsis.

Skin. Observe for skin defects or infected skin lesions that may allow for bacterial invasion of the blood stream.

PATHOPHYSIOLOGY

Escherichia coli, Klebsiella, and *Staphylococcus aureus* (gram-negative bacteria) are the most frequent causes of sepsis in adults.

The most common sites of entry for bacteria into the blood stream are the skin and the genitourinary, gastrointestinal, and respiratory tracts.

In response to pathologic bacteria or bacterial endotoxins, the body releases certain endogenous mediators.

Usually, the host response is adequate to overcome blood stream infections. On occasion, especially in debilitated patients, the immunologic response becomes overwhelmed and disordered. This incapacitation eventually leads to progressive hypotension, shock, organ failure, and possibly death.

DIAGNOSTIC STUDIES

Laboratory

Blood Culture and Sensitivity Testing. Multiple (2 to 4) blood cultures are required to confirm the presence of bacteria in the blood stream. Two sets are used for initial diagnosis, three sets are used to evaluate for continuous bacteremia, and four sets are used if the possible organism is a common contaminant (e.g., diphtheroids, *Staphylococcus epidermidis*, *Bacillus*) or if the patient has recently received antibiotics.

Sputum Culture and Sensitivity Testing. Every attempt to obtain a true sample should be made to reduce the chances of contamination with oral flora. A suction tube that bypasses the mouth can be used. Induced expectoration and bronchoscopy are also effective.

Urinalysis with Culture and Sensitivity Testing. Urinary tract infection may be the cause of sepsis. Catheterization or clean-catch technique must be used to prevent contamination.

Complete Blood Count. Usually will reveal a leukocytosis (cell counts greater than 11,000/mm^3) with a left shift.

Platelet Count. May reveal thrombocytopenia (less than 140,000/mm^3).

Serum Chemistry. May show an elevated glucose. Liver involvement may reveal elevated values on liver function tests (bilirubin, transaminases, alkaline phosphatase).

Arterial Blood Gas Analysis. Should be performed if there is any indication of respiratory impairment. May reveal hypoxemia (Pao$_2$ of less than 75 mm Hg) or respiratory alkalosis.

Serum Lactate Dehydrogenase. Elevated in the presence of end organ damage.

Radiology

Chest Film. Used to rule out pulmonary infection as the cause of sepsis. Acute respiratory distress syndrome (ARDS) may be manifested by diffuse pulmonary infiltrates. Bacterial pneumonia, obstructed pneumonia, or aspiration pneumonia may be the cause.

Other

ECG. As indicated to evaluate for arrythmias or myocardial infarction.

DIFFERENTIAL DIAGNOSIS

Traumatic
Trauma of any cause can cause communication of the bloodstream with the environment. Organisms introduced in this manner may cause fever and sepsis. Differentiated on history.

Infectious
With *meningitis*, may see nuchal rigidity, presence of Brudzinski and/or Kernig signs, leukocytosis with a shift, positive findings on cerebrospinal fluid examination.

Metabolic
Epilepsy may cause fever and mental status changes. History of generalized or focal seizure.

Neoplastic
Hypothalamic tumors may cause fever. Positive CT/MRI scan of brain.

Vascular
Stroke may cause fever. History of transient or permanent neurologic deficit, positive CT/MRI of brain, and/or focal neurologic deficit.

Acquired
Overdose or *withdrawal* may be associated with similar symptoms. Commonly implicated are phencyclidine, cocaine, amphetamines, and alcohol.

TREATMENT

Support all vital functions. Volume infusion should be performed with either Ringer lactate or colloid solutions to maintain an adequate blood pressure and urine output (greater than 0.5 mg/kg/hour). Dopamine or epinephrine may be used to support blood pressure. Pulmonary capillary wedge pressure monitoring and arterial line placement should be considered in patients in whom vital sign stability is of concern.

Supplemental oxygen should be supplied, when necessary, through nasal cannula, face mask, or mechanical ventilation. Use of anticoagulation agents may be necessary.

Strict intake and output should be documented. Oliguria (less than 0.5 mL/kg of urine output for at least 1 hour) signifies end-organ damage.

Parenteral antibiotics are preferred for a minimum of 7 to 14 days. A history to ascertain any antibiotic allergies must be obtained.

The specific cause of the sepsis should be addressed. Drain abscesses, débride necrotic tissue, discontinue or change all unnecessary intravenous (or other) lines, aspirate infected joints, drain empyemas, and consider removing all other potentially infected foreign bodies from the patient (e.g., shunts, portal catheters, prostheses).

Antibiotic coverage is begun empirically, then continued specifically (depending on culture and sensitivity results) for the causative organism. Broad-spectrum coverage, often with two or more antibiotics, is indicated after culture specimens have been obtained. Dosages should take into account the patient's age, overall health, effective serum antibiotic levels, renal/hepatic function, and clinical response. See Table 8-3.

PEDIATRIC CONSIDERATIONS

Presenting symptoms of sepsis in children are somewhat nonspecific. Children may present with fever, hypothermia, vomiting, difficulty feeding, respiratory abnormalities, irritability, abdominal distention, or jaundice. Group B streptococci and *E. coli* are the most common causes in infants. Sepsis in older children occurs most frequently with infections due to *Haemophilus influenzae, Streptococcus pneumoniae,* and *Neisseria meningitidis.* Antibiotic dosage should be adjusted for the patient's age and weight.

OBSTETRIC CONSIDERATIONS

Sepsis may result as a response to chorioamnionitis, postpartum endometriosis, or septic abortion. Aqueous penicillin, aminoglycosides, clindamycin, and cephalosporins can be used in the treatment of sepsis during pregnancy.

GERIATRIC CONSIDERATIONS

Initial symptoms may be blunted in the elderly. The patient may have a fever or hypothermia. History should include the patient's baseline mental status (e.g., dementia), as mental status changes may be a symptom of an underlying disorder. Bedridden patients are more likely to have skin breakdown or aspiration as a source of infection.

PREVENTIVE CONSIDERATIONS

Recommendations are as follows:
>   Prophylaxis with antimicrobials, either systemic or topical, for those at risk
>   Management of high-risk patients in protective environments
>   Measures to limit spread of infection within the hospital
>   Early and aggressive treatment of infections most implicated in sepsis, especially in high-risk patients

Table 8-3. Empirical Intravenous Antibiotic Selection for Severe Sepsis and Septic Shock

Source	Recommended Regimen
1. No clinically identifiable source but with likely pathogens	Antipseudomonal penicillin or cephalosporin + aminoglycoside or fluoroquinolone (if with renal insufficiency) OR
(a) Anaerobes	Imipenem (Primaxin) as a single agent
(b) *Pseudomonas aeruginosa*	Antipseudomonal penicillin or cephalosporin + aminoglycoside or fluoroquinolone + clindamycin or metronidazole (Flagyl)
	Antipseudomonal penicillin + aminoglycoside or fluoroquinolone OR
	Imipenem + aminoglycoside or fluoroquinolone
2. Community-acquired pneumonia	
(a) Immunocompetent host	Second-/third-generation cephalosporin + macrolide or quinolone OR
(b) Immunocompromised host	Beta-lactam antibiotics with beta-lactamase inhibitors
(c) Atypicals likely	Broad-spectrum coverage as with regimen for 1
	Consider empirical coverage for opportunistic infections (mycobacteria, fungi, *Nocardia*, parasites); also aggressive/invasive diagnostic workup
	2(a) or 2(b) + erythromycin or fluoroquinolone
3. Nosocomial or ventilator-associated pneumonia	Broad-spectrum coverage as with regimen for 1
4. Abdominal or intra-abdominal	
(a) *P. aeruginosa* unlikely	Imipenem or
	Ampicillin/sulbactam (Unasyn) OR
	Ticarcillin/clavulanate (Timentin) OR
	Piperacillin/tazobactam (Zosyn)
(b) *P. aeruginosa* likely or very severe infections	Ampicillin + metronidazole + aztreonam or aminoglycoside OR
	Any of the regimens in 4(a) + aminoglycoside OR
	Second-generation cephalosporin (cefoxitin, cefotetan) + aminoglycoside

Continued

Table 8–3. Empirical Intravenous Antibiotic Selection for Severe Sepsis and Septic Shock—cont'd

Source	Recommended Regimen
5. Urinary tract	
(a) *P. aeruginosa* unlikely	Third-generation cephalosporin OR
	Quinolone
(b) *P. aeruginosa* likely or very severe infections	Third-generation cephalosporin + quinolone OR
	Either regimen in 5(a) + aztreonam
6. Cellulitis or cutaneous abscess	
(a) Methicillin-resistant *Staphylococcus aureus* unlikely	Cefazolin OR
	Nafcillin
(b) Methicillin-resistant *S. aureus* or coagulase-negative staphylococci likely	Vancomycin
7. Necrotizing fasciitis	Any of the regimens in 4(a)
8. Intravascular catheter	Consider removal of catheter PLUS
(a) Outpatient-acquired infection	Third-generation cephalosporin
(b) Methicillin-resistant *S. aureus* or coagulase-negative staphylococci likely	8(a) + vancomycin
(c) Diabetes	8(b) + quinolone

From Rakel RE, Bope ET: Conn's Current Therapy 2001. Philadelphia, WB Saunders, 2001, p. 60.

PEARLS FOR THE PA

Sepsis refers to the clinical response of the patient to pathologic bacteria and toxins.

Bacteremia is defined as the presence of bacteria in the blood stream.

Sepsis leads to progressive clinical deterioration.

Empirical antibiotic therapy should be started only after specimens for culture have been obtained.

Multiple blood cultures are required to establish the diagnosis.

Syphilis

Diana Turner, PA-C

DEFINITION

An infectious disease caused by the spirochete *Treponema pallidum*, transmitted in most cases by sexual contact. Syphilis may also be congenitally acquired. There has been an increase in the incidence of syphilis since the onset of human immunodeficiency virus (HIV) disease.

HISTORY

Symptoms.   Variable, depending on stage of disease.

Primary Stage.   Clinical disease occurs during first 2 to 4 weeks after infection. Patient will have a firm, usually nontender ulcer with a well-defined margin and indurated base known as a *chancre*. The patient may have nontender regional adenopathy either unilaterally or bilaterally. Serologic tests are usually positive. This stage resolves spontaneously.

Secondary Stage.   Occurs 3 to 6 weeks after exposure. Manifestations may develop while chancre is still present. Most commonly manifests as a skin rash that can involve the entire body including the palms and soles of the feet. Patient may also present with sore throat, fever, diffuse adenopathy, mucosal ulcerations, malaise, patchy alopecia, and thinning of lateral third of the eyebrows. There may be immunotype hepatitis or nephritis. This stage resolves spontaneously. Secondary syphilis can be divided further into latent stages. In latent syphilis, the patient has positive serologic tests but no signs or symptoms of syphilis; the disease is said to be in the *early latent stage* if infection has been present for less than 1 year or in the *late latent stage* if infection has been present for more than 1 year.

Tertiary Stage. Occurs many years after infection; in this stage, the disease can affect any organ system. Patients may present with aortic aneurysm, aortic valve incompetence or coronary artery ostial stenosis, neurosyphilis (either asymptomatic or with symptoms of meningitis), optic neuritis, deafness, or general paresis. Other presenting manifestations may include tabes dorsalis consisting of lightning pains in legs, ataxia, absence of deep tendon reflexes, a Romberg sign, and Argyll Robertson pupils.

General. Ulcer of primary syphilis usually appears at site of exposure to spirochete.

Age. Can affect persons of any age, newborn to elderly.

Onset. General onset at 3 days to 3 months.

Primary Stage. Usually 2 to 4 weeks.

Secondary Stage. Usually 3 to 6 weeks.

Tertiary Stage. Years after spontaneous clearing of the secondary stage.

Duration. Variable, depending on diagnosis and treatment.

Intensity. Variable, depending on diagnosis and treatment.

Aggravating Factors. Poor patient compliance, presence of HIV infection, unreliable sexual history, and appearance of primary lesions in alternate sites.

Alleviating Factors. Spontaneous resolution of symptoms in primary and secondary stages.

Associated Factors. Concomitant sexually transmitted diseases (STDs), HIV infection, and drug use can lead to reinfection.

PHYSICAL EXAMINATION

General. Syphilis can affect all organ systems. A thorough physical examination should be performed on any patient with a positive serologic test(s).

Cardiovascular. Auscultate for the murmur of aortic stenosis and for abdominal bruits.

Extremities. In tertiary syphilis, evaluate for trophic ulcers over joints of feet or joint damage (Charcot joint).

Genitalia. Examine for the chancre of primary syphilis or condyloma latum on penis, labia, or cervix.

Head, Eyes, Ears, Nose, Throat. Examine the mucosa for ulcers or papules of the lips, mouth, or throat. Patient may present with diffuse redness of pharynx. Condylomata lata are fused, weeping papules on moist areas of the skin and mucous membranes. Look for the chancre of primary syphilis. Argyll Robertson pupils may be seen in the tertiary stage. Funduscopic examination may reveal an optic neuritis.

Lymph Nodes. Examine for involvement of regional lymph nodes when any skin manifestation of syphilis is found.

Neurologic. A complete neurologic examination should be performed in any patient with positive serologic tests to evaluate for meningeal signs, cranial nerve palsies, unequal reflexes, irregular pupils with poor light-accommodation reflexes, changes in gait, muscular hypotonia, hyporeflexia, paresthesias, Romberg sign, and analgesia. Patient may show a decrease in concentration, impairment of memory, dysarthria, or tremors of fingers or lips.

Rectum.   Examine for lesion of primary syphilis (chancre) or condyloma latum. Lesions may be wart-like or annular.

Skin.   Examine for a generalized musculopapular skin rash that is non-pruritic. If there is involvement of the palms and soles, suspect syphilis. Rash can also be pustular or follicular. In late syphilis look for gummas (painless subcutaneous nodules that may ulcerate). Patchy alopecia and thinning of lateral third of the eyebrows may be present in the secondary stage.

PATHOPHYSIOLOGY

Syphilis is caused by the spirochete *T. pallidum,* which can rapidly traverse intact mucous membranes and abraded skin. The precise mechanism of action is unknown, but *T. pallidum* evokes obliterative endarteritis, perivascular cuffing, and granulatomatous lesions called gummas. Antibodies are formed (the Wassermann antibody, or reagin, and treponemal antibody) that are useful in testing for syphilis.

DIAGNOSTIC STUDIES

Laboratory

Darkfield Examination.   For *T. pallidum,* which can be found in exudate from skin lesions or aspirates from lymph nodes. Care should be taken in collecting the specimen owing to changes in motility of the spirochete and infectiousness. This test is useful in diagnosing primary and secondary syphilis.

Fluorescent Treponemal Antibody (FTA) Test.   The tagged spirochetes will fluoresce.

FTA Absorption-Tagged Spirochetes (ABS) Test.   The tagged spirochetes will fluoresce. This test helps differentiate false positives from true syphilis. It is also useful in making a laboratory diagnosis of syphilis in the late stages of disease when results of nontrepononemal serologic tests are negative. This test is positive in primary and secondary syphilis. Positive result may revert to negative with adequate therapy. False positives may be found in systemic lupus erythematosus (SLE) and Lyme disease.

Microhemagglutination Assay.   For antibodies to *T. pallidum.*

Venereal Disease Research Laboratory (VDRL) Test.   The most widely used screening test. It is a microflocculation test that quantitatively tests for Wassermann antibody (reagin) based on titrations of diluted serum. It generally is positive 1 to 3 weeks after a primary lesion appears and is positive in secondary syphilis.

Rapid Plasma Reagin (RPR) Test.   Useful as a screening test and can be performed more easily than the VDRL test. It tests for Wassermann antibody (reagin) and is reported as positive or negative. Both the VDRL and RPR tests are used to assess adequacy of therapy.

Cerebrospinal Fluid (CSF) Examination. Recommended in secondary, latent, and tertiary syphilis. Neurosyphilis is characterized by increase in protein, increase in the number of lymphocytes, and a positive result on a CSF VDRL test. *Note:* The CSF VDRL result can be falsely negative in the patient with neurosyphilis. False-positive results on a CSF VDRL test are rare.

Radiology. Not applicable.
Other. Not applicable.

DIFFERENTIAL DIAGNOSIS

Traumatic. Not applicable.

Infectious

Lymphogranuloma venereum may appear as a small painless ulcer on the genitalia that can heal quickly in the primary stage. The patient will have a tender inguinal lymphadenopathy. Test for *Chlamydia trachomatis* by indirect fluorescent antibody titer.

Genital herpes manifests with vesicular lesions on an erythematous base on the penis, vulva, perineum, buttocks, cervix, or vagina. Culture for herpes simplex virus and look for multinucleated giant cells on Tzanck smear.

Chancroid initial lesion breaks down to a painful soft ulcer with necrotic base; may be multiple, with inguinal lymph node involvement. Positive culture for *Haemophilus ducreyi*. Patient also may have fever, chills, and malaise. Patient will have negative syphilis serology. May be confused with the chancre of primary syphilis.

In *pityriasis rosea*, fawn-colored scaly macules, pruritic, distribution along cleavage lines of trunk and proximal portions of extremities. Variants may affect axillae and groin. May mimic rash of secondary syphilis. Negative syphilis serology.

Metabolic. Not applicable
Neoplastic. With *neoplasms* of skin, liver, lung, stomach, or brain, primary occurrence, with a negative syphilis serology.
Vascular. Not applicable.
Congenital. Not applicable.
Acquired. With *drug eruptions*, the rash may mimic rash of secondary syphilis.

TREATMENT

The drug of choice for the treatment of syphilis is penicillin. Skin testing with desensitization should be done, if possible, in the penicillin-allergic patient.

Primary/Secondary/Early Latent Syphilis

Definitive therapy:

Benzathine penicillin G, 2.4 million U IM in a single dose

Alternate therapy for penicillin-allergic nonpregnant patient:

Doxycyline 100 mg PO twice a day for 2 weeks OR

Tetracycline 500 mg PO four times a day for 2 weeks OR

Erythromycin 500 mg PO four times a day for 2 weeks OR

Ceftriaxone 1 g IM or IV daily for 8 to 10 days OR

Azithromycin 2 g PO in a single dose

Therapeutic regimens other than penicillin have not been well studied. Therefore, when erythromycin, ceftriaxone, or azithromycin is used for treatment, careful follow-up is absolutely necessary to determine the efficacy of therapy.

Follow-up. At 3, 6, 12, and 24 months after therapy, a quantitative VDRL test should be performed. Adequate therapy is achieved if there is a fourfold drop in the titer at 6 months in primary, secondary, and early latent syphilis. Reinstitute treatment and test for HIV if clinical signs persist or recur, if there is a fourfold increase in the titer, or if there is a failure of an initially high titer to decrease fourfold. Some experts also recommend CSF examination.

Late Latent Syphilis/Tertiary Syphilis
(Non-Neurosyphilis)

Definitive therapy:

Benzathine penicillin G 7.2 million U total given in a dose of 2.4 million U IM every week for 3 weeks

Alternative therapy for penicillin-allergic nonpregnant patient:

Doxycycline 100 mg PO twice a day for 4 weeks OR

Tetracycline 500 mg PO four times a day for 4 weeks

Follow-up. Retest at 6, 12, and 24 months. Retreat for latent syphilis and examine CSF for signs of neurosyphilis if titers increase fourfold, if initial titer does not decrease fourfold within 12 to 24 months, or if patient has symptoms or signs of syphilis.

Indications for lumbar puncture include neurologic or ophthalmic signs or symptoms, treatment failure, serum nontreponemal antibody titer of 1:32 or greater, other evidence of active syphilis (aortitis, gumma, iritis), use of regimens other than penicillin for initial treatment, or positive assay for HIV. If CSF is abnormal or neurologic signs are present, treat for neurosyphilis. Consult with infectious disease specialist for symptomatic late syphilis.

Neurosyphilis

Definitive therapy:

Aqueous crystalline penicillin G 18 million–24 million U daily given as 3 million–4 million U every 4 hours, or as continuous infusion, IV for 10 to 14 days

Some authorities also recommend:

Benzathine penicillin G 2.4 million U IM weekly for 3 weeks follow-
ing intravenous therapy
Alternative therapy (if compliance is assured):
Procaine penicillin 2.4 million U IM daily for 10 to 14 days
PLUS
Probenecid 500 mg PO four times a day for 10 to 14 days
Some authorities also recommend:
Benzathine penicillin G 2.4 million U intramuscularly weekly for 3
weeks following intravenous therapy

HIV Infection and Syphilis

Recommendations vary. Higher doses and longer periods of therapy may be
needed. Some experts advise CSF examination and treatment with neurosyphilis regimen for all stages; some use standard penicillin therapies.

Follow-up. Careful follow-up evaluation at 1, 2, 3, 6, 9, and 12 months.
Reinfection is not uncommon. Rise or failure of titer to decrease fourfold at
6 months should elicit CSF examination and retreatment.

PEDIATRIC CONSIDERATIONS

Congenital syphilis is transmitted transplacentally to infants in mothers who
have not been treated or who have been inadequately treated. All infants
born to mothers who have reactive nontreponemal and treponemal tests
should be evaluated with a quantitative nontreponemal test performed on
infant serum (cord blood can have maternal contamination). Pathologic
examination of the placenta and umbilical cord should be performed.
Symptoms and signs include a serous nasal discharge, mucous membrane
patches, maculopapular rash, condylomata, hepatosplenomegaly, anemia,
and abnormal bone radiographs. Potential sequelae of untreated disease
include Hutchinson teeth, saddle nose, saber shins, deafness, and central
nervous system involvement. Careful follow-up evaluation by a pediatric
infectious disease specialist is required.

For management of children who are identified as having reactive serum
after the neonatal period (at 1 month of age or older), maternal serology and
records should be reviewed to assess whether the child has congenital or
acquired syphilis. Any at-risk child should have an evaluation including CSF
examination, complete blood count, chemistries, hearing and funduscopic
exam, and radiographs as indicated.

OBSTETRIC CONSIDERATIONS

Patients should receive the same penicillin therapy regimen as for a nonpregnant patient. Tetracycline and doxycycline are contraindicated in pregnancy. Erythromycin is not indicated because of risk of failure to cure the
fetus. Women treated in the second half of pregnancy are at risk for premature labor and/or fetal distress if Jarisch-Herxheimer reaction occurs.

Jarisch-Herxheimer reaction is a systemic reaction that can occur 1 to 2 hours after treatment with effective antibiotics (penicillin). Patients present with an abrupt onset of fever, chills, myalgias, headache, tachycardia, hyperventilation, vasodilatation, flushing, and mild hypotension. It is more commonly encountered in secondary syphilis but can occur during any stage. The reaction usually lasts 12 to 24 hours. Patients should be advised of the risk of reaction prior to institution of antibiotic therapy. Patient should seek medical attention if change in fetal movements is noted or contractions occur and have follow-up evaluation every month. Observe for antibody response expected in a nonpregnant patient.

GERIATRIC CONSIDERATIONS

No dosage adjustments are made for the geriatric population. The primary problem may be one of diagnosis. It is common for elderly patients to present with late complications of syphilis, and it is often difficult to differentiate them from those caused by other diseases of aging, particularly in the setting of low peripheral RPR titers and negative CSF VDRL test results.

PREVENTIVE CONSIDERATIONS

Barrier method of birth control is preferred for disease prevention.

Postexposure prophylaxis for occupational or sexual contact is not recommended. Close follow-up with periodic testing is recommended.

PEARLS FOR THE PA

Because the ulcers of primary syphilis may be atypical in appearance, any genital or oral lesion in a sexually active patient should be suspected to represent primary syphilis.

Syphilis should always be considered in the differential diagnosis for any clinical skin rash in the sexually active patient.

Central nervous system disease can appear during any stage of syphilis.

Any abnormal neurologic finding warrants a CSF examination.

All patients with syphilis should receive counseling about the risks of HIV infection and be encouraged to be tested for HIV.

Tuberculosis

Katharine Breaux, MPAS, BS, PA-C

DEFINITION

A chronic infectious disease caused primarily by *Mycobacterium tuberculosis*, transmitted through inhalation of aerosolized droplets and manifested as latent or active infection, generally in high-prevalence or high-risk groups.

HISTORY

Symptoms

Latent Disease
Generally asymptomatic.

Active Disease
Pulmonary symptoms may include fever, cough that is initially nonproductive followed by negligible mucopurulent sputum production, drenching night sweats, chills, hemoptysis, anorexia, weight loss.

Extrapulmonary symptoms vary with the clinical presentation and are listed in order of decreasing occurrence: lymphatic, pleural, skeletal, miliary or disseminated, renal, meningeal, peritoneal, and pericardial pain that is retrosternal and left precordial in location (see Physical Examination).

Less common presentations involve the following systems: gastrointestinal, genital, ocular, endobronchial, laryngeal, otic, and cutaneous (see Physical Examination).

In miliary or disseminated disease, symptoms and signs may include fever, night sweats, weight loss, fatigue, weakness, or any other accompanying pulmonary or extrapulmonary symptomatology.

General. Latent infections may progress to active infection in areas with high prevalence. Active infections are associated with chronic wasting and a general deterioration in health.

Age. Children, adults of all ages.

Onset. Latent infections begin at the time of exposure to active infection. Active infections may be insidious or acute.

Duration
Latent Disease. The patient may be infected for years.
Active Disease. Symptoms may abate as early as 2 weeks after initiation of treatment and/or cultures convert from positive to negative.

Intensity
Latent Disease. Mild.

Active Disease.   Varies, ranging from mild to severe with the clinical presentation.

Aggravating Factors.   Stress, debilitation, malnutrition (e.g., after gastric resection), substance abuse, immunosuppression, concomitant use of steroids, renal dialysis, silicosis, malignancies, major trauma, diabetes mellitus, early postpartum state.

Alleviating Factors

Latent Disease.   Systematic screening of high-risk groups, adequate ventilation of congregate living areas with high-risk groups.

Active Disease.   Early and appropriate therapy to reduce transmission, adequate ventilation in congregate living settings, masking of patients in the active disease phase, ultraviolet lighting where patients are treated, use of high-efficiency particulate air filters with administration of inhaled pentamidine to HIV-infected patients.

Associated Factors

Latent Disease.   Residence in a high-prevalence area, being in a high-risk group, occupational exposure to active disease.

Active Disease.   Congregate living settings such as prisons, homeless shelters, nursing homes; lack of native resistance.

PHYSICAL EXAMINATION

General

Latent Disease
Examination findings are normal.

Active Disease
The patient may have a wasted appearance; fever with temperatures greater than 100° F (37.8° C), fatigue, and night sweats.

Miliary or disseminated disease: Night sweats, fatigue, weakness, or any other accompanying pulmonary or extrapulmonary symptomatology.

Cardiovascular.   Pericardial friction rub and, if a constrictive pleural effusion is present, dyspnea, orthopnea, paroxysmal nocturnal dyspnea, pulsus paradoxus, pedal edema, and retrosternal and left precordial pain.

Dermatologic.   Lupus vulgaris, erythema nodosum, papulonecrotic lesions (tuberculids), any nodular or ulcerating lesion.

Gastrointestinal.   Guaiac-positive or grossly bloody stool, alternating diarrhea and constipation, anorexia, rectal ulcer, anal fistula/fissures (anorectal or perirectal abscess), jaundice, hepatomegaly, abdominal distention and/or tenderness with a palpable mass, doughy abdomen, ascites. Splenomegaly may be present in miliary or disseminated disease.

Genitourinary. May have abdominal tenderness. Tender scrotal mass with possibly a draining sinus, prostatic nodularity, or epididymal nodularity, prostatitis, epididymitis in the male; pelvic inflammatory disease, ectopic pregnancy, abnormal menstruation, and inflammation of the fallopian tubes in the female. May cause sterility in females.

Head, Eyes, Ears, Nose, Throat. Reddened conjunctivae, blurred vision, decreased visual acuity, photosensitivity. Laryngeal hoarseness and occasionally nonhealing ulcers of the tongue, oropharynx, tonsils, or epiglottis. Otorrhea, perforation of tympanic membranes, painless ear drainage, hearing deficit, facial nerve paralysis, dysphagia, odynophagia.

Lymphatic. Firm, tender (primarily cervical or supraclavicular) nodes at onset, with progression to draining lesions; with mesenteric involvement, abdominal tenderness, palpable mass.

Musculoskeletal. Painful range of motion in the weight-bearing joints (hip, knee) and, to a lesser degree, the ankle, elbow, wrist (carpal tunnel syndrome), and shoulder; with Pott's disease (thoracic spine), gibbous deformity of the spine, paralysis of the lower extremities (with neurologic compression), spinal abscess.

Neurologic. Altered mental status, headaches, lethargy, focal deficits, stupor that can progress to coma, dense paralysis, seizures, cranial nerve palsies and, less frequently, ataxia, uncontrollable movements of one lateral half of the body (hemiballismus), or decerebrate rigidity. Meningeal signs such as nuchal rigidity.

Ophthalmologic. Keratitis, chorioretinitis, uveitis, conjunctivitis, photosensitivity, decreased visual acuity.

Pulmonary. Dyspnea or pleuritic chest pain. Cough and hemoptysis. Auscultation reveals post-tussive rales in the apical posterior lung fields, distant hollow breath sounds with cavitary disease, wheeze, or friction rub. Dullness to percussion with advanced apical disease or with pleural effusion.

Renal. Flank or suprapubic tenderness, urinary frequency, dysuria, hematuria.

PATHOPHYSIOLOGY

Latent Infection

Invasion of a body site by inhaled acid-fast tubercle bacilli results in inflammation; subsequently, the tubercle bacilli are ingested by macrophages and transported to the lymphatic system (primarily regional lymph nodes). Tubercle bacilli continue to multiply, and the host develops hypersensitivity. Lymphocytes and monocytes enter the infection site and release substances that retain macrophages. Macrophages are stimulated and organized into granulomatous lesions that undergo soft tissue necrosis (caseation) followed by fibrosis, encapsulation, calcification, and scarring. Further transmission is contained in persons with normal immune function. Organisms may lie dormant indefinitely and retain the potential to reactivate if host defenses are weakened.

Active Infection
Invasion occurs in the same manner as with latent infection, but the immunocompromised host is unable to contain the spread of infection, and clinical disease develops.

DIAGNOSTIC STUDIES

Laboratory
Site-Specific Smear, Culture, and Sensitivity Testing (Sputum, Urine, Body Fluid, or Tissue).   For niacin-negative acid-fast bacilli (AFB).

Serodiagnosis.   By ELISA, polymerase chain reaction (PCR) assay, and *M. tuberculosis*–specific DNA or RNA probes applied to appropriate cultures.

Complete Blood Count.   Normochromic, normocytic anemia; occasional leukocytosis with cell counts up to 15,000/mm^3. A leukemoid reaction may occur in miliary or disseminated infections.

Serum Chemistry.   Hypoalbuminemia, hypergammaglobulinemia, hypercalcemia, abnormal liver function tests, hyponatremia.

Pleural Fluid.   Exudative fluid with increased lymphocytes, total protein greater than 3.0 g/dL, pH ranging from 7.0 to 7.3, elevated adenosine deaminase (not routinely done).

Urinalysis.   Hematuria, pyuria, and albuminuria with sterile urine cultures.

Cerebrospinal Fluid (CSF).   Increased protein, decreased glucose, and up to several hundred leukocytes (predominantly lymphocytes). Serial lumbar punctures should be performed when there is a high index of clinical suspicion.

Peritoneal Fluid.   High total protein and leukocytes (predominantly lymphocytes) in ascitic fluid.

Pericardial Fluid.   Exudative.

Gastrointestinal Tissue.   Hyperplastic or ulcerative.

Semen Sample.   Oligospermia.

Radiology
Chest Film.   Apical infiltrates and cavitary lesions are present in 25% of the cases, diffuse pulmonary infiltrates in 50%, mediastinal and hilar adenopathy in 5% to 30%, isolated middle or lower lobe infiltrates in 20% to 30%. Widened mediastinum, pericardial constriction, pericardial calcifications, atelectasis, calcified lymphatic lesions in neck and axilla, and pleural effusion may be seen, generally unilaterally. In miliary or disseminated disease, uniform small nodular (millet seed) infiltrates may be identified.

Skeletal Radiography.   Joint-specific soft tissue swelling, osteoporosis, bone and cartilage destruction.

With Pott's disease, vertebral collapse and intervertebral bone destruction in the midthoracic spine and kyphosis without scoliosis.

Intravenous Pyelography. Caliceal blunting and caliceal-interstitial reflux; later, ureteral stricture, focal calcifications, hydronephrosis.

CT Scan or MRI of the Brain. Tuberculomas, basilar meningitis, cerebral infarction, and hydrocephalus.

Other

Site-Specific Histopathologic Studies. From biopsy specimens.

Bronchoscopy. Recommended only when a diagnosis of pulmonary tuberculosis cannot readily be established by sputum culture and when chest radiograph indicates lower lobe involvement with a decreased possibility of culturing the organism from sputum culture alone.

Bone Marrow Aspiration. Recommended in HIV-seropositive patients with fever who do not have evidence of other organ involvement.

Skin Testing. Tuberculin skin testing (Mantoux method) with 0.1 mL of purified protein derivative (PPD) is indicated to detect delayed hypersensitivity. The PPD is injected intradermally on the forearm. Positive reactions are levels of induration at 48 to 72 hours based on the following cutpoints:

- Greater than or equal to 5 mm in the immunosuppressed (HIV-infected, organ transplant recipients, corticosteroid users, diabetics, the malnourished), close contacts of persons with newly diagnosed active disease, persons with chest radiographs demonstrating fibrotic lesions suggestive of old, untreated tuberculosis
- Greater than or equal to 10 mm in foreign-born from high-prevalence areas (Haiti, Southeast Asia) immigrating to the United States within the preceding 5 years, medically underserved, low income inner city populations, homeless, intravenous drug users, residents of long-term care facilities, persons with medical risk factors (renal failure, carcinoma of the head, neck, and lung, lymphoma, leukemia, following gastrectomy or jejunoileal bypass), populations in areas of increased prevalence, age younger than 4 years, mycobacteriology personnel
- Greater than or equal to 15 mm in all others
- Other skin testing considerations: The following cutpoints apply to recent converters with a change in the size of the PPD reaction within 2 years
- In persons younger than 35 years of age: increase of 10 mm or more
- In persons older than 35 years of age: increase of 15 mm or more

False negatives can occur in critically ill patients, the aged, the immunosuppressed, alcoholics, and those with any fulminant infectious process. Improper reading of the skin test and problems with the tuberculin itself can also result in false negatives.

False positives can occur in patients who have infection due to other strains of *Mycobacterium* or who have received prior bacille Calmette-Guérin (BCG) vaccination, and as a result of the booster effect.

Inability to exhibit delayed hypersensitivity indicates anergy, but anergy testing has been found to have reliability problems, particularly in the areas of standardization of controls and reproducibility of results.

DIFFERENTIAL DIAGNOSIS

Traumatic.   Not applicable.

Infectious
Pyogenic lung abscess, mycotic lung infection, community-acquired pneumonia can be differentiated on basis of chest radiograph appearance and culture.

With *fever of unknown origin*, negative cultures for AFB.

With *HIV-related illness* such as *M. avium* or *M. intracellulare* infection, *Pneumocystis carinii* pneumonia (PCP), or wasting, positive HIV assay, negative AFB cultures.

In *bacterial infections of the urinary tract*, negative AFB cultures.

In *pyogenic* or *aseptic meningitis*, negative AFB cultures.

In *viral pericarditis* or *pyogenic infection*, negative AFB cultures.

Any infectious process resulting in *chronic debilitating constitutional symptoms* may be confused with miliary or disseminated tuberculosis.

Metabolic
In *granulomatous* and *connective tissue disease*, negative AFB cultures.

In *Crohn's disease*, positive history, negative AFB cultures.

Neoplastic
With *pulmonary* or *laryngeal malignancy*, positive biopsy, identification of primary tumor (in metastatic disease), negative AFB cultures.

Vascular.   Not applicable.
Congenital.   Not applicable.
Acquired.   In *alcoholic liver disease*, negative AFB cultures.

TREATMENT

See Tables 8-4 through 8-10. All antituberculosis drugs have potential toxicity, and baseline pretreatment laboratory workup should include a complete blood count, platelet count, uric acid, and renal and liver function tests. These tests should be monitored at regular intervals and drugs withheld, discontinued, or changed as appropriate. Potential toxicity is increased in persons 35 years of age and older, alcoholics, active intravenous drug users, and postpubescent black and Hispanic females.

PEDIATRIC CONSIDERATIONS

Infants have a greater risk of developing active disease when exposed and should receive prophylaxis if they have had close contact with an active case.

Tuberculin skin testing should be performed on a routine basis in children attending daycare centers and school.

Table 8–4. Antituberculosis Regimens for the Non–HIV-Infected: Latent Infection

Drug	Interval and Duration	Adult Dosage [max]
Isoniazid*	Daily for 9 mo†	5 mg/kg [300 mg]
	Biweekly for 9 mo†	15 mg/kg [900 mg]
Isoniazid*	Daily for 6 mo†	5 mg/kg [300 mg]
	Biweekly for 6 mo†	15 mg/kg [900 mg]
Rifampin PLUS	Daily for 2 mo	Rifampin 10 mg/kg [600 mg]
Pyrazinamide‡		Pyrazinamide 15-20 mg/kg [2.0 g]
Rifampin	Daily for 4 mo	10 mg/kg [600 mg]

Children: The only recommended treatment regimen for latent infection in children is isoniazid for 9 mo (10 mg/kg daily or 20-40 mg/kg biweekly via directly observed therapy).

*Pyridoxine (vitamin B_6) should be used (25 mg daily or 50 mg biweekly) with isoniazid in HIV-infected children, pregnant women, or persons with seizure disorders or conditions in which neuropathy is common (i.e., diabetes, uremia, alcoholism, malnutrition). Although pyridoxine intake in a healthy individual's normal diet should be adequate, the preference is to give pyridoxine to all patients on isoniazid.

†These regimens should be given by directly observed therapy.

‡Severe and even fatal liver injuries have been reported with this regimen. It is not recommended for patients on other potentially hepatotoxic drugs, alcoholics, or persons with a history of liver disease. Liver function tests should be measured at baseline and at 2, 4, and 6 wk of treatment. Treatment should be stopped permanently for AST >5× upper limit of normal, AST > normal with symptoms of hepatitis, bilirubin > normal.

AST, aspartate transaminase; HIV, human immunodeficiency virus; max, maximum dose.

OBSTETRIC CONSIDERATIONS

From 1% to 3% of pregnancies in the United States will be associated with tuberculosis. Tuberculosis does not affect the pregnancy course, although reactivation can occur during pregnancy in 5% to 10% of patients with prior tuberculous infection. Congenital tuberculosis occurs rarely; the infection is most often acquired at the time of delivery. Infants of untreated mothers should be immediately isolated from the mother and should receive isoniazid (isonicotinoylhydrazine [INH]) therapy or BCG vaccination. BCG vaccine should also be administered to infants of inadequately treated mothers. Antituberculosis prophylaxis can usually be deferred until after delivery in the asymptomatic patient who has a positive result on skin testing, even in HIV-positive patients. If the indications are strong for instituting prophylaxis prior to delivery, INH can be administered for 6 to 9 months starting after the first trimester.

Table 8–5. Antituberculosis Regimens for the Non–HIV-Infected: Active Infection

Drug	Daily Dose [max]	Biweekly Dose* [max]	Thrice-Weekly Dose* [max]
Initial Treatment Phase, Months 1-2			
Isoniazid	C: 10 mg/kg	C: 20-40 mg/kg	C: 20-40 mg/kg [900 mg]
PO, IM, IV	A: 300 mg [300 mg]	A: 15 mg/kg [900 mg]	A: 15 mg/kg [900 mg]
Rifampin	C: 10-20 mg/kg	C: 10-20 mg/kg	C: 10-20 mg/kg
PO, IV	A: 10 mg/kg [600mg]	A: 10 mg/kg [600 mg]	A: 10 mg/kg [600 mg]
Pyrazinamide	C: 20-30 mg/kg	C: 50-70 mg/kg	C: 50-70 mg/kg
PO	A: 25 mg/kg [2 g]	A: 50-70 mg/kg [4 g]	A: 50-70 mg/kg [3 g]
Ethambutol	C: 15-25 mg/kg	C: 50 mg/kg	C & A:† 25-30 mg/kg
PO	A:†15-25 mg/kg	A:†50 mg/kg	
Continuation Phase, Months 3-6			
Isoniazid	C: 10 mg/kg	C: 20-40 mg/kg	C: 20-40 mg/kg [900 mg]
PO, IM, IV	A: 300 mg [300 mg]	A: 15 mg/kg [900 mg]	A: 15 mg/kg [900 mg]
Rifampin	C: 10-20 mg/kg	C: 10-20 mg/kg	C: 10-20 mg/kg
PO, IV	A: 10 mg/kg [600 mg]	A: 10 mg/kg [600 mg]	A: 10 mg/kg [600 mg]
Pyrazinamide	C: 20-30 mg/kg	C: 50-70 mg/kg	C: 50-70 mg/kg
PO	A: 25 mg/kg [2 g]	A: 50-70 mg/kg [4 g]	A: 50-70 mg/kg [3 g]
Continue until laboratory results document susceptibility to INH and RIF and/or sputum is AFB negative.			
Ethambutol	C: 15-25 mg/kg	C: 50 mg/kg	C & A:†25-30 mg/kg
PO	A:†15-25 mg/kg	A:†50 mg/kg	

Continued

Table 8–5. Antituberculosis Regimens for the Non–HIV-Infected: Active Infection—cont'd

Drug	Daily Dose [max]	Biweekly Dose* [max]	Thrice-Weekly Dose* [max]
Continue until laboratory results document susceptibility to isoniazid and rifampin and/or sputum is acid fast bacillus negative.			
Continuation Phase, Months 7-9: for patients who are still culture positive at 2 mo and who are at high risk for relapse			
Isoniazid PO, IM, IV	C: 10 mg/kg A: 300 mg [300 mg]	C: 20-40 mg/kg A: 15 mg/kg [900 mg]	C: 20-40 mg/kg [900 mg] A: 15 mg/kg [900 mg]
Rifampin PO, IV	C: 10-20 mg/kg A: 10 mg/kg [600 mg]	C: 10-20 mg/kg A: 10 mg/kg [600 mg]	C: 10-20 mg/kg A: 10 mg/kg [600 mg]

*These regimens should be given by directly observed therapy only.

†Ethambutol dosing should be based on ideal body weight determined using the following formulas: *males*: 50 kg + 2.3(height in inches – 60); *females*: 45 kg + 2.3(height in inches – 60).

A, adult; C, child; max, maximum dose.

Table 8–6. Active Infection (Drug Resistance or Drug Intolerance)*

Drug	Daily Dose [max]
Streptomycin†: IM	**C:** 20-40 mg/kg **A:** 15 mg/kg [1 g]
Levofloxacin: PO	**A:** 750 mg
Ofloxacin: PO	**A:** 600-800 mg
Ciprofloxacin: PO	**A:** 750-1500 mg
Amikacin: IV, IM	**C:** 15-30 mg/kg **A:** 15 mg/kg
Kanamycin, Capreomycin: IM/IV	**C:** 15-30 mg/kg **A:** 15 mg/kg [1 g]
Ethionamide: PO	**C:** 15-20 mg/kg **A:** 500-1000 mg [1 g]
Cycloserine: PO	**C:** 15-20 mg/kg **A:** 150 mg/kg [1 g]
Para-aminosalicylic acid: PO	**C:** 150 mg/kg **A:** 150 mg/kg [12 g]
Clofazimine: PO	**C:** 50-200 mg **A:** 100-300 mg

*Substitution of any of these drugs for standard therapy should be made only after consultation with an expert in TB management. If drug-resistant tuberculosis is suspected, a four- to five-drug regimen should be used and reflect known local drug resistance patterns. The fifth drug used should be streptomycin. Final treatment regimen should be based on final sensitivity results

†First-line medication; can be substituted for ethambutol (EMB) in initial regimen.

max, maximum dose.

Special Considerations:

Meningeal or Miliary (Disseminated) Disease

1. Isoniazid (INH) and pyrazinamide (PZA) penetrate the blood-brain barrier, and cerebrospinal fluid concentrations parallel blood concentrations. Rifampin (RIF) is less effective, but all three drugs should be used. Corticosteroids may be used for adjunctive therapy in the first 6 wk and tapered appropriately in patients with neurologic deficits.

2. If INH or RIF cannot be used, two-drug therapy should continue for minimum of 18 mo *and* at least 12 mo after culture conversion. PZA should be substituted for whichever drug cannot be used.

3. Treatment should be continued for a minimum of 9 mo and at least 6 mo after culture conversion noted by three negative cultures.

Pregnant Women

INH plus EMB is considered first-line treatment. RIF may also be used in a 9-mo treatment regimen. Streptomycin (SM) should be avoided (as noted later) owing to the potential for ototoxicity in the fetus. There are insufficient data regarding the teratogenic potential of PZA for it to be used safely. Ethionamide has known teratogenic potential and should not be used.

Patients with Renal Disease

INH and RIF should be administered after dialysis with no dosage adjustment necessary. Dose adjustments should be made for EMB and PZA. SM should be avoided if possible.

Table 8–7. Antituberculosis Regimens for Persons Co-infected with HIV: Latent Infection*

Drug*	Interval and Duration
Isoniazid	Daily for 9 mo
Isoniazid	2 times/wk for 9 mo
Rifamycin and Pyrazinamide†	Daily for 2 mo

*See Table 8-10 regarding HIV medications.

†For patients with intolerance to pyrazinamide, some experts recommend the use of rifamycin or rifabutin alone for preventive treatment. Most experts agree that available data support the recommendation that this treatment can be administered for as short a duration as 4 mo, although some experts would treat for 6 mo.

HIV, human immunodeficiency virus.

GERIATRIC CONSIDERATIONS

Rates of tuberculosis are highest for people 65 years of age or older.

The primary presentation in 84% of affected elderly patients is pulmonary.

In large elder care facilities, an appropriate tuberculosis control and prevention program should be in place.

PREVENTIVE CONSIDERATIONS

Educational efforts should be directed toward inhabitants of poor urban areas, where tuberculosis occurs disproportionately among persons who are members of racial and ethnic minorities.

The management of contacts of patients with multiple drug–resistant tuberculosis should involve referral to a physician with expertise in tuberculous disease when treatment is indicated and should be determined by the susceptibility pattern of the source isolate.

Public health departments should remain at the forefront of training and education and be provided with adequate funding to accomplish this effectively.

The potential for nosocomial spread of infection must be taken seriously and appropriate measures (negative-pressure rooms, particulate respirator masks, ultraviolet irradiation of the air) implemented to prevent development of new cases.

Agents of choice for treatment of active tuberculosis in the pregnant patient are INH and ethambutol. If necessary, rifampin can also be given. Pyridoxine should be given to prevent peripheral neuritis if INH is used. Streptomycin, capreomycin, kanamycin, and cycloserine all should be avoided owing to potential fetal ototoxicity or central nervous system side effects.

Table 8–8. Antituberculosis Regimens for Persons Co-infected with HIV*: Active Infection

	Induction Phase		Continuation Phase	
Drug	Interval and Duration		Drug	Interval and Duration
INH, RFB, PZA	Daily for 2 mo (8 wk)		INH RBF	Daily or 2 times/wk for 4 mo (18 wk)
OR			OR	
INH RFB	Daily for 2 wk, then 2 times/wk for 9 mo		INH RFB	2 times/wk for 4 mo (18 wk)
Nine-month SM-based therapy† (may be prolonged‡ to 12 mo)				
INH, SM, PZA	Daily for 2 mo (8 wk)		INH, SM, PZA	2-3 times/wk for 7 mo (30 wk)
Six-month RIF-based therapy (may be prolonged§ to 9 mo)				
INH, RIF‖ PZA,¶ EMB¶ (or SM)	Daily for 2 mo (8 wk)		INH RIF	Daily or 2-3 times/wk for 4 mo (18 wk)
OR			OR	
INH, RIF, PZA,¶	Daily for 2 wk, then 2-3 times/wk for 6 wk		INH RIF	2-3 times/wk for 4 mo (18 wk)

Continued

Table 8–8. Antituberculosis Regimens for Persons Co-infected with HIV*: Active Infection—cont'd

	Induction Phase		Continuation Phase	
Drug	Interval and Duration		Drug	Interval and Duration
EMB‖ (or SM) OR INH, RIF, PZA, EMB (or SM)	3 times/wk for 2 mo (8 wk)		OR INH, RIF, PZA, EMB	3 times/wk for 4 mo (18 wk)

*See Table 8-10 for considerations regarding HIV medications.

†SM is contraindicated for pregnant women.

‡Every effort should be made to continue administering SM for the total duration of treatment. When SM is not used for the recommended 9 mo, EMB should be added to the regimen and the treatment duration should be prolonged from 9 mo (38 wk) to 12 mo (52 wk).

§Duration of therapy should be prolonged for patients with delayed response to therapy. Criteria for delayed response should be assessed at the end of the 2-mo induction phase and include (a) lack of conversion of the *Mycobacterium tuberculosis* culture from positive to negative and (b) lack or resolution or progression of signs or symptoms of tuberculosis.

‖Continue PZA and EMB for the total duration of the induction phase (8 wk).

¶Continue PZA for the total duration of the induction phase (8 wk). EMB can be stopped after susceptibility test results indicate *Mycobacterium tuberculosis* susceptibility to INH and RIF.

EMB, ethambutol; INH, isoniazid; PZA, pyrazinamide; RFB, rifabutin; RIF, rifampin; SM, streptomycin.

Table 8–9. Antituberculosis Medications

Drug	Daily Dose [max]	Biweekly Dose [max]*	Thrice-Weekly Dose [max]*	Administration Route
IHN	C: 10-20 mg/kg A: 5 mg/kg [300 mg]	C: 20-40 mg/kg A: 15 mg/kg [900 mg]	C: 20-40 mg/kg A: 15 mg/kg [900 mg]	PO or IM
RIF†	C: 10-20 mg/kg A: 10 mg/kg [600 mg]	C: 10-20 mg/kg A: 10 mg/kg [600 mg]	C: 10-20 mg/kg A: 10 mg/kg [600 mg]	PO or IV
OR				
RFB†	C: 10-20 mg/kg A: 5 mg/kg [300 mg] OR C&A: NA†[150 mg] OR C&A: NA†[450 mg]	C: 10-20 mg/kg A: 5 mg/kg [300 mg] OR C: 10-20 mg/kg† A: 5† OR C&A: NA†[450 MG]	C&A: Not known OR C&A: Not known [300 mg] OR C&A: Not known	PO or IV
PZA	C&A 15-30 mg/kg [2.0 g]	C&A: 50-70 mg/kg [3.5 g]	C&A: 50-70 mg/kg [2.5 g]	PO
EMB	C&A: 15-25 mg/kg [1600 mg]	C&A: 50 mg/kg [4000 mg]	C&A: 25-30 mg/kg [2000 mg]	PO
SM‡	C: 20-40 mg/kg A: 15 mg/kg [1 g]	C&A: 25-30 mg/kg [1.5 g]	C&A: 25-30 mg/kg [1.5 g]	IM/IV

*All intermittent dosing should be administered with directly observed therapy.

†Not applicable. See Table 8-10 regarding HIV medications.

‡Maximum dose for patients 60 years of age or older is limited to 10 mg/kg [750 mg].

A, adult; **C**, child; EMB, ethambutol; INH, isoniazid; max, maximum dose; PZA, pyrazinamide; RFB, rifabutin; RIF, rifampin; SM, streptomycin.

Table 8–10. Recommendations for Coadministering Selected Antiretroviral (Anti-HIV) Drugs with the Antimycobacterials Rifabutin and Rifampin

Antiretroviral*	Use in combination with rifabutin	Use in combination with rifampin	Comments
Saquinavir* Hard-gel capsules (HGC)	Possibly,† if antiretroviral regimen also inclues ritonavir	Possibly, if antiretroviral regimen also includes ritonavir	Coadministration of saquinavir SGC with usual-dose rifabutin (300 mg daily or 2-3 ×/wk) is a possibility. However, the pharmacokinetic data and clinical experience for this combination are limited.
Soft-gel capsules (SGC)	Probably‡	Possibly, if antiretroviral regimen also inludes ritonavir	The combination of saquinavir SGC or saquinavir HGC and ritonavir, coadministered with (1) usual-dose rifampin (600 mg daily or 2-3 ×/wk), or (2) reduced-dose rifabutin (150 mg 2-3 ×/wk) is a possibility. However, the pharmacokinetic data and clinical experience for these combinations are limited. Coadministration of saquinavir HCG or saquinavir SGC with rifampin (in the absence of ritonavir) is not recommended because rifampin markedly decreases concentrations of saquinavir.
Ritonavir	Probably	Probably	If the combination of ritonavir and rifabutin is used, then a substantially reduced-dose rifabutin regimen (150 mg 2-3 ×/wk) is recommended. Coadministration of ritonavir with usual-dose rifampin (600 mg daily or 2-3 ×/wk) is a possibility, though pharmacokinetic data and clinical experience are limited.
Indinavir	Yes	No	There is limited, but favorable, clinical experience with coadministration of indinavir§ with a reduced daily dose of rifabutin (150 mg) or with the usual dose of rifabutin (300 mg 2-3 ×/wk). Coadministration of indinavir with rifampin is not recommended because rifampin markedly decreases concentrations of indinavir.
Nelfinavir	Yes	No	There is limited, but favorable, clinical experience with coadministration of nelfinavir∥ with a reduced daily dose of rifabutin (150 mg) or with the usual dose of rifabutin (300 mg 2-3 ×/wk).

Amprenavir	Yes	No	Coadministration of nelfinavir with rifampin is not recommended because rifampin markedly decreases concentrations of nelfinavir. Coadministration of amprenavir with a reduced daily dose of rifabutin (150 mg) or with the usual dose of rifabutin (300 mg 2-3 ×/wk) is a possibility, but there is no published clinical experience. Coadministration of amprenavir with rifampin is not recommended because rifampin markedly decreases concentrations of amprenavir.
Nevirapine	Yes	Possibly	Coadministration of nevirapine with usual-dose rifabutin (300 mg qd or 2-3 ×/wk) is a possibility based on pharmacokinetic study data. However, there is no published clinical experience for this combination. Data are insufficient to assess whether dose adjustments are necessary when rifampin is coadministered with nevirapine. Therefore, rifampin and nevirapine should be used in combination only if clearly indicated and with careful monitoring.
Delavirdine	No	No	Contraindicated because of the marked decrease in concentrations of delavirdine when administered with either rifabutin or rifampin.
Efavirenz	Probably	Probably	Coadministration of efavirenz with increased-dose rifabutin (450 or 600 mg qd or 600 mg 2-3 ×/wk) is a possibility, although there is no published clinical experience. Coadministration of efavirenz¶ with usual-dose rifampin (600 mg qd or 2-3 ×/wk) is a possibility, although there is no published clinical experience.

*Usual recommended doses are 400 mg two times a day for each of these protease inhibitors and 400 mg of ritonavir.

†Despite limited data and clinical experience, the use of this combination is potentially successful.

‡Based on available data and clinical experience, the successful use of this combination is likely.

§Usual recommended dose is 800 mg every 8 hours. Some experts recommend increasing the indinavir dose to 1000 mg every 8 hours if indinavir is used in combination with rifabutin.

‖Usual recommended dose is 750 mg three times a day or 1250 mg twice daily. Some experts recommend increasing the nelfinavir dose to 1000 mg if the three-times-a-day dosing is used and nelfinavir is used in combination with rifabutin.

¶Usual recommended dose is 600 mg daily. Some experts recommend increasing the efavirenz dose to 800 mg daily if efavirenz is used in combination with rifampin.

HIV, human immunodeficiency virus.

PEARLS FOR THE PA

Anyone with latent or active tuberculosis should receive HIV testing and counseling.

Empirical treatment with multidrug regimens for suspected active tuberculosis should be initiated early and continued until culture results are available.

Directly observed therapy (DOT) is the method of choice for treatment of active tuberculosis. DOT should also be considered for treatment of latent tuberculosis in persons at high risk for noncompliance.

As chemotherapy for tuberculosis expands, a careful review of all drugs a patient is taking for comorbid conditions should be performed to reduce the risk of serious drug interactions.

The single etiologic agent responsible for most deaths worldwide is Mycobacterium tuberculosis.

Further Reading

American Thoracic Society and Centers for Disease Control and Prevention: Diagnostic standards and classification of tuberculosis in adults and children. Am J Respir Crit Care Med 161:1376-1395, 2000.

Braunwald E, Fauci AS, Kasper DL, et al (eds): Harrison's Principles of Internal Medicine, 15th ed. New York, McGraw-Hill, 2001.

Centers for Disease Control: Screening for tuberculosis and tuberculous infection in high-risk populations and the use of preventive therapy for tuberculous infection in the United States: Recommendations of the Advisory Committee for Elimination of Tuberculosis. MMWR 39(RR-8):1-12, 1990.

Centers for Disease Control and Prevention: Prevention and treatment of tuberculosis among patients infected with human immunodeficiency virus: Principles of therapy and revised recommendations. MMWR 47(RR-20):1-51, 1998.

Centers for Disease Control and Prevention: Update: Fatal and severe liver injuries associated with rifampin and pyrazinamide for latent tuberculosis infection and revisions in American Thoracic Society/CDC recommendations—United States 2001. MMWR 50(RR-34):733-735, 2001.

Centers for Disease Control and Prevention: Progressing Toward Tuberculosis Elimination in Low-Incidence Areas of the United States: Recommendations of the Advisory Council for the Elimination of Tuberculosis. MMWR Recomm Rep 51 (RR-5):19-20, 2002.

Georgia Division of Public Health and the Atlanta TB Prevention Coalition: Georgia TB Reference Guide. Available at http://www.ph.dhr.state.ga.us/epi/manuals/tbguide

Goldman L, Ausiello D (eds): Cecil Textbook of Medicine, 22nd ed. Philadelphia, Saunders, 2004.

Guidelines for the Use of Antiretroviral Agents in HIV-Infected Adults and Adolescents. U.S. Department of Health and Human Services and the Henry J. Keiser Family Foundation, Feb 4, 2002.

Guidelines for the Use of Antiretroviral Agents in Pediatric Infection. National Pediatric and Family HIV Resource Center, Health Resources and Services Administration, and the National Institutes of Health, Dec 14, 2001.

Haas W: *Mycobacterium tuberculosis. In* Mandell GL, Bennett JE, Dolin R (eds): Principles and Practice of Infectious Diseases, 5th ed. Philadelphia, Churchill Livingstone, 2000.

Labus JB, Lauber AA: Patient Education and Preventive Medicine. Philadelphia, WB Saunders, 2001.

Mandell GL, Douglas RG Jr, Bennett JE (eds): Principles and Practice of Infectious Disease, 5th ed. New York, Churchill Livingstone, 2000.

Tierney LM Jr, McPhee SJ, Papadakis MA: Current Medical Diagnosis and Treatment. New York, McGraw-Hill, 2003.

Updated US Public Health Service Guidelines for the Management of Occupational Exposures to HBV, HCV, and HIV and Recommendations for Postexposure Prophylaxis. MMWR 50(RR-11), 2001.

NEPHROLOGY

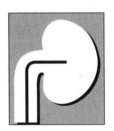

9

Acid-Base Disturbances

Sandra Lynn Roberts, MMSc, PA-C

DEFINITION

Under certain clinical conditions, there may be a generation of excess acid or base in the body that may result in a medical emergency. *Acidosis* is a state in which there is a net accumulation of acid that may result in acidemia (blood pH less than 7.36). *Alkalosis* is a state in which there is a net accumulation of base that may result in alkalemia (blood pH greater than 7.44).

Both acidosis and alkalosis can be divided into respiratory and metabolic causes. Metabolic acidosis can be further divided into anion gap and non-gap (hyperchloremic) forms.

The kidney plays a major role in maintaining hydrogen ion homeostasis through various mechanisms, including reabsorbing and regenerating acid-buffering agents. With kidney disease, these mechanisms can be impaired, resulting in varying degrees of metabolic acidosis (e.g., acid retention or bicarbonate wasting).

HISTORY

Symptoms
Acidosis.   Nausea, vomiting, diarrhea, rapid (Kussmaul) respirations.
Alkalosis.   Nausea, vomiting, and mental status depression.

General
Acidosis.   The patient may have a history of diabetes, trauma, or ingestion of ethylene glycol, methanol, high-dose aspirin, or paraldehyde. Ascertain a history of kidney failure, prior episode of acidosis, failure to take prescribed medications (e.g., insulin); assess for central nervous system changes, blurred vision, abdominal pain, malaise (with methanol or ethylene glycol ingestion), or tinnitus (with ingestion of salicylates).

Alkalosis.   The patient may have a history of ingestion of bicarbonate, diuretic use, hypokalemia, dehydration, muscle cramps, licorice consumption (the glycyrrhizic acid found in licorice acts as a mineralocorticoid, and high levels can cause an alkalosis), steroid intake, and cardiac arrhythmias.

Age.   Any.
Onset.   Gradual to acute.
Duration.   Acute with short or prolonged duration.
Intensity.   Clinically inapparent to life-threatening.

Aggravating Factors
Acidosis.   Ingestion of drugs that cause acidosis or worsening of the underlying cause (e.g., worsening kidney/pulmonary function).

Alkalosis.   Continued diuretic use, hypokalemia, vomiting, excess mineralocorticoid from adrenal tumors or adrenocorticotropic hormone (ACTH)-producing tumors, high-renin states (such as renal artery stenosis), and correction of hypercapnia.

Alleviating Factors.   Correction of the underlying factors.

Associated Factors.   Respiratory alkalosis or acidosis can exist in combination with metabolic alkalosis or acidosis. It is common to find a compensatory change in respiratory pattern directed at minimizing the effect of the metabolic process and keeping the pH near normal (e.g., a patient may hyperventilate to compensate for a metabolic acidosis).

PHYSICAL EXAMINATION

General.   The patient may be in acute distress or appear quite normal. Clinical presentation will be determined by the severity of acidemia or alkalemia and underlying medical disorders.

Cardiovascular
Acidosis.   The patient may have hypotension, cardiovascular decompensation, and tachycardia.

Alkalosis.   The patient may experience cardiovascular collapse with a very high pH.

Gastrointestinal
Acidosis.   Abdominal tenderness.

Neurologic
Acidosis.   Patients with certain ingestions (e.g., ethylene glycol) may have stupor, slurred speech, or coma progressing to heart failure.

Alkalosis.   Manifestations of neuromuscular irritability such as tetany, muscle cramps, and depressed central nervous system function are associated with respiratory alkalosis.

Ophthalmologic
Acidosis.   Methanol may cause hyperemia of optic disc and retinal edema that can progress to fixed pupils.

Pulmonary
Acidosis.   Kussmaul respiration (rapid deep breathing). Fruity breath noted with diabetic ketosis.

Alkalosis.   Low respiratory rate.

Renal
Acidosis.   Costovertebral angle tenderness may be noted with acute renal failure; urinary bladder may be distended.

Skin
Acidosis. Patients with toxic ingestions (e.g., ethylene glycol) may be cyanotic.

PATHOPHYSIOLOGY

Acidosis: Metabolic
Metabolic acidosis can generally be divided into gap acidosis and nongap (hyperchloremic) acidosis.

Gap acidosis can occur when unmeasured anions increase in the serum, causing a drop in the concentration of bicarbonate (HCO_3). The normal anion gap (the difference between measured and unmeasured anion concentrations) is approximately 12 mEq/L (anion gap = $Na^+ - [HCO_3^- + Cl^-]$). This normal gap is due to phosphates, proteins, and sulfates normally present in serum but not measured in the electrolytes. The gap may increase as a result of increased amounts of these acidic substances; this can occur in only a few clinical states: ketoacidosis, lactic acidosis, renal failure (due to inability to excrete sulfates or phosphates), and ingestion of drugs such as methanol, ethylene glycol, salicylates, and paraldehyde. An easy mnemonic is MUDPILES, for Methanol, Uremia, Diabetes, Paraldehyde, Ingestants, Lactic acidosis, Ethylene glycol, Salicylates.

Nongap acidosis results when an elevation in chloride occurs with a drop in bicarbonate, causing acidosis but without an increase in the gap. Causes for nongap (hyperchloremic) acidosis include drugs (acidifying salts in hyperalimentation, acetazolamide), gastrointestinal causes (diarrhea, uterosigmoidostomy), low plasma aldosterone, and renal causes (interstitial nephritis, proximal/distal renal tubular acidosis resulting from tubular secretory defect secondary to resistance to effects of aldosterone). Essentially, the underlying problem is either retention of hydrochloric acid (HCl) or loss of HCO_3, resulting in acidosis.

Alkalosis
Alkalosis can be classified according to whether the cause is generation or maintenance of elevated HCO_3. *Generating* causes include loss of acid (upper gastrointestinal losses with vomiting, renal losses), HCO_3 addition (with intravenous or oral administration of sodium bicarbonate [Na^+ HCO_3]), contraction (contraction prevents the kidney from being able to excrete HCO_3 and by stimulating renin/aldosterone, thus generating new HCO_3), and posthypercapnia (in patients who have a compensatory increase in HCO_3 in response to chronic respiratory acidosis).

Maintenance causes include volume contraction (increased proximal tubule reabsorption of HCO_3 and inability to excrete HCO_3), decreased serum chloride (usually same as in contraction), increased Pco_2, excess mineralocorticoid, and persistent hypokalemia.

Another type of classification for metabolic alkalosis is that of chloride-responsive (occurring with vomiting, diuretics, correction of hypercapnia, or volume contraction) versus chloride-resistant metabolic alkalosis (due to excess mineralocorticoid, Cushing's disease, licorice, potassium depletion, or Bartter syndrome), versus other causes such as milk-alkali syndrome, alkali load, or large doses of penicillin or carbenicillin.

DIAGNOSTIC STUDIES

Table 9-1 shows the categorization of simple acid-base disorders.

Laboratory
Serum Electrolytes.   Calculate anion gap; evaluate for hypokalemia, elevated serum glucose in diabetes mellitus.
Urine pH.   Indicated to help determine appropriate response by kidney to acidosis and to rule out renal tubular acidosis.
Urine Sodium and Chloride.   Used to determine volume status, as a low urine Na^+ or Cl^- is consistent with a prerenal state or volume contraction.
ACIDOSIS
Urine pH.   Should be acidic in the presence of acidosis (pH less than 5.4).
Serum Lactate.   As indicated to exclude lactic acidosis.
Urine and Serum Ketones.   Presence of ketones in the serum is consistent with ketoacidosis. Presence of ketones in urine is consistent with ketoacidosis or starvation. Salicylate level, if indicated.
Serum Osmolality (Calculated versus Measured).   Elevated in ingestions of methanol and ethylene glycol. Compare measured osmolality with calculated osmolality ($= 2 \times Na^+$ + glucose/18 + blood urea nitrogen/2.8) and if there is a large osmolar gap (measured − calculated = gap), then the diagnosis of ingestion can be made rapidly. Serum levels of ingested agents can be performed.
ALKALOSIS
Urinary Sodium and Chloride.   Low urine Na^+ or Cl^- is consistent with dehydration or a prerenal state. A urine Cl^- concentration significantly greater than the Na^+ concentration implies an increased cation gap in the urine (high urine Cl^-, large amounts of ammonium ion [NH_4^-]). A finding of large amounts of NH_4 in the urine in the presence of alkalosis is

---

Table 9–1. Simple Acid-Base Disorders

Disorder	pH	Paco$_2$	HCO$_3$
Respiratory alkalosis	Increased	Decreased	Decreased
Respiratory acidosis	Decreased	Increased	Increased
Metabolic alkalosis	Increased	Normal	Increased
Metabolic acidosis	Decreased	Normal	Decreased

HCO_3, bicarbonate; $Paco_2$, arterial partial pressure of carbon dioxide.

inappropriate. There should be absence of NH_4 and large amounts of HCO_3, as the kidney should be secreting HCO_3.

Urine pH. Used to determine if urine is acidic or alkaline in the face of systemic alkalosis.

Serum Aldosterone (for Excess Mineralocorticoid). If a possibility of chloride-resistant alkalosis exists.

24-Hour Urine for Free Cortisol. As indicated to help exclude Cushing's disease.

Radiology

In lactic acidosis, radiographic procedures may be indicated to exclude causes such as mesenteric ischemia, perforated bowel, cardiogenic shock, or malignancy.

Flat Plate Film of the Abdomen. In alkalosis, may reveal nephrocalcinosis or calcium carbonate pills in patients with calcium carbonate ingestion.

Other

If a pure metabolic acidosis is present, then the following equation pertains:
Winter's equation: $P_{CO_2} = 1.5 \times HCO_3 + 8 \pm 2$
Otherwise, the abnormality is a mixed acid-base process.

DIFFERENTIAL DIAGNOSIS

The differential diagnosis in this setting is directed at identifying the clinical state causing the acidosis or alkalosis.

Traumatic

Generalized Trauma. Can cause a lactic acidosis and precipitate ketoacidosis in a diabetic patient.

Infectious

Infection of Any Cause. Can precipitate ketoacidosis, usually in diabetics.

Metabolic

Hyperaldosteronism, Cushing's Syndrome, High-Renin States. Can cause a metabolic alkalosis.

Neoplastic

Ectopic ACTH from Tumor. Can cause Cushing's's syndrome.
Adrenal Tumor. Can cause hyperaldosteronism.

Vascular

Renal Dysfunction Due to Vascular Disease. May cause acidosis.

Vascular Renal Artery Disease. May cause secondary renin release and metabolic alkalosis.

Congenital
Bartter Syndrome. Seen in children and adults, manifested by metabolic alkalosis, hypokalemia, and normal blood pressure with high-renin state; can cause metabolic alkalosis.

Acquired
Diuretics, Licorice, Sodium Bicarbonate Ingestion, Exogenous Steroid. May cause alkalosis.
Acidifying Salts. May cause acidosis.

TREATMENT

Acidosis
GAP ACIDOSIS
Lactic Acidosis. Treat underlying cause. Restore tissue perfusion. Vasodilators such as nitroprusside may be helpful. Bicarbonate therapy controversial (unless pH is less than 7.2). May require hemodialysis.
Ketoacidosis. Treat diabetic state and correct volume depletion; correct K^+. Check blood gases and anion gap routinely. May require bicarbonate therapy (if pH is less than 7.15). If alcoholic, treat cause, institute volume and electrolyte repletion, and treat for alcohol withdrawal.
Renal Failure. Improve renal function if a correctable cause is found (e.g., obstruction). Give oral bicarbonate, or start dialysis.
Ingestions. Key is to correctly identify the agent and treat appropriately. May require hemodiaysis or alkaline diuresis.
NONGAP ACIDOSIS
Repletion therapy with bicarbonate (except in proximal renal tubular acidosis). Dosing is variable and based on the severity and duration of acidosis. One gram of $NaHCO_3$ is 12 mmol of $NaHCO_3$. Doses range from 500 mg to approximately 2 g/day. Treatment of the underlying cause is the most important component of therapy.

Alkalosis
Remove underlying stimuli to HCO_3 generation, or remove factors that sustain HCO_3 reabsorption. If alkalosis is due to alkali ingestion, cease the ingestion.
If condition is saline responsive, give adequate amount of Cl^-, either as NaCl or as KCl (if patient is potassium depleted). Amount and duration of NaCl or KCl therapy depend on volume status (state of hydration), degree of alkalosis, and clinical parameters (cardiac status, ongoing upper gastrointestinal losses).
If condition is saline unresponsive, correct abnormal metabolic state and/or block aldosterone with aldactone, starting with 25 mg three times a

day and increasing as necessary, or treat with amiloride in a dose of up to 20 mg/day.

Acetazolamide is used in patients in conditions that preclude saline infusion, as in congestive heart failure, or with volume losses (caution is advised, as urinary potassium losses may be high with acetazolamide). Begin with 500 mg.

Rarely is it necessary to give an acid load intravenously; however, acidification can be achieved with oral ammonium chloride.

Acute hemodialysis using a low-bicarbonate, high-chloride bath may be needed in cases of severely impaired renal function.

PEDIATRIC CONSIDERATIONS

Bartter syndrome can be seen in children. Diarrhea can rapidly cause a non-gap acidosis in children.

OBSTETRIC CONSIDERATIONS

Pregnant patients have a chronic, compensated respiratory alkalosis. This is often the result of chronic hyperventilation. Another acid-base parameter that is often overlooked is the effect of serum bicarbonate levels on fetal well-being. Low serum bicarbonate can lead to fetal loss. All obstetric patients with abnormally low serum bicarbonate levels should receive aggressive fluid resuscitation and oxygen supplementation even if the hemodynamic parameters are "normal." *Note*: The use of large amounts of normal saline solution has been implicated in causing hyperchloremia in both mother and fetus.

GERIATRIC CONSIDERATIONS

The elderly often are dehydrated, are on multiple medications, or have a lower glomerular filtration rate, and their general reserves (pulmonary, kidney, cardiac) are lower, especially in the presence of comorbid conditions. One must anticipate problems with these patients, as they may have multiple chronic comorbid conditions. The ability to excrete acid is somewhat impaired secondary to decreased filtration rate, and the elderly are more predisposed to osmolality disorders.

PREVENTIVE CONSIDERATIONS

The following measures are recommended:
Maintain adequate fluid levels, especially in the context of underlying medical conditions.

Maintain both pulmonary and kidney function as optimally as possible.

Optimal control of diabetes mellitus is essential.

Compliance with dosing regimens and/or supervision by a health care professional is required for medications, especially salicylates and steroids.

PEARLS FOR THE PA

In the workup of acid-base disorders, always obtain measurements of electrolyte concentrations; urine pH, Na^+, and Cl^-; and arterial blood gases.

Establish whether the patient has an acidosis or alkalosis from the blood pH.

Determine whether compensation is present (metabolic or respiratory).

Utilize Winter's equation if acidosis is present. If it adds up, then there is a simple acid-base problem. If it does not, there is a mixed acid-base problem.

Match the clinical picture with the acid-base problem to determine the etiology.

Remember MUDPILES for the causes of anion gap metabolic acidosis: Methanol, Uremia, Diabetes, Paraldehyde, Ingestants, Lactic acidosis, Ethylene glycol, Salicylates.

Acute Renal Failure

Sandra Lynn Roberts, MMSc, PA-C

DEFINITION

Acute decline in renal function. Occurs in about 5% of hospitalized patients and in up to 30% of patients requiring admission to an intensive care unit. Usually divided into prerenal, renal (most commonly manifested as acute tubular necrosis [ATN]), and postrenal causes. Prerenal factors (most common) include congestive heart failure, volume depletion, loss of renal autoregulation, blockage of renal blood flow, and sepsis. Renal factors (second most common) include injury to glomerulus, interstitium, or tubules. Postrenal factors include obstruction to urine flow. The most frequent causes of acute renal failure are prerenal azotemia and ATN.

HISTORY

Symptoms. Orthostatic hypotension, tachycardia, edema, shortness of breath, nausea, vomiting, diarrhea, anorexia, and change in mental status.

General. Patient generally feels acutely ill owing to acute metabolic derangements and accumulation of renal waste products.

Age. Any.

Onset. Acute.

Intensity. As renal function continues to decline, the symptoms worsen. A plateau is reached, and either renal function improves or the patient requires hemodialysis (time to each outcome varies).

Aggravating Factors. High protein and electrolyte intake, "effective" volume depletion, angiotensin-converting enzyme (ACE) inhibitors, nonsteroidal anti-inflammatory drugs (NSAIDs), nephrotoxic medications or illicit drug use, contrast media, systemic infections, or anesthetics.

Alleviating Factors. Increasing renal perfusion, discontinuing offending drug or medication, limiting use of contrast media, and treating the underlying cause of the acute renal failure.

Associated Factors. Comorbid conditions such as diabetes, hypertension, congestive heart failure, systemic lupus erythematosus, myocardial infarction, sepsis, or major cardiothoracic surgical procedures can complicate the medical management of patients with acute renal failure.

PHYSICAL EXAMINATION

General. Evaluate vital signs, as the patient may have hypotension. Evaluate for dehydration (dry mucous membranes, postural hypotension, tachycardia, abnormal skin turgor).

Skin. Need to examine for evidence of vasculitis, livedo reticularis, venous track marks (indicating drug use), macular/papular rash (suggesting allergic reaction or infection), rheumatic disease (e.g., malar rash with systemic lupus erythematosus), evidence for acute or chronic infection, and pallor due to anemia.

Cardiovascular. Pericardial friction rub, hypertension, hypotension, new murmur (as a cause of thromboemboli) and evidence for cardiac tamponade (check for pulsus paradoxus), and evidence for heart failure (elevated jugular venous pulsations, S_3, pulmonary rales on auscultation). Check for presence of carotid and renal bruits.

Extremities. Evaluate for pitting edema.

Genitourinary. Percuss for costovertebral angle tenderness. Palpate for enlarged kidneys and prostate or pelvic masses. Check for bladder distention and catheterize to measure post-void residual.

Head, Eyes, Ears, Nose, Throat. Evaluate for sinusitis, retinopathy, and conductive hearing loss.

Neurologic. Observe for tremor (asterixis). Carefully test mental status.

Pulmonary. May have Kussmaul respiration or rales on auscultation.

Abdominal. Evaluate for flank and sacral pitting edema.

PATHOPHYSIOLOGY

Disorders or conditions that precipitate acute renal failure are divided into prerenal, renal parenchymal, and postrenal causes.

Possible *prerenal* factors, which cause underperfusion of the kidney, are cardiac dysfunction (e.g., myocardial infarction, cardiac tamponade, congestive heart failure), volume loss (e.g., blood loss, "third spacing," diuretic use), hepatorenal syndrome, hypotension, sepsis, and loss of renal autoregulation with the use of NSAIDs or ACE inhibitors.

Renal parenchymal causes for acute renal failure can be due to involvement of the glomerulus, interstitium, or renal tubules.

Glomerular dysfunction from acute injury to the glomerulus can be seen with endocarditis, poststreptococcal glomerulonephritis, various vasculitides, cholesterol emboli, acquired immunodeficiency syndrome (AIDS), or malignant hypertension.

Interstitial injury such as acute interstitial nephritis can occur with medication use.

Tubular dysfunction (e.g., acute tubular necrosis) may occur in prolonged hypoperfusion of the kidney, shock, or aminoglycoside use.

Postrenal factors include outlet obstruction (from pelvic or prostate tumors), retroperitoneal disease (e.g., fibrosis, tumors, or hemorrhage), which causes ureter obstruction, renal tubule, or renal pelvic obstruction from blood clots, stones, or uric acid.

DIAGNOSTIC STUDIES

Laboratory
Complete Blood Count.   Elevated white blood cell (WBC) count may indicate sepsis or infectious process. Anemia may suggest chronic disease or hemorrhage. Elevated hematocrit may indicate dehydration. Elevated eosinophils may be seen with allergic interstitial nephritis or cholesterol emboli.

Hepatitis Serologic Studies.   As indicated to rule out hepatitis B.

Human Immunodeficiency Virus (HIV) Assay.   As indicated to rule out HIV infection.

Erythrocyte Sedimentation Rate (ESR).   Elevation to greater than 20 mm/hour may be seen in inflammatory diseases such as systemic lupus erythematosus, endocarditis, vasculitis, or sepsis.

Rheumatoid Factor Assay.   May be positive in endocarditis or rheumatoid arthritis.

Electrolytes.   For evidence of acidosis or hyperkalemia.

Blood Urea Nitrogen (BUN)/Creatinine.   For degree of renal dysfunction. BUN/creatinine ratio (normal 20:1) may be much higher in prerenal azotemia. The higher the rate in rise of the serum creatinine, the worse the renal dysfunction. (*Note:* A doubling of baseline creatinine, such as from 1.0 to 2.0 mg/dL, implies a 50% loss of glomerular filtration rate.) A ratio of greater than 20:1 suggests prerenal disease as long as no other cause can be found (e.g., hyperalimentation, steroid treatment, gastrointestinal bleed).

Antinuclear Antibody (ANA), Double-Stranded DNA Assays. For evidence of lupus.

Calcium. As indicated to exclude hypercalcemia with acute renal failure.

Phosphate/Creatine Kinase (CK). As indicated to exclude rhabdomyolysis.

Serum Protein Electrophoresis or Serum Immunoelectrophoresis. Used to exclude multiple myeloma.

Antineutrophil Cytoplasmic Autoantibodies (ANCA) Assay. Used to exclude Wegener's granulomatosis, vasculitis.

Anti–Glomerular Basement Membrane (Anti-GBM) Antibody Titer. Used to exclude Goodpasture syndrome.

Complement (C3, C4) Assay. Used to exclude lupus, vasculitis.

Cryoglobulin Assay. As indicated to exclude cryoglobulinemia.

Spot Urine for Sodium Concentration. Determination of sodium concentration in a random urine specimen can be used to assess volume status (provided that the patient is not currently on any diuretics). If urine Na^+ is less than 10 mEq/L, the patient is significantly volume depleted, and the fact that the renal tubules are still able to concentrate the urine suggests that the acute renal failure has not progressed to ATN. A urine sodium of greater than 40 mEq/L in the context of acute renal failure suggests progression to ATN, and in such cases determination of the fractional excretion of sodium (FENa) would be useful (see Table 9-2).

Fractional Excretion of Sodium. Based on a calculation derived from the serum/urine creatinine and the serum/urine sodium. If the FENa is less than 1%, the acute renal failure is due to a prerenal cause. If the FENa is greater than 1%, the acute renal failure is due to ATN.

Urine Sediment. Protein or cellular casts are consistent with acute glomerular or interstitial event, whereas benign urine sediment is more in line with a prerenal cause. Bland sediment or hematuria and/or pyuria is

Table 9–2. Laboratory Values: Prerenal Failure versus ATN

Analyte	Prerenal	ATN
BUN/creatinine ratio	20-40:1	10-15:1
Urine Na^+	≤10 mEq/L	>20 mEq/L
Urine concentration	Concentrated	Dilute
Osmolality	High (>500 mOsm/L)	Low (<300 mOsm/L)
Specific gravity	High (>1.020 mOsm/L)	Low (<1.010 mOsm/L)
Urine sediment	Benign	Muddy brown granular casts
FENa	≤1%	>1%

ATN, acute tubular necrosis; BUN, blood urea nitrogen; FENa, fractional excretion of sodium.

associated with postrenal causes. Muddy brown granular casts are most suggestive of ATN.

Urine Drug Screen. If indicated.

Urine Osmolality. In the context of acute renal dysfunction, a concentrated urine suggests prerenal disease, and a dilute urine suggests ATN.

Urine Eosinophils. Positive with allergic interstitial nephritis and cholesterol emboli.

24-Hour Urine for Volume, Creatinine Clearance, and Total Protein. Urine volume less than 400 mL/day indicates oliguric renal failure (common in prerenal acute failure). ATN may manifest with oliguria or nonoliguria. A baseline 24-hour creatinine clearance can allow for monitoring of renal function with time. A 24-hour protein helps to determine if the acute renal failure is due to glomerular injury (24-hour protein excretion of greater than 3 g is indicative of nephrotic syndrome).

Radiology

Renal Ultrasound Examination. As indicated to help rule out obstruction, infection. Check for hydronephrosis.

Doppler Renal Ultrasound Study. Used to evaluate renal blood flow. Check for renal artery stenosis.

Radionuclide Renal Scan. As indicated to evaluate function and blood flow to kidney.

CT Scan. As indicated to rule out obstruction, nephrolithiasis, or retroperitoneal disease.

Renal Angiography. Used to exclude renal artery lesion.

Magnetic Resonance Angiography (MRA). Evaluate renal vessels. Advantage in patients with renal failure as there is no need for exogenous contrast agent as in CT.

Other

Gallium Scan. May be positive in allergic interstitial nephritis. Negative predictive value is low.

Cystoscopy. If needed to rule out obstruction.

Echocardiography. As indicated to exclude endocarditis, tamponade, or pericardial effusion.

Kidney Biopsy. Findings on examination of glomerulus, interstitium, and tubule biopsy specimens under light and electron microscopy and immunofluorescence can be combined with the clinical presentation to help establish the diagnosis.

Swan-Ganz Pressure Monitoring. Used to determine true cardiac function and volume status.

DIFFERENTIAL DIAGNOSIS

The differential diagnosis in this setting is directed at identifying the clinical state causing the acute renal failure.

Traumatic
Acute Injury to Blood Supply (Aortal Renal Artery) or to Ureter. Positive history of blunt or penetrating trauma. May have acute abdomen, retroperitoneal blood, or hematuria.

Rhabdomyolysis. Increased CK and PO_4.

Infectious
Poststreptococcal Glomerulonephritis. Low C3 and elevated antistreptolysin O titer.

Disseminated Intravascular Coagulation. Seen with acute renal failure in conjunction with gram-positive or gram-negative infections, eclampsia, diabetic ketoacidosis, liver failure.

Bacterial Endocarditis. Low C_3, elevated rheumatoid factor.

Shunt Nephritis. Low complements, history of shunt placement.

Metabolic
Malignant Hypertension. Can be seen with scleroderma or acute nephritis.

Hypercalcemia with Nephrocalcinosis. Metabolic stone disease with obstruction.

Immunologically Mediated Disease. Examples: Goodpasture syndrome with a positive anti-GBM antibody (seen on kidney biopsy with linear deposition on immunofluorescence); Wegener's granulomatosis with lung nodules; kidney biopsy shows evidence of acute glomerulonephritis and cryoglobulinemia with low C4 and C3 (positive cryoglobulin seen with a variety of diseases including multiple myeloma, lymphoma, Sjögren's syndrome, neoplasia, and systemic lupus erythematosus).

Systemic Lupus Erythematosus. Low C3 and C4 and positive titers for ANA, anti–double-stranded DNA.

Systemic Vasculitis. Positive ANCA; in *mesangiocapillary glomerulonephritis*, low C3.

Neoplastic
Obstruction of the Ureters or Renal Artery/Vein. May be due to tumor mass, seen on CT/MRI scan or ultrasound study of the abdomen.

Multiple Myeloma. May involve the kidney.

Vascular
Cholesterol Embolization. May be seen after cardiac catheterization.

Acute Renal Artery Occlusion or Dissection. Occlusion/dissection seen on renal angiogram or MRA or lack of renal artery signal on Doppler ultrasound examination.

Congenital
Sickle Cell Disease. Causes papillary necrosis.

Acquired

Pregnancy with Obstruction. Positive human chorionic gonadotropin (HCG).

Medications. Aminoglycosides (causing acute tubular necrosis), non-steroidals and antibiotics (causing acute interstitial nephritis), and dye-induced ATN. Patients especially at risk are those with diabetes and/or chronic renal failure. Papillary necrosis can be seen in analgesic abuse.

Surgical Error. Ligation of the ureters.

TREATMENT

Generalized treatment includes controlling fluid balance; managing diet; correcting acid-base and electrolyte abnormalities; aggressively treating hypertension; and adjusting medications for degree of renal impairment. Restore adequate kidney perfusion and treat the underlying cause of the acute renal failure (e.g., give steroids for immunologically mediated acute renal failure, discontinue nephrotoxic medications, relieve obstruction.)

Prerenal

Increased urinary output plus improving serial serum BUN and creatinine values with fluid repletion indicates a prerenal cause for the acute renal failure.

Prevention is key. Correct prerenal factors (e.g., dehydration, congestive heart failure, liver failure).

Renal

Begin with volume restoration and drug level monitoring. The results of history, laboratory, and pathologic findings determine therapy. If it is an acute glomerulonephritis from endocarditis, the treatment is correcting the endocarditis. In an immunologically mediated vasculitis, the treatment may be administration of steroids or cytotoxic drugs (e.g., pulse steroid therapy with methylprednisolone at 1.0 mg/m^2 of body surface area or cytotoxic therapy with cyclophosphamide at 2.0 mg/kg/day may be given in some cases).

Acute interstitial nephritis is usually treated by removing the offending agent. Treatment with steroids is controversial.

At present there is no treatment for ATN. Use of loop diuretics, mannitol, and calcium channel blockers is controversial. Current studies are evaluating the addition of insulin-like growth factor (IGF-1) for increased tubular regeneration as well as atrial natriuretic peptide (ANP) given with dopamine to prevent systemic hypotension.

Postrenal

Relieve the obstruction by placing a Foley catheter, ureteral stents, or nephrostomy tubes, or by surgical correction of the obstructing cause.

PEDIATRIC CONSIDERATIONS

Pediatric causes of acute renal failure are similar to those in the adult. Children are prone to develop rapid dehydration.

Infants with oliguria need to be evaluated for anatomic abnormalities.

Poststreptococcal glomerulonephritis is the most common cause of acute renal failure in children. Also need to exclude Henoch-Schönlein purpura.

Nutrition and hydration are exceedingly important factors in the care of children.

OBSTETRIC CONSIDERATIONS

Eclampsia can lead to acute renal failure. If dialysis is needed for the management of acute renal failure, it poses a risk of complications (hypertension, vaginal bleeding, peritonitis) in the mother.

GERIATRIC CONSIDERATIONS

Kidney function generally declines with age. Geriatric patients are often on multiple medications. As kidney function declines, one must watch for medication reactions and be cautious in dosing medications that are cleared via the kidney. Geriatric patients are often volume depleted. Caution is advised in prescribing NSAIDs (including cyclooxygenase-2 [COX-2] inhibitors) and ACE inhibitors.

PREVENTIVE CONSIDERATIONS

Anticipating problems and minimizing kidney insults are key measures in limiting the development of acute renal failure. Although to date there have been no effective prophylactic therapies, ensuring adequate hydration is a significant prevention strategy, as well as caution in prescribing ACE inhibitors to patients who are volume depleted. There is also evidence that COX-2 inhibitors may precipitate acute renal failure in certain patients; the frequency compared with that for nonselective NSAIDs is unknown at this time. Aspirin and sulindac appear to be more "renal sparing" than other NSAIDs.

PEARLS FOR THE PA

When a patient presents with an acute decline in urine output and an elevated blood urea nitrogen/creatinine, the following measures are indicated:

Determine if it is due to acute or worsening chronic renal failure.

Evaluate for rapidly correctable causes such as volume depletion or obstruction.

Continued

Chronic Renal Failure

Sandra Lynn Roberts, MMSc, PA-C

DEFINITION

Gradual decline in renal function.

HISTORY

Symptoms. Anorexia, pruritus, weight loss, lethargy, fatigue, change in sleep pattern, depression, nocturia, anemia, nausea, edema, and shortness of breath. These symptoms occur in the setting of decreased urine output, with increased bleeding tendencies secondary to platelet abnormalities.

General. Often, patients may be asymptomatic or have only minimal symptoms of fatigue. Family members may note changes in the patient. Severity of renal dysfunction will determine symptomatology. The patient may have a history of long-standing diabetes mellitus, hypertension, arteriosclerotic disease, analgesic abuse, gout, amyloid, ureteral reflux during childhood, or polycystic kidney disease.

Age. Any age, but usually affects older patients.

Onset. Gradual, although acute renal failure can occur in patients with chronic renal failure.

Duration. Progressive.

Intensity. Mild at first, worse as renal function declines.

Aggravating Factors. Dehydration, high-protein diet, increased fluid intake with oliguria, nephrotoxic medications, drugs, and acute renal failure.

Alleviating Factors.   Low-protein and low-electrolyte diet, dialysis, renal transplantation.

Associated Factors.   Decline in general health, uncontrolled systemic illnesses (e.g., diabetes, heart disease, hypertension, lupus).

PHYSICAL EXAMINATION

General.   The patient may appear thin or cachectic, depressed, or fatigued.

Cardiovascular.   Peripheral edema, symptoms of heart failure (e.g., shortness of breath, orthopnea), pericardial friction rub.

Neurologic.   Tremor, asterixis, surprising mental clarity even with elevated blood urea nitrogen (BUN) and creatinine. "Stocking-glove" paresthesias suggest peripheral neuropathy.

Ophthalmologic.   Diabetic eye changes (e.g., proliferative retinopathy) or hypertensive eye changes.

Skin.   Dry, evidence of scratching due to pruritus, yellowish brown discoloration in Caucasian patients. "Uremic frost" in very late stages (unusual).

PATHOPHYSIOLOGY

Chronic injury to the kidney may be the result of a single event (rarely with poststreptococcal glomerulonephritis) leading to inflammation and injury significant enough to eventually cause scarring of the kidney. More commonly, chronic insults such as those incurred with uncontrolled diabetes mellitus, hypertension, or obstruction may result in chronic renal failure. As with acute injury, chronic injury is divided into prerenal, renal, and postrenal causes.

Possible *prerenal* causes are vascular disease and arterionephrosclerosis.

Renal factors include glomerular or interstitial scarring from long-standing diabetes (Kimmelstiel-Wilson glomerulosclerosis), sclerosis associated with hypertension, interstitial scarring from drugs (nonsteroidals, analgesics), frequent ureteral reflux, gout, and uncontrolled lupus.

Postrenal factors include long-standing obstruction from stones, tumor, or prostatism.

DIAGNOSTIC STUDIES

Laboratory

Complete Blood Count.   May have severe anemia (hematocrit less than 25 mg/dL) suggesting chronic injury with subsequent decrease in erythropoietin production.

Calcium, Phosphate Levels.   In advanced stages, high phosphate (range 6 to 8 mg/dL) with low calcium may indicate chronic injury due to inability of kidney to filter PO_4.

Parathyroid Hormone (PTH). High level due to chronic low calcium and high phosphate (intact PTH level greater than 65 pg/mL). Results in secondary hyperparathyroidism and renal osteodystrophy.

Increased Potassium. Potassium levels of greater than 5.0 mEq/L may result from chronic distal tubular injury.

Blood Urea Nitrogen (BUN) and Creatinine. Progressively increasing levels of BUN and creatinine in the absence of acute illnes. May also be elevated with gastrointestinal bleed, steroid therapy, or hyperalimentation secondary to the inability of the kidney to filter metabolites.

Low Serum Bicarbonate. From chronic metabolic acidosis (HCO_3 level approximately 10 to 20 mEq/L range) due to inability of kidney to filter/neutralize acid load.

Alkaline Phosphatase. Mild to moderate increase secondary to renal osteodystrophy.

Radiology

Renal Ultrasound Examination. Shows small scarred kidneys that are echodense.

Renal Doppler Scan. Poor function and flow of both kidneys.

Hand Radiographs. Evidence of subperiosteal bone resorption with erosion of phalanges is single most sensitive radiographic sign of secondary hyperparathyroidism.

DIFFERENTIAL DIAGNOSIS

The differential diagnosis in this setting is directed at identifying the clinical state causing the chronic renal failure.

Traumatic

Not applicable.

Infectious

Low-Grade Skin Infections. Causing secondary amyloid.

Chronic Subacute Bacterial Endocarditis. Can cause acute and chronic renal failure by an immune-mediated glomerular injury.

Metabolic

Gout. Produces uric acid deposits; elevated serum uric acid; intratubular obstruction and injury.

Nephrocalcinosis. Will cause intratubular injury. Exclude medullary cystic or sponge disease.

Long-Standing Systemic Lupus Erythematosus. Positive antinuclear antibody (ANA) titer, systemic signs such as joint pains or malar rash.

Neoplastic
Long-Standing Low-Grade Obstruction.   Will cause interstitial scarring.
Multiple Myeloma with Amyloid.   Will cause glomerular damage.

Vascular
Arterionephrosclerosis with Scarring.   Can result in glomerular injury.

Congenital
Reflux Nephropathy.   Occurs primarily in children, causes interstitial scarring.
Medullary Cystic Disease.   May cause renal interstitial injury.
Polycystic Kidney Disease.   An inherited disorder that can cause end-stage renal disease by middle age.

Acquired
Analgesic Neuropathy.   Chronic use of analgesics may cause interstitial scarring. Chronic use of NSAIDs may cause interstitial nephritis.

TREATMENT

Prevention of end-stage renal disease requiring dialysis is the goal in treatment of chronic renal failure. Patients are placed on kidney transplant lists as soon as possible and treated medically for as long as possible provided that there is an acceptable quality of life to the patient. There are no absolute BUN or creatinine values that necessitate initiation of dialysis. Each patient is treated on an individual basis, and dialysis is initiated as indicated to preserve an acceptable quality of life for the patient.

Key measures may include low-protein (60-70 g/day protein restriction) and low-phosphate diet, parathyroidectomy, oral or intramuscular calcium supplementation, oral HCO_3, oral phosphate binders, lipid-lowering drugs, and ACE inhibitors.

Dialysis may be either hemodialysis or chronic ambulatory peritoneal dialysis.

Renal transplantation is the only remaining option for patients with end-stage renal disease. Once patients start on a form of renal replacement therapy, they are immediately evaluated for kidney transplantation and placed on a kidney transplant waiting list.

PEDIATRIC CONSIDERATIONS

Need to exclude ureteral reflux as a cause of renal scarring. Nutritional support is essential if early dialysis is indicated.

OBSTETRIC CONSIDERATIONS

Only a few pregnant patients with chronic renal failure who are undergoing dialysis will successfully carry a pregnancy to full term. With dialysis, there is the possibility of maternal complications such as hypertension, vaginal bleeding, or peritonitis.

GERIATRIC CONSIDERATIONS

The elderly are at least five times more likely to develop end-stage renal disease than are younger adults. Many patients with chronic renal failure take multiple medications. This becomes an issue with the elderly, in terms of both affordability of the medications and the ability to comply with prescribed regimens.

Many elderly patients with CRF have multiple comorbid conditions, which must be taken into consideration in determining treatment of end-stage renal disease. As a patient gets older, it becomes more difficult to qualify for kidney transplantation.

Vascular disorders should always be considered in the elderly patient with renal failure. Smoking has been identified as an independent risk factor in progression of microvascular and macrovascular disease in the elderly.

PREVENTIVE CONSIDERATIONS

Prevention of chronic renal failure requires aggressive treatment of both diabetes and hypertension, the two main causes of end-stage renal disease and need for hemodialysis in the United States. Early and consistent intervention in treating any potential cause for renal damage is necessary. Also important is cessation of smoking as early as possible.

High-protein diets, popular for weight loss, should be avoided in persons with renal disease.

PEARLS FOR THE PA

When evaluating the patient with chronic renal failure, it is imperative to exclude reversible causes such as low-grade chronic obstruction, analgesic or NSAID use, and underlying medical conditions such as chronic infections or myeloma.

Exclude medications that can cause a chronic interstitial nephritis such as long-term use of diuretics or NSAIDs.

Exclude renovascular stenosis in patients with hypertension.

Obtain a baseline renal ultrasound study in all patients.

If no treatable cause is found, frequent follow-up evaluation is indicated to check for signs of uremia.

Continued

PEARLS FOR THE PA—cont'd

Involve the family members in evaluating for potential serious symptoms.

Remember the mnemonic AEIOU for the five main reasons for hemodialysis: Acidosis, Electrolyte disturbance, Ingestants, volume Overload, Uremia.

Treat diabetes and hypertension aggressively. Diabetes is the primary cause and hypertension is the next most common cause for hemodialysis in the United States.

Electrolyte Imbalance: Na⁺ and K⁺

Sandra Lynn Roberts, MMSc, PA-C

DEFINITION

Alteration in the normal electrolyte (Na^+, K^+) composition of the serum.

HISTORY

Symptoms

Hyponatremia. Change in mental status, seizures, hypothermia, agitation, nausea, vomiting, weakness, headache.

Hypernatremia. Lack of water intake, thirst, polyuria.

Hypokalemia. Weakness, diarrhea, vomiting, polyuria, periodic paralysis.

Hyperkalemia. Only 25% of patients have symptoms, usually muscle weakness, cardiac arrhythmia, or decrease in urine output.

General

Hyponatremia. Syndrome of inappropriate antidiuretic hormone secretion (SIADH) due to lung cancer/smoking, metastatic cancer, recent central nervous system problems (e.g., infection, tumor), recent new medications, thyroid disease, adrenal problems, ascites, heart failure, thiazide diuretics, nonsteroidal anti-inflammatory drugs (NSAIDs), chlorpropamide, or narcotics.

Hypernatremia. History of adrenal problems, low blood pressure, diuretic use, hyperalimentation or interruption of access to free water by mouth.

Hypokalemia. Recent new medication (e.g., diuretics), hypertension (from mineralocorticoid-producing tumor); symptoms of Cushing's disease or excessive steroid use (e.g., muscle weakness, easy bruisability, hirsutism, buffalo hump).

Hyperkalemia.   Recent new medication (e.g., potassium-sparing diuretics, angiotensin-converting enzyme [ACE] inhibitors, NSAIDs, beta blockers, digitalis), history of gastrointestinal bleeding, use of salt substitute.

Age.   Any.

Onset.   Acute or chronic.

Duration.   Brief or chronic.

Intensity.   Very high or low serum concentrations of Na+ or K+ can have severe clinical consequences.

Aggravating Factors

Hyponatremia.   Additional water intake.

Hypernatremia.   Diuretics, lack of water intake.

Hypokalemia.   Diuretics, gastrointestinal or renal losses of K+, alkylosis.

Hyperkalemia.   Increased potassium intake, renal failure, potassium-sparing medications, medications resulting in decreased aldosterone production (ACE inhibitors or angiotensin II receptor blockers), acidosis.

Alleviating Factors.   Correction of underlying process.

Associated Factors.   Impaired renal function, thyroid and adrenal abnormalities, alcoholism, pneumonia, certain medications, and lung cancer.

PHYSICAL EXAMINATION

General

HYPONATREMIA

Need to evaluate volume status as accurately as possible to determine whether the patient is hypovolemic, euvolemic, or hypervolemic.

HYPERNATREMIA

Need to exclude clinical evidence for dehydration such as dry mucous membranes, hypotension, poor skin turgor, or absence of axillary sweating. Check for altered mental status.

HYPOKALEMIA

Dehydration from polyuria, diuretics, or vomiting.

Cardiovascular

HYPONATREMIA

Evaluate volume status. Examine neck veins for increased jugular venous pulsation and blood pressure (including orthostatic measurements).

HYPOKALEMIA

Irregular heart rate (especially in a patient on digoxin).

Endocrinologic

HYPONATREMIA

Evaluate for evidence of hypothyroidism (absence of lateral eyebrow hair, deep voice, hypothermia, delayed deep tendon reflexes, thin skin, altered mental status, neck scar from previous thyroid surgery), and adrenal insufficiency (Addison disease) (low blood pressure, hyperpigmentation of palm creases due to decreased adrenocorticotropic hormone).

HYPOKALEMIA
Evidence for excess steroid use or production (Cushingoid state) (e.g., buffalo hump, weakness, easy bruisability, abdominal striae).

Neurologic

HYPERKALEMIA/HYPOKALEMIA
Neuromuscular irritability (flaccid paralysis, weakness).
Hypernatremia/Hyponatremia. Altered mental status (rapidity of electrolyte change is a very important therapeutic and prognostic indicator).

Renal

HYPERKALEMIA
Need to exclude evidence for renal failure (e.g., tremor, pericardial friction rub, uremic signs).

PATHOPHYSIOLOGY

HYPONATREMIA
Primarily a disorder of maintaining water load, not salt loss, except in rare settings involving increased salt loss with use of thiazide diuretics or salt-losing nephropathy.

The inability to maintain a water load can be assessed as follows:

The most common approach is the iso-osmolar (serum osmolality of 280 to 285 mOsmol/L) versus hypo-osmolar (285) classification. After the osmolality is established, assess whether the patient is euvolemic, hypervolemic, or hypovolemic.

With hyperosmolar hyponatremia, glucose or mannitol must be present. With iso-osmolar hypernatremia, consider lipids, proteins, or isotonic glucose. With hypo-osmolar hypernatremia, evaluate volume status.

A patient who is *hypovolemic* tends to have H_2O and salt losses (gastrointestinal/renal losses, diuretics, Addison disease) and drinks excess water, thereby decreasing serum sodium. In the *euvolemic* patient, need to exclude hypothyroidism, SIADH (due to tumor or any of variety of drugs, usually centrally acting drugs or narcotics). In the *hypervolemic* patient, consider heart, liver, or renal failure or nephrotic syndrome.

HYPERNATREMIA
Usually due to excessive H_2O loss (dehydration) as seen with central or nephrogenic diabetes insipidus, diuretics, increased H_2O losses not adequately replaced such as with burns, fever in infants, or elderly persons without access to water (e.g., stroke patients, those receiving hyperalimentation with decreased water intake). Rarely due to increased Na^+ administration (e.g., use of 3% saline in adults).

HYPERKALEMIA
Pseudohyperkalemia may exist with high platelet count or high white blood cell count. True hyperkalemia occurs with rapid infusion or intake of

KCl, decreased renal excretion, or altered cellular shifts. Decreased renal excretion may occur with renal failure, distal tubular dysfunction, or drugs that affect distal tubular function (e.g., amiloride, spironolactone, triamterene). K^+ is primarily intracellular (only 65 to 70 mEq/L KCl is present in extracellular fluid); thus, any process that impairs K^+ transfer into cell, or increases K^+ transfer out of cell, will cause hyperkalemia. Inorganic acidosis, lack of insulin, beta-adrenergic blockade can cause hyperkalemia. Drugs that affect the renin-angiotensin system or that impair response to aldosterone can increase K^+ (e.g., potassium-sparing diuretics, beta blockers, ACE inhibitors, angiotensin II receptor blockers).

HYPOKALEMIA

Increased renal or gastrointestinal losses, cellular shifts of K^+ into cell (alkalosis, insulin, beta-adrenergic stimulation), or inadequate potassium intake can cause hypokalemia (e.g., the elderly and alcoholics).

DIAGNOSTIC STUDIES

Laboratory

HYPONATREMIA

Serum Sodium.   Decreased (less than 136 mEq/L).

Serum Glucose.   Serum Na^+ will decrease by 1.6 mEq/L for every 100 mg/dL increase over the normal blood glucose of 100 (e.g., a glucose level of 1000 mg/dL is 900 above 100; thus, the Na^+ would be decreased by 9×1.6 or 14, so serum $Na^+ = 140 - 14 = 126$).

Blood Urea Nitrogen (BUN)/Creatinine.   As indicated to exclude renal dysfunction.

Serum Osmolality.   Normal level is 280 to 285 mOsm/L. Used to determine if the patient is hyperosmolar.

Urine Osmolality.   A value of greater than 300 mOsm/L implies antidiuretic hormone (ADH) effect present.

Triglycerides.   Normal level is less than 215 mg/dL. Used to exclude hypertriglyceridemia (greater than 1000) as a cause of hyponatremia (pseudohyponatremia).

Cortisol.   Normal baseline or stimulated level is greater than 20 μg/dL. As indicated to exclude Addison disease.

Thyroid Function Test.   As indicated to exclude hypothyroidism.

Urine Sodium.   Normally, the urine Na^+ reflects fluid intake. A low urine Na^+ (less than 10 mEq/L) suggests renal hypoperfusion. A level greater than 20 suggests euvolemia, volume expansion, high salt intake, diuretics, or salt wasting.

HYPERNATREMIA

Serum Sodium.   Increased (greater than 144 mEq/L).

BUN/Creatinine.   As indicated to exclude renal failure or dehydration.

Serum and Urine Glucose.   Indicated to exclude an osmotic diuresis.

Serum Osmolality.   Used to help document hyperosmolarity in the serum.

Urine Osmolality.   Should be higher than the serum osmolarity; otherwise, there is evidence of insufficient levels or effect of ADH on the kidney to preserve water.

Urine Electrolytes. Na$^+$ and Cl$^-$ should be low (less than 10 mEq/L), as hypernatremia usually implies dehydration except in persons with a high sodium intake.

HYPERKALEMIA

Serum Potassium. Increased (greater than 5.0 mEq/L).

BUN and Creatinine. To exclude renal dysfunction.

Serum pH. Useful if the HCO$_3$ is low to determine the degree of acidosis.

Lactate Dehydrogenase (LDH). Used to rule out pseudohyperkalemia.

Platelet Count. If elevated (greater than 1,000,000 per mm^3), may cause a pseudohyperkalemia. Plasma K$^+$ should be obtained if there is any question of a pseudohyperkalemia.

Serum Phosphate. If high, may indicate rhabdomyolysis or renal failure.

Complete Blood Count. If white blood cell count is elevated, may have a pseudohyperkalemia.

Urine Potassium and Osmolality, Serum Osmolarity. Osmolarity and K$^+$ in serum and urine can be used to measure transtubular potassium gradient (TTKG), to indicate whether the renal response to serum potassium changes is appropriate. Calculation of TTKG is as follows: urine K$^+$ /plasma K$^+$ × serum osmolality/urine osmolality. A high TTKG indicates large renal K$^+$ loss, and a low TTKG suggests small renal K$^+$ loss.

Serum Renin or Aldosterone. Occasionally may be helpful to document hyporenin state, hypoadrenal state (aldosterone should be high in the presence of hyperkalemia).

HYPOKALEMIA

Serum Potassium. Decreased (less than 3.5 mEq/L).

Electrolytes. If HCO$_3$ is high, may indicate an alkalosis.

Serum Osmolality. As indicated to calculate TTKG.

Blood pH. As indicated to determine the degree of alkalosis if HCO$_3$ is high.

Renin, Aldosterone. Used to exclude inappropriately high aldosterone if the diagnosis is unclear.

Urine Potassium. Used to measure the TTKG to help determine if the hypokalemia is from urine losses (high TTKG) or from gastrointestinal losses (low TTKG).

Urine Osmolality. Used to calculate the TTKG.

Radiology

HYPONATREMIA

CT Scans, MRI, Plain Radiographs. Indicated if tumor or central nervous system event is suspected, especially in cases of SIADH. Pneumonia may also cause SIADH.

HYPERNATREMIA

Pituitary CT/MRI Scans. Indicated if central diabetes insipidus is suspected.

Renal Ultrasound Examination. As indicated to exclude obstruction, which can cause distal tubular injury and consequent nephrogenic diabetes insipidus.

HYPERKALEMIA
Renal Ultrasound Examination.   As indicated to exclude obstruction.
HYPOKALEMIA
Adrenal CT Scan or MRI.   Useful to exclude adrenal tumor.

Other
HYPERNATREMIA
Fluid Deprivation Test with Exogenous ADH.   Useful to differentiate central from nephrogenic diabetes insipidus. *To test*: Withhold fluids until urine osmolality varies less than 30 mOsm/L and then give ADH. A normal response is a further rise in urine osmolality with exogenous ADH. In central diabetes insipidus, response should be normal because the kidney is normal. In nephrogenic diabetes insipidus, response will be impaired because the defect is at the renal collecting duct (end-organ injury).
HYPERKALEMIA
ECG.   Performed to exclude peaked T waves.

DIFFERENTIAL DIAGNOSIS

Traumatic
HYPONATREMIA
Central Nervous System Trauma.   Can cause SIADH.
HYPERKALEMIA
Rhabdomyolysis.   Can be caused by trauma or electrical injury.
HYPERNATREMIA/HYPOKALEMIA
Not applicable.

Infectious
HYPONATREMIA
Lung Infection.   Can cause SIADH.
Central Nervous System Infection.   Can cause SIADH.
HYPERNATREMIA
Infections That Cause Fever.   May cause hypernatremia.
HYPERKALEMIA
Sepsis.   May cause renal failure.
HYPOKALEMIA
Not applicable.

Metabolic
HYPONATREMIA
Hypothyroidism.   May cause hyponatremia.
Addison Disease.   May cause hyponatremia.
HYPERNATREMIA
Diabetes Insipidus.   A result of a central lack of ADH, resulting in hypernatremia.
HYPOKALEMIA
Cushing's Syndrome.   Can result in hypokalemia.

Mineralocorticoid Excess.   Can result in hypokalemia.
HYPERKALEMIA
Addison Disease.   Can result in hyperkalemia.
Inorganic Acidosis.   Can result in hyperkalemia.

Neoplastic
HYPONATREMIA
Central Nervous System or Lung Tumor.   Can cause SIADH.
Renal Failure.   Can result in hyponatremia.
HYPOKALEMIA
Tumors Producing ACTH or Mineralocorticoid.   Can result in hypokalemia.
HYPERKALEMIA
Cancers.   Can result in renal failure.
HYPERNATREMIA
Not applicable.

Vascular
HYPONATREMIA
Vascular Disease.   Can result in renal failure.
HYPERNATREMIA/HYPOKALEMIA
Not applicable.
HYPERKALEMIA
Renal Failure From Any Cause.   Can cause hyperkalemia.

Congenital
HYPERKALEMIA
Childhood Reflux.   Can cause renal injury.
HYPONATREMIA/HYPERNATREMIA/HYPOKALEMIA
Not applicable.

Acquired
HYPONATREMIA
Medications.   Can cause SIADH or renal failure
Diuretic Use.   Can result in hyponatremia
HYPERNATREMIA
Diuretic Use.   Can result in hypernatremia.
HYPOKALEMIA
Diuretic and Steroid Use.   Can result in hypokalemia.
HYPERKALEMIA
Potassium-Sparing Diuretics.   Can actually cause a hyperkalemia.

TREATMENT

HYPONATREMIA
Correct the underlying cause if possible. Evaluate fluid status.

HYPOVOLEMIA

Administer saline. It is important to increase the serum sodium to 120 mEq/L. This can be done with normal saline or 3% saline. Replacement depends on the degree of dehydration and severity of hyponatremia. If condition is acute and symptomatic, correct more rapidly (up to 20 mEq Na$^+$/L/24 hours); if chronic, correct more slowly.

EUVOLEMIA

Restrict water intake to 1000-1500 mL/day and monitor serum sodium values.

HYPERVOLEMIA

Restrict water intake; administer loop diuretics such as furosemide (dose dependent on degree of volume expansion, renal function, and severity of hyponatremia). If serum sodium is very low, there is a danger of correcting too fast, which may cause severe central nervous system injury. Thus, if serum Na$^+$ is 110, correct to 120 rapidly (up to 20 mEq Na$^+$/L/24 hours) and then slowly over the next few days to normal.

In the case of SIADH, may fluid restrict or use demeclocycline (600-1200 mg/day) without fluid restriction (except in patients with liver cirrhosis). Vasopressin antagonists may be available in the future. They appear to block action of ADH, causing water diuresis without change in filtration rate or solute excretion.

HYPERNATREMIA

Replace with H$_2$O, not too rapidly. Correct one-half of the deficit in the first 12 hours and the remainder of the deficit in the next 24 hours. H$_2$O can be given orally or intravenously as 5% dextrose in water (D$_5$W) or in one-fourth or one-half normal saline (D$_5${¼}NS or D$_5${½}NS). The rate of replacement can be estimated after calculating the H$_2$O deficit. For example, in a 70-kg patient with an Na$^+$ of 140 mEq/L, normal total body H$_2$O would be $(0.6 \times 70) \times (140/140) = 42$ L. If the Na$^+$ is 170, the total body H$_2$O would be $(0.6 \times 70) \times (140/170) = 34.6$ L. The H$_2$O deficit would be $42 - 34.6$ or 7.4 L.

In neurogenic diabetes insipidus, prescribe oral or nasal desmopressin (DDAVP), chlorpropamide, clofibrate, or thiazide diuretics. For nephrogenic diabetes insipidus, restrict water intake, treat underlying cause, and use thiazide diuretics.

HYPOKALEMIA

Administer KCl, orally or intravenously, to achieve serum K$^+$ level of greater than 3.5 mEq/L. Most of the K$^+$ is intracellular. A drop in K$^+$ of 1.0 mEq/L implies approximately a 10% drop in total body K$^+$ (approximately 300 mEq). Replacement therapy should proceed carefully; give less with renal failure with close monitoring of the serum K$^+$ (especially if replacement therapy is given intravenously).

HYPERKALEMIA

For emergency therapy of acute hyperkalemia:
1. Stabilize cardiac membrane with 10-20 mL of 10% calcium gluconate given over 10 minutes.
2. K$^+$ removal: Loop diuretics such as intravenous furosemide (40 mg) and increase dose if there is renal failure, or with hemodialysis.

3. Cellular shift: One ampule of dextrose (50 g intravenously) with 10 U of regular insulin. In severe acidosis, intravenous $NaHCO_3$ 1 or 2 ampules may be beneficial. To stabilize cardiac membrane, 10-20 mL of calcium gluconate may be helpful.

For nonemergency therapy:

1. May use sodium polystyrene sulfonate (Kayexalate) 25-50 g orally with 20% sorbitol or as a rectal enema.
2. Loop diuretics can also be used. Give furosemide 40 mg initially and increase dose as necessary.

PEDIATRIC CONSIDERATIONS

HYPONATREMIA/HYPOKALEMIA/HYPERKALEMIA
Same as in adult.

HYPERNATREMIA
Undiluted formula can give hypernatremia. Can occur rapidly with diarrhea.

OBSTETRIC CONSIDERATIONS

Large amounts of normal saline solution should be avoided because of possible hyperchloremia in mother and fetus. Chlorpropamide and clofibrate are contraindicated.

GERIATRIC CONSIDERATIONS

Ensure adequate fluid (free water) intake. Ensure proper intake of medications such as diuretics. Elderly persons are more predisposed to osmolality disorders. Therefore, in an elderly person with altered mental status, always check the sodium level.

PREVENTIVE CONSIDERATIONS

Anticipate problems. Ensure adequate intake of free water, especially in the elderly, stroke patients, and patients receiving hyperalimentation. Treat the underlying cause (e.g., pneumonia or lung cancer in SIADH), or remove offending agent (lithium) in nephrogenic diabetes insipidus or remove pituitary tumor and replace with ADH in central diabetes insipidus). Periodically check electrolyte levels when changing medications or medication doses that can alter the serum Na^+ or K^+.

PEARLS FOR THE PA

All patients with the following symptoms need to undergo electrolyte screening to avoid potentially serious medical consequences.

HYPONATREMIA: *Change in mental status, seizures, hypothermia, agitation, nausea, vomiting, weakness, headache.*

HYPERNATREMIA: *Lack of water intake, thirst, polyuria, seizures.*

HYPOKALEMIA: *Weakness, diarrhea, vomiting, polyuria, periodic paralysis.*

HYPERKALEMIA: *Only 25% of patients have symptoms, usually muscle weakness, cardiac arrhythmia, or decrease in urine output.*

Patients on digoxin and diuretics should be closely monitored for K^+ values. A low potassium can augment digoxin toxicity. Most of these patients should be on potassium supplementation.

Glomerular Disease

Sandra Lynn Roberts, MMSc, PA-C

DEFINITION

Glomerular injury that may cause renal dysfunction. The injury may be due to a known disease such as lupus nephritis or may be idiopathic. The most common form of glomerular disease, other than diabetic glomerulonephropathy, is immunoglobulin A (IgA) nephropathy (Berger disease).

HISTORY

Symptoms.　Hematuria, edema, decrease in urine output, foamy urine, dark urine, hypertension, hemoptysis, malaise, lethargy, nausea, and anorexia.

General.　The patient usually feels ill if the clinical presentation is one of renal failure with symptoms of uremia. Patient may present with decrease in urine output (if acute glomerulonephritis is present), hypertension, or edema. If the process is chronic, the patient may be asymptomatic or may notice only foamy urine and edema.

Age. Any.

Onset. Usually acute, although a gradual onset may also be seen.

Intensity. Edema is worse with large protein losses. Blood pressure may be quite high.

Aggravating Factors. Massive proteinuria, renal failure.

Alleviating Factors. Treatment of underlying process that is causing injury to the glomeruli.

Associated Factors. Underlying medical problems.

PHYSICAL EXAMINATION

General. Hypertension due to renal vasospasm and salt retention.

Cardiovascular. Auscultation may reveal pericardial friction rubs (sign of uremia) or a new murmur.

Extremities. Look for evidence of pitting edema.

Neurologic. Tremor, seizures.

Pulmonary. Kussmaul respiration (rapid, deep respiration seen with acidosis) may be present.

Skin. May show evidence of vasculitis, rheumatic disease, or infection (e.g., cellulitis, abscess).

PATHOPHYSIOLOGY

Glomerular lesions are a group of pathologic disorders in which the glomerulus is the sole or main site of injury. These disorders have been classified *histologically* as follows:

1. Minimal-change disease: glomerular epithelial foot process fusion causing proteinuria (IgA nephropathy, nephrotic syndrome, solid tumors, diabetes, nonsteroidal anti-inflammatory drugs [NSAIDs])
2. Focal glomerular sclerosis: may have superimposed disease with minimal change (hypertension, diabetes, sickle cell disease, lupus, IgA nephropathy, NSAID and analgesic nephropathy)
3. Membranous glomerulonephritis: thickening of basement membrane or glomerulus with or without immune deposits (hepatitis B, lupus, rheumatoid arthritis, sarcoid, carcinoma, NSAIDs)
4. Proliferative glomerulonephritis, including mesangiocapillary, mesangial, and crescentic glomerulonephritis: proliferative lesions that actively injure and damage the glomerulus, which may demonstrate cell proliferation, migration of polymorphonuclear cells, and actual necrosis involving part of or the entire glomerulus (endocarditis, hepatitis B and C, lupus, poststreptococcal glomerulonephritis, cryoglobulinemia, rheumatoid arthritis, Henoch-Schönlein purpura)

These disorders have been classified *clinically* as follows:

Acute glomerulonephritic syndrome: hematuria, proteinuria, red blood cell casts, hypertension, and oliguria (usually infectious etiology)

Rapidly progressive glomerulonephritis: rapid, progressive loss of renal function with oliguria (lupus)

Chronic glomerulonephritis: relentless, progressive loss of renal function; hematuria, proteinuria, and hypertension

Persistent urinary abnormalities with few or no symptoms

Nephrotic syndrome: heavy proteinuria (protein excretion of greater than 3.5 g/day), edema, hypertension, and lipidemia

DIAGNOSTIC STUDIES

Laboratory

Electrolytes.   For evidence of acidosis, hyperkalemia.

Blood Urea Nitrogen (BUN)/Creatinine.   For estimating degree of renal dysfunction. BUN/creatinine ratio (normal 20:1) may be much higher in prerenal azotemia. The higher the serum creatinine, the worse the renal dysfunction. (*Note*: A doubling of baseline creatinine, such as from 1.0 to 2.0 mg/dL, implies a 50% loss of glomerular filtration rate.)

24-Hour Urinary Protein, Creatinine Clearance, and Volume.   If nephrosis is present, there would be greater than 3.0 g/day of protein or decrease in creatinine clearance with renal failure.

Lipid Panel.   Elevated lipids found in nephrotic syndrome.

Urinalysis.   Sediment may be "active" with proteinuria, hematuria, red blood cell or white blood cell casts. Gross hematuria may be present with IgA nephropathy.

Antinuclear Antibody (ANA), Double-Stranded DNA Assays.   For evidence of lupus.

Rheumatoid Factor Assay.   May be positive in endocarditis, rheumatoid arthritis.

Cryoglobulin.   As indicated to exclude cryoglobulinemia and may be found early in acute glomerulonephritis and immune-mediated glomerulonephritis but absent in IgA nephropathy.

Hepatitis Serologic Studies.   As indicated to rule out hepatitis B or C.

Complete Blood Count.   Elevated white blood cell count may indicate sepsis. Anemia may suggest chronic disease or hemorrhage. Elevated hematocrit may indicate dehydration. Elevated eosinophils can be seen with allergic interstitial nephritis or cholesterol emboli. Fragmented red blood cells may be present. Platelet abnormalities manifest with acute glomerulonephritis and other proliferative glomerulonephropathies.

Complement (C3, C4).   Will be low in endocarditis, lupus, acute glomerulonephritis, and immune-mediated glomerulonephropathies.

Erythrocyte Sedimentation Rate (ESR)/C-Reactive Protein.   Increase of ESR to greater than 20 mm/hour may be seen in diseases such as systemic lupus erythematosus, endocarditis, vasculitis, or sepsis. May be significantly elevated in certain proliferative glomerulonephropathies.

Antistreptolysin O (ASO) Titer.   Increase is associated with acute streptococcal glomerulonephritis.

Microbiology Tests. Throat and skin cultures for group A streptococci in acute glomerulonephritis.

Serum IgA. May be increased in 50% of patients with IgA nephropathy.

Anti–Glomerular Basement Membrane (Anti-GBM) Antibody/Antineutrophil Cytoplasmic Antibody (ANCA) Titers. Increased in patients with certain types of proliferative glomerulonephropathies (Goodpasture syndrome, Wegener granulomatosis).

Radiology

Gallium Scan. Sometimes positive in minimal-change disease.

Other

Kidney Biopsy. Sample should be reviewed by light microscopy, electron microscopy, and immunofluorescence methods. Evidence for immune-mediated injury would be the presence of "deposits" in the glomerulus seen on electron microscopy and with immunofluorescence techniques. The deposits may be present in the subepithelial space (with postinfectious glomerulonephritis), intramembranous (in membranous nephropathy), or subendothelial (with disorders such as systemic lupus erythematosus). Extensive crescent formation may suggest rapidly progressive glomerulonephritis.

DIFFERENTIAL DIAGNOSIS

Glomerular injury is classified as primary or secondary. Primary lesions are those of unknown etiology; secondary lesions are those for which the cause is known. The classification is based on the pathogenetic mechanism.

Infectious

Postinfectious (Poststreptococcal) Glomerulonephritis. Associated with a history of streptococcal infection.

Shunt Nephritis. Seen in patients with ventriculovascular shunts who have chronic, low-grade infections.

Bacterial Endocarditis. Either acute or subacute, can manifest with glomerulonephritis.

Viral Infection. May cause glomerular injury. Hepatitis B and C and human immunodeficiency virus (HIV) infection are the most common.

Visceral Bacterial Infections. May contribute to the development of glomerulonephritis.

Metabolic

The lesion in these metabolic states may be a proliferative glomerulonephritis or a membranous lesion mediated through immune complex deposits derived from a systemic source.

Rheumatoid Arthritis with Positive Rheumatoid Factor Assay. Not in itself a common cause of renal dysfunction, but renal dysfunction may be related to therapy (e.g., gold, penicillamine, NSAIDs).

Mixed Cryoglobulinemia. Positive cryoglobulin assay.
Systemic Lupus Erythematosus. Positive ANA titer.

Neoplastic
Hodgkin's Disease or Lymphoma. May cause a minimal-change lesion.
Carcinomas/Solid Tumors. May be seen as mass on MRI or CT scan of affected organ. Associated with membranous lesions.

Vascular
Systemic Vaculitis (e.g., Polyarteritis Nodosa). May be associated with glomerular injury.
Goodpasture's Syndrome. May be associated with sinusitis, granulomas, and glomerulonephritis, as these conditions may cause small- and medium-artery vasculitis. Associated with anti-GBM antibody. May be associated with pulmonary hemorrhage.
Wegener's Granulomatosis. May be associated with sinusitis, granulomas, and glomerulonephritis, as these conditions may cause small- and medium-artery vasculitis.
Henoch-Schönlein Purpura. Seen mostly in children and can cause an immune complex glomerulonephritis with predominantly IgA immune complexes.
IgA Nephropathy (Berger's Disease). Causes IgA deposits in the glomerulus.

Acquired
Medications (e.g., Gold, Captopril, D-Penicillamine, Probenecid). May cause a membranous lesion.
NSAIDs. Have been associated with minimal-change disease.

Traumatic
Congenital. Not applicable.

TREATMENT

Treatment is based on the type and severity of the renal lesion, the state of the lesion, and associated medical illnesses. IgA nephropathy patients with poor prognosis should receive angiotensin-converting enzyme (ACE) inhibitors and oral high-dose omega-3 fatty acids (fish oil).

Steroids such as prednisone (dose dependent on degree of inflammation and type of lesion) are used to decrease the inflammation in proliferative lesions and decrease proteinuria in minimal-change disease. They also help treat membranous, focal, and segmental glomerulosclerosis. Cyclosporine has been found to be helpful in steroid-resistant presentations of minimal-change disease.

Cytotoxic agents such as cyclophosphamide (dose dependent on the type of renal lesion and its severity and concomitant systemic disease) are also used in proliferative lesions in conjunction with steroids with or without plasmapheresis (best when started early in disease course).

Antibiotics and symptomatic treatment are used for acute glomerulonephritis. Antibiotics are also indicated to reduce frequency of group A streptococcal carrier state.

For long-term benefit, strict control of hypertension and hyperlipidemia is strongly recommended.

PEDIATRIC CONSIDERATIONS

All glomerular lesions found in adults may also be seen in children. Idiopathic nephrotic syndrome in children is most commonly associated with minimal-change disease. IgA nephropathy and focal and segmental glomerulosclerosis also are common. Hemolytic-uremic syndrome can be quite devastating and cause acute renal failure. Presenting symptoms usually are microangiopathic hemolytic anemia, thrombocytopenia, and renal failure, often associated with fever and central nervous system changes.

OBSTETRIC CONSIDERATIONS

Acute Glomerulonephritis. Acute glomerulonephritis is rare in pregnancy. A possible complication to notice is the development of pregnancy-induced hypertension in the pregnant patient with acute glomerulonephritis, which can increase perinatal morbidity. If the blood pressure is well controlled and the patient maintains a low-salt diet, the pregnancy should progress without difficulty.

Chronic Glomerulonephritis. In chronic glomerulonephritis, the outcome of the pregnancy hinges on whether hypertension is present along with severe renal disease. If this is the case, the fetal survival rate is only approximately 55%. The presence of azotemia will also adversely affect the pregnancy outcome. Maternal risks include chronic hypertension, preeclampsia, and anemia. With nephrotic syndrome, there is an increased risk of thromboembolism and other coagulation changes associated with pregnancy owing to existing hyperlipidemia and edema.

Corticosteroids are excreted in breast milk and can cause untoward effects in an infant (e.g., water and salt retention).

GERIATRIC CONSIDERATIONS

Elderly persons are much less likely to develop acute poststreptococcal and IgA glomerulonephropathy. They are much more likely to develop membranous and vasculitic nephropathies.

PREVENTIVE CONSIDERATIONS

Important measures include early diagnosis and treatment of streptococcal infections, maintenance of vaccination protocols, and limiting intake of drugs known to cause glomerular/membranous nephropathies (i.e., gold, NSAIDS, lithium).

PEARLS FOR THE PA

The presence of acute or chronic renal failure, hypertension, proteinuria, edema, and active urine sediment suggests a glomerular lesion.

Workup should be directed at excluding a secondary cause (e.g., infection, systemic lupus erythematosus, vasculitis).

Obtain a renal biopsy if indicated.

Appropriate therapy should be initiated early to minimize irreversible renal injury.

Limit use of NSAIDs.

Nephrolithiasis

Sandra Lynn Roberts, MMSc, PA-C

DEFINITION

Nephrolithiasis (presence of kidney stones) is due to a variety of metabolic or renal disorders. From 75% to 80% of stones are composed of calcium oxalate (pure or mixed). Incidence is highest in the southeastern United States. Less commonly found in African Americans, American Indians, and Asians. Recurrence rate is up to 75%.

HISTORY

Symptoms. Flank pain that may radiate to groin; dysuria, nausea, vomiting, and, if infection is present, fever with chills.

General. Obtain a history of risk factors (e.g., dehydration, family history of stones, hypercalciuria, hyperoxaluria, hyperuricosuria, hypocitruria). The patient may have a history of urinary tract infections, hematuria, pyuria, gout, gastrointestinal problems (e.g., chronic diarrhea, malabsorption, small bowel surgery) or may be taking new vitamins or drugs. Also significant is dietary intake of calcium, high protein, foods containing oxalate, sodium, and water.

Age. Generally in the adult population.

Onset. May be asymptomatic or acute.

Duration. Varies with size and number of stones.

Intensity. From asymptomatic to very intense pain.

Aggravating Factors. Any of the risk factors for stone disease (as listed under General earlier).

Alleviating Factors. Passage of stone, destruction of stone via ultrasound, medical therapy, or surgical removal.

Associated Factors. Risk factors (as noted), chronic acidosis (metabolic), chronic alkalosis (metabolic), sarcoid, hyperparathyroidism, and hyperthyroidism.

PHYSICAL EXAMINATION

General. Determine blood pressure. Patient may be hypotensive, suggesting dehydration.

Costovertebral angle tenderness may be elicited. Flank or abdomen may be tender to palpation.

Skin. Look for evidence of dehydration: dry mucous membranes, flat neck veins, absence of axillary sweat.

PATHOPHYSIOLOGY

Theories of stone formation include the following:
- Crystallization/precipitation of stone-forming constituents due to:
   Hypercalciuria: From absorptive hypercalciuria due to elevated 1,25-dihydroxycholecalciferol, renal leak hypercalciuria, and resorptive hypercalciuria.
   Hyperoxaluria: Uncommon, but seen with enteric hyperoxaluria in patients with inflammatory bowel disease or following intestinal bypass surgery.
   Hyperuricosuria: Seen in patients with gout, increased protein intake. The oxalate or uric acid can act as nidus for calcium stone formation. These constituents have to be in concentrations above their solubility product.
- Matrix: Other factors such as glycoproteins act as a matrix source.
- Inhibitors: Stones can form if inhibitors of stone formation, including citrate, pyrophosphates, and magnesium, are decreased.

Other types of stones also can occur, such as cystine stones in hypercystinuria and magnesium-ammonium-phosphate (MAP) stones in infection. These MAP stones can take the form of staghorn calculi.

DIAGNOSTIC STUDIES

Laboratory

Complete Blood Count. Elevated white blood cell count with infection.

Blood Urea Nitrogen (BUN)/Creatinine. Elevated BUN/creatinine ratio (greater than 20:1) suggests dehydration. Creatinine greater than 1.6 mg/dL indicates renal dysfunction.

Urine pH. If acid (pH less than 5.5), uric acid stones are more common. If alkaline (pH greater than 6.5), infection stones, calcium phosphate stones are more common.

Urinalysis. Red blood cells, if present, may signify infection or renal parenchymal injury. Microscopic techniques to evaluate crystals.

24-Hour Urine. Measure calcium (upper limits 300 mg for men and 250 mg for women), cystine (men, 300 mg; women, 300 mg), oxalate (men, 50 mg; women, 50 mg), uric acid (men, 800 mg; women, 750 mg), and sodium to determine dietary intake, volume (less than 1 L of volume increases risk).

Serum Calcium, Phosphate, Uric Acid, Electrolytes. As indicated to help exclude acidosis and hypokalemia (low potassium will decrease citrate secretion).

Parathyroid Hormone (PTH). Intact PTH (greater than 65 mEq/L) with a high or normal serum calcium.

Urinary Cyclic Adenosine Monophosphate. If high, consistent with elevated PTH.

Radiology
Flat Plate of the Abdomen (with or without Tomography). As indicated to help determine location of stone and stone burden.

Spherical (helical) CT. To visualize radiolucent or radiopaque stones.

Intravenous Pyelography. As indicated to determine presence of stone and stone location. Caution needed in patients allergic to dye.

Other
Stone analysis to determine type of stone.

DIFFERENTIAL DIAGNOSIS

Traumatic
Renal Injury. Hematuria may set up nidus for later stone formation.

Infectious
Urease-Producing Organisms. Most commonly *Proteus, Klebsiella*, and *Pseudomonas*. May cause infection predisposing to stone formation.

Metabolic
Hyperparathyroidism. Increased urinary calcium.

Sarcoid. Increased 1,25-vitamin D_3, leading to increased calcium absorption.

Hyperthyroidism. Increased bone calcium loss.

Neoplastic
Tumors. May cause obstruction to renal flow, increasing chance of infection. Tumors may cause hypercalcemia chronically with hypercalciuria.

Vascular
Not applicable.

Congenital
Inherited Tubular Defect. Cystine stones can form.

Acquired
Medications (e.g., Triamterene). May cause stones.

TREATMENT

Correct underlying problems, if possible, (e.g., infection, hyperparathyroidism, hyperthyroidism) and increase fluid intake (to greater than 2 L/day orally to help dilute the urine).

For absorptive hypercalciuria (increased gastrointestinal absorption of Ca^{2+}), give sodium cellulose phosphate, thiazide diuretics 25-50 mg/day, neutrophosphates 500 mg four times a day.

For renal leak, give hydrochlorothiazide 25-50 mg/day.

For subtle hyperparathyroidism, treatment may include oral phosphates, 500 mg four times a day, surgery, or shock wave lithotripsy.

For *sarcoid*, treat with steroids.

For management of infection-related *struvite "staghorn" stones*, may need long-term appropriate antibiotic therapy effective against *Proteus* species (dose depends on renal function), or surgery to remove stone. Recurrence is frequent.

For *hyperuricemia* (uric acid stones), increase fluid intake, decrease purine intake (meats) and add allopurinol 300 mg/day. Add allopurinol for both patients with hyperuricosuria and patients predisposed to formation of calcium-containing stones, because uric acid may be a nidus. Increase renal stone inhibitors in the urine with $NaHCO_3$ (can start with 600 mg twice a day).

For *hyperoxaluria* (calcium oxalate stones), attempt to decrease oxalate intake by decreasing intake of nuts, cocoa, spinach, cranberries, colas, and teas.

Surgical management may involve basket catch, open procedure, or extracorporeal shock wave lithotripsy if needed.

PEDIATRIC CONSIDERATIONS

Same workup and treatment as for adults. Exclude reflux, infections, anatomic defects.

OBSTETRIC CONSIDERATIONS

The normal physiologic changes that occur with pregnancy predispose women to ureteral reflux and stone formation within the upper urinary tract. This is due to dilatation of the renal pelvis and ureters with associated decrease in peristalsis, which in turn is secondary to increased progesterone secretion and possibly to the mechanical obstruction of the ureters from the enlarging uterus. Renal calculi occur in approximately 1 out of every 1000 pregnancies.

If nephrolithiasis is suspected, an intravenous pyelogram may be performed. The presence of renal calculi should always be ruled out in cases of acute pyelonephritis that do not resolve with appropriate antibiotics. Most renal stones are composed of calcium; therefore, hyperparathyroidism should be ruled out. Workup should also include serum urate determination.

If there is complete obstruction of a ureter in the pregnant patient, the blockage should be removed expeditiously. During the first two trimesters, the stones can be removed surgically. Nephrostomy is advisable as a temporizing measure if treatment is needed during the third trimester, until after delivery, when definitive treatment can be carried out.

GERIATRIC CONSIDERATIONS

Chronic bladder catheterization promotes infection, which can result in struvite stone formation. Ensure adequate fluid intake in elderly persons.

PREVENTION

Important measures include dietary counseling/modification; maintenance of adequate fluid levels; anticipation of situations causing an increase in calcium or uric acid (e.g., malignancies and their treatment); limiting intake of vitamin D; parathyroidectomy, if warranted; and chemoprophylaxis in patients with infected renal calculi.

PEARLS FOR THE PA

Kidney stones should be ruled out in all patients with unexplained gross or microscopic hematuria.

In the patient with nephrolithiasis, it is important to obtain a full medical history including dietary habits, fluid intake, and family history.

Obtain baseline laboratory analysis including blood urea nitrogen, creatinine, calcium, uric acid, and electrolytes.

Perform a urinalysis including pH, and 24-hour urine for volume, calcium, uric acid, and culture.

Send the stone for analysis.

Flat plate of the abdomen with tomograms should be obtained to evaluate the "stone burden."

Therapy should be aimed at pain control and hydration and should include measures specific to the type of stone.

Pyelonephritis: Upper Tract Infection

Sandra Lynn Roberts, MMSc, PA-C

DEFINITION

Infection and subsequent inflammation of the kidney and pelvis. Acute pyelonephritis is usually caused by acute bacterial infection of the kidney. Chronic pyelonephritis is usually caused by renal tract abnormalities with chronic infection and subsequent renal parenchymal scarring. More common in women than in men.

HISTORY

Symptoms.   Can range from dysuria and hematuria to acute flank pain associated with fever, chills, colicky abdominal pain, nausea, and vomiting.

General
Acute Pyelonephritis.   Patients are usually quite ill, presenting with flank or loin pain, high fever, or nausea.

Chronic Pyelonephritis.   The course is more insidious. Patients commonly present with symptoms of lower tract infection (dysuria, frequency). Other common presenting signs of chronic pyelonephritis are related to chronic renal injury, hypertension, salt wasting, and dehydration. Ascertain a history of previous urinary tract infections in childhood and during pregnancy.

Age.   No specific age group except with xanthogranulomatous pyelonephritis, which is usually seen in elderly women with renal calculi or obstructive uropathy. Young children may have accompanying vesicoureteral reflux.

Onset.   In acute pyelonephritis the symptoms are acute, whereas in chronic pyelonephritis the onset may be gradual over a period of months to years.

Duration.   Depends on underlying anomaly. Simple infections respond rapidly. Abnormalities such as stone, tumor, trauma, or abscess will prolong the process.

Intensity.   Mild to severe.

Aggravating Factors.   Factors predisposing to infection include urinary tract obstruction, neurogenic bladder, pregnancy, diabetes mellitus, vesicoureteral reflux, and instrumentation of the urinary tract.

Alleviating Factors.   Appropriate antimicrobial therapy, correction of underlying pathology (e.g., relief of obstruction, stone, or drainage of abscess).

Associated Factors.   Neurogenic bladder, analgesic nephropathy, sickle cell disease or trait, immunosuppression, and virulence factors found in bacteria (e.g., K antigen, hemolysis).

PHYSICAL EXAMINATION

General
Hypertension may be present in renal failure with volume overload.
   Acute Pyelonephritis.   Usually a sick-appearing patient with fever.
   Chronic Pyelonephritis.   The patient may appear quite normal, with normal findings on examination.

Extremities
Edema may be present in renal failure with volume overload.

Renal
   Acute Pyelonephritis.   Tender kidney anteriorly or painful costovertebral angle to deep palpation.
   Chronic Pyelonephritis.   The patient may have absent to minimal symptoms.

Skin
Dehydration may be present with tubular injury. Dry mucous membranes, flat neck veins, absence of axillary sweating.

PATHOPHYSIOLOGY

Escherichia coli is the most common pathogen (in 75% or more of all cases). Other organisms include gram-negative rods (e.g., *Klebsiella, Proteus, Enterobacter*) and rarely *Candida,* gram-positive cocci, and *Mycobacterium tuberculosis.*
   Acute Pyelonephritis.   Histologic hallmarks of acute pyelonephritis include edema of parenchymal tissue, areas of patchy infection or abscess formation, and accumulation of polymorphonucleocytes around and in tubules. The renal cortex is usually spared.
   Chronic Pyelonephritis.   In chronic pyelonephritis, scarring and fibrosis of the renal parynchema are the most common pathologic findings.

DIAGNOSTIC STUDIES

Laboratory
Urine Culture.   For causative organisms.
Urinalysis.   May show proteinuria, secondary to renal injury.

Electrolytes. May show hyperkalemia (due to distal tubular injury) or elevated blood urea nitrogen (BUN) and creatinine (due to renal injury).

Arterial Blood Gas Analysis. May show acidosis, due to tubular and interstitial destruction.

Radiology

ACUTE PYELONEPHRITIS

Renal Ultrasound Study. May find stone, abscess, enlarged kidney.

CT with Contrast. Can clearly identify areas of infection within kidney.

Gallium or Indium Radionuclide Scans. Will determine if there are still foci of infection present in the kidney or collecting systems.

CHRONIC PYELONEPHRITIS

Chronic pyelonephritis is a radiologic diagnosis based on clubbed calyces found with scarring (due to chronic infection or reflux) seen on intravenous pyelogram or retrograde studies.

Other

Not applicable.

DIFFERENTIAL DIAGNOSIS

Infectious

Infections Due to Gram-Positive Cocci, Candida, or Mycobacterium tuberculosis. Rare causes of pyelonephritis.

Prostatitis. May predispose the patient to developing pyelonephritis.

Metabolic

Metabolic Stone Disease. May cause injury or obstruction, thus creating a site for infection to occur.

Neoplastic

Renal or Abdominal Neoplasm. May cause obstruction with the possibility of infection. Positive CT scan of abdomen.

Congenital

Vesicoureteral Reflux. Seen especially in children predisposed to pyelonephritis.

Acquired

Analgesic Abuse or NSAID Abuse. History of medication use. May be associated with papillary necrosis.

Instrumentation. History of ureteral or renal procedure.

Traumatic. Not applicable.

Vascular. Not applicable.

TREATMENT

Correct any underlying pathology if present. Then institute antimicrobial therapy as follows:
- For mild infections, oral therapy with one of the following:
  Ciprofloxacin 500-750 mg every 12 hours
  Amoxicillin 500 mg every 8 hours
  Cephalexin 500 mg every 6 hours
  Amoxicillin–clavulanic acid 500 mg every 8 hours
  Trimethoprim-sulfamethoxazole 160/800 mg twice a day
- For moderate to severe infections, parenteral therapy (IM or IV) including:
  Standard:
  Ampicillin 1 g every 4 hours. May include one or more of the following:
  Aminoglycoside 1.5 mg/kg every 8 hours
  Alternate:
  Ceftriaxone 1 g every 24 hours
  Ceftazidime 1 g every 8 hours
  Aztreonam 1-2 g every 8 hours
  Imipenem 0.5 g every 6 hours
  Azlocillin 1 g every 8 hours
  Ampicillin 1-2 g PLUS sulbactam 0.5-1.0 g every 6 hours
- For suspected *Chlamydia trachomatis* infection (pyuria without bacteriuria):
  Doxycycline 100 mg every 12 hours for 7 days
  Erythromycin 500 mg every 6 hours for 7 days

The duration of therapy for acute pyelonephritis is usually 2 weeks, unless there is an underlying anatomic defect or obstruction preventing adequate drainage of urine.

Treatment of chronic pyelonephritis may necessitate therapy for months.

PEDIATRIC CONSIDERATIONS

Vesicoureteral reflux probably is a major cause of renal impairment/scarring in conjunction with bacteriuria or recurrent infections in infants. It is important to evaluate for urinary infection in all young children with fever.

OBSTETRIC CONSIDERATIONS

Pyelonephritis occurs in 1% to 2 % of pregnant patients. A common etiologic factor in pyelonephritis during pregnancy is asymptomatic bacteriuria. This is present in 4% to 7% of pregnant women and often leads to pyelonephritis if left untreated. Pregnancy is associated with an increased risk of progression to upper urinary tract infection owing to progressive dilatation of the renal calcyes, renal pelvis, and ureters along with mechanical obstruction of the ureters, all of which predispose to vesicoureteral reflux. The most common pathogen is *Escherichia coli.*

The mother with pyelonephritis is at risk for multiple organ system abnormalities including anemia, acute respiratory distress syndrome, endotoxic shock, and premature labor. There is also the possibility of perinatal fetal death and delivery of a low birth weight infant. All pregnant women with acute pyelonephritis should be hospitalized for close observation, parenteral hydration, and intravenous antibiotics. After consultation with the obstetrician, if a patient has more than one episode of acute pyelonephritis during the same pregnancy, prophylactic antibiotics should be strongly considered. Nitrofurantoin is considered a safe option.

GERIATRIC CONSIDERATIONS

Urinary tract infections are a significant cause of morbidity in elderly persons (usually secondary to chronic or intermittent Foley catheterization or neurogenic bladder). Urinary tract infections can cause a decrease in the glomerular filtration rate, predisposing the patient to chronic pyelonephritis.

PREVENTION

Prophylaxis with antibiotics and use of sterile technique and short-term catheterization. A vaccine is currently being evaluated against the common type I pilus antigen of *E. coli.*

PEARLS FOR THE PA

If a patient presents with fever and flank pain, rapid workup of the cause and institution of appropriate therapy are essential to prevent renal parenchymal injury.

If obstruction is present, rapid correction is required.

The possibility of pyelonephritis must be considered in all patients undergoing intermittent or chronic bladder catheterization.

Renal and Vascular Hypertension

Sandra Lynn Roberts, MMSc, PA-C

DEFINITION

Elevated blood pressure (hypertension) is classified as either essential (most common form, with blood pressure greater than 140/90 mm Hg) or secondary. Renal hypertension is considered a form of secondary hypertension. Other causes of secondary hypertension include endocrine disorders, coarctation of the aorta, toxemia, drugs, and increased intracranial pressure. Renovascular hypertension is the most common curable form of hypertension. It is usually due to fibromuscular disease in young people and to atherosclerosis in elderly persons.

HISTORY

Symptoms. Often no symptoms are present. If blood pressure is very high, headaches may occur.

General. Factors that suggest renal and vascular hypertension include family history, renal failure, renal dysfunction as a result of treatment with angiotensin-converting enzyme (ACE) inhibitors, or unprovoked hypokalemia. Ascertain a history of oral contraceptive use in women.

Age. Any, but hypertension with onset before age 30 or after age 50 years merits further investigation into secondary causes.

Onset. May have gradual onset or acute worsening of otherwise acceptable blood pressure control.

Duration. Usually chronic.

Intensity. Mild to severe.

Aggravating Factors. Oral contraceptives, nonsteroidal anti-inflammatory drugs (NSAIDs), renal failure, preexisting atherosclerotic disease, presence of multiple cardiovascular risk factors (e.g., smoking, essential hypertension, and increased cholesterol).

Alleviating Factors. Appropriate antihypertensive medication, correction of underlying medical condition (which may require surgical intervention).

Associated Factors. Preexisting essential hypertension or other secondary causes of hypertension including endocrine disorders, toxemia, coarctation of the aorta, drugs, and increased intracranial pressure.

PHYSICAL EXAMINATION

General. Need to evaluate all organ systems for end-organ damage.

Cardiovascular

Blood Pressure
Measure with patient supine, sitting, and upright (2 minutes apart), and document initial blood pressure in both arms. Blood pressure should be similar in both arms; if it is not, consider coarctation of the aorta.

Pulse
Postural changes can occur with dehydration and in patients on antihypertensive medication and those on fludrocortisone (Florinef) who develop elevated blood pressure when supine.
Evaluate for congestive heart failure.
Evaluate pulses in neck, over femoral artery, and in distal legs and auscultate for bruits (carotid/abdominal/renal bruits in particular).

Gastrointestinal
Rectal Examination. As indicated to exclude enlarged prostate causing urinary obstruction.

Head, Eyes, Ears, Nose, Throat
Funduscopic Examination. Indicated to evaluate vessels, exclude papilledema, and classify hypertensive retinal changes (normal to grade IV).

Neurologic
Perform a full neurologic examination to evaluate for focal deficits associated with a primary neurologic condition.

PATHOPHYSIOLOGY

Activation of renin-angiotensin system can occur in a variety of settings and cause hypertension. Any disorder that causes decreased blood flow to the kidney or causes injury to the kidney will cause release of renin. Elevated renin levels will increase angiotensin II levels, which will cause hypertension through its vasoconstrictive properties, and stimulation of aldosterone to help conserve sodium. The etiology for these clinical findings in renal and vascular hypertension includes the following.

Renal Hypertension. Vasculitis (e.g., lupus), obstruction, renal aretery stenosis, acute glomerular injury and enlarged kidneys (e.g., polycystic kidney disease).

Vascular Hypertension. Arteriosclerosis (in approximately 75% of all cases), fibromuscular dysplasia (in approximately 15% of all cases), intrarenal arterial branch narrowing, dissection of aorta and renal artery, arteritis, renal thrombosis or embolism, coarctation of the aorta, and rarely an extrinsic compression of the renal artery by a mass.

DIAGNOSTIC STUDIES

Laboratory
Chemistry Profile. Hypokalemia is consistent with activated renin-angiotensin-aldosterone system (less significant if patient is on diuretic therapy); blood urea nitrogen (BUN) and creatinine indicated to evaluate renal function, and bicarbonate (HCO_3) to assess for alkalosis seen with low potassium and high aldosterone.

Urinalysis. May have proteinuria, but not a specific feature.

24-Hour Urine. For protein, creatinine clearance. Decreased creatinine clearance is seen in renal failure, and nephritic-range proteinuria can be seen with cases of accelerated or malignant hypertensive crisis.

Serum Antinuclear Antibody (ANA), Rheumatoid Factor, C3, C4 Assays. As indicated to exclude vasculitis.

Peripheral/Renal Vein Renin Levels (with or without Captopril). Performed to exclude renal hypertension secondary to renal artery stenosis. Increased peripheral renin levels do not provide information about which kidney is involved. Individual renal vein renin levels can give information on which kidney is involved if unilateral renal artery stenosis is present.

Radiology
Captopril Provocation Test. Look for rise in peripheral renin level after administration of ACE inhibitor (captopril), suggesting renovascular disease.

Captopril Renography (Radionuclide Scanning). Look for decreased uptake of radioisotope by affected kidney after administration of captopril. This test is less reliable in African Americans and in patients with preexisting renal dysfunction.

Renal Doppler Ultrasound Study (Duplex Scanning). Direct renal artery study may demonstrate increased velocity at the area of stenosis. Useful in evaluating patients after angioplasty with renal stent placement and detection of renal artery stenosis in transplanted kidneys. Currently being evaluated using captopril to improve accuracy.

Renal Angiography. The definitive test to visualize the renal artery (invasive). Correlation between angiographic picture and degree of renal ischemia is poor. Risk for dye-induced renal failure or cholesterol embolization has been decreased with the use of smaller-lumen catheters.

Renal Digital Subtraction Angiography (DSA). Images can be recalled immediately and digitalized images can be computer enhanced. Uses half the amount of contrast material as in conventional renal angiography.

Magnetic Resonance Angiography. Helpful with proximal renal artery lesions. Not as effective in patients with fibromuscular disease. Noninvasive and does not require potentially nephrotoxic contrast agent.

CT Angiography (Spiral [Helical] CT). Gives the diagnostic accuracy of angiography with the low risk of DSA (very little dye).

CO_2 Angiography. In this method, currently under evaluation, CO_2 is used as an arterial contrast (instead of dye), and DSA is used for the imaging. This combination allows diagnostic imaging of the renal arteries and is used to guide angioplasty procedures and does not require any nephrotoxic dye for contrast purposes.

Intravenous Pyelography. No longer used as a screening test. If one kidney is visualized sooner than the other or if size disparity is present, it may indicate the presence of a renal artery lesion. Unreliable in detecting branch or bilateral artery stenosis.

Other
Echocardiography. Used to determine cardiac end-organ damage.

DIFFERENTIAL DIAGNOSIS

Traumatic
Acute Renal Artery or Vein Injury. History of trauma. Elevated lactate dehydrogenase with renal infarction. Renal injury seen on renal angiogram or venogram.

Infectious
Chronic Pyelonephritis. Presence of small, scarred kidneys. May have a history of kidney stones or infections. In *chronic ureteral reflux*, hypertension may be a feature, especially in children with a history of reflux and subsequent renal failure.

Metabolic
Pheochromocytoma. Releases norepinephrine, causing hypertension.

Cushing's Syndrome. Patients can present with hypokalemia and hypertension due to excessive glucocorticoid and mineralocorticoid effect.

Hyperthyroidism/Hypothyroidism. Hypertension is a possible finding. Abnormal thyroid function studies.

Hyperaldosteronism. Elevated levels of aldosterone will cause sodium retention and hypertension.

Acromegaly. Elevated growth hormone level, increased size of hands and feet, and acromegalic facies. Usually mild hypertension.

Vascular
Not otherwise applicable.

Congenital
Coarctation of the Aorta. Abnormalities on blood pressure measurements between the arms.

Acquired
Drugs. A common cause of hypertension. NSAIDs, glucocorticoids, cocaine, licorice, mineralocorticoids, birth control pills, sympathomimetic drugs, monoamine oxidase inhibitors.

Toxemia of Pregnancy.   Hypertension and edema are hallmarks.
Obesity.   Hypertension is a frequent finding.

TREATMENT

Correct underlying pathology. *Note*: Renal artery stenosis in a hypertensive patient is not necessarily the cause of the hypertension. If renal ischemia is present along with the renal artery stenosis, the diagnosis of renovascular hypertension is much more conclusive. Remember that a patient can have both essential and secondary hypertension at the same time.

Surgical

If renal artery stenosis is present, angioplasty of the renal artery can be considered; however, restenosis is much more common in patients with atheromatous stenosis (compared with those with fibromuscular dysplasia). Often, renal angioplasty does not correct the hypertension to a large degree if pre-existing essential hypertension is present (which is often the case in the elderly). Renal angioplasty is a viable option in patients who cannot undergo a major surgical procedure (e.g., nephrectomy.)

If a renal parenchymal process is present, correct obstruction and treat vasculitis or the glomerular lesion.

Pharmacologic

If invasive procedures pose too much risk, medical/pharmacologic therapy may be tried. Diuretics such as thiazide or loop diuretics may be contraindicated in renal artery stenosis because such agents may decrease glomerular filtration rate and increase renin release.

ACE inhibitors, such as captopril or enalapril, may also be contraindicated because they may decrease glomerular filtration rate. These medications are contraindicated in patients with bilateral renal artery stenosis or unilateral renal artery stenosis in a solitary kidney.

Calcium channel blockers (e.g., nifedipine 10 mg three times a day as initial dose), beta blockers (e.g., propranolol 40 mg twice a day as initial dose), and vasodilators (e.g., hydralazine 10 mg four times a day as initial dose) are appropriate drugs for medical therapy. Drop in blood pressure may decrease perfusion pressure and decrease glomerular filtration rate if the stenosis is significant.

PEDIATRIC CONSIDERATIONS

Secondary causes of hypertension in children are parenchymal disease in approximately 80% of the cases, renal artery disease in approximately 15% (usually due to fibromuscular disease), and coarctation of the aorta in approximately 2%.

OBSTETRIC CONSIDERATIONS

Hypertension and edema are the hallmarks of toxemia of pregnancy. Patients may require renal ultrasound if the hypertension is not responsive to conventional therapies.

GERIATRIC CONSIDERATIONS

Renovascular disease is a major cause of end-stage renal disease in the elderly. Elderly persons are more likely to have coexistent essential and renovascular hypertension. One should routinely check the BUN and creatinine and blood pressure of elderly patients placed on ACE inhibitors. If an elevation occurs with therapy with ACE inhibitors, consider renovascular etiology.

PREVENTIVE CONSIDERATIONS

Strict attention to monitoring and reducing cardiovascular risk factors to reduce the risk of atherosclerosis. Routine blood pressure screenings are also recommended.

PEARLS FOR THE PA

The possibility of renal or vascular hypertension must be considered if a patient presents with new-onset hypertension, hypokalemia (in the absence of diuretics), or sudden difficulty with control of stable hypertension, or with sudden development of pulmonary and/or peripheral edema after treatment with an ACE inhibitor (consider renal artery stenosis).

Tubulointerstitial Diseases

Sandra Lynn Roberts, MMSc, PA-C

DEFINITION

Any process that damages the tubules or interstitium, or both (does NOT include the glomerulus).

HISTORY

Symptoms. History of fever, rash, and recent intake of new medication makes allergic interstitial injury a distinct possibility. The patient may present with polyuria, dehydration, or mental status changes.

General. Obtain a history of new medication intake, heavy metal exposure, ethylene glycol, chemotherapy, or poison ingestion. Additional history of infections, antibiotic intake, episodes of low blood pressure, exposure to dye, possible renal obstruction due to stones (cystine, uric acid, or infectious), gout, sickle cell disease, muscle injury, malignancy, and history of sarcoidosis or multiple myeloma. Chronic intake of analgesics, nonsteroidal anti-inflammatory drugs (NSAIDs), or cancer medications can invoke a chronic process. It is essential to get the best history from family, patient, charts, and other caregivers to help determine the etiology of the tubulointerstitial process.

Age. Any.

Onset. Acute or gradual.

Duration. May be brief or chronic.

Intensity. Can be severe with acute renal failure or mild with no change in renal function.

Aggravating Factors. Old age, underlying chronic renal failure, continued use of offending agents.

Alleviating Factors. Recovery of renal function, discontinuance of offending agents.

Associated Factors. Underlying medical problems, dehydration, hyperkalemia, acidosis.

PHYSICAL EXAMINATION

General. Include all organ systems and evaluate for evidence of tumors.

Cardiovascular. The patient may be hypotensive.

Extremities. Tender muscles may suggest rhabdomyolysis.

Gastrointestinal. Palpate for masses or tenderness. Observe for signs of infection.

Genitourinary. Palpate for tenderness. Perform rectal examination to rule out an enlarged prostate.

Neurologic. Evaluate mental status (may be altered with poisons, alcohols).

Pulmonary. Auscultate for rales, rhonchi. Observe for hemoptysis, which may be consistent with infection or tuberculosis.

Skin. Observe for rash, skin infections, dehydration.

PATHOPHYSIOLOGY

Acute interstitial nephritis is considered a common cause of renal dysfunction. Chronic interstitial nephritis has been shown to be responsible for up to 25% of cases leading to permanent renal failure.

Injury to the interstitium and tubules can occur through a variety of mechanisms including infection, drugs, immune disorders, neoplasms, genetic factors, and irradiation. Much of the inflammation associated with these mechanisms is immunologic in nature, often requiring a combination of inciting insult and immune response genes. Any of these disorders can cause acute tubulonecrosis or an interstitial destructive process (allergic interstitial nephritis, scarring of the interstitium, or an inflammatory process with white cell infiltration). If the process is chronic, it will eventually affect the glomeruli and cause renal failure.

Chronic tubulointerstitial processes may cause the patient to present with impaired concentrating ability due to interstitial injury causing polyuria, dehydration, decreased reabsorption of sodium due to tubular injury (salt wasting), hyperkalemia due to distal tubular injury, or a metabolic acidosis due to distal tubular injury or impaired ammonia generation in the medullary interstitium. Tubule defects and tubule syndromes (e.g., Fanconi syndrome) are more common in chronic interstitial nephritis than in acute interstitial nephritis.

DIAGNOSTIC STUDIES

Laboratory
Complete Blood Count. Elevated white blood cell count may be found with infections, cancers; anemia may indicate (although not always) chronic disease or cancer; abnormal red cells may indicate sickle cell disease.

Serum Calcium. Elevations may suggest hypercalcemic nephropathy.

Uric Acid. Elevations may suggest urate nephropathy.

Heavy Metal Levels. For lead, mercury levels.

Electrolytes. May show hyperkalemia. Hypernatremia may be present if patient is dehydrated or acidotic. Nongap acidosis may be seen (low bicarbonate [HCO_3] with high chloride).

Blood Urea Nitrogen (BUN)/Creatinine. As indicated to evaluate renal function. Abnormality is usually the first indication of tubulointerstitial disease.

Urinalysis. Shows red and white blood cells with occasional red or white blood cell casts. Mild to moderate proteinuria and hematuria. Occasionally gross hematuria is seen. Check pH to determine the ability to acidify the urine and specific gravity to determine concentrating ability of the kidney.

24-Hour Urine. For protein and creatinine clearance. Total protein excretion usually less than 3 g/24 hours.

Fractional Excretion of Sodium (FENa). Usually greater than 1% secondary to concentrating defect.

Urine Eosinophils. Eosinophiluria has been reported with interstitial nephritis, but negative predictive value is low.

Urine Electrolytes and Osmolality. As indicated to determine whether the kidney has the appropriate response to hyperkalemia (urine potassium should be high in hyperkalemia), volume loss (urine osmolality should be high with dehydration), or acidosis (urine should be acidic, or urine chloride should be much higher than the sodium consistent with a large amount of ammonia [NH_3]).

Serum and Urine Immunoelectrophoresis.   As indicated to help exclude myeloma.

Anti–Glomerular Basement Membrane (Anti-GBM) Antibody, Cryoglobulin, Antinuclear Antibody (ANA), Double-Stranded DNA Assays.   For immune disorder workup.

Radiology

Renal Ultrasound Examination.   Performed to evaluate cystic disease, chronic obstruction. The kidney may be normal or slightly increased in size (in contrast to smaller kidneys seen in chronic renal failure).

Intravenous Pyelography.   In the absence of renal failure, may be indicated to rule out obstruction or stones. Retrograde study may be beneficial if reflux is a possibility, especially in children.

Other

Kidney Biopsy.   Useful to establish the tissue pathology. Often needed for definitive diagnosis of tubulointerstitial disease.

Gallium Scan.   May have positive uptake in allergic interstitial nephritis. Negative predictive value is low and often requires follow-up kidney biopsy if negative.

DIFFERENTIAL DIAGNOSIS

Traumatic

Rhabdomyolysis.   May cause acute tubular injury (e.g., myoglobin causing acute tubulonecrosis).

Infectious

Acute Tubulointerstitial Nephritis.   May result from bacteriuria (pyelonephritis or chronic infection from reflux). Rarely, tuberculosis, malaria, or syphilis.

Metabolic

Hypercalcemia and Hyperuricosemia.   May occur with calcium or urate deposition.

Chronic Hypokalemia.   May cause tubular injury.

Kidney Stones and Obstruction.   May be visualized on CT (with dilated collecting system), ultrasound study, or intravenous pyelogram.

Immune Disorders: Lupus, Anti-GBM Disease, Mixed Cryoglobulinemia.   All can cause renal failure.

Neoplastic

Multiple Myeloma, Light Chain Disease, Leukemia, and Lymphomatous Infiltration.   Long-term obstruction from tumor: Can manifest with renal dysfunction.

Vascular
Not applicable.

Congenital
Medullary Sponge Disease, Polycystic Kidney Disease. May cause chronic renal failure.

Acquired
Chronic Medication Use: NSAIDs, Aspirin. May cause tubulointerstitial disease.
Acute Medication-Induced Disease. Drugs causing primarily interstitial damage: penicillins (most frequently associated medication), cephalosporins, sulfa drugs, rifampin, nonsteroidals, diuretics, cimetidine, allopurinol, tetracycline. Drugs causing primarily tubular injury: aminoglycosides, cephalothin.

TREATMENT

Identify and correct underlying process; remove inciting factor(s).
If allergic interstitial nephritis is present, steroids may be used. Begin with prednisone 40 mg/day and taper rapidly over a few days. Benefit of steroid therapy has not been clearly established. Treatment of acute interstitial nephritis without infection consists of corticosteroids (1 mg/kg/day) and/or cyclophosphamide (2 mg/kg/day) for up to 1 year. Discontinue both if no improvement is seen after 6 weeks of therapy.

PEDIATRIC CONSIDERATIONS

Exclude chronic reflux with chronic or acute infection. Fanconi syndrome causing proximal tubular injury may be seen in childhood.

OBSTETRIC CONSIDERATIONS

No specific indications.

GERIATRIC CONSIDERATIONS

Minimize or anticipate problems in elderly patients who are taking NSAIDs and/or diuretics.

PREVENTIVE CONSIDERATIONS

Minimize use of offending medications (i.e., antibiotics and NSAIDs). Identify and treat pyelonephritis as soon as possible and anticipate renal problems on the basis of primary disease diagnosis and treatments.

PEARLS FOR THE PA

Half of the patients with chronic tubulointerstitial disease usually present with hypertension, normal findings on urine sediment analysis, and a nongap metabolic acidosis.

History is essential to exclude medications (especially antibiotics), excessive use of analgesics, or acute medical illness as the cause.

Treatment is directed at correcting the underlying disorder.

Further Reading

Brenner BM,: The Kidney, 7th ed. Philadelphia, Saunders, 2004.

Davidson AM, Cameron JS, Grünfeld JP, et al: Oxford Textbook of Clinical Nephrology. Oxford, Oxford University Press, 1998.

Kiningham RB: Asymptomatic bacteriuria in pregnancy. Am Fam Physician 47:1232, 1993.

Schrier RW: Renal and Electrolyte Disorders, 4th ed. Boston, Little, Brown, 1992.

Schrier RW, Gottschalt CW: Diseases of the Kidney, 7th ed. Boston, Little, Brown, 2001.

Scorpio RJ, Esposito TJ, Smith LG: Blunt trauma during pregnancy: Factors affecting fetal outcome. J Trauma 32:213, 1992.

Goldman L, Ausiello D (eds): Cecil Textbook of Medicine, 22nd ed. Philadelphia, Saunders, 2004.

NEUROLOGY

10

Dementia

William A. Mosier, EdD, MPAS, LMFT, PA-C (Major-USAFR)
and William M. Hardy, PhD, MS, PA-C

DEFINITION

Dementia is a disorder of the brain characterized by a progressive intellectual decline, eventually leading to deterioration in self-care and social functioning. The onset is insidious, with memory impairment, personality changes, and behavior problems becoming more pronounced over time. A cause for the dementia may be measurable with laboratory or radiographic studies, or the dementia may be a diagnosis of exclusion (Alzheimer disease).

HISTORY

Symptoms. Impaired ability to learn new information or to remember previously learned information, language disturbance, difficulty carrying out motor activities (despite intact motor function), trouble recognizing objects (despite intact sensory function), problem with staying organized, forgetfulness, emotional lability, progressively increasing confusion, personality changes, inability to perform complex tasks, impaired judgment, hallucinations, and physical deterioration.

General. It is common for someone other than the patient (e.g., family member) to be the first to seek medical advice concerning the patient's condition. The afflicted person may be unaware of any mental deterioration. Common early presenting complaints include the patient's neglecting personal responsibilities and hygiene. Marked personality changes may also be a chief complaint of family members.

Age. Elderly, usually beginning in the fifth decade and increasing with advancing age.

Onset. Gradual, months to years.

Duration. Slow and progressive.

Intensity. Initially mild, but may be incapacitating in later stages of the illness.

Aggravating Factors. Some medications, illicit drugs, alcohol, and deteriorating physical health.

Alleviating Factors. Generally none; however, early intervention can slow the progression of symptoms. Early symptoms may not be recognized if the patient is performing routine, simple tasks. Therefore, diagnosis may not be timely enough to make a significant impact on slowing the progression of symptoms.

Associated Factors. General physical deterioration.

PHYSICAL EXAMINATION

General. The patient may display hostility about being brought to see a health care provider. The patient may be repetitive in response to questions asked during the initial evaluation and may act confused and defensive. A thorough physical examination, to include all organ systems, is necessary, as the patient may be unaware of or unable to communicate symptoms of any underlying illnesses.

Neurologic. Perform a complete mental status examination evaluating the patient's insight into the condition; orientation to person, place, time, and surroundings; memory of remote, intermediate, and immediate events; identification of common objects; simple mathematic calculations; and ability to interpret abstract thoughts. A complete neurologic examination must be performed including assessment of cranial nerves, motor function, gait, all sensory modalities (touch, temperature, two-point discrimination, pain, proprioception), and cerebellar function. The extremities may be rigid or spastic, and the reflexes may be symmetrically increased. The neurologic examination findings are typically nonfocal, and the diagnosis is generally derived from the history and mental status examination. See Table 10-1. A focal neurologic finding may indicate a neoplasm, stroke, or other cause of the patient's symptoms.

PATHOPHYSIOLOGY

Dementia involves a general deterioration of the cerebrum and diencephalon. The frontal lobes suffer the greatest damage. Any disease that alters cerebral metabolism can cause symptoms of dementia. The most common form of dementia, Alzheimer disease, results from a degeneration and loss of neurons and formation of senile plaques.

DIAGNOSTIC STUDIES

Laboratory

Serum Chemistry Profile. Used to rule out hyponatremia (normal sodium 136 to 145 mEq/L); liver function abnormalities as indicated by elevated levels of lactate dehydrogenase (LDH), alanine aminotransferase (ALT) (formerly serum glutamic-oxaloacetic transaminase [SGOT]), aspartate aminotransferase (AST) (formerly serum glutamic-pyruvic transaminase [SGPT]); renal failure with elevated blood urea nitrogen (BUN) (normal 10 to 20 mg/dL) and creatinine (normal 0.6 to 1.2 mg/dL); and nutritional abnormalities with decreased albumin (normal 3.5 to 5.0 g/dL) or prealbumin.

24-Hour Urine for Albumin. Used to determine nutritional status.

Complete Blood Count. Elevated white blood cell count (normal 4500 to 11,000/mm³) in infection; decreased hemoglobin (normal range in males

Table 10–1. Folstein Mini-Mental State Examination

Task	Instructions	Scoring	
Date orientation	"Tell me the date." Ask for omitted items.	One point each for year, season, date, day of week, and month	5
Place orientation	"Where are you?" Ask for omitted items.	One point each for state, county, town, building, and floor or room	5
Register 3 objects	Name three objects slowly and clearly. Ask the patient to repeat them.	One point for each item correctly repeated	3
Serial sevens	Ask the patient to count backwards from 100 by 7. Stop after five answers. (Or ask patient to spell "world" backwards.)	One point for each correct answer (or letter)	5
Recall 3 objects	Ask the patient to recall the objects mentioned above.	One point for each item correctly remembered	3
Naming	Point to your watch and ask the patient: "What is this?" Repeat with a pencil.	One point for each correct answer	2
Repeating a phrase	Ask the patient to say "no ifs, ands, or buts."	One point if successful on first try	1
Verbal commands	Give the patient a plain piece of paper and say: "Take this paper in your right hand, fold it in half, and put it on the floor."	One point for each correct action	3
Written commands	Show the patient a piece of paper with "CLOSE YOUR EYES" printed on it.	One point if the patient's eyes close	1
Writing	Ask the patient to write a sentence.	One point if sentence has a subject, has a verb, and makes sense	1
Drawing	Ask the patient to copy a pair of intersecting pentagons onto a piece of paper.	One point if the figure has ten corners and two intersecting lines	1
Scoring	A score of 24 or above is considered normal.		30

Adapted with special permission of the Publisher, Psychological Assessment Resources, Inc., 16204 North Florida Avenue, Lutz, Florida 33549, from the Mini-Mental State Examination, by Marshal Folstein and Susan Folstein, Copyright 1975, 1998, 2001 by Mini Mental LLC, Inc. Published 2001 by Psychological Assessment Resources, Inc. Further reproduction is prohibited without permission of PAR, Inc. The MMSE can be purchased from PAR, Inc. by calling (800) 331-8378 or (813) 968-3003.

14 to 18 g/dL, in females 12 to 16 g/dL) and hematocrit (normal males 40 to 54 mg/dL, females 37 to 47 mg/dL) in anemia.

Serum Vitamin B_{12} Level. Normal 200 to 1100 pg/mL. Decreased in deficiency states (pernicious anemia).

Toxicology Screen or Serum Drug Levels of Prescribed Medications. As indicated to rule out toxicity or intoxication.

Thyroid Function Tests. May be elevated or depressed.

Cerebrospinal Fluid Examination. Venereal Disease Research Laboratory (VDRL) test positive in neurosyphilis; cultures for bacteria, fungi, mycobacteria, and yeast as indicated to rule out meningitis. In meningitis, glucose (normal 40 to 80 mg/dL) is reduced, protein (normal 15 to 45 mg/dL) is increased, and cell count with differential white count (white blood cell count normal 0 to 10 mg/L) is elevated.

Dexamethasone Suppression Test. Indicated if Cushing disease is suspected. Urine and plasma free cortisol are normally suppressed with low-dose dexamethasone (0.5 mg every 6 hours). Levels are also suppressed with higher-dose dexamethasone (2 mg every 6 hours) in pituitary-dependent Cushing disease. There is no suppression of levels in nonpituitary Cushing disease.

Human Immunodeficiency Virus (HIV) Testing. If positive, opportunistic neurologic infection with normal to low white blood count or neoplasm should be ruled out.

Radiology

CT, MRI, and Positron Emission Tomography (PET). As indicated to rule out focal neurologic lesion, hydrocephalus, or demyelinating disease (MRI only). Brain atrophy on CT/MRI is not a reliable indicator of impaired intellectual function. However, PET, when available, can be used as an adjunct to the clinical evaluation in patients with suspected Alzheimer type dementia because the glucose usage pattern observed in these cases is relatively specific.

Other

Electroencephalogram (EEG). Used to evaluate for occult seizure, or focal finding not apparent on CT or MRI.

Cardiac Evaluation. Used to rule out a cardiogenic source for cerebral emboli (e.g., valvular heart disease or arrhythmia). Should include echocardiogram and electrocardiogram.

Cerebral Angiography or Noninvasive Cerebral Blood Flow Studies. As indicated to evaluate patency of the internal carotid arteries and intracerebral circulation.

Psychologic Evaluation. Including Wechsler Adult Intelligence Scale, a standard memory test, and a depression inventory (to rule out depression masking as dementia).

DIFFERENTIAL DIAGNOSIS

Traumatic

Chronic/Acute Subdural Hematoma. Usually associated with a history of head trauma. May have headache, confusion, or focal neurologic finding such as hemiparesis; positive CT/MRI.

Infectious

Brain Abscess. Focal neurologic abnormality; patient may have nuchal rigidity or other signs of meningeal irritation, febrile, elevated white blood cell count (may be absent in HIV infection), positive CT/MRI.

Neurosyphilis. History of untreated syphilis, positive serum or cerebrospinal fluid (CSF) VDRL test.

Meningitis. Nuchal rigidity, fever. Elevated white blood cell count, elevated CSF protein and low CSF glucose, positive CSF cultures.

Metabolic

Hepatic Failure. Elevated values on liver function studies, with history of hepatitis or alcohol abuse; may have asterixis.

Renal Failure (Uremia). Elevated BUN and creatinine; may have hypertension, muscle wasting, purpura.

Hypothyroidism/Hyperthyroidism. Abnormal thyroid function tests.

Cushing Disease. Central obesity, diabetes mellitus, moon facies, easy bruisability, striae, abnormal dexamethasone suppression test.

Hypoglycemia. Decreased serum glucose.

Neoplastic

Primary or Metastatic Brain Tumor. Headache, signs of increased intracranial pressure, and focal neurologic findings; positive CT/MRI.

Vascular

Multi-Infarct Dementia. Causes stepwise decrease in mental function (as each infarct takes place); may have focal neurologic findings, cardiogenic source of emboli, atherosclerosis, positive angiogram, or cerebral blood flow study.

Pernicious Anemia. Low serum vitamin B_{12}. Decreased hemoglobin and hematocrit. May have associated nutritional deficiency.

Congenital

Demyelinating Disease. Patient may present at a young age with waxing and waning neurologic symptoms over months to years.

Acquired

Alcoholic Dementia. History of alcohol abuse; may have abnormal liver function tests.

Chronic Drug Intoxication. History of ongoing use/abuse of drugs; elevated drug levels or positive toxicology screen.

Depression. Patient is oriented; close examination will reveal cognitive functioning within normal limits.

TREATMENT

The goal of therapy is to correct any identifiable potentially reversible condition. If no potentially causative agent is found, supportive care is arranged for the patient and family. In the late stages of dementia, placement in a long-term care facility may be necessary. Many patients with dementia develop comorbid depression. These patients should be considered for a trial on one of the selective serotonnin reuptake inhibitors (SSRIs) or related antidepressants such as citalopram, fluoxetine, fluvoxamine, mirtazapine, nefazodone, paroxetine, sertraline, or venlafaxine. Another important consideration is disruptive behavior such as agitation, aggression, or delusions. Patients who manifest any of these behaviors should be considered candidates for antipsychotic medication. The newer antipsychotics such as risperidone, quetiapine, olanzapine, and ziprasidone are safe and effective for use in this population.

In the case of Alzheimer type dementia, specific drugs have demonstrated considerable efficacy. (See Table 10-2.)

PEDIATRIC CONSIDERATIONS

The patient who presents at a young age with signs of dementia requires a thorough workup to evaluate the cause of the symptoms. An underlying cause will almost always be found for memory and intellectual decline in the child.

OBSTETRIC CONSIDERATIONS

No specific indications.

GERIATRIC CONSIDERATIONS

Dementia is a disease of the elderly. It is very important to rule out potentially reversible causes of dementia in order to treat the patient effectively. Over 80% of persons manifesting symptoms of dementia will experience a progressive loss of intellectual functioning and memory sufficients to eventually cause a loss of independent living skills. Vital to effective management of a patient's dementia is the identification of any comorbid conditions and implementation of proper interventions. The provision of ongoing care is especially important to ensure an optimal quality of living as the dementia progresses.

Table 10–2. Pharmacologic Treatment of Alzheimer Dementia

Drug	Dosing	Risks/Precautions	Contraindication(s)
Donepezil (Aricept)	Initial 5 mg qd Then 10 mg after 4-6 wk	Supraventricular conduction disturbances, GI bleed, asthma, seizure	None
Tacrine (Cognes)	Initial 10 mg qid; can be increased at 4-wk intervals to max of 160 mg daily	Liver function, asthma, GI bleed	Hx of jaundice Elevated bilirubin
Rivastigmine (Exelon)	Initial 1.5 mg bid with food Then 3 mg bid if well tolerated after 2 wk; increase to tolerance; max dose 12 mg/daily	Nausea, vomiting, GI bleed, supraventricular conduction disturbances, seizures, asthma	None
Galantamine (Reminyl)	4 mg bid with food; may be increased at 4-wk intervals to max of 12 mg bid	AV block, GI bleed, asthma, seizures	None

AV, atrioventricular; GI, gastrointestinal; Hx, history.

PREVENTIVE CONSIDERATIONS

There is no way to prevent dementia. Secondary prevention involves patient safety issues to prevent injury secondary to the dementia. Medication should be monitored with sufficient frequency to ensure optimal dosing for maximal efficacy and minimal side effects. Once dementia is diagnosed, the goal of management must be to use medication to target symptoms and provide adequate education about the disease to the patient and family. A proactive approach to intervention should be taught to the patient and the family. It will be important to sustain independent living as long as possible by making environmental adjustments that facilitate self-help. Estrogen, vitamin E, and aspirin have demonstrated some protective effect against the development of Alzheimer type dementia. However, to be effective they must be started before the onset of symptoms. Persons with a positive family history for Alzheimer type dementia may consider the use of one or more of these agents.

PEARLS FOR THE PA

The history is the key to the diagnosis of dementia.

Findings on physical examination may be unremarkable.

Dementia results from a general deterioration of the cerebrum and diencephalon.

A thorough search for potentially reversible underlying conditions is required.

Encephalitis

Catherine R. Judd, MS, PA-C

DEFINITION

Encephalitis is a viral infection of the brain or spinal cord, most commonly due to herpesviruses or arboviruses. Encephalitis can produce mental status changes, seizures, and motor and sensory deficits.

HISTORY

Symptoms. Fever may or may not be present. May be associated with nuchal rigidity, headache, nausea, vomiting, photophobia, myalgia, tremor, seizures, mental status changes, delirium, speech impairment, hemiparesis, involuntary movements, gait disturbance, diplopia, or facial weakness.

General.   The presence of encephalitis in the summer or fall suggests a potential epidemic due to arthropod-borne viruses. Diagnostic clues are provided by any of the following:

- History of viral inoculation (e.g., mosquito or tick)
- Presence of respiratory and/or gastrointestinal disturbance
- History of recent epidemic
- Travel in an endemic region
- Increased frequency in infants and children

Patients with a history of herpes simplex virus (HSV) infection, latent or active, are at risk for herpes encephalitis. Immunocompromised patients and those with acquired immunodeficiency syndrome (AIDS) are at increased risk for AIDS encephalitis or central nervous system (CNS) infection with cytomegalovirus or papovaviruses. La Crosse encephalitis is the most common form of *endemic* encephalitis in North America. It is mosquito-borne and generally affects children. Occurrence of *epidemic* encephalitis depends on region and season of the year. Most common in North America is mosquito-borne St. Louis encephalitis. In other parts of the world, encephalitis associated with poliovirus infection is among the most common, along with retroviral encephalitis.

Age.   Any.

Onset.   May be acute or preceded by a febrile illness and malaise of several days' duration.

Duration.   May be short-lived (10 to 21 days) or leave permanent residual defects such as cognitive and memory impairment, personality changes, or hemiparesis.

Intensity.   May be relatively mild or fatal. HSV encephalitis and eastern equine encephalitis (EEE) are the most severe.

Aggravating Factors.   Immunocompromised states.

Alleviating Factors.   Early supportive care. Treatment with acyclovir in HSV encephalitis.

Associated Factors.   Living in endemic areas of arthropod-borne viruses and/or mosquito-infected areas, history of recent viral infection, infection with HSV.

PATHOPHYSIOLOGY

Viruses that cause encephalitis can be categorized as those occurring in seasonal and potentially epidemic patterns (arboviruses), those occurring in patients with a preexisting viral illness (HSV, Epstein-Barr virus [EBV], mumps virus, varicella virus, measles virus), and those occurring in immunocompromised patients (as in human immunodeficiency virus [HIV] infection). Other viruses such as papovaviruses, cytomegalovirus, and slow viruses may cause encephalitis, but a review of all of the causative viruses is beyond the scope of this book.

Arboviruses

Arboviruses (*arthropod-borne viruses*) are spread from an infected source (e.g., horse or bird) to humans via arthropod bites (e.g., mosquitoes or ticks). Infection tends to follow a seasonal pattern when mosquitoes and ticks are more active (summer and early autumn) as well as a geographic distribution. Common arbovirus infections are EEE; western equine encephalitis (WEE); St. Louis encephalitis; Venezuelan encephalitis (VE), which is more common in Florida and the southwestern United States; California virus encephalitis (CVE); and Japanese B encephalitis (JBE), which is the most common worldwide. EEE is the most severe.

Herpes Simplex Virus

HSV encephalitis is the most common form of encephalitis in those with pre-existing viral illness and also the most severe. In adults, it is usually due to infection with the herpes simplex virus type 1 (HSV-1), which also causes oral lesions. Herpes simplex virus type 2 (HSV-2) is usually encountered in neonates. Inoculation with virus is from infected genital lesions in the mother.

HSV may cause hemorrhagic, necrotizing lesions in the brain, usually located in the inferior and medial temporal and frontal lobes. This may be from seeding of latent infection via trigeminal or olfactory nerve pathways. Skin and genital lesions usually are not evident at clinical presentation. Mortality rates are 50% to 80% in untreated patients and 20% to 30% in treated patients.

Epstein-Barr Virus; Mumps, Varicella, Measles Viruses

Infection with EBV may result in recurrent or prolonged bouts of meningitis. Encephalitis due to mumps, varicella, or measles virus is rare. It tends to occur in the winter and spring, which coincides with the period of increased incidence of these infections. Complications of varicella and measles include subacute sclerosing panencephalitis (SSPE) and acute disseminated encephalitis (ADE). SSPE may appear several years following inoculation, causing neuronal loss, gliosis, and demyelination. ADE is usually encountered 1 to 3 weeks after infection or vaccination and can result in rapid clinical deterioration as a result of acute demyelination.

Human Immunodeficiency Virus

HIV is a retrovirus that can affect the peripheral or central nervous system. Infection with the virus causes AIDS dementia, due to atrophy, axonal loss, demyelination, gliosis, and cellular infiltration with multinucleated giant cells. It occurs in approximately 60% of AIDS patients. Up to 10% of previously undiagnosed AIDS patients will present with only neurologic complaints.

PHYSICAL EXAMINATION

General. Fever (temperature greater than 101°F or 38.5°C) may be present. Seizures or frank delirium may be seen on clinical presentation.

Neurologic. A full mental status examination should be performed to evaluate for subtle or apparent changes. Evaluate the patient's speech content for dysphasia (word-finding problems or slow, pausing speech). The motor examination may reveal evidence of a hemiparesis. Observe for involuntary movements. Intention tremor may be elicited when the patient attempts to grasp an object just out of reach. Evaluate the gait for imbalance. Deep tendon reflexes may be asymmetrical, and a Babinski sign (upturning of the toes on stroking the plantar aspect of the foot) may be present. Check the cranial nerves for any irregularity. Ocular paresis and facial weakness are the most commonly encountered abnormalities. Nystagmus may be present on evaluation of extraocular movements. Meningeal signs such as nuchal rigidity (extreme discomfort on passive flexion of the neck), flexion of the hip and knee with flexion of the neck (Brudzinski sign), and the inability to fully extend the legs (Kernig sign) may be present. Evaluate for frontal release signs such as grasp or suck reflex. The suck reflex is elicited by stroking the patient's cheek. If the patient's mouth moves to suckle on the finger, the test is positive. Grasp reflex test is performed by gently stroking the patient's palm. The test is positive if the patient grasps the hand and is unable to let go.

DIAGNOSTIC STUDIES

Laboratory

Cerebrospinal Fluid (CSF) Examination. May show elevated opening pressure (normal 50 to 175 mm H_2O). Findings on CSF studies may initially be normal and not show any change for up to a week. CSF findings are typically similar to those in aseptic meningitis with a pleocytosis, usually with lymphocytes predominating. Glucose may be normal (normal 40 to 80 mg/dL) and protein is elevated (normal 15 to 45 mg/dL). Specimens should be obtained for viral isolation but are rarely diagnostic.

Other Body Fluids. Blood, stool, and nasopharyngeal swab specimens should be obtained as indicated for viral, bacterial, acid-fast bacillus, and fungal cultures. Isolation of virus is rare. Enteroviruses that are identified from sources other than CSF probably are not the causative agent.

Serologic Studies. Performed in the acute and convalescent periods. A fourfold rise in titer to a specific viral agent is diagnostic.

Chemistry Profile. Used as a baseline and to identify any abnormalities.

HIV Assay. May be positive in patients who do not have other symptoms of AIDS.

Radiology

CT/MRI of the Brain. Patients with suspected encephalitis should undergo neuroimaging. CT is often normal early in the disease course but may show cerebral edema, atrophy, hemorrhagic lesions, or focal, low-density lesions surrounded by edema. MRI is more sensitive than CT. T_1-weighted images may show low-density lesions surrounded by edema that do not initially enhance with the administration of gadolinium. T_2-weighted images may show increased signal of the lesions. Gyral edema may be seen. Lesions may be unilateral or bilateral and generally affect the white matter. HSV infection has a predilection for the temporal lobes and HIV infection, the frontal lobes.

Serial CT/MRI scans are recommended to exclude a progressive process such as cerebral abscess.

Other

Brain Biopsy. Done only in cases in which cause cannot be found through other means. Valuable to rule out nonviral causes of brain injury. Careful sampling of leptomeninges and areas of neurophil should be examined for intranuclear viral inclusion, immunofluorescence, and viral isolation, and by electron microscopy. Brain biopsy is diagnostic for HSV encephalitis but there are other less invasive techniques available to diagnose HSV infection.

Electroencephalography (EEG). May be normal initially and later reveal focal abnormalities.

DIFFERENTIAL DIAGNOSIS

Traumatic

Cervical Disk Herniation/Cervical Stenosis. Symptoms in a radicular or myelopathic distribution.

Infectious

Nonviral CNS Infections. Including bacterial/spirochetal infections such as tuberculosis or other mycoplasmal infection, syphilis, leptospirosis, borreliosis, brucellosis, legionnaires' disease, cat-scratch disease, rickettsiosis, toxic shock syndrome.

Fungal Infections. Cryptococcosis, coccidioidomycosis, candidiasis, histoplasmosis, blastomycosis, and parasitic infections: differentiated on diagnostic studies.

Non-CNS Infections. Viral, bacterial, fungal infections of cranium, epidural space, sinuses, eye, ear, oropharynx: differentiated on diagnostic studies.

Metabolic

Complicated Migraine, Low-Pressure Headache. Differentiated on history and examination.

Neoplastic

Malignancy, Especially Involving the Meninges. Cells may be seen in CSF.

Impending Herniation. may be associated with acute hydrocephalus, mass lesion, seen on CT/MRI.

Vascular
Subarachnoid or Subdural Hemorrhage. More acute presentation. Differentiated on CT/MRI.
Vasculitis. Examples: Kawasaki disease, polyarteritis nodosa, primary CNS vasculitis, rheumatoid arthritis, systemic lupus erythematosus (SLE), temporal arteritis.

Congenital
Not applicable.

Acquired
Vaccination Reaction. Acute disseminated encephalitis may be seen following vaccination for rabies, diphtheria, smallpox, tetanus, typhoid, or influenza. Symptoms begin 1 to 3 weeks following inoculation and can lead to rapid clinical deterioration. Early symptoms include headache, fever, and lethargy followed by seizures and/or focal neurologic deficits, coma, and death. Recovery can be complete, or the patient may be left with residual deficits.
Complicated Irritants. Radiopaque dye, lead, mercury.
Drugs. Azathioprine, cytosine, arabinoside, isoniazid, penicillin, trimethoprim, NSAIDs, caffeine (withdrawal), amantidine, rimantidine, vidarabine.
Immune-mediated. Serum sickness, graft-versus-host disease, post–cardiac transplantation syndrome, intravenous immunoglobulin (IVIG), OKT3.
Post–Lumbar Puncture. History of recent procedure.

TREATMENT

Diagnosis may be elusive. It is expedient to obtain an infectious disease consultation to help in identifying the causative agent. Monitor vital signs (respiration, blood pressure, pulse). Management and supportive therapy should include monitoring of intracranial pressure, fluid restriction, avoidance of hypotonic intravenous solutions, and suppression of fever. Initiate specific anitiviral therapy as soon as possible. Attention to fluid and electrolytes is imperative. If the patient has CT/MRI or clinical evidence of increased intracranial pressure, give dexamethasone 2 to 10 mg intravenously or orally every 6 hours for the first four days of therapy. Mannitol may be given. Patients with decreased level of consciousness should be protected from aspiration.

Consider antiviral medications (see Table 10-3).

Table 10–3. Pharmacotherapy for Viral Encephalitis

Drug	Pathogen	Dosing	Complication
Acyclovir (Zovirax)	HSV	10 mg/kg IV q8h × 10 days	Renal toxicity
Ganciclovir (Cytovene)	CMV	5 mg/kg IV q12h	Renal toxicity
Ribavirin (Virazole)	Myxovirus	15-25 mg/kg/day	Bone marrow
Rimantadine (Flumadine)	Influenza A virus	3.3 mg PO q12h	CNS

CMV, cytomegalovirus; CNS, central nervous system; HSV, herpes simplex virus.

PEDIATRIC CONSIDERATIONS

Infants may present with convulsions or fever of acute onset. Perform lumbar puncture for CSF analysis to exclude other, potentially related disorders, such as meningitis.

OBSTETRIC CONSIDERATIONS

HSV-2 infection is primarily a disease of infants due to genital transmission from the mother to the neonate.

VEE
Pregnant women infected with this disease during the first and second trimesters are at risk for fetal encephalitis and fetal death.

WEE
Congenital infections have been documented, and can result in severe and progressive neurologic deterioration in the infant.

JBE
Fetal death and abortion due to transplacental JBE infection have been reported.

GERIATRIC CONSIDERATIONS

When elderly patients with complicated medical illness who are also debilitated and immunocompromised present with signs and symptoms of encephalitis, the causative agent must be sought and the disease treated aggressively.

PREVENTIVE CONSIDERATIONS

Patients living in geographic areas where encephalitis has been identified or is prevalent should be educated about risk of transmission from mosquitoes and ticks. Areas in which rainwater collects and provides a breeding medium for mosquitoes should be identified and the water emptied.

PEARLS FOR THE PA

The presence of encephalitis in the summer or fall suggests a potential epidemic due to arthropod-borne (mosquito and tick) viruses.

HSV is the most common cause of viral encephalitis.

HSV encephalitis and EEE are the most severe forms of the disease.

It is important to treat suspected cases of HSV encephalitis with antiviral medication because of the higher morbidity and mortality rates for this type.

A meningitis associated with only meningeal signs, headache, and photophobia is termed **aseptic meningitis.** *When other neurologic signs and symptoms are associated with the process, the disorder is called meningoencephalitis.*

Intracranial Neoplasm

James B. Labus, PA-C

DEFINITION

A neoplasm that arises inside the skull from cells of, supporting, and surrounding the central nervous system (CNS). Gliomas, which arise from the glial supporting cells of the brain and spinal cord, account for 50% to 65% of primary brain tumors. Gliomas are graded I to IV, depending on the degree of anaplasia. Gliomas are classified as astrocytoma, anaplastic astrocytoma, or glioblastoma multiforme. Other primary tumors include meningioma, ependymoma, ganglioneuroma, juvenile pilocytic astrocytoma, oligodendroglioma, craniopharyngioma, lymphoma, schwannoma, medulloblastoma, pineal tumor, pituitary adenoma, vascular tumors, and germ cell tumors.

HISTORY

Symptoms. Patients may present with new-onset seizure, focal neurologic findings, or symptoms of increased intracranial pressure. A lesion may be found incidentally on CT or MRI.

Seizures may be focal in nature (without loss of consciousness) or generalized (with loss of consciousness). Focal neurologic findings are due to compression or invasion of neural structures. Specific abnormalities depend on the portion of the CNS involved and include hemiparesis, hemisensory loss, cranial nerve deficits, ataxia, partial visual loss, diplopia, hearing loss, dysphagia, dysphasia, and/or mental status changes.

Symptoms of increased intracranial pressure include headache, nausea/vomiting, lethargy, and/or blurred vision.

General. Inquire about the progression of symptoms. Intracranial lesions can grow slowly or can be very aggressive. The intracranial compartment is a closed space; lesions can grow slowly and the brain will accommodate until there is no more space available. At that time symptoms can become rapidly progressive. If the lesion is fast-growing, the brain cannot accommodate, and edema will ensue and symptoms will develop more quickly.

Symptoms may be vague (e.g., personality change, lethargy) and noticed by a family member rather than the patient.

Brain tumors are classified as intrinsic or of the CNS (e.g., glioma) and extrinsic or arising from adjacent structures (e.g., meningioma).

Age. Any, but cell types vary with age. See Pathophysiology later on.

Onset. May be gradual or acute, with seizure or increased intracranial pressure.

Intensity. If intracranial pressure is elevated, lesion can be life-threatening.

Aggravating Factors. Patient's becoming overheated and alcohol use can increase intracranial pressure.

Alleviating Factors. Reducing intracranial pressure.

Associated Factors. Patients with neurofibromatosis are at increased risk for development of intracranial lesions. There is an increased risk in workers in oil refineries and with rubber and drug manufacturing.

PHYSICAL EXAMINATION

General. Observe the patient for overall appearance. The patient may be disheveled, lethargic, responsive, or normal in affect. While obtaining a history, evaluate for subtle changes in mental status and insight into the condition.

Neurologic. A full neurologic examination is performed on the initial and subsequent visits. Treatment and/or tumor progression can cause regression or worsening of abnormalities noted on the examination.

A full mental status examination is performed including orientation, calculation, and abstraction.

Motor, sensory, cerebellar, and cranial nerve examinations are performed and results documented.

Ophthalmologic. Funduscopic examination should be performed to evaluate for papilledema. Visual field testing should be performed with confrontation or formally by opthalmology if abnormality is suspected.

PATHOPHYSIOLOGY

There is no known cause of primary intracerebral neoplasms. Tumors cause symptoms by pressure on the brain through external pressure and/or edema formation.

Tumors of Glial Cell Origin

Astrocytoma: Arise from the supportive structures (astrocytes) of the brain.

Anaplastic astrocytoma: Rapidly growing, more aggressive astrocytoma.

Glioblastoma multiforme: May also be called a grade IV astrocytoma. Very aggressive.

Ependymoma: A neoplasm of the ependymal cells that line the ventricles. It may manifest with obstructive hydrocephalus. Usually benign, ependymomas comprise about 5% of adult and 10% of children's tumors.

Juvenile pilocytic astrocytoma: A relatively common tumor of childhood. The lesion tends to occur in the cerebellum and exhibits cyst formation. Patients present with cerebellar symptoms of ataxia, nausea, vomiting, and headache.

Mixed glioma: A tumor type in which there are several types of glial cells.

Oligodendroglioma: Accounts for 5% of gliomas. These tumors occur mostly in young adults.

Optic nerve glioma: Occurs in or near the optic nerves. More prevalent in patients with neurofibromatosis.

Ganglioneuroma: The rarest glioma. The lesion is generally slow growing and is composed of both glial cells and mature neurons.

Non–Glial Cell Tumors

Meningioma: Generally benign lesion that arises from the meninges that cover the brain and spinal cord. Symptoms are due to compression of neural structures. These tumors account for about 27% of primary brain tumors.

Craniopharyngioma: Occurs at the base of the brain near the optic nerves, optic chiasm, and hypothalamus. Patient presents with visual changes if the optic nerves are involved, hormonal changes if the hypothalamus is compressed, or diabetes insipidus. The lesion is more common in children.

Medulloblastoma: A primitive neuroectodermal tumor that tends to be very aggressive. It accounts for greater than 25% of childhood tumors. Symptoms include ataxia, nausea, vomiting, and headache. Other types of primitive neuroectodermal tumors are neuroblastoma, pineoblastoma, medulloepithelioma, ependymoblastoma, polar spongioblastoma.

Pineal tumors: Arise in the area of the pineal gland. Constitute about 1% of brain tumors. Can occur in children.

Pituitary adenoma: See "Pituitary Adenoma" in Chapter 4, Endocrinology.

Schwannoma (neurofibroma): A generally benign tumor that arises from the Schwann cells. If it affects CN VIII it is called an acoustic neuroma.

Vascular tumors: Lesions that are composed of vascular tissue. Hemangioblastoma may be associated with Von Hippel–Lindau disease.

Germ cell tumors: Include germinomas, embryonal carcinomas, choriocarcinomas, and teratomas.

DIAGNOSTIC STUDIES

Laboratory

Complete Blood Count. White blood cell (WBC) count elevated in cerebral abscess or meningitis.

Chemistry Profile. Hyponatremia can cause seizures. Liver functions may be abnormal with anticonvulsant use. Hepatic disease can also cause neurologic changes. Also used as a baseline.

Radiology

CT/MRI of the Brain. Performed with and without contrast/gadolinium. MRI is preferred, to show the location of the lesion and presence/absence of edema.

Cerebral Angiography. Indicated if vascularity of the lesion must be evaluated preoperatively or if a vascular lesion needs to be ruled out.

Other

Electroencephalogram (EEG). Can be performed to measure cerebral irritability and possibility of seizure.

DIFFERENTIAL DIAGNOSIS

Traumatic

Head Trauma. Cerebral injury can manifest with increased intracranial pressure (ICP), seizure, and focal neurologic changes. Differentiated on CT/MRI.

Infectious

Cerebral Abscess. Can appear as a ring-enhancing lesion. May be differentiated on MRI or on biopsy/surgery.

Metabolic
Seizure. Can be caused by a variety of metabolic disorders (see topic Seizure Disorders).

Neoplastic
Metastatic Tumor. Metastatic cancer frequently seeds in the brain (usually breast or lung cancer). Patients may present with metastatic cancer with a brain lesion. May require histologic confirmation.

Vascular
Intracranial Aneurysm. Can cause focal neurologic abnormalities with or without hemorrhage. Differentiated on angiography.
Arteriovenous Malformation. Tend to have distinct appearance on CT/MRI. Differentiated on angiography.

Congenital. Not applicable.
Acquired. Not applicable.

TREATMENT

Treatment depends on patient's age, tumor type and location, and the patient's medical condition.

Pharmacologic. Steroids may be given initially for symptoms of increased intracranial pressure. Dexamethasone (Decadron) 2-10 mg every 6 hours can be used. Mannitol may be required for acute decrease in intracranial pressure. Anticonvulsant medication is given to control seizures when present, or as a prophylactic measure preoperatively.

Surgical. Surgery to remove the lesion is generally the treatment of choice. Most tumors are surgically accessible. Patients may require temporary or permanent ventricular catheterization (shunt placement) to drain CSF from the ventricles before or during the surgical procedure.

Radiotherapy
Radiotherapy focuses on residual tumor that could not be surgically excised. Generally recommended for aggressive tumors (such as glioblastoma multiforme), as these tumors are infiltrative and cannot be removed completely. Irradiation begins after surgical wound healing is complete.

Traditional External Beam Radiotherapy
Hyperfractionated. Small, frequent radiation dosages that result in a higher overall daily dose.
Stereotactic Radiotherapy. Delivers a high dose of focal external beam radiation precisely to the tumor site using multiple angles. The route is varied to reduce exposure of the surrounding tissue to radiation and increase radiation to the target.

Interstitial Brachytherapy. Radioactive implants or seeds placed in the tumor bed.

Chemotherapy
Usually given in combination with another modality to inhibit tumor growth. May be given orally, intravenously, intrathecally, or directly into the tumor bed.

Other
Antiprogesterone Agents. Have a role in treatment of some meningiomas.

Angiogenesis Inhibitors. Interfere with growth of tumor-associated blood vessels.

Differentiating Agents. Used to convert immature tumor cells into mature cells.

Immunotherapy. Treatment includes interferons (which may be toxic to many tumor cells), lymphocytes that are injected into the tumor to boost an immune response.

Tumor Vaccines. Modified tumor cells that are reintroduced into the patient to elicit an immune response.

Gene Therapy. Transfer of genetic material into a tumor cell to destroy or stop tumor growth. Tumors are coded to self-destruct, make cells more mature; genes to strengthen the immune system, increase the tumor cell's responsiveness to drugs.

Viral Modification
Used to deliver a therapeutic agent to modify the tumor.

PEDIATRIC CONSIDERATIONS

Gliomas tend to occur in the cerebellum and brainstem in children. Juvenile pilocytic astrocytomas tend to be very low grade and medulloblastoma very aggressive.

Symptoms in children include nausea, headache, speech and balance problems, difficulty swallowing, hemiparesis, and hemisensory loss. Radiation therapy is used for tumors that cannot be resected.

Brain tumor is the second leading cause of cancer death in children younger than 15 years of age.

Children with a history of successfully treated leukemia are at increased risk of brain tumor.

OBSTETRIC CONSIDERATIONS

Attention to increased intracranial pressure with Valsalva maneuvers during delivery is imperative in a patient with a known intracranial lesion. See "Seizure Disorders" later in this chapter for anticonvulsant considerations.

GERIATRIC CONSIDERATONS

Glioma and meningioma are more common in the adult and elderly populations.

PREVENTIVE CONSIDERATIONS

No behavioral factors have been associated with the development of brain tumors.

PEARLS FOR THE PA

Glioma is the most common intrinsic brain tumor.

Meningioma is the most common extrinsic brain tumor.

Childhood tumors tend to occur in the cerebellum and brainstem.

Meningitis

Keith W. Kettell, MPAS, PA-C

DEFINITION

Meningitis is an inflammation of the leptomeninges (the arachnoid and pia mater) and the cerebrospinal fluid (CSF). The inflammatory process extends throughout the subarachnoid space of the brain and spinal cord and commonly involves the ventricles. Irritation of the meninges may be due to blood, bacteria, viruses, or tumor cells.

HISTORY

Symptoms. Fever, severe headache, vomiting, seizure, change in mental status, neck stiffness (nuchal rigidity), photophobia, and the inability to extend the legs are the most common presenting complaints. The symptoms may be accompanied by a rash, ecchymosis, or arthritis.

Symptoms referable to a primary infectious source, such as sinusitis, pneumonia, or upper respiratory infection, may also be present. Infants, small children, and elderly persons may not present with classic findings (see Pediatric Considerations and Geriatric Considerations).

General. Inquiry should be made about recent history of infectious disease (e.g., upper respiratory infection, pneumonia, sinusitis, ear infection, mastoiditis, gastrointestinal infection), the presence of a foreign body (e.g., heart valve or ventriculoperitoneal/ventriculoatrial shunt), the possibility of meningitis in persons in close contact with the patient, and recent invasive procedures (e.g., neurosurgical or ear-nose-throat procedures, lumbar punctures).

Age. Because vaccination has markedly decreased the incidence of childhood *Haemophilus influenzae* type b infections, acute meningitis, previously most common in children, has become predominantly a disease of young adults and the elderly. The median age at diagnosis is 25 years.

Onset. Symptoms may develop over several hours or several days.

Duration. Progressive.

Intensity. Frequently fatal if left untreated. Even with treatment, the mortality rate for bacterial meningitis ranges from 10% to 30%.

Aggravating Factors. Prognosis is worse in those patients with concurrent disorders such as diabetes mellitus, head trauma, alcoholism, systemic infections, and immunocompromised status. Prognosis worsens with advancing age (older than 60 years), onset of seizures during the first 24 hours after infection, hypotension, and coma or obtundation on hospital admission.

Alleviating Factors. Early diagnosis and timely, appropriate treatment.

Associated Factors. Upper respiratory infections, sinusitis, mastoiditis, pneumonias, gastrointestinal and systemic infections, and foreign bodies that communicate directly with the CSF all may lead to bacterial meningitis. Any disorder that allows bacteria to enter the CSF (e.g., skull fracture, congenital conditions) puts the patient at high risk for developing meningitis. Persons who are exposed to crowded conditions (e.g., in dormitory situations) are at an increased risk of contracting the disease.

PHYSICAL EXAMINATION

General. A patient may appear to be in mild distress or significant distress, lethargic, or in a coma. Fever is present in approximately 95% of patients and typically lasts 4 to 8 days after appropriate therapy has begun. Stiff neck is apparent in about 90% of patients. Hypotension and/or tachycardia may be present and indicate potential vascular collapse. The most common features of bacterial meningitis are headache, fever, nuchal rigidity, and neurologic abnormalities. Seizures, either focal or generalized, occur in about 10% to 30% of patients, usually within 24 hours of hospital admission. Papilledema occurs only occasionally; its absence does not exclude the possibility of dangerously increased intracranial pressure.

Neurologic. Meningitis is usually manifested by signs of meningeal irritation. Physical findings of meningeal irritation and impaired neuromuscular response include nuchal rigidity, Kernig sign (when the hip is flexed at 90 degrees, attempted extension of the knee meets resistance at 135 degrees), and Brudzinski sign (passive flexion of the neck causes knee and hip flexion). These signs may not be present in infants, small children, the elderly, and persons in a coma.

Focal neurologic signs may include cranial nerve palsies, aphasia, and hemiparesis as a consequence of infection-induced vasculitis or pressure from purulent exudate on neurologic structures. These focal signs are present in approximately 30% of patients. A full mental status examination should be performed to evaluate for subtle changes that could signal a worsening of the patient's condition.

Skin. May show evidence of petechial or purpuric rash or ecchymosis.

PATHOPHYSIOLOGY

The most common organism causing bacterial meningitis in adults is *Streptococcus pneumoniae* (the pneumococcus). It is the causative pathogen in 58% to 62% of adult cases in the United States. Bacteremia is nearly always present. Other major organisms in community-acquired cases of meningitis are:

- *Neisseria meningitidis,* occurring primarily in young adults
- *Listeria monocytogenes,* especially in immunocompromised or elderly patients
- *H. influenzae*
- Group B streptococci (*Streptococcus agalactiae*)

Any organism gaining entrance to the CSF may cause meningitis. Infection with meningococci should be suspected if there are associated skin findings such as petechial or purpuric rash or ecchymosis, and in epidemics of meningitis. Epidemics are caused by airborne spread of nasopharyngeal organisms, with subsequent infection that may develop into meningitis.

The most common port of bacterial entry into the CSF is via the bloodstream. Other means of infection include bacterial spread from adjacent structures (e.g., sinuses) and direct implantation (e.g., with lumbar puncture). Bacterial infection of the meninges results in inflammatory changes in blood vessel walls, which may lead to thrombosis and decreased cerebral perfusion, and/or accumulation of exudate within the CSF pathways, which may result in hydrocephalus.

Cerebral edema may lead to herniation and death. Injury to the blood-brain barrier causes congestion of the choroid plexus, resulting in disturbed CSF dynamics. Late complications include adhesive arachnoiditis, meningomyelitis, subdural hygroma, and intracerebral abscess.

Viral meningitis is most often caused by enteroviruses, mumps virus, arboviruses, and herpes simplex virus (HSV) and may be preceded by an upper respiratory or other illness.

Chemical meningitis may be caused by irritants entering the CSF such as blood or instilled agents (contrast dye or anesthetic agents). An uncommon complication is adhesive arachnoiditis.

DIAGNOSTIC STUDIES

Laboratory
CSF Examination. Lumbar puncture should be performed expeditiously to avoid delay in diagnosis of meningitis, which may have serious consequences. Headache and fever remain the primary indications for lumbar puncture. Contraindications to lumbar puncture include increased intracranial pressure, skin infection at the lumbar puncture site, uncorrected bleeding dyscrasias, and severe cardiorespiratory distress (in the neonate). If there is any question of a space-occupying intracranial lesion, CT or MRI of the brain should be performed and neurosurgical consultation should be obtained before performing the lumbar puncture. Patients should be apprised of the complications of performing the procedure.

For this test, 3 to 4 tubes of CSF are drawn via lumbar puncture:

Tube 1 (the least likely to be contaminated) is sent for *stat* Gram stain and culture and sensitivity testing for acid-fast bacilli, anaerobes, mycobacteria, fungi, and viruses. May include complete blood count if subarachnoid hemorrhage is suspected.

Tube 2 is sent for determination of glucose and protein.

Tube 3 is used for complete blood count (as the specimen is obtained after any blood from a traumatic lumbar puncture has cleared).

Tube 4 can be kept in reserve or can be used for special studies such as immunoassay or multiple sclerosis profile.

The classic findings in bacterial meningitis are:

1. An elevated white blood cell count (normal 0 to 10/mm^3) with a predominance of polymorphonucleocytes
2. Elevated protein (normal 15 to 45 mg/dL)
3. Reduced glucose level to values of 40 mg/dL (normal 40 to 80 mg/dL) or less (or less than 50 % of the simultaneous blood level) in 50% of patients with bacterial meningitis—a valuable finding for distinguishing bacterial meningitis from most viral meningitides or parameningeal infections

The lumbar puncture should be repeated if there is any doubt about the findings on the initial lumbar puncture or if the patient fails to improve in 1 to 3 days and meningitis is suspected. The CSF findings in viral meningitis are of a CSF pleocytosis, usually with lymphocytes predominating. Glucose may be normal to reduced, and protein is usually not markedly elevated. If tumor cells are identified, a thorough search for the primary cause should be instituted.

CSF Immunoassay. Should be ordered if cultures are negative and meningitis is suspected or if the patient has been administered antibiotics before the lumbar puncture.

CSF Serology. Indicated if a viral cause is suspected.

Complete Blood Count. Frequently will show an elevated white blood cell count with a left shift.

Erythrocyte Sedimentation Rate (ESR). May be elevated. Normal: in males, 0 to 9 mm/hour; in females, 0 to 20 mm/hour, may be as high as 42, adjusted for age and sex.

Electrolytes. May show an elevation in the blood urea nitrogen (BUN) (normal 10 to 20 mg/dL) and creatinine (normal 0.6 to 1.2 mg/dL) with dehydration. Sodium (normal 136 to 145 mEq/L) may be decreased owing to the syndrome of inappropriate antidiuretic hormone secretion (SIADH).

Blood Cultures. Should be performed in all patients and may lead to the identification of the causative organism if the CSF examination is negative.

Nasopharyngeal Cultures. Cultures of the upper respiratory tract usually are not helpful in establishing an etiologic diagnosis.

Coagulation Profile: Prothrombin Time (PT), Partial Thromboplastin Time (PTT), Bleeding Time. Normal values: PT 10 to 15 seconds, PTT 30 to 45 seconds, bleeding time less than 9 minutes. May be abnormal owing to disseminated intravascular coagulation.

Radiology

Chest Film. As indicated to evaluate for pneumonia as a causative source.

Skull and Sinus Films. As indicated to evaluate for sinusitis, mastoiditis, or osteomyelitis as a causative source.

CT or MRI Scan of the Brain. CT is not indicated in most patients with bacterial meningitis. If a mass lesion (cerebral abscess, subdural empyema, or hygroma (especially in children) is suspected on the basis of history, clinical setting, or physical findings (papilledema, focal cerebral signs), then CT should be performed.

CT Scanning with Radionuclide-Labeled Albumin or Magnetic Resonance Cisternography. Used to determine the site of CSF leak when indicated. Magnetic resonance cisternography is noninvasive and rapid; seems highly accurate in detecting fistulas.

Cerebral Angiography. Used to diagnose arteritis or venous sinus thrombosis.

DIFFERENTIAL DIAGNOSIS

Traumatic

Cervical Spine Injury. May cause stiff neck. Not usually associated with a fever or mental status changes except with a head injury or substance abuse. Unlike in nuchal rigidity due to meningeal irritation, neck rotation is also limited.

Skull Fracture. Fractures occurring at the base of the skull that result in CSF rhinorrhea can lead to bacterial colonization of the CSF.

Infectious

Brain Abscess. May be due to meningitis or rupture into the CSF to cause a meningitis. Will classically appear as a ring-enhancing lesion on CT/MRI of the brain.

Meningism Due to Other Causes. Such as head and neck infections, pneumonia, and septicemia. CSF examination is normal.

Metabolic

Behçet Disease. Associated with mouth and genital ulcers, uveitis, skin lesions, arthritis, and irritability. Cause of recurrent meningitis. Uncommon.

Mollaret Meningitis. Repeated febrile episodes of mild meningeal symptomatology, usually without neurologic abnormalities. CSF examination initially may demonstrate large endothelial cells, along with polymorphonuclear leukocytes, which are subsequently replaced by lymphocytes. Uncommon.

Vogt-Koyanagi-Harada Syndrome. Recurrent meningitis associated with uveitis, meningoencephalitis, deafness, vitiligo, and alopecia. The disorder affects different systems at different times. Uncommon.

Neoplastic

Posterior Fossa Tumors. May cause a stiff neck. Usually not associated with a fever and the onset is more gradual. Lumbar puncture should not be performed if this type of tumor is suspected as it may cause herniation. CT or MRI of the brain should be performed first.

Erosive Skull Base Lesions. Can lead to CSF leaks and predispose the patient to develop meningitis.

Dermoid Cysts. May leak and cause recurrent aseptic meningitis.

Vascular

Subarachnoid Hemorrhage. Associated with severe headache and stiff neck of acute onset. Usually not associated with fever. CT scan of the brain will show blood in the subarachnoid space, and fluid obtained at lumbar puncture will be bloody. The blood will not clear as more CSF is withdrawn (when subarachnoid hemorrhage is suspected, the red blood cell count of tube 1 will be roughly equal to the red blood cell count of tube 4, thus ruling out a traumatic lumbar puncture).

Congenital

Menigomyelocele (Spina Bifida) and Other Anatomic Defects. Can expose the CSF to the external environment, leading to meningitis.

Congenital Dermal Sinus. Can expose the CSF to the external environment, leading to meningitis.

Acquired

Alcohol Intoxication. May cause confusion similar to that seen in meningitis. If this is associated with fever, lumbar puncture should be performed to rule out meningitis.

Chemical Meningitis. May be due to contrast media or agents (e.g., used in spinal anesthesia) injected into the subarachnoid space.

TREATMENT

Vital signs should be supported with volume replacement or pressors.

Lumbar puncture CSF specimens (and all other appropriate culture specimens) should be obtained before initiation of any antibiotic therapy. Complications of lumbar puncture include injury to a nerve root, introduction of infection, cerebellar herniation, bleeding into the CSF, seeding of the CSF with an epidermoid tumor, and diplopia.

If the procedure cannot be performed, pancultures are obtained (blood, urine, sputum, nasopharyngeal) and antibiotic therapy based on a presumptive diagnosis is instituted. Prophylactic antibiotic therapy should be instituted until results of cultures are obtained. Choice of antibiotics should be based on spectrum of action and ability to penetrate the blood-brain barrier (see Table 10-4).

Viral and chemical meningitis are managed symptomatically. If the cause of the meningitis is unknown, assume it to be bacterial and institute antibiotic therapy.

The causative factor for the meningitis (e.g., mastoiditis, sinusitis, infected shunt) should be properly managed.

Cerebral edema may be managed with osmotic diuretics such as mannitol, mechanical respiration with hyperventilation (maintaining a partial pressure of carbon dioxide [P_{CO_2}] of 25 mm Hg) or, in severe instances, CSF drainage via ventriculostomy.

Anticonvulsants are given if the patient experiences seizures. Anticonvulsants include:

Diazepam: administered slowly intravenously in a dose of 5-10 mg in the adult patient; indicated in the acute seizure setting

Phenytoin (Dilantin): loading dose of 15 mg/kg (not to exceed 50 mg every 3 minutes) followed by 100 mg intravenously three times a day until the patient can tolerate oral dosing three times a day to a serum level of 10 to 20 µg/mL

Phenobarbital: consider 30 mg three times a day, adjusting to a serum level of 15 to 40 µg/L

Carbamazepine (Tegretol): slowly increase dose to 200 mg twice a day to a serum level of 4 to 12 mg/L

If an epidemic of meningitis is suspected, mass vaccinations and medical prophylaxis may be indicated. Contact local and regional health authorities to institute such measures.

PEDIATRIC CONSIDERATIONS

Infants may not exhibit meningeal signs and present with only nonspecific findings such as irritability, fever, lethargy, vomiting, or seizure. The fontanel should be palpated for bulging, which suggests meningitis or raised intracranial pressure. Lumbar puncture should be performed in any child in whom the cause of symptoms is not readily apparent. Contraindications to immediate lumbar puncture include:

- Evidence of increased intracranial pressure with neurologic dysfunction
- Hypertension and bradycardia with respiratory abnormalities

Table 10–4. Antimicrobial Regimens for Selected Pathogens

Organism	Regimen
Streptococcus pneumoniae	*Adults and children >1 m old*: If the pneumococcus is known to be susceptible to penicillin (MIC ≤ 0.1 µg/mL), use penicillin as below; otherwise, begin therapy with: Vancomycin 15 mg/kg IV q6h PLUS *Adults*: Ceftriaxone 2 g IV q12h *Infants 8-28 d old*: Cefotaxime 50-75 mg/kg IV q6h *Infants >28 d old*: Ceftriaxone 100 mg/kg IV q12h at diagnosis, then qd
Neisseria meningitidis	*Adults*: Pen G 4 million U by Volutrol over 30 min q4h *Children >28 d old*: Pen G 50,000 U/kg IV q6h *Children ≤7 d old*: Pen G 50,000 U/kg IV q12h *Penicillin-allergic patients*: Chloramphenicol *Note*: Penicillin may cure the meningitis but fail to eradicate the nasal carrier state of the patient. To prevent postdischarge transmission of meningococci from the patient to siblings or other contacts, eradicate the carrier state of the patient with rifampin before discharge: *Children >1 m old*: Rifampin 10 mg/kg (max dose 600 mg) PO q12h for a total of 4 doses in 2 d *Children ≤28 d old*: Rifampin 5 mg/kg PO q12h for a total of 4 doses in 2 d *Teenagers or adults*: Rifampin 600 mg PO q12h for a total of 4 doses in 2 d
Group B streptococci	*Adults*: Ampicillin 2.0 g IV q4h PLUS cefotaxime 2.0 g IV q6h *Neonates*: Ampicillin 50 mg/kg IV q12h PLUS cefotaxime 50 mg/kg IV q12h

Haemophilus influenzae type b	With either regimen, repeat CSF examination/culture 24-36 h after start of therapy.
	There are three major components of therapy:
	1. Antibiotics
	    Adults: Cefotaxime 2 g IV q4-6h
	    Children >28 d old: Ceftriaxone 100 mg/kg/IV qd

Continued

Table 10–4. Antimicrobial Regimens for Selected Pathogens—cont'd

Organism	Regimen
	Children 8-28 d old: Cefotaxime 50 mg/kg/IV q8h
	Ampicillin may be used for therapy of Hib meningitis only if the infecting strain is demonstrated not to produce beta-lactamase.
	2. Inhibition of TNF-α production
	Data from studies in children with *Haemophilus influenzae* meningitis indicate that an inhibitor of TNF-α production, dexamethasone, 0.4 mg/kg IV q12h for 2 d of antibiotic therapy, reduces the neurologic sequelae of meningitis. There are no completely comparable data for adults or regarding meningitis caused by other pathogens, but in the absence of a specific contraindication, such as a history of tuberculosis, consider dexamethasone in meningococcal, pneumococcal, and other bacterial meningitides in which the inflammatory reaction seems to be more deleterious than helpful to the patient.
	3. Eradication of Hib carrier state
	Treated patients should be given rifampin prior to discharge:
	Children >1 mo old: Rifampin, 20 mg/kg (max dose 600 mg) PO daily × 4 d
	Adults or teenagers: Each dose is 600 mg. This therapy may not be necessary if the patient was treated with cefotaxime or ceftriaxone, either of which eradicates nasal carriage of Hib.
Listeria monocytogenes	*Adults:* Ampicillin 2 g IV q4h (consider adding gentamicin 2 mg/kg loading dose, then 1.7 mg/kg q8h)
	Children >28 d old: Ampicillin 50 mg/kg q6h PLUS gentamicin, 2.5 mg/kgIV per 8 h
	Neonates: Ampicillin 50 mg/kg IV q12h PLUS gentamicin, 2.5 mg/kg IV q8-24 h
Staphylococcus aureus	*Adults:* Nafcillin OR oxacillin (2 g IV every 4 h) OR vancomycin 1.0 g IV q6-12h PLUS rifampin 600 mg PO qd
	Children >28 d old: Nafcillin OR oxacillin 37 mg/kg IV q6h OR vancomycin 40-60 mg/kg IV divided q12h
	Neonates: Nafcillin OR oxacillin 25 mg/kg IV q12h

Gram-negative bacilli (not *H. influenzae*): *Klebsiella* spp., *Escherichia coli*, etc. *Pseudomonas, Enterobacter, Acinetobacter* species	*Adults:* Ceftazidime 2.0 g IV q8h PLUS gentamicin 2 mg/kg IV loading dose, then 1.7 mg/kg q8h thereafter *Children:* Seek pediatric infectious disease consultation. Often develop resistance to cephalosporins during therapy; therefore, susceptibility testing should be done on each successive isolate, and if cephalosporin resistance arises, older children, teenagers, and adults may be treated with systemic plus intraventricular aminoglycosides as follows (an infectious disease consultation is recommended): Give intraventricular gentamicin 0.03 mg/mL of CSF volume OR intraventricular amikacin 0.1 mg/mL of CSF volume PLUS Standard intravenous therapy with the same aminoglycoside

CSF, cerebrospinal fluid; Hib, *Haemophilus influenzae* type b; MIC, minimum inhibitory concentration; Pen G, penicillin G; TNF, tumor necrosis factor.

• Severe cardiopulmonary compromise

Factors such as premature birth, prolonged labor, premature rupture of fetal membranes, and maternal infections play a role in the development of meningitis in the first 28 days of life. Infants will be more prone to the development of subdural effusions, which may require aspiration.

OBSTETRIC CONSIDERATIONS

No specific indications.

GERIATRIC CONSIDERATIONS

Elderly patients may have a nonclassic presentation with a chief complaint of only decreased mental status, seizures, or focal neurologic deficits. The pathogens that most frequently cause meningitis in older adults are *S. pneumoniae, L. monocytogenes,* and gram-negative bacilli. As is the case with small children, meningitis carries higher morbidity and mortality rates in this age group. Atypical presentation may delay diagnosis and intervention. Coexisting diseases and altered physiologic responses to infection may contribute to an atypical presentation of symptoms. Existing chronic disease may mask an acute infection. Febrile response may be nonexistent or blunted in older adults with a bacterial infection. In the elderly, an acute unexplained functional deterioration should prompt suspicion of an acute infectious process.

PREVENTIVE CONSIDERATIONS

The institution of routine *H. influenzae* vaccination has played a major role in the marked decline in *H. influenzae* meningeal infections. Patients should be encouraged to actively participate in annual vaccination programs. Infant immunization against *H. influenzae* should be encouraged. Adult immunization in persons at high risk for contracting meningococcal and pneumococcal infections is also warranted. Any HIV-positive patient presenting with fever, headache, and/or focal neurologic signs should be evaluated immediately for meningitis. In cases of exposure to persons with meningitis, prophylactic treatment may be indicated.

PEARLS FOR THE PA

Bacterial meningitis is a medical emergency requiring immediate diagnosis and rapid institution of antimicrobial therapy. Delay in performing a diagnostic lumbar puncture should be avoided.

Continued

PEARLS FOR THE PA—cont'd

Broad-spectrum antibiotics with adequate CSF penetration should be given after CSF culture specimens are obtained.

If the cause of meningitis is unknown, assume it to be bacterial and institute antibiotic therapy.

If a cerebral mass lesion is suspected, a CT or MRI study of the brain should be performed and consultation sought, before performing a lumbar puncture.

Migraine

Charlene M. Morris, MPAS, PA-C

DEFINITION

Migraine is a disorder characterized by paroxysmal attacks of headache pain secondary to an unknown derangement of cranial circulation causing vasodilatation. Theories include a cascade of 5-hydroxytryptamine (5-HT) (serotonin) activation of the trigeminal nerve and subsequent vasoactive reaction with prostaglandin release and pain. (See Table 10-5.)

HISTORY

Symptoms. Headache may be preceded by a prodrome—a short period of irritability or depression followed by a severe, throbbing, often initially unilateral headache with associated nausea, vomiting, and photophobia. Some patients may experience an aura of transient neurologic symptoms involving the visual, auditory, olfactory, sensory, or motor system. Transient visual auras are the most common and include flashing lights, shapes, or hemianopsia. Typically, the visual symptoms spread over the visual field. Auras may occur without headache as well (acephalgic migraine).

Basilar migraines manifest with symptoms of vertebrobasilar ischemia (e.g., vertigo, diplopia, sycope). They may be preceded by an aura. Other subtypes include hemiplegic migraines and ophthalmoplegic migraines. These subtypes require a full neurologic evaluation to rule out primary neurologic disorders.

General. The condition is often familial, and 75% of the cases occur in females.

For evaluating a headache, use the mnemonic DANGER to identify an underlying neurologic process, rather than a migraine:

Table 10–5. Diagnostic Criteria For Migraine Headache

Migraine Without Aura

A. At least five attacks fulfilling Criteria B through D
B. Headache lasting 4-72 hours
C. At least two of the following characteristics:
    1. Unilateral location
    2. Pulsating quality
    3. Moderate to severe intensity
    4. Aggravated by routine activities such as walking upstairs
D. During the headache at least one of the following apply:
    1. Nausea or vomiting
    2. Photo/phonophobia

Migraine With Aura

A. At least two attacks fulfilling the characteristics under B
B. At least three of the following four characteristics:
    1. One or more fully reversible aura symptoms
    2. At least one aura symptom over more than 4 min or two or more symptoms occurring in succession
    3. No single aura symptom lasts more than 60 min
    4. Headache follows aura with a free interval of less than 60 min (headache may begin before or simultaneously with the aura)

From Headache Classification Subcommittee of the International Headache Society: International Headache Society Classification, 2nd ed. Oxford, UK, Blackwell Publishing, 2003. Available at www.I-H-S.org.

    D   disc choked or diplopia
    A   alertness or thinking impaired
    N   neck stiffness
    G   gait abnormality
    E   epileptic seizure or syncope
    R   recent onset or recent history of "the worst headache of my life"

    Age.   Patients usually have their first migraine headache between ages of 10 and 30 years. May occur at any age. Most cases occur in females after menarche. There is a tendency toward remission after age 50.

    Onset.   Infrequent or secondary to "trigger" factors.

    Duration.   Can persist up to 48 hours without treatment.

    Intensity.   Severe, debilitating pain with headache, but patients completely recover after pain ceases. Not life-threatening.

    Aggravating Factors.   Biologic factors: Hormonal influences associated with menses, pregnancy, menopause, and birth control pills. Diet factors: Cheese, aspartame, chocolate. Substance abuse: Caffeine, alcohol, over-the-counter (OTC) sympathomimetics. Environmental irritants: Chemicals, smoke. Body rhythm changes: Sleep disturbances.

Increased sensory input, systemic disease, emotional factors, stress, and "let-down" periods.

Alleviating Factors.   Appropriate pharmacologic and treatment management. Prophylaxis when indicated.

Associated Factors.   Strong family history of similar headaches. May be directly related to *CACNA1A* genes.

There is a comorbidity with epilepsy, seizures, depression, and stroke.

PHYSICAL EXAMINATION

General.   The patient may be irritable, may squint or demonstrate mild diaphoresis. Nausea and vomiting are possible with an acute headache. Evaluate for signs of trauma.

Head, Eyes, Ears, Nose, Throat.   The patient may have objective evidence of diplopia, photophobia, fortification spectra or loss of peripheral visual fields. These resolve with the onset of headache.

Neurologic.   Rarely, patients will have transient, focal neurologic deficits with an aura. These disappear with the onset of headache. Reported transient neurologic deficits include vertigo, paresthesias, light-headedness, and alterations in the level of consciousness. Findings on the neurologic examination in association with a headache should be normal.

PATHOPHYSIOLOGY

The cause of migraine headache is thought to be a 5-HT receptor mediated by the serotonin system, which produces prostaglandins and vasoactivity. Symptoms associated with migraine are related to cerebral blood flow and, more specifically, to vessel caliber. Aura is associated with the vasoconstrictive phase and headache with the vasodilatory phase. Nitric oxide may be an important trigger.

DIAGNOSTIC STUDIES

Specific diagnostic procedures are performed in ambiguous cases or when the diagnosis is not definite based on history and physical examination.

Laboratory
Complete Blood Count.   Indicated to rule out infectious conditions or anemia.

Chemistry Profile.   Used to evaluate glucose, electrolytes, dehydration as a cause of the headaches.

Erythrocyte Sedimentation Rate.   As an indicator of underlying inflammatory process.

Thyroid Profile. As indicated to rule out hyperthyroidism/hypothyroidism.

Drug Screen. Used to evaluate for toxic or illicit medication levels.

Radiology

CT/MRI of the Brain. As indicated to rule out mass lesion or other intracranial pathology. This may be reassuring to the patient if negative.

Cerebral Angiography. As indicated to rule out aneurysm, arteriovenous malformation, or carotid artery or cerebrovascular disease.

Other

Electroencephalography (EEG). Rule out seizure disorder.

Visual Evoked Potentials. Used to evaluate for discrete lesions or demyelinating disease not apparent on CT/MRI.

Lumbar Puncture. Will rule out meningitis and neurosyphilis.

DIFFERENTIAL DIAGNOSIS

Traumatic

Postconcussion. Patient has onset of headaches following a known head injury.

Costen syndrome. Pain in the temporomandibular joint. Pain is present during mastication and palpation.

Infectious

Meningitis. Patient may be febrile, have nuchal rigidity and Kernig and Brudzinski signs. CSF examination reveals an elevated protein associated with a decreased glucose and, possibly, the causative organism.

Neurosyphilis. May have psychiatric features.

Sinusitis. May have a history of seasonal allergies or of sinusitis. Frequently associated with an upper respiratory infection. Sinuses may be tender to palpation. Plain skull radiographs or CT will reveal an air-fluid level in the sinuses.

Postherpetic Neuralgia. Patient will have pain in the distribution of a previous herpetic eruption.

Metabolic

Thyroid disease. Positive thyroid function studies.

Diabetes mellitus. Positive history or elevated serum glucose levels.

Glaucoma. In acute glaucoma, the patient may complain of unilateral eye pain and redness and decreased vision. In chronic glaucoma, the patient may notice a visual field deficit or a general deterioration in visual acuity.

Benign Intracranial Hypertension (Pseudotumor Cerebri). Papilledema and signs of increased intracranial pressure (e.g., abducens nerve palsy) without neurologic impairment.

Neoplastic
Intracranial Lesion.   Headaches progressively increase in intensity. May have focal neurologic deficits in association with headache. CT/MRI reveals the lesion.

Vascular
Subarachnoid Hemorrhage.   Classically an acute, severe headache associated with profound nuchal rigidity. Blood is present in the basilar cisterns on CT; CSF is bloody.
Carotidynia.   May follow dental trauma.
Cluster Headache.   Severe, unilateral, orbital, temporal, or supraorbital pain, lacrimation, nasal stuffiness, rhinorrhea. Occurs daily for days, weeks, or months with remissions.

Congenital
Not otherwise applicable.

Acquired
Medication withdrawal. Alcohol, caffeine may cause transient headache. History of withdrawal.

TREATMENT

Treatment is defined as either abortive or prophylactic. Abortive medications are taken only for an episode of headache. Prophylactic therapies are used on a daily basis to prevent the onset of headache. Narcotics are not recommended owing to the possibility of a "rebound" phenomenon (e.g., if patients miss a dose of narcotic, they will have a headache, so they become dependent on regular use of narcotics). Reassurance about the benign nature of the process (e.g., "you don't have a brain tumor") can help relieve symptoms.

Abortive Therapy
NSAIDs are used at the onset of a headache. They are effective first-line medications for mild to moderate migraine. Agents include ibuprofen (Advil, Motrin) and preparations such as butalbital-acetaminophen-caffeine (Esgic, Phrenilin), acetaminophen-aspirin-caffeine (Excedrin Migraine), barbiturate/acetaminophen/caffeine (Fioricet), and isometheptene mucate–dichloralphenazone–acetaminophen (Midrin).
Triptan drugs stimulate 5-hydroxytryptamine type 1 ($5HT_1$) receptors and are typically used at the onset of moderate to severe headaches resistant to NSAIDs. They are *not* for use in basilar or hemiplegic migraine. The dose may be repeated for persistent headaches up to a maximum dose. Triptan drugs include:
Naratriptan (Amerge) 1-2.5 mg, maximumum dose 5 mg/24 hours
Almotriptan (Axert) 6.25-12.5 mg, maximumum dose 2 doses/
    24 hours

Sumatriptan (Imitrex) 25-100 mg, maximumum dose 200 mg/24 hours (also available as injectable 6 mg, with a maximum of 2 injections in 24 hours, OR nasal spray 5-20 mg, maximum dose 40 mg/day)

Rizatriptan (Maxalt) 5-10 mg, maximumum dose 30 mg/24 hours

Zolmitriptan (Zomig) 2.5-5 mg, maximumum dose 10 mg/24 hours

Another drug from the same class may be tried if one is not effective.

Ergot derivatives have alpha-adrenergic blocking and serotonin antagonist activity. These drugs include:

Ergotamine tartrate (Cafergot) 2 tablets initially, maximumum dose 6 tablets per attack and 10 tablets/week

Dihydroergotamine mesylate 4 mg/mL nasal spray, maximumum dose 6 sprays/24 hours and 8 sprays/week

Prophylactic Therapy

This is indicated if the headache occurs more often than once per week. Treatment is less necessary if abortive therapy is effective.

Beta blockers are effective, inexpensive, and beneficial in the comorbid condition of hypertension. The effects may not be apparent for 3 months; also, weaning is required when the medication is discontinued. These agents include:

Timolol maleate (Blockadren) 10-30 mg twice daily

Propranolol HCl 160-240 mg/day in divided doses

Anticonvulsants also may be useful:

Divalproex sodium (Depakote) 250 mg twice daily, maximumum dose 1 g/24 hours; titrate dose to effect

Adjunctive medications include:

Metoclopramide, promethazine, chlorpromazine: for nausea

Caffeine: may potentiate other medications

Nonpharmacologic Treatments

Biofeedback, exercise, yoga, acupuncture, manipulation including osteopathy, chiropractic, and massage therapy.

Alternative medications may be of benefit:

Riboflavin 400 mg/day

Magnesium 400-600 mg/day

Butterbur (*Petasites hybridus*)

Feverfew (*Tanacetum parthenium, Chrysanthemum parthenium*)

PEDIATRIC CONSIDERATIONS

Use NSAID. Triptan drugs not currently approved for use in persons younger than 18 years of age. Referral to a pediatric neurologist may be necessary for refractory headaches.

OBSTETRIC CONSIDERATIONS

Many women with migraine experience clinical improvement during pregnancy. However, a small percentage may become worse, especially during the first trimester.

Migraines may increase in the postpartum period.

For pharmacologic treatment, see Table 10-6.

GERIATRIC CONSIDERATIONS

Migraine headaches tend to subside after the age of 50. In women, severity and frequency of migraines are reduced with the onset of menopause. If a patient older than 50 complains of new-onset headache, a full investigation is warranted to rule out primary neurologic disease as the cause.

Table 10–6. Pregnancy Risk Categories* of Migraine Medications

Medication	Risk Category
Acetaminophen	B
Meperidine	B, D (third trimester)
Metroclopramide	B
NSAIDs	B†
Mefenamic acid	C
Triptans	C (pregnancy registry for sumatriptan is under way‡)
Barbiturates	C/D
Propranolol	C
Amitriptyline	D
Ergotamine	X

* Categories: A: safety established using human studies; B: presumed safety based on animal studies; C: uncertain safety; D: unsafe; X: highly unsafe.

† Avoid if possible because NSAID use could lead to premature closure of the ductus arteriosus.

‡ Call the Sumatriptan Pregnancy Registry at (800) 722-9292, extension 39441, with questions concerning the use of sumatriptan during pregnancy.

NSAIDs, nonsteroidal anti-inflammatory drugs.

From Newman LC, Lay CL: Menstruation-Associated Migraine. West Conshohocken, PA, Meniscus Educational Institute, 1999. Available at www.meniscus.com.

PREVENTIVE CONSIDERATIONS

Appropriate diagnosis and management is of primary importance. Many patients suffer with migraines because they are under the impression that nothing can be done.

Identification and subsequent avoidance of known trigger factors constitutes an important measure.

Patients should be reassured that, in all likelihood, there is no brain tumor. Only about 1 in 2000 migraine patients will prove to have an intracerebral lesion if the neurologic examination is normal.

PEARLS FOR THE PA

Effective treatment is available for migraine.

Use the IHS criteria to diagnose migraine headaches.

Do not use triptan medications for basilar migraine.

Weaning off narcotic medication is recommended to reduce the chance of rebound headache.

In all likelihood, the migraneur does not have a brain tumor.

Multiple Sclerosis

M. Katherine Reynolds, BS, PA-C

DEFINITION

Multiple sclerosis (MS) is a disease that is characterized by disseminated areas of demyelination and sclerosis of the brain and/or spinal cord. Periods of exacerbation and remission of neurologic symptoms occur in approximately 75% of persons afflicted with the condition.

HISTORY

Symptoms. Classic clinical symptoms include optic neuritis, paresthesias in one or more extremities or one side of the face, focal weakness, numbness, impaired visual acuity, double vision, difficulty with speech, intentional tremor, bladder dysfunction (e.g., urgency or hesitancy), sexual dysfunction, gait imbalance, the sense of an electric shock radiating down the spine or into the limbs when the neck is flexed (Lhermitte phenomenon), tonic spasms, clumsy unilateral hand and arm movements, and vertigo. Heat may accentuate symptoms.

General. The initial attack is usually insidious and may be discounted by the patient. The initial attack is followed by virtually complete recovery lasting anywhere from 1 to more than 25 years. Subsequent exacerbations of symptoms are characterized by less complete recovery with progressive disability. Exacerbations are associated with one or more new lesions or the enlargement of established lesions. These lesions can be verified with MRI scanning.

Age. Predominantly a disease of young adults, with peak for age at onset of 18 to 35 years. During the peak age period, MS affects women more than men (5:1). However, the incidence is the same for both men and women after age 40. A more progressive course occurs in patients whose MS is diagnosed after the age of 40.

Onset. The first episode may be acute or subclinical and may last only hours to days (depending on the size and location of the lesion). As a rule, the onset is gradual. Relapses (exacerbations) vary markedly and depend on the site of the lesion within the central nervous system.

Duration. The disease is lifelong. Exacerbations in the early stages may resolve spontaneously, resulting in what would appear to be a complete recovery. This is due to the ability of the central nervous system (CNS) to recover after the initial inflammatory demyelination. However, recovery becomes less complete with recurrent inflammatory demyelination. The average patient has approximately two exacerbations every 3 years. A relapse is arbitrarily defined as recurrence of symptoms lasting at least 24 hours.

Intensity. Varies from an absence of symptoms to debilitating symptoms that cause significant functional impairment. Most new lesions occur in areas of the CNS that are clinically silent, producing no symptoms initially. Recurrent lesions or recurrent inflammatory demyelinations may result in gliotic scarring, axonal injury, and neuronal loss producing significant decline in neurologic function.

Aggravating Factors. The severity and length of periods of exacerbation are more pronounced during times of emotional or physical stress, such as during pregnancy and for 3 months post partum. The use of alcohol can aggravate and augment active neurologic symptoms.

Alleviating Factors. Appropriate interventions.

Associated Factors. MS is prevalent in temperate zones, with 0.1% to 0.3% of the population being affected. MS is virtually nonexistent near the equator. With increasing latitude, the prevalence of MS increases from 50 to 150 per 100,000, with some rare exceptions. MS is uncommon in blacks. MS demonstrates a familial tendency. Twin studies reveal that persons with a positive family history for MS are at a 15% to 20% higher risk for developing the disease.

PHYSICAL EXAMINATION

General. A complete physical examination is important. It should include assessing active and passive range of motion of all extremities.

Observe tandem gait for ataxia. Also observe the patient changing positions and performing fine motor skills to assess coordination.

Neurologic. A complete detailed neurologic examination is crucial. Funduscopic examination should be performed to evaluate the integrity of the optic nerve. Perform confrontation testing and, if indicated, visual mapping for visual field defects. Test extraocular movements for nystagmus and ocular palsies. Test visual acuity and pupillary reactivity. All cranial nerves should be carefully examined for subtle findings. Cranial nerves I (olfactory), III (oculomotor), VI (abducens), and V (trigeminal) are commonly affected in MS. Deep tendon reflexes may be hyperactive, with presence of Babinski sign or sustained ankle clonus. Abdominal reflexes may be absent. Sensory modalities should be evaluated including vibratory sensation, touch, pinprick, and proprioception.

Paraparesis or paraplegia may occur in later stages of the disease.

Marked increase in muscle tone may preferentially affect upper extremities over lower extremities.

Sphincter tone is commonly affected.

PATHOPHYSIOLOGY

The signs and symptoms of MS are directly related to the number and location of CNS lesions. Demyelination occurs during the inflammatory process affecting the myelin and the underlying axon. Myelin is the lipid-rich plasma membrane that surrounds and insulates axons and augments action potential formation and completion. Areas of demyelination are seen as plaque on MRI. The appearance is of sharp contrast compared with the surrounding tissue.

Demyelination interrupts current flow. In short segments, distal transmission can still occur. However, in longer segments, distal flow is decreased or absent. Thus, the longer the demyelinated segment, the fewer the action potentials and the more clinically evident the neurologic deficit.

Some neurologic symptoms occur secondary to surrounding plaque edema and inflammation. These plaques release toxic factors from immunocompetent cells that are an irritant to the brain and may even contribute to symptoms.

DIAGNOSTIC STUDIES

Laboratory
Diagnosis of MS is based primarily on history and physical examination. There is no single laboratory test that is pathognomonic for MS; however, some laboratory tests and results support the diagnosis.

Cerebrospinal Fluid (CSF) Examination. Albumin levels are elevated in 20% to 30% of patients. Immunoglobulin (IgG) may be elevated, with an IgG index elevation seen in 90% of MS cases identified by clinical evidence.

Oligoclonal bands, which indicate synthesis of IgG, may be found on CSF electrophoresis in 85% to 95% of patients with MS (see Table 10-7).

Radiology

MRI of the Brain and/or Spinal Cord. This is the single best neuroimaging technique used to assist in diagnosis. MRI is able to identify lesions in 85% to 95% of patients with clinically identifiable MS. Lesions (plaques) are seen best on T_2-weighted images. The scan will typically show plaques grouped around the lateral and third ventricles, but may also be seen in the cerebrum, cerebellum, brainstem, and spinal cord. On serial MRI studies, plaques may appear to disappear or increase in size without onset of new clinical symptoms. MRI should also used to rule out other intracranial or intraspinal pathology (see Table 10-7).

Other

Evoked Potential Monitoring. Evoked potentials are electrical events emanating from an afferent system in the CNS. Abnormalities in evoked potentials help in detection and diagnosis of subclinical lesions. Most frequently used are somatosensory evoked potentials, visual evoked responses, and brainstem auditory evoked potentials.

Somatosensory evoked potentials are obtained by transcutaneous electrical stimulation of peripheral nerves. Dysfunction of the sensory pathway causes conduction delays. Somatosensory evoked potentials are abnormal in 70% to 90% of MS patients.

Visual evoked potentials are obtained through repetitive flashes of light or pattern shift stimulation. These are abnormal in 90% of MS patients with optic neuritis.

Brainstem auditory evoked potentials use auditory stimuli. They have a much lower sensitivity rate and are less useful in the identification of MS.

DIFFERENTIAL DIAGNOSIS

Any neurologic condition that manifests with transient neurologic symptoms can be confused with MS. A review of all of these potential conditions is beyond the scope of this discussion. Only the more commonly encountered conditions are listed here.

Table 10–7. Cerebrospinal Fluid Protein Abnormalities in Multiple Sclerosis

	Albumin	IgG/Total Protein	IgG/ Albumin	IgG Index	Oligoclonal Bands
Clinically definite disease	23%	67%	73%	92%	95%
Normal	3%	NR	3%	3%	7%

NR, not recorded.

Traumatic
Herniated Disk. Symptoms confined to a radicular distribution. Seen on MRI.

Infectious
Acute Disseminated Encephalomyelitis. Usually following onset of measles, rubella, smallpox. Manifests with decreased tendon reflexes, sensory impairment, paralysis of bowel and/or bladder.

Acute Epidural Abscess. May manifest with unilateral weakness of the extremities.

Acute Myelitis. Evaluate for evidence of Epstein-Barr virus (EBV) or herpesvirus B infection.

Meningovascular Syphilis. Differentiated with positive rapid plasma reagin (RPR) assay/Venereal Disease Research Laboratory (VDRL) test.

Cryptococcosis. Lumbar puncture specimen shows CSF-encapsulated yeast, increased protein, decreased glucose, positive-encapsulated antigen in CSF.

Sarcoidosis. Positive biopsy, noncaseating epithelioid granulomas, bilateral hilar adenopathy on chest film.

Toxoplasmosis. Isolate *Toxoplasma gondii* from body fluids. Trophozoites from tissue.

Lyme Disease. Spirochetal etiology. Disappears when treated with penicillin.

Metabolic
Systemic Lupus Erythematosus (SLE). Sixty percent of cases of SLE are due to Sjögren-Larsson syndrome; positive antinuclear antibody, positive lupus erythematosus cell test, leukopenia, pernicious anemia.

Progressive Multifocal Leukoencephalopathy. May appear to be exacerbation of MS; look for leukemia or lymphoma as causative factor.

Spinocerebellar Ataxias. Explore family history. Hereditary factors may be suggestive. Look for cerebellar degeneration on MRI.

Vitamin B_{12} Deficiency. Muscular weakness, positive Schilling test.

Behçet Disease. Recurrent iridocyclitis and meningitis. Evaluate for recurrent mouth ulcers, genital sores, and eye inflammation.

Myasthenia Gravis. Progressive weakness as day progresses (see "Myasthenia Gravis" next in this chapter).

Amyotrophic Lateral Sclerosis. Patient will present with lower motor neuron and pyramidal symptoms. Patient will not have abnormal sensory findings.

Mitochondral Encephalopathies. Difficult to diagnose. Common finding is hyperlacticacidemia.

Neoplastic
Optic Nerve Glioma. Gradual monocular visual loss. Symptoms are progressive and do not remit. MRI/CT scanning will confirm lesion.

Vascular

Thrombotic Event.   May cause acute monocular visual loss. Funduscopic examination may reveal the thrombus.

Transient Ischemic Attack (TIA).   May cause neurologic symptoms that go into remission. Angiogram or ultrasound examination of the carotid or vertebral arteries may reveal a stenosis. MRI/CT scanning may reveal small infarcts. All MS studies will be negative.

Congenital

Malformation of the Cervical Spine or Skull Base.   May cause symptomatic relapses. CT studies with bone windows may help in diagnosis.

Cervical Spondylosis.   May cause pain and/or weakness in one extremity. MRI/CT and plain films of the cervical spine will help to identify lesion.

Hereditary Ataxias.   Degeneration of spinocerebellar tracts, corticospinal tracts. Familial history is commonly the key to diagnosis.

Acquired

Postinfectious Encephalomyelitis, Postvaccine Encephalomyelitis.   Onset of symptoms will occur 2 to 4 weeks after vaccination. May be extremely difficult to differentiate between a first attack of MS and postinfectious or postimmunization encephalomyelitis.

TREATMENT

MS is a chronic progressive process without a demonstrated cure. The goal of therapy is to decrease length and number of relapses, decrease intensity of acute episode, and attempt to slow disease process.

Long-term supportive care is essential to the patient's psychologic outlook. Thus, a multidisciplinary approach may be helpful. Patients should be encouraged to keep physically fit and avoid smoking, as respiratory musculature can be affected. Avoidance of alcohol is recommended, as it augments preexisting cerebellar deficits.

Treatment of Specific Symptoms

Fatigue.   Rest seems to be the most beneficial. Reevaluate any sedating medications the patient may be taking. Trials of amantadine (100 mg every morning and early afternoon) and modafinil (400 mg or less every morning) are under way; however, their efficacy has not been proved.

Spasticity.   Depending on degree of spasticity, pharmacologic therapies include:

Baclofen, a GABA agonist: Drug of first choice. Initial dose 5 mg three times a day with increase of 5 to 10 mg every 3 days as needed.
   Mild: 5 mg three times a day–10 mg four times a day
   Moderate: 10-20 mg four times a day
   Severe: doses up to 120 mg a day as tolerated

Zanaflex (creates less weakness than baclofen but has a higher incidence of somnolence): 2 mg at bedtime, up to maximum of 36 mg in divided doses three to four times a day.

Gabapentin (Neurontin): Does not interact with GABA receptors. The mechanism of action is unknown; however, it is a useful third-line agent for spasticity, especially nocturnal spasms. Initial dose 100 mg three times a day; may be gradually increased to a maximum of 900 mg three times a day.

Benzodiazepam: Usually a third- or fourth-line agent. Bedtime doses for nocturnal spasms refractory to treatment with baclofen or gabapentin.

Diazepam: 5-15 mg at bedtime.

Dantrolene: Usually third-line agent used in nonambulatory patients, owing to potential hepatotoxicity and tendency to aggravate muscle weakness.

Tremor and Ataxia. Both are poorly responsive to drug therapy. Rehabilitation with occupational therapy can provide adaptive equipment to maintain independence. Physical therapy can aid with gait training. The following regimen can be tried:

Klonopin: May be dosed to an endpoint of effective control or unacceptable sedation. Begin with 0.5 mg at bedtime, with morning and evening doses added over a 2-week period. Daily dose to be increased by 0.5 mg every 5 days beginning with bedtime dose.

Urinary Bladder Dysfunction. Anticholinergics tend to work well:

Ditropan 2.5 mg twice a day–5.0 mg three times a day

Propantheline 15 mg three times a day up to 30 mg four times a day

Intermittent catheterization 4 to 6 times a day may be needed because of the atonic bladder.

Bowel Dysfunction. Constipation may be common both to the disease state and as a side effect of medication. Patients should avoid laxatives. A high-fiber diet should be stressed. Adequate oral fluids and stool softeners should be encouraged.

Sexual Dysfunction. Erectile dysfunction secondary to MS may respond to sildenafil citrate (Viagra) 50 to 100 mg as needed.

Pain Syndromes. The most common found with MS are neuralgia, meningeal irritation, dysesthesias, and secondary muscle pain.

For neuralgia, begin with gabapentin 100 mg three times a day and increase as tolerated to a maximum of 3600 mg/day in three or four divided doses. Use of carbamazepine (Tegretol) in conjunction with gabapentin may be beneficial for second-line intervention. Other alternatives are phenytoin (Dilantin), amitriptyline, and baclofen.

Meningeal irritation usually occurs with acute inflammation and is treated with high-dose corticosteroids.

Dysethesias are difficult to treat but tend to respond to tricyclic antidepressants and carbamazepine. Doses are increased gradually to allow the patient to develop tolerance to the side effects.

Muscle pains are common owing to MS-induced abnormal gait, weakness in upper extremities, and poor sitting posture. Treatment should be directed at the underlying cause. Nonsteroidal anti-inflammatory drugs (NSAIDs) and physical therapy are beneficial.

Disease Therapy

Corticosteroids are used in patients with acute onset of neurologic impairment. Long-term use does not affect the overall course of the disease process. Adrenocorticotropic hormone (ACTH), 40 units intravenously or intramuscularly for 5 days with a gradual taper, or methylprednisolone, 1 g daily for 5 to 7 days, may be beneficial in somatic relapses.

Currently, three drugs are approved in the United States market for preventive therapy for relapsing MS: interferon beta-1a (Avonex), interferon beta-1b (Betaseron), and glatiramer acetate (Copaxone).

PEDIATRIC CONSIDERATIONS

MS is rare in the pediatric population. Only 0.2% to 2% of cases present before 10 years of age. The prognosis for childhood MS is similar to that in adults.

OBSTETRIC CONSIDERATIONS

There is a remarkable increase in exacerbations of preexisting MS during pregnancy and for 9 months post partum (most marked in the first 3 months). Evidence supports hormonal influence. Women with MS complicating childbirth should be counseled appropriately.

GERIATRIC CONSIDERATIONS

A particularly difficult problem for older patients with MS is urinary retention. Patients may have suprasacral spinal cord lesions and eventually develop detrusor-sphincter dyssynergy, which can be a source of considerable discomfort and inconvenience. In some instances a sphincterotomy is necessary. Supportive measures are critical. The appropriate use of toilet substitutes, incontinence undergarments, modification of fluid intake patterns, and environmental adjustments can be of benefit. Patient comfort can be enhanced with both behavioral measures and drug therapy.

PREVENTIVE CONSIDERATIONS

There is no primary prevention of MS. However, counseling patients about avoiding emotionally and physically stressful situations can assist with control of symptoms. Patients should be educated about the importance of taking steps to minimize exacerbation of the disease. Because living with MS can be difficult, patients should be encouraged to join a support group or contact the National MS Society (see chapter Resources).

PEARLS FOR THE PA

Headache is not a symptom of MS.

Trigeminal neuralgia in patients younger than age 40 years represents MS until proven otherwise.

Diagnosis of MS is not secure unless there is a history of remission and relapses and evidence on examination of more than one CNS lesion.

Long-term, supportive care of the patient is essential.

The classic finding in MS is white matter plaques seen on T_2-weighted MRI scans of the brain or spinal cord.

Myasthenia Gravis

William A. Mosier, EdD, MPAS, LMFT, PA-C (Major-USAFR)

DEFINITION

Myasthenia gravis (MG) is the most common disorder affecting neuromuscular junctions. It is an autoimmune disorder, characterized by fluctuating muscle weakness and fatigue.

HISTORY

Symptoms. Extraocular muscle weakness with resultant diplopia and ptosis are frequently the earliest symptoms. Oropharyngeal and/or facial muscle weakness can cause dysphagia andproblems in speaking and/or chewing. The patient feels a generalized fatigue with weakness of the extremities. The trunk muscles and diaphragm can be affected. Bowel and bladder sphincters may be affected as the disease progresses. Pain is rarely a primary complaint. The symptoms of physical weakness tend to be less severe in the early morning and become more pronounced as the day progresses. Rest tends to help a patient regain strength.

General. The onset of MG may be either gradual or sudden. Patients may, on retrospective analysis, be found to have had symptoms for quite some time prior to seeking medical attention. The condition may not have been apparent when certain activities that worsened the patient's weakness were avoided. It is important to obtain a detailed history of activities that produce weakness in specific muscle groups. Diplopia and ptosis may become worse during periods of eyestrain such as reading or driving. Extremity weakness may become evident after repeated lifting. Oropharyngeal symptoms include choking and exit of fluid from the nose during swallowing. Hoarseness or a nasal quality to the voice may become increasingly noticeable to the patient or family members as the day progresses. It may disappear each morning, only to reappear each afternoon. The patient may find it necessary to manually hold the jaw closed after talking or eating, owing to muscle weakness.

Age.   May appear at any age.

Women.   Most prevalent in the third decade of life.

Men.   Most prevalent in the fifth and sixth decades.

Onset.   Slow and progressive.

Duration.   The disease course is variable. Some patients may experience a rapid progression, whereas others may experience several months of relative stability. Progression to a generalized disease usually occurs within the first year after the onset of symptoms. Remission, when it occurs, may last months to years.

Intensity.   The disease may be limited to the extraocular muscles throughout the course or progress to involve the oropharyngeal and extremity musculature. Varying periods of remission may occur early in the course of the disease. Death is most common in the first year of the disease.

Aggravating Factors.   Emotional stress, hyperthyroidism, hypothyroidism, systemic illness, pregnancy, menses, elevations in temperature (seasonal, fever, hot water), and certain drugs (e.g., *d*-penicillamine, quinidine, quinine, procainamide, aminoglycoside antibiotics, timolol maleate [ophthalmologic], beta blockers, calcium channel blockers, neuromuscular blocking agents such as succinylcholine or *d*-tubocurarine).

Alleviating Factors.   Rest and appropriate treatment.

Associated Factors.   MG is associated with other conditions that have an assumed immunologic cause (e.g., rheumatoid arthritis, systemic lupus erythematosus, hyperthyroidism). Owing to the intermittent nature of the symptoms, many patients are incorrectly perceived as having a psychiatric illness.

PHYSICAL EXAMINATION

General.   The patient may appear generally fatigued. The patient may exhibit a surprised or snarled facies as a result of chronic contracture of the frontalis muscle to compensate for ptosis or from overall facial muscle weakness.

Head, Eyes, Ears, Nose, Throat.   Testing the oropharyngeal musculature is imperative. Listen to the voice character. The patient may have a nasal quality to the voice, especially after talking for a prolonged period (more pronounced in the evening than in the morning). Testing of the laryngeal muscles can be accomplished by asking the patient to make a high-pitched sound, which may produce a pronounced hoarseness. Test jaw strength manually by attempting to open the patient's mouth against resistance; normally, this cannot be done.

Neurologic. As muscle weakness may vary, a specialized muscle strength examination is required. Test muscle strength repeatedly while the patient attempts maximal resistance. Allow the patient to rest, and repeat the maneuver. A false-positive examination may be encountered if the repetitive testing elicits pain. Pain is not a common symptom of MG. Any extremity or trunk muscle can be affected, but muscles primarily affected include the neck flexors, deltoid, wrist extensors, and fingers. Atrophy of the extremities is present in only 10% to 20% of patients. Deep tendon reflexes and sensory examination are typically normal.

Ophthalmologic. Most patients will exhibit a bilateral, asymmetrical weakness of several extraocular muscles, not in a specific cranial nerve distribution. Pupillary reactivity is normal. Ptosis is usually present if extraocular muscle weakness is present. It is typically asymmetrical and variable during sustained activity. Test eyelid closure by attempting to open the eyelid. Weakness may be elicited by asking the patient to look at the ceiling (ptosis) or holding the gaze in the lateral position for several minutes (diplopia).

PATHOPHYSIOLOGY

MG is an autoimmune disease that results from the destruction of postganglionic acetylcholine (ACh) receptors located at neuromuscular junctions. These junctions serve as the interface between nerve fibers and muscle fibers. The destruction is caused by circulating antibodies attacking the acetylcholine receptors. Normally, acetylcholine is released by the motor nerve terminal in packages (quanta). The quanta then diffuse across the synaptic cleft and bind to receptors on the muscle end plate, which eventually results in muscle contraction. In MG, the motor end plate loses its normal folded shape, widens, and is bound with antibodies, so that a lower concentration of acetylcholine reaches the receptor sites. The amount of acetylcholine released is not diminished. It is only the receptors for acetylcholine that are affected.

Abnormalities of the thymus occur in as many as 75% of patients with MG. Up to 50% of patients with a diagnosed thymoma have or will eventually develop MG. The role of the thymus in MG is unknown, but it is postulated that both the thymus and the neuromuscular junction are affected by an immunologic reaction to an antigen common to both sites. The spinal cord and brain are not affected.

DIAGNOSTIC STUDIES

Laboratory
Serum Antibodies That Bind to the Human Acetylcholine Receptor Antibody (AChRAb). Presence of antibodies is noted in 54% of patients

with ocular weakness only, in 74% of those with clinical disease, and in 74% to 99% of those with acquired MG. Elevated levels are virtually confirmatory. However, negative levels do not rule out the disease. The level of AChRAb does not correlate with the severity of disease. Usually not present in those who do not have MG, but antibody presence has been reported in other systemic diseases. False positives may be seen if the blood specimen is drawn 48 hours after general anesthesia.

Radiology

Chest Film. Because of the relationship between thymomas and MG, a plain chest radiograph should be obtained to look for a smooth or lobulated soft tissue mass near the origin of the great vessels at the base of the heart.

Chest CT. The most sensitive technique for detecting small thymomas. However, small tumors cannot always be distinguished from a normal thymus. A CT scan is useful for demonstrating local invasion of tumor through thymic capsule into lung, chest wall, diaphragm, great vessels, pericardium, or pleura.

Other

Edrophonium Hydrochloride (Tensilon) Test. Edrophonium is administered intravenously in incremental doses beginning with 2 mg and evaluating response at 45 to 60 seconds up to a maximum dose of 10 mg (infant dose is 0.15 mg/kg given subcutaneously); this is followed by a motor examination. If the patient's weakness is due to abnormal neuromuscular transmission, there should be improvement. Dramatic improvement may be noticed in strength of the ocular and pharyngeal muscles. Improvement in extremity strength is an objective physical finding on motor examination. This test is not specific to MG, as improvement may occur in patients with other motor neuron diseases. To prevent potential gastrointestinal side effects, dosing at 10 mg should be avoided, if possible. It is often the case that an adequate response is achieved without dosing beyond 8 mg.

Electromyography (EMG). Repetitive nerve stimulation may show decreasing amplitude (approximately 10% from the initial measurement). This finding is more often encountered in the proximal musculature. Needle EMG may show variability in the amplitude or shape of action potentials and is also used to rule out other diseases that may mimic MG. In as many as 99% of patients with MG, single-fiber EMG is the most sensitive test. Increased neuromuscular jitter (a sign of impaired neuromuscular transmission) may be seen when testing specific muscles. However, increased neuromuscular jitter is not specific for MG. It may also be encountered in diseases of the anterior horn cell, nerve, or muscle.

Stapedial Reflex Fatigue. This technique can be used to evaluate fatigue of the stapedius muscle. Sustained contraction of the muscle (which exerts tension on the tympanic membrane) is obtained by emitting sound to the ear, stimulating the tympanic membrane. Acoustic impedance is measured and will significantly decrease in the presence of MG owing to stapedius muscle fatigue. The test is painless and is useful in patients in whom cooperation is difficult. It is particularly useful in the pediatric population. This test is used in confirming rather than diagnosing neuromuscular transmission disorders.

Ocular Muscle Function Tests. Include EMG of the ocular muscles, tonometry, and Lancaster red-green tests of ocular motility. Used in confirming rather than diagnosing neuromuscular transmission disorders.

DIFFERENTIAL DIAGNOSIS

Traumatic

Head injury. May produce extraocular muscle weakness. Patients will have a history of trauma, and the deficit will not wax and wane.

Insect and Snake Bites. May contain neurotoxins that affect neuromuscular transmission. The venom of cobras, sea snakes, rattlesnakes, black widow spiders, and scorpions all can produce symptoms similar to those of MG. A history of bites needs to be obtained in indigenous areas.

Infectious

Botulism. Due to ingestion of *Clostridium botulinum*, found in seafood or in inadequately sterilized canned foods. Patients usually have a history of ingestion of such foods and experience nausea and vomiting 12 to 36 hours before the onset of symptoms. Symptoms include dilated pupils, blurred vision, dysphagia, dry mouth, constipation, and urinary retention followed by severe muscle paralysis with possible respiratory arrest. Weakness may also involve the ocular muscles and tongue. The toxin blocks release of acetylcholine.

Metabolic

Persons with systemic lupus erythematosus, inflammatory neuropathy, amyotrophic lateral sclerosis, rheumatoid arthritis (in persons receiving D-penicillamine), and unaffected persons related to MG patients may have AChRAb present in the serum.

Systemic Lupus Erythematosus. Does not involve the extraocular muscles.

Multiple Sclerosis (MS). Presents with waxing and waning neurologic findings. Differentiated through physical examination findings and history of specific neurologic symptoms. A complete MS workup is necessary to rule out MS as a diagnosis.

Polymyositis. Does not involve the extraocular muscles.

Disorders of the Anterior Horn Cell, Nerve or Muscle. Can be differentiated from MG on EMG.

Diabetes Mellitus. May cause ptosis and/or extraocular muscle weakness (due to small-vessel disease) or extremity numbness and weakness. Patients will have a history of diabetes mellitus. Deficit will not wax and wane. Differentiated on EMG.

Lambert-Eaton Myasthenic Syndrome. Is a rare condition associated with small cell lung cancer in two-thirds of cases. Differentiated by the clinical presentation. Proximal muscles are affected symmetrically, and oropharyngeal and ocular symptoms are less conspicuous. Response to cholinesterase inhibitors is poor.

Amyotrophic Lateral Sclerosis. May have EMG findings similar to those in MG.

Thyrotoxicosis. May occur simultaneously with MG and create a myopathy. Frequently associated with exophthalmos and does not respond to neostigmine.

Neoplastic
Thymoma. May have elevated levels of AChRAb.

Intracerebral Neoplasm. May cause ptosis and/or extraocular muscle weakness and dysphagia. Deficit will not wax and wane. Lesion usually visible on CT/MRI of brain.

Vascular
Intracerebral Aneurysm (of the Posterior Communicating Artery). May cause a cranial nerve III palsy, which includes ptosis and extraocular muscle weakness. Deficit will not wax and wane. Lesion seen on cerebral angiogram.

Congenital. Not applicable.

Acquired
Postoperative (Complication of General Anesthesia). May give false-positive AChRAb.

D-Penicillamine. Used to treat rheumatoid arthritis, Wilson disease, and cystinuria. Symptoms of MG may develop. However, symptoms will resolve after discontinuation of the drug.

Hysteria or Emotional Illness. MG may be misdiagnosed as hysteria, depression, or somatization disorder. Ptosis and dysphagia are absent, and no objective findings can be demonstrated. The patient may report improvement with neostigmine.

Nutritional Deficiency. Characterized by ptosis and bulbar weakness in patients with nutritional deprivation. Reported to respond to parenteral thiamine. (Often alcohol abuse related.)

TREATMENT

There is no generally recognized monotherapy for MG. Each patient must be treated individually with regard to severity of disease, functional impairment, and age. Improvement or remissions can occur in the absence of therapy; therefore, response to a specific therapy must be determined over the course of time.

Cholinesterase Inhibitors
Allow for prolonged effect of acetylcholine at the neuromuscular junction by inhibiting enzymatic hydrolysis. If the medication produces

decrease in strength, the dose is too high. Dose should be adjusted for optimal effect.

Drugs include:

Pyridostigmine bromide (Mestinon) at an initial dose of 30-90 mg every 6 hours. Dose can be gradually increased to 180 mg every 3 to 4 hours, with sustained-release pyridostigmine 180 mg given at bedtime. (Initial dose in infants and children should start at 1.0 mg/kg.) Pyridostigmine is the mainstay of medical therapy.

Neostigmine bromide (Prostigmin) 7.5-45 mg every 2 to 6 hours, with an average maintenance dose of 150 mg/d (in infants and children; 0.3 to 0.5 mg/kg).

Ambenonium chloride (Mytelase) for moderate to severe MG 5-25 mg 3-4 times a day, beginning with a low dose and slowly titrating upward every 2 days.

A cholinergic crisis may occur with large doses of cholinesterase-inhibiting drugs. Symptoms include nausea, vomiting, sweating, salivation, colic, diarrhea, miosis, bradycardia, and increased weakness. Hypotension can be treated with atropine.

Thymectomy

Following thymectomy, 80% of patients will experience long-lasting relief of their symptoms, with no known chronic sequelae. Thymectomy can be considered in persons with a life expectancy of greater than 10 years and in those with a thymoma. Younger patients and those patients early in the course of their disease seem to benefit most.

Corticosteroids

Recommended regimen is:

Prednisone 60-70 mg/day (children: 1.5-2.0 mg/kg/day), administered as alternate-day dosing. This should be carefully monitored and decreased over a period of months to the lowest effective dose, usually not less than 5-10 mg on alternating days.

Hospitalization is required when prednisone therapy is instituted, as approximately 50% of patients will experience a transient worsening of symptoms. Seventy-five percent of patients will experience significant improvement and 15% may have some improvement in their condition. Significant weakness may recur if treatment is withdrawn.

Immunosuppressant Drugs

Recommended regimen is:

Azathioprine (Imuran) 50 mg/day for initial dose, increased by 50 mg/day every 3 to 10 days, to a maximum dose of 150 mg/day.

Improvement takes 4 months in most patients but may take up to 8 months. Weakness recurs 2 to 3 months after the drug is withdrawn. Considered for patients with late-onset MG, in those in whom corticosteroids are contraindicated, as secondary treatment in patients resistant to corticosteroids or thymectomy, and in association with corticosteroids. Side effects include gastrointestinal upset, leukocytopenia, and elevation of liver enzymes. Alternative regimen is:

Cyclophosphamide (Cytoxan) 150-200 mg/day orally, to a maximum total dose of 5-10 g, OR 200 mg intravenously for 5 days.

Alopecia (common), leukopenia, nausea, vomiting, anorexia, and discoloration of the nails or skin all may be encountered with use of cyclophosphamide.

Plasma Exchange
Almost all patients will experience improvement following plasma exchange. It can be used for sudden deterioration in MG patients and to achieve improvement preoperatively for thymectomy. Improvement can be seen immediately and may continue for months after the treatment. Weakness returns unless adjunctive therapy is begun with immunosuppression or thymectomy.

Other Treatments
Other treatments include gamma globulin, splenic and total body irradiation, splenectomy, guanidine hydrochloride, and aminopyridines. Respiratory assistance may be required during a myasthenic crisis that might be brought on by emotional or physical disturbance.

PEDIATRIC CONSIDERATIONS

Only 10% of cases occur in children younger than 10 years of age. Congenital MG should be suspected in any infant presenting with bilateral ptosis. The deficit primarily affects the extraocular and facial muscles and does not significantly involve the extremities. Plasma exchange and thymectomy do not result in improvement. The only appropriate treatment is with oral anticholinesterase medications. It is an autosomal recessive trait with a male-to-female ratio of 2:1.

Transient neonatal MG occurs in 15% of infants born to mothers with MG. The disorder results from the transplacental interaction between the mother's IgG antibodies with fetal acetylcholine receptors. Infants tend to recover spontaneously within 2 to 3 months after birth. There seems to be no relation between the severity of the disease of the mother and that of the infant. Fetal anomalies have been reported in small study groups of mothers with MG. These include flexion/contracture anomalies and pulmonary hypoplasia. Neonates with this condition have no greater risk of developing MG later in life than persons in the general population. The diagnosis is made utilizing the same tests as employed for testing adults. Treatment is with age-appropriate doses of anticholinesterase drugs.

OBSTETRIC CONSIDERATIONS

Azathioprine should not be used in females of childbearing age owing to the possibility of teratogenicity.

GERIATRIC CONSIDERATIONS

More common in men than in women at this period in life, and the symptoms of muscle weakness and fatigue that becomes more pronounced with activity and decreases with rest should prompt diagnostic testing for MG. Any geriatric patient presenting with a complaint of weakness and fatigue should be assessed for signs of impaired ocular movement and ptosis. If physical examination uncovers these findings, MG should be high on the list of suspected conditions responsible for the symptoms.

PREVENTIVE CONSIDERATIONS

Avoidance of stressful stimuli and ample rest are critical to controlling symptoms of MG. For this reason, stress management training and MG support groups can be useful for empowering patients to take control of their response to the disease process. A diet containing foods high in potassium should be encouraged.

PEARLS FOR THE PA

MG is characterized by fluctuating muscle weakness.

Ptosis and diplopia are frequently the earliest symptoms.

Patients may be incorrectly perceived as having a psychiatric illness.

MG is an autoimmune disease.

Incorrect diagnosis of MG may have serious consequences for the patient. A myasthenic crisis can result from not maintaining medication at an adequate dose Exacerbation of symptoms can also occur from emotional stress, infection, or physical injury. Overmedicating can produce a cholinergic crisis. The greatest risk from underdosing or overdosing medication is respiratory failure.

Parkinson Disease

Catherine R. Judd, MS, PA-C

DEFINITION

Parkinson disease (PD) is a chronic, progressive, neurodegenerative disorder resulting from loss of pigmented brainstem nuclei prevalent in the substantia nigra, a pigmented nucleus containing dopaminergic neurons projecting to the putamen and caudate. The resultant loss of inhibitory dopaminergic activity results in the motor symptoms that characterize Parkinson disease including tremor, rigidity, bradykinesia, and postural instability. Parkinson disease is the most common movement disorder encountered in primary care.

HISTORY

Symptoms. A pill-rolling tremor with frequency of 3 to 6 Hz in one hand is the first manifestation observed in over half of all patients with Parkinson disease. Tremor, usually unilateral at onset, is exaggerated by stress and anxiety, increases at rest, decreases with movement, and is absent during sleep. Slowness of movements (bradykinesia) results in difficulties in dressing, maintaining hygiene, and eating. As the disorder progresses, stiffness, decreased movement (hypokinesia), postural instability, and disturbance in equilibrium increase risk of falling. Posture becomes stooped, with festinating gait and difficulty initiating movement (akinesia). There is decrease in spontaneity and decrease in facial expression, resulting in "masked facies." Speech is affected, with difficulty forming words, increased salivation, and drooling. Patients experience significant difficulty with handwriting. Autonomic symptoms that commonly occur include orthostatic hypotension, constipation, hyperhidrosis, muscle cramps, micrographia, hypophonia, and monotonous speech. Bladder abnormalities may be a feature of Parkinson disease or may be due to side effects from medications used to treat the disorder. A decline in intellect may also be present, and dementia is found in over half of patients.

General. The diagnosis of Parkinson disease is not difficult owing to the characteristic features of the disorder and response to medication. However, a full history of contributing factors must be obtained. Consider family history of neurodegenerative diseases (e.g., Huntington disease), occupational exposure to heavy metals, infectious diseases (e.g., human immunodeficiency virus [HIV] infection, syphilis, encephalitis), medication use or abuse, and mental health issues.

Age. Onset is between 40 and 70 years of age, mean age 54 (peak onset in mid-50s). Rarely occurs in patients younger than 30 and declines after age 70. Affects 1% of patients older than 65. In rare cases it may begin in childhood or adolescence.

Onset. Insidious. Patients most often present with unilateral hand tremor, bradykinesia, muscular rigidity, postural instability, and clumsiness.

Duration. Parkinson disease is a chronic, progressive degenerative disease.

Intensity. Symptoms are initially mild, with little functional impairment. As the disease progresses, symptoms frequently become debilitating and incapacitating.

Aggravating Factors. Emotional stress may exacerbate tremors.
Alleviating Factors. Appropriate medication.
Associated Factors. Fall injuries caused by unstable gait. Depression is common and should be treated aggressively with appropriate antidepressants.

PATHOPHYSIOLOGY

Symptoms of Parkinson disease are due to degeneration of the corpus striatum and substantia nigra. The subsequent reduction in dopaminergic neurons reduces the availability of the neurotransmitter dopamine. Decreases in other neurotransmitters occur, including norepinephrine, serotonin, acetylcholine (may contribute to dementia), somatostatin, cholecystokinin-8, substance P, met-enkephalin, and leu-enkephalin. The etiology of Parkinson's disease is unknown, but environmental factors may play a role. No gender, ethnic, or geographic predilections are known. Some families have demonstrated an autosomal dominant risk factor.

PHYSICAL EXAMINATION

General. Hallmark signs include a resting tremor that decreases with movement. The tremor may be confined to one limb or one side or may be bilateral. The patient's face may show a lack of facial expression ("masked facies"), with exaggerated glabellar reflex (Myerson sign): blinking that does not stop or diminish while tapping forehead. A fine tremor may be present that involves the mouth. Other findings include sialorrhea and a moist, oily face with seborrheic dermatitis.

Neurologic. "Cogwheel" rigidity, which is demonstrated when passive movement of a joint produces a jerking or successive "catching." Voluntary movements are slowed and gait is unsteady (especially on turning) and shuffling, owing to bradykinesia. Ability to perform rapid alternating movements will generally be reduced. Handwriting analysis may show a micrographia that is characterized by progressively smaller writing (e.g., when writing a sentence, the initial words are larger and then progressively decrease in size). Reflexes are variable.

DIAGNOSTIC STUDIES

There are no diagnostic tests for Parkinson disease. Diagnosis is clinical.

Laboratory
Liver Function Tests and Serum Copper and Ceruloplasmin Determinations. Performed in younger patients to rule out Wilson disease.
Serologic Studies. As indicated to diagnose neurosyphilis or acquired immunodeficiency syndrome (AIDS).

Radiology
CT/MRI of Brain.   Usually normal, but may show nonspecific cortical atrophy. Useful when diagnosis is uncertain or patient fails to respond to pharmacotherapy, to detect lacunar infarcts and brainstem or cerebellar atrophy.
Single Photon Emission Computed Tomography (SPECT).   Using the isotope 6-[18F]fluorolevodopa reveals decreased uptake in the corpus striatum.

Other
Electroencephalography (EEG).   Typically normal
ECG.   Typically normal. However, in patients with tremor; an atrial flutter artifact may be present.

DIFFERENTIAL DIAGNOSIS

Traumatic
Head Trauma.   Rare and due to midbrain hemorrhage. Associated with a history of trauma and other brainstem abnormalities.
Dementia Pugilistica.   Seen in boxers as a result of repetitive trauma and diffuse neuronal injury.

Infectious
Creutzfeldt-Jakob Disease.   Symptoms are accompanied by dementia, myoclonic jerking, pyramidal signs, and specific EEG abnormalities.
HIV Infection or Neurosyphilis.   Exhibit symptoms similar to those of Parkinson disease. Differentiated on serologic studies.
Postencephalitic Parkinsonism.   May have a history of immediate or remote encephalitis (febrile illness with lethargy). Symptoms may be the same as those seen with idiopathic Parkinson disease. Differentiated by history and the presence of mental changes, oculomotor dysfunction, sleep abnormalities, and other movement disorders.

Metabolic
Wilson Disease.   Tremors of early onset with other abnormal movements not consistent with Parkinson disease will be present.
Huntington Disease.   Positive family history of Huntington disease and the presence of dementia will differentiate.
Shy-Drager Syndrome.   Symptoms similar to Parkinson's disease, but are accompanied by autonomic symptoms and more diffuse neurologic findings (e.g., lower motor neuron and cerebellar).
Progressive Supranuclear Palsy.   Symptoms similar to those of Parkinson disease, but accompanied by abnormalities in eye movements along with pseudobulbar paralysis and loss of axial tone.

Neoplastic
Brain Tumors.   Due to compression or invasion of the corpus striatum. Seen on CT/MRI of brain.

Vascular
Lacunar Infarct. Involving the corpus striatum. Uncommon and primarily affects the lower limbs to a greater extent than the upper limbs.

Congenital
Juvenile Parkinson Disease. Patients will commonly have a positive family history of the disorder.

Acquired
Toxic Exposure. Caused by exposure to toxins such as manganese dust, carbon disulfide, cyanide, carbon monoxide, insecticides, and herbicides.

Drug-Induced. May be caused by high-potency neuroleptic drugs (e.g., phenothiazines, fluphenazine, haloperidol); reserpine; antiemetics, especially prochlorperazine and metoclopramide; *N*-methyl-4-phenyl-1,2,3,6-tetrahydropyridine (MPTP), present in the street drug "synthetic heroin"; lithium; and α-methyldopa (rarely).

Tremor of Advancing Age. May be confusing if the tremor and bradykinesia are mild. Other findings (e.g., rigidity) are absent.

Depression. Patient may exhibit flat blunted affect with decreased facial expression, psychomotor retardation. Frequently coexists with Parkinson disease and should be treated aggressively with appropriate antidepressants with minimal dopaminergic activity. Other findings (e.g., rigidity) are absent.

Other
Hydrocephalus. From any cause. CT/MRI of brain will reveal enlarged ventricles. Symptoms respond to a shunting procedure.

TREATMENT

Medical Therapy
Parkinson disease is progressive and unremitting. No curative treatment is currently available. Treatment is palliative and directed at reducing symptoms. All of the dopaminergic agents used in the treatment of Parkinson disease act by increasing the activity of central dopamine receptors. They all share similar side effects including anorexia, vomiting, dizziness, dyskinesia, psychosis, depression, and dementia. Associated medication side effects may outweigh benefits.

Drugs
When to institute pharmacotherapy is controversial.

Carbidopa-levodopa (Sinemet) is the mainstay of pharmacotherapy. It can produce a significant decrease in bradykinesia, rigidity, and tremor. Patients with relatively mild symptoms are frequently restored to near normal level of functioning. Carbidopa-levodopa is available in several formulations (10 mg/100 mg, 25 mg/100 mg, and 25 mg/250 mg) as well as extended-release (50 mg/200 mg and 25 mg/100 mg) tablets. Starting dose is one 25/100-mg tablet three times daily. Extended-release formulations (Sinemet CR) are particularly beneficial in patients with wide fluctuations in symptoms, providing for more even blood levels, but have slower onset of action. Medication-induced psychosis (hallucinations and paranoia) can be treated with low-dose atypical antipsychotics such as risperidone or quetiapine or aripiprazole.

The addition of carbidopa to levodopa increases the availability of levodopa, which crosses the blood-brain barrier where it is converted to dopamine. Side effects of levodopa alone include cardiac arrhythmia and orthostatic hypotension. These side effects are rare in preparations that include carbidopa. Dyskinesia, confusion, or fluctuating symptoms during the day may necessitate a drug "holiday" for which the drug is gradually decreased over several days; after approximately 2 weeks, it is restarted. Following the drug holiday, some patients may require a lower dose to manage symptoms. During the drug holiday, patients should be informed of the risk of depression, aspiration pneumonia, and deep vein thrombosis. Levodopa should not be given to patients with psychosis, glaucoma, malignant melanoma, or peptic ulcer disease, or to persons taking monoamine oxidase inhibitors (MAOIs). As Parkinson disease progresses, effectiveness of levodopa decreases.

Dopamine agonists (bromocriptine, pergolide, pramipexole, ropinirole) control symptoms in the early stages of Parkinson's disease, with carbidopa/levodopa added as the disease progresses.

Bromocriptine (Parlodel) is a direct dopamine (D_2) receptor agonist. It allows for lower doses of levodopa, with improvement in side effect profile and fewer symptomatic fluctuations and reduction in dyskinesia. Initial dose is 2.5 mg/day, increased by 2.5 mg in daily increments as tolerated up to 10-30 mg twice a day; however, there is little improvement beyond 20 mg/day in most patients.

Bromocriptine should be avoided in patients with peripheral vascular disease, recent myocardial infarction, or peptic ulcer disease and in those with comorbid mental health diagnosis.

Pergolide (Permax) is a direct dopamine agonist (D_1 and D_2 receptors). Benefits and side effects are similar to those of bromocriptine. Starting dose is 0.05 mg/day for 3 days and increasing in 0.05-mg increments every 3 days. On average, optimal response is achieved at 0.75-1.5 mg/day to a maximum dose of 5 mg/day.

Pramipexole 0.375 mg three times a day, increase by 0.25 mg every 7 days for 7 weeks to 0.5 to 1.5 mg three times a day.

Ropinirole 0.25 mg three times a day and increase by 0.75 mg per week until dose is 1 mg three times a day, then increase by 1.5 mg per week. Maximum dose is 24 mg/day. Take with food. If medication needs to be discontinued, taper over 7 days.

Selegiline (Eldepryl) is an MAO-B inhibitor. It increases levels of intrinsic and extrinsic dopamine by blocking its catabolism. Selegiline may be considered in younger patients and in those with mild symptoms. It may decrease the progression of Parkinson disease. It can be used in addition to other medical therapies, but efficacy remains unproved. Dosing is 5 mg with morning meal and 5 mg with afternoon meal.

Amantadine 100 mg taken twice a day is useful in patients with mild symptoms. It enhances synthesis and release of dopamine. Administered as monotherapy or with levodopa. Recommended in patients younger than age 60 and in older patients with mild symptoms. Available in liquid and tablet forms. Lower extremity and ankle edema is most common side effect.

Anticholinergic drugs (muscarinic receptor blockers) may decrease tremor, rigidity, and sialorrhea in some patients. Caution should be used in administering these drugs to patients with glaucoma, prostatic hypertrophy, or poor intestinal motility. Use with considerable caution in the elderly. Potential side effects include confusion, hallucinations, urinary retention, dry mouth, and constipation. Benztropine mesylate (Cogentin) can be dosed at 1 to 6 mg daily. Trihexyphenidyl (Artane) can be prescribed at 6 to 20 mg daily.

Surgical Intervention

Ablative Therapy: Thalmotomy and Pallidotomy. This procedure places stereotactic lesions in the pallidum or thalamus. Pallidotomy provides marked improvement with decreases in tremor, rigidity, and bradykinesia. Potential complications of pallidotomy include visual impairment, facial paresis, hemiparesis, and speech and memory impairment, and swallowing and balance may be affected. Thalamotomy can significantly decrease tremors. Unilateral lesions have fewer complications. Bilateral thalamotomy has been associated with speech problems and is rarely performed. Candidates are those patients who are levodopa responders but continue to have progressive disease. This procedure may decrease rigidity but does not affect bradykinesia. The procedure is contraindicated in patients who have dementia, complicated medical illnesses, or coagulopathy.

Deep-Brain Stimulation (DBS). DBS is a reversible procedure used in patients with bilateral symptoms. An electrode is placed in the brain and connected to a pulse generator inserted subcutaneously below the clavicle. Electrical impulses interrupt neuronal pathways responsible for tremor.

Tissue Implantation. Transplant of adrenal medullar tissue or fetal substantia nigra into the caudate nucleus has achieved improvement in symptoms in approximately one-fourth of patients undergoing the procedure. Duration of symptom improvement on average is over 2 years, but this approach is considered less successful than ablative therapy of DBS.

Gene Therapy

This modality is in the experimental stage. Research is exploring ways to increase dopamine levels and increase longevity of nigrostriatal cells.

PEDIATRIC CONSIDERATIONS

Symptoms of Parkinson disease in children should alert the clinician to the possibility of other neurodegenerative and hereditary diseases.

OBSTETRIC CONSIDERATIONS

Parkinson disease is rare in women in their reproductive years. The medications used in treatment of Parkinson disease have not been established as being safe for the pregnant patient. Teratogenic risk has been demonstrated in animal studies.

GERIATRIC CONSIDERATIONS

Parkinson disease is a common neurologic disorder and increases in frequency with aging. Average age at onset is in the sixth decade.

PREVENTIVE CONSIDERATIONS

Patients and their families should be encouraged to participate in local and national support groups. These groups provide supportive patient education and literature. Patients should participate in a regular exercise program focusing on maintaining range of motion and muscle strength. Patients who experience a delayed response to medications should be instructed to take medication before meals to improve efficacy. They should also be cautioned to reduce dietary protein to enhance medication effectiveness. For patients who have difficulty swallowing, thickened liquids such as milkshakes and nectars can be helpful. Pudding can be used to aid in swallowing pills. Consultation and follow-up with physical, occupational, and speech therapy can enhance the quality of life and allow for increased function as the disease progresses.

Patients should be educated and strongly encouraged to take all medications as prescribed and not stop any medications abruptly. They should use caution when walking on uneven or unfamiliar terrain to avoid falling. They should not drive or operate dangerous machinery unless approved by health care provider. Climbing stairs or stepladders should be avoided.

PEARLS FOR THE PA

Parkinson disease is a progressive neurodegenerative disease due to a reduction in levels of the neurotransmitter dopamine.

Hallmark symptoms of the disorder include tremors, rigidity, bradykinesia, and postural instability.

Mainstay of treatment is carbidopa-levodopa.

All medications used in the treatment of Parkinson disease have associated side effects and risks. The risk-benefit ratio must be carefully considered before institution of pharmacotherapy.

Peripheral Neuropathy

Mona M. Sedrak, PhD, PA-C

DEFINITION

Diseases of the peripheral nervous system, peripheral neuropathies, range in severity from mild sensory abnormalities to life-threatening paralytic disorders. Anatomically, disorders of the peripheral nervous system can affect spinal nerve roots (radiculopathy), the brachial or lumbar plexus (plexopathies), and/or single or multiple nerves.

Polyneuropathy is a generalized process that results in widespread and symmetrical effects on the nervous system. *Focal* or *multifocal neuropathy*, also referred to as mononeuropathy or mononeuropathy multiplex, is the local involvement of one or more individual peripheral nerves.

HISTORY

Symptoms. Symptoms are dependent on the nerves affected and may affect motor, sensory, and/or autonomic systems.

- Motor: Weakness is the main symptom. Difficulty with activities of daily living; muscle cramping and fasciculation. Distal muscles are affected initially, then proximal muscles, except with inflammatory neuropathy.
- Sensory: Numbness and tingling (paresthesias); burning sensations (dysesthesias); loss of proprioception.
- Autonomic: Postural hypotension, abnormal sweating, constipation, and urinary retention.

General. Correctly identifying and diagnosing peripheral neuropathies can be challenging. Damage to peripheral nerves can be caused by greater than 100 different disease processes and toxins. A complete medical history is important in evaluating contributing systemic illnesses, predisposing hereditary factors, and occupational exposure to toxins or heavy metals. Using a systematic approach to evaluation will lead to the identification and diagnosis of many treatable causative disorders.

Age. Dependent on the etiology of the neuropathy. Incidence increases with advancing age and the development of chronic systemic conditions.

Onset. Generally gradual over months to years, unless due to trauma.

Duration. Dependent on the etiology but may be permanent.

Intensity. Varies from intermittent paresthesias in one extremity to severe dysesthesia. In the case of Guillain-Barré syndrome, may affect the muscles of respiration, necessitating the use of ventilatory assistance.

Aggravating Factors. If the neuropathy is due to entrapment, repetitive use may increase symptoms. Poor control of blood glucose in the diabetic patient may hasten progression of symptoms. Some chemotherapeutic agents and toxins may also increase symptoms.

Alleviating Factors. Heat and ice may alleviate some of the symptoms. Avoidance of alcohol and repetitive trauma. Strict control of blood glucose may slow down the progression of the neuropathic process and even reverse some of the existing damage.

Associated Factors. Exposure to heavy metals (e.g., lead, arsenic, thallium, mercury, copper). Disorders such as Charcot-Marie-Tooth, Dejerine-Sottas, and Refsum diseases and porphyric neuropathy may be of genetic origin. Certain drugs may induce or exacerbate a neuropathy.

PHYSICAL EXAMINATION

A complete physical examination should be performed to evaluate for possible systemic processes that may be contributing to the neuropathic process.

Neurologic

Motor Examination. Distal muscle groups are affected initially. Loss of muscle tone progresses from distal to proximal. Look for signs of decreased muscle tone. Deep tendon reflexes are diminished to absent. Muscle strength is decreased in the distribution of the affected peripheral nerve.

Sensory Examination. Assess proprioception, response to vibration (using 128-Hz tuning fork), temperature, light touch, sharp/dull touch. Examination characteristically shows decreased sensation to sharp or light touch in a "stocking-glove" or peripheral nerve distribution.

Autonomic Examination. Take blood pressure measurements. Look for signs of orthostatic hypotension; check post-void residuals.

PATHOPHYSIOLOGY

The axon, myelin sheath, or Schwann cell may be affected. On the basis of clinical features alone, it is difficult to predict whether a patient has a predominantly axonal or demyelinating pattern of peripheral nerve injury. Damage to small unmyelinated and myelinated fibers can result in loss of temperature and pain sensation. Damage to large myelinated fibers results in motor or proprioceptive defects. Some neuropathies affect the motor fiber. Others affect the dorsal root ganglia (sensory fibers), producing sensory symptoms. Occasionally, cranial nerves may also become involved.

Peripheral neuropathies may be associated with any of numerous underlying disorders and can be categorized as follows:

Immune-Mediated Neuropathies
- Guillain-Barré syndrome
- Chronic inflammatory demyelinating neuropathy
- Multifocal motor neuropathy
- Vasculitic neuropathies

Guillain-Barré syndrome (GB) is characterized by reduced nerve conduction velocities and focal segmental demyelination on the peripheral nerves, nerve roots and/or cranial nerves. Microscopic examination may reveal concentrations of monocytes, lymphocytes, or macrophages. GB is thought to be of viral etiology.

Hereditary Neuropathies
- Charcot-Marie-Tooth disease
- Amyloid neuropathies

Of the hereditary causes, Charcot-Marie-Tooth disease is the most common familial motor and sensory abnormality. It is transmitted in an autosomal dominant fashion. It is characterized by motor and sensory conduction loss of less than 65% of normal and prolonged distal latencies on nerve conduction velocity. Type I is characterized by segmental demyelination, partial remyelination, and Schwann cell proliferation seen on microscopic examination of the nerve. Type II exhibits motor conduction of less than 65% of normal but reduced evoked potential amplitudes. Microscopic examination reveals a fatty degeneration of nerve fibers (wallerian degeneration).

Metabolic Neuropathies
- Diabetic neuropathies
- Diabetic polyneuropathy
- Hepatic neuropathy
- Uremic neuropathy
- Porphyric neuropathy

Diabetic peripheral neuropathy commonly occurs as a distal, symmetrical, predominantly sensory neuropathy that causes sensory deficits marked by a stocking-glove distribution. Symptoms include numbness, tingling, and paresthesias in the extremities.

Toxic Neuropathies
- Alcohol-nutritional neuropathy
- Toxic chemicals: lead, arsenic, cyanide, thallium, organophosphates

- Drugs: isoniazid (INH), lithium, gold, metronidazole, dapsone, cisplatin, vincristine, hydralazine, phenytoin (Dilantin)

Alcoholic and nutritional neuropathies are caused by malabsorption, decreased nutritional uptake, and increased thiamine requirement. Deficiencies of thiamine, folic acid, and vitamin B_{12} affect the posterior and lateral columns of the spinal cord. Symptoms include numbness, paresthesias of the extremities, weakness, ataxia, and loss of vibration sense.

Neuropathies Associated with Infectious Disease
- Human immunodeficiency virus infections
- Lyme disease
- Leprous neuropathy
- Entrapment and compressive neuropathies
- Carpal tunnel syndrome
- Bell palsy
- Trigeminal neuralgia

Entrapment neuropathy can occur secondary to ligamentous inflammation due to overuse. Common sites include the wrist (carpal tunnel syndrome) due to inflammation of the volar carpal ligament, and the elbow (ulnar nerve palsy), due to local trauma of the ulnar nerve or hypertrophy of the transverse ligament.

DIAGNOSTIC STUDIES

Laboratory
Complete Blood Count. As indicated to rule out infection, anemia.

Erythrocyte Sedimentation Rate. Nonspecific but can screen for systemic, inflammatory processes.

Antinuclear Antigen, Rheumatoid Factor Assays. As indicated to evaluate for connective tissue disease.

Lyme Titer. As indicated to evaluate for Lyme disease.

Human Immunodeficiency Virus (HIV) Assay. In patients with risk factors.

Thyroid-Stimulating Hormone (TSH) Assay. In suspected hypothyroidism.

Vitamin B_{12} and Folate Levels. In suspected nutritional deficiency or if macrocytosis is noted or deficiencies are present on complete blood count.

Glucose, Creatinine, Blood Urea Nitrogen (BUN). As indicated to evaluate for possible diabetes mellitus or renal disease.

Radiology
Chest Film. Used to rule out sarcoidosis and lung carcinoma.

Radiographs of Affected Body Part. In suspected trauma or nerve compression.

CT/MRI of the Spine. If radiculopathy or neoplasm is suspected.

Other

Neurophysiologic Testing. Used to differentiate among longstanding neuropathies, demyelination, entrapments, and acute processes. Autonomic nerves and small unmyelinated fibers cannot be tested. The examination can assess an isolated nerve. It measures the amplitude and velocity of nerves.

Nerve Conduction Velocity. The nerve is stimulated via a skin electrode. This creates an action potential. Motor nerve testing requires distal placement of electrodes and sensory nerve testing requires proximal placement. The action potential is quantified to determine abnormalities. Demyelinating lesions will show slow nerve conductions and prolonged distal latencies. F waves and focal demyelinating blocks may also be seen.

Electromyography (EMG). A needle is placed in a skeletal muscle to assess its function at rest and with stimulation. An axonal process produces spontaneous activity on the EMG and low amplitude evoked responses with preserved conduction velocities. Results can be altered by the use of narcotics, muscle relaxants, and anticholinergic medication.

Nerve Biopsy. Used for analyzing the extent of demyelination. However, it is rarely indicated. Utilized when vasculitis, amyloidosis, or sarcoidosis is suspected. Sural (calf) nerve samples are rarely needed.

Genetic Testing. Becoming more available to identify hereditary neuropathies.

Serum Protein Electrophoresis. Used for evaluating inflammatory conditions in motor neuropathies.

Heavy Metals. Screening with exposure history only.

Lumbar Puncture. Elevated cerebrospinal fluid protein level may be suggestive of chronic inflammatory demyelinating polyradiculopathy.

Metastatic Workup. In a patient with ataxia, consider evaluation for occult malignancies.

DIFFERENTIAL DIAGNOSIS

Traumatic
Compression or Entrapment. Due to herniated spinal disk or due to direct trauma to the nerve.

Infectious. Not otherwise applicable.
Metabolic. Not otherwise applicable.

Neoplastic
Tumor of the Nerve (e.g., Schwannoma). Manifests with peripheral nerve symptoms.

Vascular. Not otherwise applicable.
Congenital. Not otherwise applicable.

Acquired
Radiation Therapy. History of radiation to the area.

TREATMENT

Identification of any contributing systemic illness or condition is essential. Treatment of all systemic disorders may help relieve symptoms and halt progression. However, patients must be advised that recovery may be a slow process.

Entrapment neuropathies may require steroid injection and/or surgical decompression.

Diabetic patients should be placed on strict management of the serum glucose. Nutritional support services should be consulted to aid in this effort. Close follow-up and routine serum glucose testing are mandatory.

Alcoholic patients should be given appropriate support and/or referral to cease alcohol intake.

For patients with heavy metal exposure, it is important to remove the toxin.

For GBS, the primary treatment is to support vital functions. If the paralysis ascends, ventilatory support may be necessary. Plasmapheresis is helpful if given early in the course of the disease and is usually reserved for those patients with rapidly progressive disease. Intravenous immunoglobulin is also considered.

Nonspecific immunomodulating treatments may include corticosteroids, plasmapheresis, immunosuppressants, and intravenous immunoglobulins.

Painful neuropathies may respond to tricyclic antidepressants (amitriptyline) or anticonvulsants (carbamazepine, phenytoin, gabapentin).

Supportive treatments should include physical therapy, occupational therapy, and counseling, as needed.

PEDIATRIC CONSIDERATIONS

Common peripheral nerve conditions in children include:
  Bell palsy (idiopathic facial nerve dysfuction): Manifests with unilateral paralysis of the face. The seventh nerve may become compressed and demyelinated in response to inflammation within the facial canal. Diagnosis is based on clinical findings. Treatment is usually not indicated.
  Acute and chronic inflammatory demyelinating polyneuropathy (GBS): An acute monophasic illness characterized by demyelination of the peripheral nerves. Treatment involves plasmapheresis.
  Hereditary polyneuropathies: These motor and sensory neuropathies are a group of genetic disorders. Most common are Charcot-Marie-Tooth disease, Dejerine-Sottas disease, and Refsum disease.

OBSTETRIC CONSIDERATIONS

Pregnancy can put the patient at risk for developing carpal tunnel syndrome. This is due to swelling of the median nerve, which results from the edema commonly associated with pregnancy. Treatment can include flexion splinting and cortisone injections, as needed. Entrapment of the posterior tibial nerve below the medial malleolus may also occur during pregnancy.

GERIATRIC CONSIDERATIONS

Peripheral neuropathy is a serious and common complication of many chronic illnesses in older patients. Neuropathies can be due to long-standing diabetes mellitus, hypothyroidism, neoplasms, and inflammatory processes such as systemic lupus erythematosus (SLE). Older patients may experience vitamin deficiencies and drug-associated sensory neuropathy with a greater frequency than in younger patients. Eliciting a full history is often difficult in this population but is vital for ensuring an accurate diagnosis and treatment.

PREVENTIVE CONSIDERATIONS

Patients should be educated regarding risk reduction: controlling diabetes, avoiding toxins, and avoiding alcohol abuse. Compliance with medication dosing and timing is imperative. Compliance with occupational safety measures and physical therapy regimens, as well as home exercise programs, must be stressed.

Patients should be encouraged to report changes in health status, worsening of symptoms, and chronic health problems to their health care providers on an ongoing basis.

PEARLS FOR THE PA

The etiology of peripheral neuropathy involves any of numerous pathologic processes.

Peripheral neuropathies are usually due to systemic illness.

A full history plus comprehensive physical examination is key to proper disease identification, diagnosis, and treatment.

Seizure Disorders

Catherine R. Judd, MS, PA-C

DEFINITION

A *seizure* is an abnormal, paroxysmal discharge of cerebral cortical neurons leading to immediate alterations in level of consciousness, sensory and motor function, and/or mental status. Seizures may be caused by a number of acute or chronic injuries or disorders affecting the central nervous system (CNS). The term *epilepsy* is generally reserved for a disorder in which the patient has experienced at least two recurrent seizures without any identifiable precipitating cause. Treatment of any underlying disorder can often prevent further seizures. Seizures occur in two forms: convulsive and nonconvulsive. Convulsive forms are easily recognized and are characterized by generalized tonic-clonic muscle activity followed by alternating relaxation and tonic activity. Nonconvulsive forms, characterized by alterations of consciousness and unusual stereotyped, repetitive behaviors (automatisms), often go unrecognized. Seizures are classified according to observable behavioral and electroencephalographic changes.

HISTORY

Symptoms

Generalized Seizures

Primary generalized tonic-clonic seizures include grand mal and petit mal type seizures. They manifest with sudden loss of consciousness and violent generalized tonic muscle contractions followed by rhythmic clonic (jerking) movements of the extremities, head, and trunk. They may be associated with tongue biting and incontinence. A postictal state of drowsiness lasting several minutes follows each seizure.

Absence seizures manifest with unresponsive staring and cessation of activity, with intermittent eye flutter lasting less than 20 seconds.

Myoclonic seizures manifest with rapid jerking of extremities, trunk, and/or facial muscles. The seizures may be focal or widespread. Loss of consciousness is not typical.

Atonic seizures result in sudden brief loss of muscle tone that may result in a head drop or a fall and may or may not occur with loss of consciousness.

Partial Seizures

Partial seizures can be subclassified as simple partial (consciousness maintained) or complex partial (loss of consciousness or awareness, frequently with blank stare and automatisms). Partial seizures are typically defined as seizures with a focal onset. Partial seizures are sometimes preceded by an aura such as unpleasant taste or feelings of panic lasting no longer than 2 or 3 minutes. Patients are frequently amnestic for the event. Partial seizures may progress to generalized tonic-clonic seizures.

Seizure presentation depends on the spread of the ictal discharge. When the primary motor strip is involved, there are clonic (jerking) movements of the contralateral side. Seizures of the sensory cortex consist of paresthesias. Olfactory hallucinations may occur when the medial temporal cortex is involved. Experiences such as déjà vu occur when the limbic cortex is affected.

Unclassified (Special) Seizures: Reflex and Febrile Seizures
Reflex seizures occur in response to a stimulus such as a flashing light or specific sound.

Febrile seizures generally are seen in children 6 months to 5 years of age. The seizure usually occurs as a generalized seizure during a fever spike. Heredity appears to play a role, and the event is generally benign. Findings on electroencephalography (EEG) are usually normal after the event. The risk of developing a seizure disorder later in life is the same as in the population at large. Febrile seizures may be confused with a primary CNS infection manifesting with seizures. (Seizures that are secondary to infection may be focal or prolonged, are associated with EEG abnormalities, and may be recurrent.) (See Table 10-8.)

General
A thorough medical history must be obtained, including information on the use of alcohol or drugs, to assess for presence of systemic disorders that may contribute to the development of seizures. A careful review of systems with attention to neurologic symptoms is imperative to evaluate for diseases that may cause seizures. Symptoms such as headache, nausea, vomiting, focal and subtle neurologic deficits, or photophobia may be present with cerebral mass lesions. Inquire about a history of head trauma, recent infections, whether the patient (especially children) was febrile during the seizure, family members with a seizure disorder, nutritional deficiencies, vascular diseases, and other neurologic diseases.

To assist in classifying the seizure type and to identify any localized focus of the seizure, the patient and any observers of the seizure event should be interviewed to determine if there was any aura or localizing signs.

Inquire about symptoms that occur during sleep. The patient may awake incontinent or may have bitten the tongue while asleep. These

---

Table 10–8. International Classification of Epileptic Seizures

Generalized seizures (bilaterally symmetrical and without focal onset)
    Generalized tonic-clonic
    Absence (petit mal)
    Myoclonic
    Akinetic
    Infantile spasms
    Atonic
Partial seizures (seizures beginning focally)
    Simple partial (without impairment of consciousness)
    Complex partial (with alteration of consciousness)
    Partial with secondary generalization
Unclassified seizures
    Reflex seizures (stimulus-induced: e.g., photic-induced)
    Febrile

nocturnal events may not be initially diagnosed because they are not witnessed.

Age.   Approximately 1% of the population has a seizure disorder. The incidence is bimodal, higher in both children and the elderly.

Onset.   Variable (depending on seizure type).

Duration.   Variable (depending on seizure type).

Intensity.   The seizure may be barely perceptible (absence seizure) or so severe that it results in continuous seizure activity, cerebral oxygen deprivation, and death (status epilepticus).

Aggravating Factors.   Any irritant to the cerebral cortex can be a possible precipitant. An existing seizure disorder may be aggravated with noncompliance with anticonvulsant medications. Sleep deprivation can precipitate a seizure.

Alleviating Factors.   Identify and treat any underlying condition. Ensure compliance with taking the appropriately prescribed anticonvulsant medication.

Associated Factors.   Injuries may occur during a grand mal seizure. Occasionally, the contractions are so intense as to cause vertebral compression fractures, tongue lacerations, tooth damage, or airway compromise (e.g., dentures may become dislodged and block the airway).

PHYSICAL EXAMINATION

General.   Physical examination findings will depend, in large part, on the underlying cause of the seizure.

In the postictal period (following a seizure), the patient may be lethargic or have focal neurologic signs (e.g., hemiparesis). Full evaluation of vital signs should be performed to rule out hyperthermia or hypotension. Observe the patient for obvious signs of drug or alcohol use or withdrawal. A complete physical examination should be performed after a generalized tonic-clonic seizure to look for injuries resulting from the seizure.

Head, Eyes, Ears, Nose, Throat.   Funduscopic examination may reveal papilledema (a sign of increased intracranial pressure). Assess for signs of head trauma such as contusion, Battle sign (retroauricular hematoma), or "raccoon eyes."

Neurologic.   A full and complete neurologic examination is essential for all patients presenting with history of recent seizure. Neurologic examination may be normal. Intracerebral neoplasms may cause focal neurologic deficits. Perform full mental status, cranial nerve, motor, sensory, and reflex examinations. Meningitis manifests with signs of meningeal irritation such as nuchal rigidity (Brudzinski sign) and the inability to fully extend the legs (Kernig sign). Meningeal signs may not be present in infants, small children, elderly persons, and comatose patients.

If the seizure is witnessed, observe for localizing signs (e.g., unilateral extremity movement or automatisms existing alone or followed by a generalized seizure), and document time of the event. After the event, perform a neurologic examination to note any focal deficits.

PATHOPHYSIOLOGY

Seizures may result from idiopathic factors or may be produced by disease processes or brain trauma. Under the appropriate chemical and electrical stimuli, seizure activity can occur. Certain regions of the brain are particularly sensitive to seizure activity. Irritation to the cerebral cortex caused by trauma, infectious processes, hyperthermia, neoplasms, metabolic disorders, electrolyte abnormalities, vascular diseases, degenerative diseases, congenital anomalies, substance abuse and withdrawal, or hereditary factors can result in seizure activity. However, the amygdala and hippocampus are also very susceptible to biochemical disturbances.

The precipitating cause of a seizure is not always apparent or identifiable. Causes can be divided into two broad categories:

- Toxic/metabolic
  Electrolyte abnormalities (hyponatremia, hypomagnesemia, hypocalcemia)
  Drugs (cocaine, theophylline, phenothiazines and atypical antipsychotics, lithium, tricyclic antidepressants, isoniazid, and penicillins)
  Acute drug withdrawal (alcohol, benzodiazepines, barbiturates, cocaine)
  Metabolic (hypoglycemia, uremia, hepatic encephalopathy, anoxia, porphyria)
- Associated with other systemic conditions
  Eclampsia
  Cardiac disease (syncope, arrhythmias)
  Hyperthermia
  Infections (*Shigella* infection, cholera, infections leading to shock or hypoxia)

DIAGNOSTIC STUDIES

Laboratory
Chemistry Profile.   May show hyponatremia (normal sodium 136 to 145 mEq/L), elevated glucose (normal 70 to 105) or altered calcium, albumin, magnesium, blood urea nitrogen (BUN) (normal 10 to 20), creatinine (normal 0.6 to 1.2), or liver function tests (lactate dehydrogenase [LDH], serum aspartate transaminase [AST] and alanine transaminase [ALT] [formerly SGOT and SGPT]).

Complete Blood Count.   White blood cell (WBC) count (normal 4500 to 11,000/mm^3) may be elevated in presence of infection.

Arterial Blood Gas Analysis.   Performed if airway compromise or hypoxia is a concern.

Blood Cultures.   If infectious process/sepsis is suspected.

Anticonvulsant Levels.   If a patient has a history of taking anticonvulsant medication or if no history is available, blood to assess levels should be drawn. If an anticonvulsant is started, levels should be monitored from the outset.

Toxicology Screen. Should be obtained in all patients when cause of seizure cannot be identified.

Urinalysis with Culture and Sensitivity Testing. May reveal a urinary tract infection.

Lumbar Puncture. Cell count, glucose (normal 40 to 80 mg/dL), and protein (normal 15 to 45 mg/dL). *Stat* Gram stain, culture, and sensitivity testing to rule out meningitis. Pleocytosis may be seen after a prolonged, generalized seizure. Follow-up of culture results is essential.

Radiology

MRI/CT/Positron Emission Tomography (PET) of the Brain. Should be performed as indicated in all patients with focal neurologic signs and in adults with new-onset seizures to rule out neoplasm, abscess, or other focal cause for the seizure.

MRI is the most sensitive technique for detecting underlying cerebral abnormality. MRI is indicated in all adults with an unexplained seizure. If the initial MRI study fails to detect a source of the seizure disorder, follow-up MRI is recommended in 3 to 6 months.

CT (without contrast), although less sensitive than MRI, is recommended as the initial study in trauma and when the patient is in an immediate post-ictal state. It is also appropriate if the patient is showing residual neurologic deficit at the time of imaging.

PET (with ^{18}F-deoxyglucose) is useful for localizing the seizure focus. It is especially useful in a patient with complex partial seizures that do not respond to medication and with negative findings on MRI.

Other

EEG. EEG can provide precise definition of the nature of an abnormal neural discharge and is useful for identifying seizure type 60% of the time. EEG can differentiate between partial and primary generalized seizures. A focal EEG abnormality points to a partial seizure disorder whereas a generalized abnormality indicates a primary generalized seizure. Twenty-four-hour ambulatory monitoring or continuous video-recorded monitoring can distinguish epileptic from nonepiletic events. The two typical patterns to look for are slowing of the wave pattern and classic epileptiform activity (brief, abrupt stopping and starting of spikes). Forty percent of seizure disorders are not identifiable on EEG.

DIFFERENTIAL DIAGNOSIS

Traumatic

Brain Trauma. Can cause loss of conscousness. May be the cause of seizure.

Infectious
Shivering. In a febrile patient with impaired mental status, may be confused with seizure.

Metabolic
Syncope. May be due to metabolic cause or due to arrhythmias, valvular heart disease, vasovagal syndromes, or orthostatic hypotension. May require full evaluation to differentiate from seizure.
Migraine. May cause transient neurologic symptoms. May require full evaluation to differentiate from seizure.

Neoplastic. Not otherwise applicable.

Vascular
Transient Ischemic Attacks. Cause transient neurologic symptoms. May require full evaluation to differentiate from seizure.

Congenital. Not otherwise applicable.
Acquired. Not otherwise applicable.

Other
Sleep Disorders: Narcolepsy/Cataplexy or Night Terrors. Differentiated on history or may require full evaluation to differentiate from seizure.
Psychiatric Disorders: Panic Attacks, Fugue States, and Psychogenic (Nonepileptic) Seizures. May require full evaluation to differentiate from seizure.
Childhood Breath-Holding Spells. Directly correlated on history.

TREATMENT

During a generalized tonic-clonic seizure, a patient must be protected from potential for harm incurred during uncontrolled movements. Move furniture or any other potentially harmful items from the immediate area, as appropriate. Seizure precautions should include padded bed rails, frequent observation, and monitoring of vital signs; NEVER place the fingers into a patient's mouth during a seizure. Maintain a clear airway.

Anticonvulsant medications should be instituted immediately on obtaining a diagnosis of seizure disorder (see Table 10-9).

Monotherapy is preferable to increase compliance, reduce cost, and minimize side effects. If monotherapy is not effective in controlling seizures, addition of a second or third drug may be necessary.

Close monitoring of serum anticonvulsant levels is important to avoid toxicity in the older medications. Always check for drug interactions, as they may alter serum anticonvulsant levels. The acute use of anticonvulsant medication during the seizure episode is usually not necessary unless the seizure is prolonged or recurs within 1 hour.

Anticonvulsants may be discontinued if the patient remains seizure free for a period of 2 to 5 years. EEG is performed while the patient is taking the

Table 10-9. Table of Common Antiepileptic Drugs

Generic Name	Trade Name	Usual Daily Dosage		Principal Therapeutic Indications	Effective Blood Level* (µg/mL)
		Children	*Adults (mg)*		
Phenobarbital	Luminal	5-6 mg/kg (8 mg/kg in infants) in divided doses	100-300 per day	Tonic-clonic seizures; partial motor seizures, active convulsions	10-40
Phenytoin	Dilantin	5-7 mg/kg/day in 2 divided doses	300-500 per day	Tonic-clonic seizures; focal motor and complex partial seizures	10-20
Carbamazepine	Tegretol	15-20 mg/kg/day	600-1200 in divided doses bid or tid	Tonic-clonic seizures; complex partial seizures; focal motor seizures	4-12
Primidone	Mysoline	10-25 mg/kg in 3 or 4 divided doses	500-1500	Tonic-clonic seizures; focal motor and complex partial seizures	5-15
Ethosuximide	Zarontin	15-30 mg/kg	750-2000	Absence	50-100
Diazepam	Valium	0.15-2 mg/kg IV	10-150	Status epilepticus (ONLY)	
Lorazepam	Ativan	0.03-0.22 mg/kg IV	0.1 mg/kg	Status epilepticus (ONLY)	
ACTH gel		20-80 U/d IM (6-8 wk)	not applicable	Infantile spasms	
Valproate	Depakote	30-60 mg/kg	1000-3000	Absence and myoclonic seizures; petit mal; infantile spasms; as an adjunctive drug in tonic-clonic and complex partial seizures	50-100

Continued

Table 10-9. Table of Common Antiepileptic Drugs—cont'd

Generic Name	Trade Name	Usual Daily Dosage		Principal Therapeutic Indications	Effective Blood Level* (μg/mL)
		Children	Adults (mg)		
Clonazepam	Klonopin	0.01-20 mg/kg	1.5-2.0	Myoclonus; petit mal; akinetic; infantile spasms, complex partial seizures	0.01-0.07
Felbamate	Felbatol	15-45 mg/kg/day	1200-3600	Partial seizures	Level not established
Gabapentin	Neurontin	10-50 mg/kg/day	900-1800	Partial, simple, complex seizures	Level not established
Lamotrigine	Lamictal	0.15-15 mg/kg/day	200-400	Partial seizures	Level not established
Oxcarbazepine	Trileptal	age 4-16, 4-5 mg/kg bid, max 600 mg/day	300-600 mg bid, max 1200 mg/day	Partial seizures	Level not established
Tiagabine	Gabitril	Not recommended	32-56	Partial seizures	Level not established
Topiramate	Topamax	NA	200-400 in divided doses tid	Partial seizures	Level not established

*Average trough values.

ACTH, adrenocorticotropic hormone; bid, twice a day; NA, not applicable; tid, three times a day.

(From Wiederholt WC: Neurology for Non-Neurologists, 4th ed. Philadelphia, WB Saunders, 2000, with permission.)

medication and, if findings are normal, the drug is tapered. A second EEG examination is then performed with the patient off anticonvulsants to evaluate for cerebral irritability.

Anticonvulsants should be given for seizure prophylaxis to patients undergoing intracranial procedures.

Status Epilepticus

Defined as continuous, generalized seizure activity. This condition may be fatal, or result in significant neurologic impairment, if left untreated, owing to cerebral oxygen depletion.

It is important to maintain a patent airway with an oral device or endotracheal intubation. Cardiac monitoring should be instituted. If the patient is hypotensive, 0.5-1 mg of atropine is given. *Stat* laboratory studies are performed including electrolytes, complete blood count, calcium, arterial blood gas analysis, toxicology screen, and anticonvulsant levels.

Intravenous thiamine 100 mg, 50% glucose 25-50 mL, and normal saline 50-100 mg are given.

Diazepam 10-20 mg or 10.15 mg/kg is given at 3- to 5-minute intervals until the seizure is controlled.

Intravenous phenytoin is given in a loading dose of 20 mg/kg, not to exceed 50 mg every 3 minutes.

Intravenous lorazepam 2-8 mg IV can be considered if phenytoin or diazepam is unsuccessful at controlling seizure.

If seizures persist, the patient should be intubated and phenobarbital given in a dose of 15 mg/kg IV at 100 mg/min.

General anesthesia ultimately may be required to control the seizures.

PEDIATRIC CONSIDERATIONS

Neonatal Seizures (Age 0 to 1 month)

Seizures in infants present somewhat differently than in adults, presumably owing to the lack of development of the cerebrum. Seizures may be manifested by respiratory pause, brief movement of a limb, body stiffening, or lip smacking. This activity may be difficult to distinguish from normal infantile movements. Seizures occurring in the immediate postpartum period of a difficult birth (24 to 48 hours) may signify significant cerebral injury. If a seizure occurs within days to weeks post partum, it may be due to either hereditary or acquired factors. Causes of neonatal seizures include congenital anomalies, hypoxia, birth injury, and metabolic disorders.

Infantile Seizures (Age 1 to 6 months)

The usual seizure pattern in this age group is a myoclonic jerk of the head and arms that may involve the entire body. This jerking is termed *infantile spasms*. These spasms may be benign or due to encephalopathies, metabolic diseases, or developmental disorders. Causes of infantile seizures include factors that cause neonatal seizures.

Seizures in Early Childhood (Age 6 months to 3 years)

Etiologic factors include those described for younger patients as well as trauma and fever. This is the age group in which status epilepticus and benign febrile seizures may become manifest. Epilepsies associated with mental retardation (e.g., Lennox-Gastaut syndrome) may occur as myoclonus, grand mal events, or petit mal seizures. Petit mal seizures rarely begin before age 4. Relatively benign partial seizures may also occur in this age group. CT/MRI scans of the brain are generally not required for the first episode of a generalized febrile seizure unless focal neurologic signs are present or the seizure is prolonged or recurrent. Lumbar puncture should be performed to rule out meningitis.

Seizures in Late Childhood/Adolescence

Consider full workup including CT/MRI, EEG, and lumbar puncture to evaluate the cause of an initial seizure. Usually the seizure will be due to idiopathic factors. If the patient has a history of one or more seizures in the past, a developmental disorder should be suspected. Correct identification of seizure type is imperative so that appropriate therapy can begin at an early age. Patients with petit mal seizures may complain only of difficulty in school, and patients labeled with benign febrile seizures may actually have temporal lobe epilepsy, which carries a risk of diminished intellectual function. Adolescents involved with substance abuse may present with seizures.

OBSTETRIC CONSIDERATIONS

Patients with a prior history of epilepsy who become pregnant can vary widely on how the seizure activity occurs during pregnancy. Fifty percent of patients will have no change in their seizure activity; one-third will have increased frequency of seizures; and the remainder will have decreased seizure activity. Factors associated with pregnancy that can increase the possibility of increased seizure activity are fatigue, sleep deprivation, and frequent vomiting; also associated with increased risk of seizure is male gender of the fetus. Serum anticonvulsant drug levels are likely to decrease owing to increased blood volume during pregnancy, decreased protein binding, and inconsistent intestinal absorption.

Fetal effects from epilepsy include premature delivery and an increased frequency of epilepsy and congenital anomalies. An epileptic patient has a 6% to 10% chance of having an abnormal baby. Even though all anticonvulsant medications have been associated with adverse fetal outcomes, the risk to the fetus from uncontrolled maternal seizures is generally greater than the risk from the medications.

Because of the possible effects of anticonvulsants on the fetus causing neural tube defects, monotherapy with the lowest dose possible is the most prudent treatment choice. Use of phenytoin, phenobarbital, carbamazepine, and primidone is associated with lower risk during pregnancy than that due to use of trimethadione and valproic acid, which are contraindicated because of higher incidence of neural tube defects. Pregnancy termination may be recommended in patients who were taking trimethadione at the time of conception and during the first trimester. Ethosuximide and clonazepam also increase the risk of birth defects.

Phenytoin use has been associated with fetal hydantoin syndrome (craniofacial abnormalities, mental retardation, growth retardation, and other anomalies). However, it has been suggested that phenytoin should be considered a first-line agent in status epilepticus secondary to eclampsia. Diazepam, phenytoin, phenobarbital, and pentobarbital all have been recommended for treatment of status epilepticus in the obstetric patient. All anticonvulsants will predispose the pregnant patient to bleeding because of pregnancy-associated coagulation changes. Epileptic patients should also be maintained on folic acid, iron, vitamin D, and vitamin K supplementation during pregnancy.

If a woman's first seizure occurs during pregnancy, and there is no history of preeclampsia, a complete seizure workup should be performed immediately.

GERIATRIC CONSIDERATIONS

Elderly patients with multiple medical problems treated with polypharmacy must be monitored carefully regarding potential drug-drug interactions that can induce metabolic states that can potentially affect anticonvulsant levels and lower seizure threshold.

PREVENTIVE CONSIDERATIONS

Patients should be counseled regarding risk of seizures and those factors increasing the risk of seizure such as trauma and head injury, alcohol consumption, sleep deprivation, stress, infections and fever, and drugs known to lower seizure threshold. Issues regarding driving and operating dangerous machinery also need to be addressed. All states have regulations regarding seizure disorders and driving.

Patients should know the warning signs and symptoms of impending seizure, medication side effects, and need for lifestyle modification. Understanding that anticonvulsants are prophylaxis and not a cure is a vital consideration for patient education.

PEARLS FOR THE PA

Seizures are defined as partial (focal onset), generalized, or special.

Epilepsy refers to chronic, recurrent seizures without an identifiable underlying disease process.

It is important to differentiate benign forms of seizures from those due to an underlying disease process, so that appropriate intervention can be initiated.

Transient Ischemic Attack/Stroke

Catherine R, Judd, MS, PA-C

DEFINITION

A *transient ischemic attack* (TIA) is a brief period of neurologic deficit resolving within 24 hours (usually in less than 10 minutes) caused by vascular disease that produces areas of cerebral ischemia. A *stroke* results in focal or multifocal deficits persisting more than 24 hours. TIAs and strokes may be caused by ischemia (in 80% of cases) from arteriosclerosis or emboli or by hemorrhage (in 20%). Key features of TIAs and stroke are as follows:

Signs and symptoms occur suddenly.

Signs and symptoms can help determine the site of the lesion.

It is unlikely that symptoms developing over days and weeks are due to a stroke. When this occurs, other causes must be sought (e.g., space-occupying lesion).

HISTORY

Symptoms. Neurologic signs depend on the location of the lesion. Carotid (anterior) artery involvement manifests with contralateral upper and/or lower extremity symptoms and/or face, contralateral hemiparesis or numbness, or dysarthria and may include speech disturbance or amaurosis fugax (perception of a curtain or veil descending over one eye on the side of the lesion). Vertebrobasilar (posterior) artery lesions manifest with hemiparesis, dysarthria, dysphagia, vertigo, and loss of balance, clumsiness, weakness, diplopia, and homonymous hemianopsia (opposite visual field).

Symptoms lasting longer than 24 hours rule out TIA; cessation of symptoms within 10 minutes increases the likelihood of TIA. Onset of headache as symptoms resolve is suggestive of migraine.

General. A complete medical history must be obtained. It is valuable to include witness accounts of the events occurring at the onset of symptoms. The progression of symptoms is also important to note. To help predict the clinical course, it is important to document frequency of episodes, date of first event, presence of underlying coronary or heart disease, and cardiovascular risk factors. Patients experiencing TIAs are at risk for a subsequent stroke if they have hypertension or cardiac disease or are older than 65 years of age. Incapacitating strokes are more likely in patients with carotid symptoms than in those with vertebrobasilar dysfunction. Patients are at increased risk for stroke within the first 3 months following onset of TIAs.

Age. Patients younger than 45 account for less than 5% of strokes. Incidence doubles each decade over age 60.

Onset. Abrupt (within minutes).

Duration. Symptoms resulting from TIAs usually last less than 10 minutes and by definition not longer than 24 hours, with minimal residual deficits. Deficits from strokes may resolve but tend to persist, leaving the patient with some degree of permanent disability.

Intensity. Minimal symptoms to life-threatening.

Aggravating Factors. Hypertension, uncontrolled atrial fibrillation, valvular heart disease, diabetes mellitus, polycythemia vera, drug abuse, and acquired immunodeficiency syndrome (AIDS).

Alleviating Factors. Stroke prevention through risk factor identification and reduction is imperative and may be a major factor in the rapid decline over the past two decades in mortality. Early identification and aggressive treatment of risk factors such as hypertension, diabetes, coronary artery disease, carotid bruits, atrial fibrillation, and smoking can help to minimize risk.

Associated Factors. Cardiac arrhythmia, cardiomyopathy, contraceptive use, nicotine, excessive alcohol use, valvular heart disease, vasculitis, hyperlipidemia, hypercoagulable state, hyperviscosity, illicit drug use, hypertension, and genetic predisposition.

PHYSICAL EXAMINATION

General. Patients who have experienced a TIA, which by definition is brief, may appear asymptomatic at the time they are examined. It is important to determine the location of the causative lesion. Patients may be markedly paretic or have other observable neurological deficits. Blood pressure should be measured in both arms to rule out subclavian steal syndrome.

Neurologic. Assessment of patient's level of consciousness is important to document. Note if the patient is alert, somnolent, stuporous, or comatose. Depressed level of consciousness points to multifocal, bihemispheric, or brainstem lesion. Thorough evaluation of cerebral functions must be performed. The patient's motor function, speech, language, sensory processes, emotional status, and thought content must be assessed. A complete evaluation of each cranial nerve, cerebellar function, and reflexes is necessary.

Vascular. Auscultate for bruits at the carotid arteries, aorta, and femoral arteries. Palpate for peripheral pulses, as atherosclerotic vascular disease is usually diffuse.

PATHOPHYSIOLOGY

Cerebrovascular disease resulting in a cerebrovascular accident is the most common cause of neurologic disability in Western countries. Each year approximately a half million Americans suffer a new or recurrent event, and nearly one-fourth of those die. Stroke is the third leading cause of death in the United States.

The major types of cerebrovascular disease are:
- Cerebral insufficiency due to transient disturbance of blood flow (e.g., hypertensive encephalopathy)
- Cerebral infarction from either an embolism or thrombosis of the intracranial or extracranial arteries
- Cerebral hemorrhage including hypertensive parenchymal hemorrhage and subarachnoid hemorrhage from an aneurysm
- Cerebral arteriovenous malformation that can cause symptoms of either a mass lesion, infarction, or hemorrhage

DIAGNOSTIC STUDIES

Laboratory
Complete Blood Count with Differential and Platelet Count. As indicated to rule out polycythemia vera or infection.

Coagulation Studies: Prothrombin Time (PT), Partial Thromboplastin Time (PTT). To rule out bleeding dyscrasias and to monitor levels in patients taking warfarin or heparin.

Serum Chemistry Profile. Electrolytes to identify any abnormalities, especially hyponatremia. Glucose levels should be monitored to rule out or assess status of diabetes mellitus. Renal and liver function tests, cholesterol and triglyceride levels must be checked for risk factors and complications.

Homocysteine Level. Should be determined because of the link between elevated homocysteine levels and stroke risk.

Vitamin B_{12} and Folate Levels. Used to monitor homocysteine levels. (Persons with low serum B_{12} or folate tend to have increased homocysteine levels.)

Rapid Plama Reagin (RPR) Assay. As indicated to rule out syphilis.

Erythrocyte Sedimentation Rate. May be elevated with inflammatory conditions or infections.

Human Immunodeficiency Virus (HIV) Assay. If patient is in a high-risk group.

Toxicology Screen. If the patient is comatose or diagnosis is not apparent.

Radiology
Chest Film. This study should be obtained to evaluate pulmonary status, search for primary lung tumors, and rule out cardiovascular abnormalities. Calcifications surrounding the aorta may be a significant finding.

MRI and CT. These studies can help to identify the cause of the stroke and to assess damage. CT is preferred for acute hemorrhage. With cerebral infarct, CT findings can be negative for several days. MRI is useful to identify silent infarcts, old infarcts, and nonvascular disease entities such as tumors.

Magnetic Resonance Angiography (MRA). This is a useful noninvasive assessment of the vertebrobasilar system.

Cerebral Angiography. Performed when diagnosis is in doubt, a vascular obstruction is suspected, or surgical intervention is being considered. Useful to identify degree of carotid, verebrobasilar, or interacerbral vessel stenosis. Preferred when searching for source of infarcts (more sensitive for small lesions). May also identify suspected or incidental aneurysms.

Ultrasonography. Used when carotid lesions are suspected. Doppler and B-mode ultrasound techniques provide a noninvasive tool for determining lumen size and identifying carotid arterial lesions. Transcranial Doppler examination provides a minimally invasive way to assess ophthalmic circulation, carotid stenosis, intracranial vessels, and posterior circulation.

Other

ECG. Used to identify arrhythmias as a cause of embolus formation.

Echocardiography (ECG). Used to assess for valvular heart disease and to search for vegetations as a source of emboli.

Holter Monitoring. Should be used to evaluate for intermittent arrhythmia.

DIFFERENTIAL DIAGNOSIS

Traumatic

Subdural Hematoma (Acute or Chronic). May cause focal neurologic deficits, especially hemiparesis or dysphasia. Patient may have a history of trauma. Elderly patients with chronic subdural hematoma often have only a distant history of trauma or no memory of a traumatic event. A hematoma may be visible on CT of brain.

Infectious

Brain Abscess. Patient may have a history of recent dental or invasive procedure or sinusitis. A ring-enhancing lesion may be visible on CT/MRI of brain.

Neurosyphilis. Positive RPR assay.

Encephalitis. Patient may live in an endemic area. See "Encephalitis" earlier in this chapter.

AIDS. Positive HIV assay.

Endocarditis. Septic emboli are the source of the neurologic deficit. Positive echocardiogram and/or blood cultures.

Metabolic

Hyperinsulinism. History of poorly controlled diabetes mellitus. Low blood glucose will be apparent.

Toxic Encephalopathy. History of industrial or environmental exposure to toxins. History of drug use/abuse. CT/MRI reveals diffuse changes.

Lupus Cerebritis. History of systemic lupus erythematosus.

Neoplastic

Primary or Metastatic Intracerebral Lesions. Progressive symptoms of increased intracranial pressure and/or focal neurologic deficits. Mass seen on CT/MRI of brain.

Vascular

Migraine Headache. Patient may have a personal or family history of migraines. Transient neurologic symptom (e.g., visual scotoma, hemiparesis) followed classically by a unilateral headache. May have repeated similar events. Usually seen in younger age groups.

Temporal Arteritis. May cause blindness if left untreated. Associated with an elevated erythrocyte sedimentation rate.

Aneurysm. Can be congenital or acquired from atherosclerotic disease and cause subarachnoid hemorrhage. Aneurysm usually identified on cerebral angiography.

Arteriovenous Malformation. May cause "intracerebral steal" and transient neurologic deficits due to high flow. Large arteriovenous malformations will be seen on CT. Smaller arteriovenous malformations will be more visible on MRI study or cerebral angiogram.

Acquired

Alcoholic Encephalopathy. History of alcohol abuse. Liver function studies will be elevated. Asterixis may be present ("flapper tremor").

TREATMENT

The following measures are essential to ensure adequate and timely intervention:

Education of patients at risk

Early recognition of signs and symptoms

Prompt transport to hospital

Rapid triage, evaluation, and treatment

Thrombolytic agents and other emerging therapies provide opportunity to limit neurologic damage and improve outcomes. However, to be effective, these agents must be administered within 3 hours of the neurovascular event. Therefore, rapid evaluation and intervention are imperative.

Administration of thrombolytic agents such as TPA, streptokinase, and urokinase constitutes first-line intervention.

Patients with evidence of hemorrhage, internal bleeding, serious head trauma, recent intracranial surgery or lumbar puncture, history of arteriovenous malformation or recent myocardial infarction, or elevated blood pressure, or who have had a witnessed seizure, are not candidates for thrombolytic therapy.

At-risk patients should be anticoagulated with aspirin 325 to 1300 mg/day. If the patient is intolerant of aspirin, or if symptoms persist despite aspirin therapy, consider ticlopidine hydrochloride 250 mg twice a day. If more aggressive anticoagulation is required, consider treatment initially with heparin, then with low-dose warfarin (Coumadin). Close laboratory monitoring of prothrombin time and partial thromboplastin time with warfarin and heparin therapy is essential.

Treat anterior circulation TIAs by identifying the degree (or presence) of carotid artery stenosis. If occlusion with ipsilateral stenosis is greater than 70%, carotid endarterectomy should be considered in addition to medical therapy. Combining endarterectomy with medical therapy is more beneficial than medical therapy alone.

Obtain imaging studies to evaluate for infarct any time there is a transient or persistent neurologic deficit. Because an infarct may not be immediately apparent on CT, a follow-up study should be ordered in 48 hours.

If no hemorrhage is apparent and the infarction is small to moderate in size, consider anticoagulation or thrombolytic therapy as described.

If the infarct is large or there is hemorrhagic transformation, postpone anticoagulation for 5 to 7 days and reevaluate with CT or MRI.

Patients with deteriorating neurologic status must be evaluated for metabolic disorders (see Differential Diagnosis).

Calcium channel blockers such as nifedipine or cerebral-specific calcium channel blockers (nimodipine) can be used to theoretically reduce secondary neurologic injury.

Immediate care of the patient consists of support of vital functions including airway management, adequate oxygenation, intravenous fluids to maintain hydration, consideration of parenteral nutrition, attention to bowel and bladder functions, and measures to prevent decubitus ulcers.

Treat hypotension aggressively. Treat hypertension conservatively. The goal is to maintain cerebral perfusion. Use intravenous antihypertensives for better titration control.

Cardiac monitoring is required for at least the first 5 days.

Daily electrolyte values are obtained to assess hyponatremia.

PEDIATRIC CONSIDERATIONS

Stroke is uncommon in children. When it does occur, it is seen most frequently between the ages of 1 and 5, but it may occur at any age. Potential causes include underlying cardiopulmonary, hematologic, systemic, valvular, and intracranial vascular disorders. Congenital cyanotic heart disease is the most common underlying systemic disorder predisposing children to stroke. Sickle cell anemia, meningitis, trauma, and acute and congenital hemiplegias of childhood are other possible etiologic factors. Because many conditions leading to childhood stroke produce emboli, multifocal neurologic involvement is common. Clinical assessment is aimed at identifying specific deficits related to impaired cerebral blood flow and identifying predisposing disorders. Initial treatment should provide support for pulmonary, cardiovascular, and renal function as well as correction of the underlying problem. The prognosis for neurologic recovery is excellent for most children. Seizures occur in approximately 30% of patients, and chronic learning and behavior problems are common sequelae.

OBSTETRIC CONSIDERATIONS

Cerebrovascular accidents account for 8.5% of maternal deaths during pregnancy. In these patients, arterial occlusions rather than venous occlusions are the most common cause of stroke. In cerebrovascular accidents due to embolic events, most of the emboli in pregnancy originate from the heart. Atrial fibrillation carries an increased risk of embolus formation in the pregnant patient. Existing intracerebral aneurysms or intracranial vascular malformations can result in intracranial hemorrhage in the obstetric patient. These patients are at risk during Valsalva maneuvers, particularly during labor and delivery.

GERIATRIC CONSIDERATIONS

Stroke is a disease most closely associated with the geriatric population. Risk of TIAs and stroke increases with age and with history of previous TIA or stroke. Although the incidence of stroke has been declining in recent years, it still affects over 50,000 senior citizens a year. Seventy-five percent of all strokes occur in persons older than 75 years of age. Unfortunately, the symptoms of cerebral ischemia in older adults are often overlooked or misinterpreted. Stroke rehabilitation should be started as early as possible after the event. The prognosis for regaining of functional independence is related to the patient's mentation, motivation, and energy level and the availability of an aggressive program for rehabilitation. Depression is a very common comorbid condition following stroke. Patients should be monitored for symptoms of depression and if present, antidepression medication should be initiated as appropriate.

PREVENTIVE CONSIDERATIONS

Smoking cessation, adequate blood pressure control, lowering of serum cholesterol and triglycerides, and adequate control of diabetes, hypercoagulopathy, and sickle cell anemia all are important for primary prevention of TIA/stroke. Identification and treatment of patients with carotid stenosis and increased red blood cell count also are useful.

A daily aspirin for at-risk patients is advised, unless contraindicated by other medical conditions.

Prophylactic anticoagulation should be considered for patients with thrombus, prosthetic heart valve, recent myocardial infarction, or chronic arrhythmia. Anticoagulation therapy should be continued for 3 to 6 months.

Secondary prevention efforts (after an event has occurred) include anticoagulation and patient education regarding future risk. Expectations of recovery should be discussed with patient, caretakers, and family members. Planning for intermediate care and rehabilitation should begin immediately in a facility experienced with working with stroke patients. Early physical therapy is imperative to improve mobility, provide training in transfer techniques, promote ambulation, and maximize ability to perform activities of daily living.

PEARLS FOR THE PA

TIA is a temporary condition that results in little or no residual neurologic deficit.

Stroke is a fixed neurologic deficit resulting from infarction or hemorrhage.

Thrombolytic therapy must be administered within 3 hours of the neurovascular event.

Primary prevention is the key.

Further Reading

Adelman AM, Daly MP: Geriatrics: 20 Common Problems. New York, McGraw-Hill, 2001.

Advanced Cardiac Life Support Provider Manual. Dallas, Texas, American Heart Association, 2001.

Albers GW, Amarenco P, Easton JD, et al: Antithrombotic and thrombolytic therapy for ischemic stroke. Chest 119:300S, 2001.

Beers MH, Berkow R (eds): The Merck Manual of Diagnosis and Therapy, 17th ed. Rahway, NJ, Merck Research Laboratories, 1999.

Braunwald E, Fauci AS, Kasper DL, et al (eds): Harrison's Principles of Internal Medicine, 15th ed. New York, McGraw-Hill, 2001.

Campbell WW, Pridgeon RM: Practical Primer of Clinical Neurology. Philadelphia, Lippincott Williams & Wilkins, 2002.

Chapuis T: Parkinson's disease: Manifestations and management. Clinician Rev 12:63-68, 2002.

Diamond S: Herbal headache remedies: What to tell your patient. Consultant 41(12):1618-1620, 2001.

Eisenberg RL, Margulis AR: What to Order When: Pocket Guide to Diagnostic Imaging, 2nd ed. Philadelphia, Lippincott Williams & Wilkins, 2000.

Follett KA. The surgical treatment of Parkinson's disease. Annu Rev Med 51:135-147, 2000.

Goldman L, Ausiello D (eds): Cecil Textbook of Medicine, 22nd ed. Philadelphia, Saunders, 2004.

Goroll AH, Mulley AG: Primary Care Medicine: Office Evaluation and Management of the Adult Patient, 4th ed. Philadelphia, Lippincott Williams & Wilkins, 2000.

Kane RL, Ouslander JG, Abrass IB: Essentials of Clinical Geriatrics, 4th ed. New York, McGraw-Hill, 1999.

Labus JB, Lauber AA: Patient Education and Preventive Medicine. Philadelphia, WB Saunders, 2001.

Mathew NT: Pathophysiology, Epidemiology, and Impact of Migraine. Houston Headache Clinic, Houston. Contact at www.houstonheadacheclinic.com.

McDonough DL, Goldstein LB: Assessing the patient with suspected stroke. Emerg Med 34:32-43, 2002.

Mendis T, Suchowersky O, Lang A, Gauthier S: Management of Parkinson's disease: A review of current and new therapies. Can J Neurol Sci 26:89-103, 1999.

Mohr JP, Thompson JLP, Lazar RM, et al: A comparison of warfarin and aspirin for the prevention of recurrent ischemic stroke. N Engl J Med 345:1444-1451, 2001.

Physician Assistants Prescribing Reference, Spring 2002. Available at www.prescribingreference.com

Rakel RE, Bope ET (eds): Conn's Current Therapy 2004. Philadelphia, Saunders, 2004.

Rakel RE: Saunders Manual of Medical Practice, 2nd ed. Philadelphia, Saunders, 2000.

Rolak LA: Neurology Secrets, 3rd ed. Philadelphia, Hanley & Belfus, 2001.

Rowland LP: Merritt's Neurology, 10th ed. Philadelphia, Lippincott Williams & Wilkins, 2000.

Gilbert DN, Moellering Jr RC, Sande MA: The Sanford Guide to Antimicrobial Therapy, 33rd ed. Hyde Part, VT, Antimicrobial Therapy, Inc, 2003.

Schuchat A, Robinson K, Wenger JD, et al: Bacterial meningitis in the United States in 1995. N Engl J Med 337:970, 1997.

Sigurdardottir B, Bjornsson OM, Jonsdottir KE, et al: Acute bacterial meningitis in adults: A 20-year overview. Arch Intern Med 157:425, 1997.

Webb KMA: Headache. Scientific American Medicine CD-ROM 2000, Ch V111.

Weinert WJ, Goetz CG: Neurology for the Non-neurologist, 4th ed. Lippincott Williams & Wilkins, Philadelphia, 1999.

Wiederholt WC: Neurology for Non-Neurologists, 4th ed. Philadelphia, WB Saunders, 2000.

Resources

National Multiple Sclerosis Society, 205 East 42nd St., New York, NY 10017; telephone (800) 624-8236.

ONCOLOGY

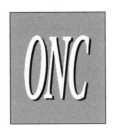

11

Adrenal Carcinoma

Charles W. Reed, MEd, MPAS, PA-C

DEFINITION

A primary endocrine carcinoma of the adrenal gland.

HISTORY

Symptoms. Patient may present with acute obstructive symptoms or systemic symptoms related to hormone production (see Physical Examination section, General).

General. Two-thirds of adrenal carcinomas occur in women.

Age. May appear at any age, most commonly at 40 years.

Onset. Usually acute.

Duration. Aggressive and rapidly progressive.

Intensity. Subacute or acute.

Aggravating Factors. None specific.

Alleviating Factors. Treatment of symptoms related to overproduction of hormones.

Associated Factors. None specific.

PHYSICAL EXAMINATION

General. Patients may present in hypertensive crisis or with hypokalemic alkalosis or ketoacidosis, precocious puberty, or hirsutism.

Abdominal. Adrenal masses are large and may be palpable.

Thorax. Gynecomastia, supraclavicular, or axillary lymphadenopathy.

PATHOPHYSIOLOGY

Adrenal carcinomas usually metastasize to the lungs and liver and may metastasize to bone. Fifty percent produce corticosteroids including aldosterone, androgens, cortisol, and estrogen. The hormone production is usually the cause of systemic symptoms.

Untreated adrenal carcinoma is generally fatal 2 to 4 months after diagnosis. Even with treatment, the 5-year survival rate is poor.

DIAGNOSTIC STUDIES

Laboratory

24-Hour Urine and Dexamethasone Suppression Test. If evidence of cortisol overproduction.

Radiology
Chest Film. For evidence of metastasis.
CT/MRI of the Abdomen. As indicated to confirm presence of lesion and evaluate size and location.
Metastatic Workup. Including radiographs of any area to reveal metastatic lesions, but CT of chest, abdomen, and pelvis is usually done even if the patient is asymptomatic.
Bone Scan. For evidence of metastasis.

Other
Biopsy. Performed on the most superficial site of metastasis. Metastatic disease will be histologically identical to the primary tumor. If the tumor is intra-abdominal only, exploratory laparotomy is the diagnostic procedure of choice.

DIFFERENTIAL DIAGNOSIS

Traumatic. Not applicable.
Infectious. Not applicable.

Metabolic
Ectopic adrenocorticotropic hormone (ACTH) secretion.

Neoplastic
Pituitary Cushing Syndrome. No intra-abdominal lesion. Pituitary lesion seen on MRI of the brain.
Adrenal Adenoma. Differentiated on biopsy; resection.
Multiple Endocrine Neoplasia (MEN). A cluster of genetic abnormalities occurring as multiple tumors of various endocrine glands in the same patients.
Other Intra-abdominal Masses. Differentiated on biopsy; resection.

Vascular. Not applicable.
Congenital. Not applicable.
Acquired. Not applicable.

TREATMENT

Surgical. Removal of primary tumors is always the first choice. Because adrenal tumors are often large and have metastasized at presentation, complete resection may not be possible. In those cases, palliative resection of as much of the tumor as possible is recommended.
Radiotherapy. Not effective as a primary treatment, but may be used to decrease tumor burden.
Chemotherapy. Mitotane may help reduce tumor bulk. There are no effective primary chemotherapeutic regimens.

PEDIATRIC CONSIDERATIONS

Adrenal carcinoma may occur in childhood and may be associated with precocious puberty. Patient may present with marfanoid body habitus.

OBSTETRIC CONSIDERATIONS

None specific.

GERIATRIC CONSIDERATIONS

None specific.

PREVENTIVE CONSIDERATIONS

None.

PEARLS FOR THE PA

Never assume a tumor is an isolated lesion. Many neoplasms can be part of a cluster of neoplastic processes. Evidence of an endocrine disorder should raise suspicion for other associated neoplasms.

Bladder Cancer

Charles W. Reed, MEd, MPAS, PA-C

DEFINITION

Cellular atypia of variable degree in the urinary bladder.

HISTORY

Symptoms. Hematuria with or without dysuria may be seen in 75% of cases. Vesical irritability may be seen in 30% of cases.

General. There is no pathognomonic sign or symptom of bladder cancer. There is a male-to-female ratio of 3:1.

Age. Incidence increases with advancing age. The peak incidence is in the seventh decade of life.

Onset. A long latency period is observed.

Duration. Early diagnosis can lead to 5-year survival rates of greater than 75%. Patients with regional and distant disease have a poor prognosis, with 5-year survival rates of 46% and 9%, respectively. However, for disease that is local (muscle-invasive only), the survival rate is now greater than 70%.

Intensity. Initially mild but may be incapacitating in terminal stages.

Aggravating Factors. Cigarette smoking is the biggest risk factor, with rates 2 to 3 times that of the nonsmoking population.

Alleviating Factors. None.

Associated Factors. Occupational exposure has been implicated in the development of bladder cancer in aniline dye workers, painters, printers, leather workers, and those working with dry cleaning solvents or rubber. Schistosomiasis and squamous cell carcinoma of the bladder have a close association.

PHYSICAL EXAMINATION

General. A thorough and complete physical examination is necessary to rule out the presence of metastatic lesions.

Genitourinary. A bimanual examination at the time of biopsy is performed to evaluate the extent of the tumor. Palpate for flank tenderness, suggesting nephrolithiasis as a cause for hematuria.

PATHOPHYSIOLOGY

Most bladder cancers are of the transitional cell variety. They are usually papillary and multicentric. These tumors have pushing borders that do not invade the muscularis layer and usually carry a better prognosis. Squamous cell tumors account for only 6% to 8% of bladder cancers. Two percent of bladder cancers are adenocarcinomas; these lesions usually arise from the dome of the bladder.

DIAGNOSTIC STUDIES

Laboratory

Complete Blood Count. White blood cell count (WBC) elevated in infection.

Renal Function Tests. Creatinine and blood urea nitrogen (BUN) may be elevated in metastatic disease.

Liver Function Studies. Lactate dehydrogenase (LDH) and alkaline phosphatase may be elevated in metastatic disease.

Urinalysis. May reveal an asymptomatic hematuria.

Radiology

Excretory Urography. Intraluminal filling defect can sometimes be seen.

Abdominal CT/MRI and Bone Scan. Performed in any patient where suspicion for tumor and metasasis is high.

Intravenous Pyelography. Used in staging of bladder cancer and used to rule out nephrolithiasis.

Other

Urinary Cytology. As indicated to evaluate for abnormal cells.

Cystoscopic Examination. As indicated to visualize changes in the bladder lining.

Transurethral Biopsy. Biopsy of suspected lesions both adjacent to and distant from the main lesion.

DIFFERENTIAL DIAGNOSIS

Traumatic. Not applicable.

Infectious

Urinary Tract Infection. May mimic early symptoms of hematuria and vesical irritability. Urine culture is usually positive.

Metabolic

Neprolithiasis. May manifest with hematuria. Usually associated with flank pain. Positive intravenous pyelogram.

Neoplastic

Benign Papilloma. Has a delicate fibrovascular core covered by normal transitional cell epithelium less than six layers thick.

Vascular. Not applicable.
Congenital. Not applicable.
Acquired. Not applicable.

TREATMENT

Once the diagnosis of bladder cancer is made, staging must be undertaken in order to determine a treatment plan. Staging consists of evaluation with intravenous pyelography, bimanual examination, and cystoscopy with biopsy or resection of suspected lesions. Results of the pathologic examination are critical to accurate staging.

Radiotherapy, chemotherapy, and biologic therapies are used in the treatment of bladder cancer.

PEDIATRIC CONSIDERATIONS

No specific indications.

OBSTETRIC CONSIDERATIONS

Antineoplastic medications may pose grave risks to the fetus. However, their use is recommended if absolutely required during pregnancy.

GERIATRIC CONSIDERATIONS

Screening for hematuria in healthy men age 50 and older may decrease morbidity and mortality rates and is cost-effective.

PREVENTIVE CONSIDERATIONS

Approximately 50% of all bladder cancers result from tobacco exposure and about 25% from occupational exposure. The incidence of bladder cancer in workers exposed to aromatic amines is very high. Aniline dyes used in the textile and rubber industries are also well-known contributors.

Avoidance of tobacco and of exposure to known environmental causes would markedly reduce the incidence of bladder carcinoma.

PEARLS FOR THE PA

There is no sign or symptom pathognomonic for bladder cancer.

The degree of hematuria in no way correlates with the severity of the disease.

Early diagnosis can lead to 5-year survival rates of greater than 75%.

Breast Cancer

Charles W. Reed, MEd, MPAS, PA-C

DEFINITION

Tumor in the glandular ducts or lobes of the breast.

HISTORY

Symptoms. Breast mass found on palpation is most frequently located in the upper, outer quadrant. Patient may only complain of a lump in the axilla. Occasionally there may be erythema, nipple retraction, or pain.

General. The patient often finds breast masses and lumps incidentally.
Age. Mean age at diagnosis is 60.
Onset. Insidious.
Duration. From 1 to 60 months.
Intensity. Often asymptomatic.
Aggravating Factors. None.
Alleviating Factors. Decrease in dietary fat intake.
Associated Factors. Family history of breast cancer in first-degree relatives, early age at menarche, nonparity or late child-bearing (after the age of 30 years), higher education and socioeconomic status, smoking, increased age, history of radiation to the chest or neck, alcohol consumption, late menopause (older than 55), or genetic carrier of *BRCA1* or *BRCA2* genes.

Presence of *BRCA1* poses the greatest risk at 8 to 42 times that in the general population, depending on age. Indications for genetic testing for *BCRA1* and *BCRA2* in patients with breast or ovarian cancer include family history of two or more first-or second-degree relatives with breast or ovarian cancer; one or more first-degree relatives with history of breast or ovarian cancer before age 45; presence of bilateral disease or multiple primary sites; presence of breast and ovarian cancer in premenopausal patients; and known *BRCA* mutations in relatives.

PHYSICAL EXAMINATION

General. Patient is usually in no acute distress, with normal findings on general examination.
Breast. Breast mass on palpation.
Extremities. Palpate for bone tenderness and evaluate range of motion of the joints to detect bone metastases.
Lymphatic. Evaluate for adenopathy by palpating the cervical, supraclavicular, and axillary nodes.
Neurologic. Evaluate for focal neurologic deficit (including extremity strength) to evaluate for metastases or compression of the central nervous system.
Pulmonary. Auscultate for rales or rhonchi, which may indicate infiltrate with a metastatic lesion. Percuss for mass.

PATHOPHYSIOLOGY

Infiltrating ductal carcinoma accounts for 80% of female breast cancers. Papillary and noninvasive ductal carcinoma is seen in only 5% of cases. Paget disease and medullary, tubular, metaplastic, apocrine and adenoid cystic, and mucinous carcinomas are the other histologic tumor types encountered.

Research surrounding the *HER2* gene and tumor expression of the growth factor receptor HER2 is providing for improved treatment outcomes in certain patients with aggressive breast cancer. The *HER2* gene codes for

HER2, which is overexpressed in 25% to 30% of breast cancers, increasing tumor aggressiveness.

DIAGNOSTIC STUDIES

Laboratory
Electrolytes. Used as baseline prior to instituting therapy.
Liver Function Studies. Elevated values in hepatic or bone metastases.
Complete Blood Count. Thrombocytopenia or pancytopenia may be seen in metastatic disease. Anemia of chronic disease may also be present.
Serum Calcium. Elevated in metastatic disease.
CA 15-3, CA 27-29, CA 549, MAM-6, MSA. Any of these antigens will be elevated in metastatic disease.

Radiology
Mammography. Used as a screening test in women 40 and older. Multiple recommendations exist, with no clear standard. The American Cancer Society recommends annual screening at age 40 and older. Some authorities recommend earlier mammograms for women who have a first-degree relative with a breast cancer diagnosis at age younger than 35 years.
Bone Scan. As indicated to rule out metastasis.
Abdominal Ultrasound Examination or CT. As indicated to rule out metastasis.
Chest Film. As indicated to rule out metastasis.

Other
Bone Marrow Aspiration. As indicated to rule out metastasis.
Biopsy of Mass. As indicated to determine the cell type, rule out malignancy, and assess hormone receptor activity.

DIFFERENTIAL DIAGNOSIS

Traumatic
Hematoma. History of breast trauma. Mass will resolve with time.

Infectious
Lactational Mastitis. History of breastfeeding.

Metabolic
Gynecomastia. Secondary to steroid use or hormonal dysfunction (e.g., pituitary adenoma), may have galactorrhea.

Neoplastic. Not otherwise applicable.
Vascular. Not applicable.

Congenital

Fibrocystic Breast Disease. Multiple, often bilateral painful masses in the breast, with worsening of symptoms during the premenstrual phase. Biopsy or aspiration of suspicious lesions is advised. It is often difficult to differentiate fibrocystic breast lesions from carcinoma. Ultrasound examination may be helpful in differentiating solid from cystic masses.

Acquired

History of Previous Ionizing Radiation. Is a risk factor for the development of breast cancer.

TREATMENT

Treatment is largely dependent on the stage of the tumor. Whether a lumpectomy or a mastectomy is performed depends on the patient's desire for breast conservation surgery, tumor size, age of patient, presence or absence of axillary node involvement, and whether the tumor is palpable. Generally, stage I or II cancers can be managed with lumpectomy and sentinel node biopsy, plus axillary node dissection if biopsy findings are positive. Lumpectomy is preferred in older patients, who will be unable to tolerate chemotherapy and will therefore be given postoperative radiation with subsequent hormonal treatment.

Adjuvant systemic chemotherapy is given to those patients whose disease is node-positive stage II or III. Patients receive postoperative radiation to the affected breast if they have undergone lumpectomy. Hormonal therapy is reserved for those who have positive assays for estrogen or progesterone receptors in their tumors. They are generally treated with tamoxifen or a tamoxifen-like drug. Patients can also receive postoperative radiation if they have chest wall involvement.

Tumors are checked for overexpression of the HER2 receptor. Patients with aggressive HER2-positive tumors have the option of recombinant monoclonal antibody (anti-HER2) treatment. This treatment has shown promising results, with increased time to tumor progression, higher response rates, lower mortality rates at 1 year, and longer overall survival. Research is ongoing.

PEDIATRIC CONSIDERATIONS

Not applicable.

OBSTETRIC CONSIDERATIONS

Diagnosis is a challenge because of pregnancy-related changes in breast tissue. Mammography contributes little information owing to the increased water density of the breast. Ultrasonography is the most useful diagnostic tool in this population. Biopsy of suspected lesions poses little risk to mother or fetus.

Breast cancer is the most common malignancy associated with pregnancy. There is a higher frequency of metastasis to the axillary nodes and a shorter length of survival in pregnant patients. This has been attributed mainly to delays in the diagnosis and treatment in the obstetric patient. Overall, treatment is the same as in the nonpregnant patient.

Chemotherapy is a relative contraindication during pregnancy, and radiation therapy is not recommended. However, particularly in invasive or disseminated breast cancer that is detected during the first two trimesters of pregnancy, mastectomy is recommended, with prompt institution of chemotherapy and radiation therapy as appropriate. A delay in starting radiation treatment to allow for fetal maturity is not advised. Often, termination of the pregnancy due to the use of chemotherapeutic agents and radiation treatment is encouraged. If the cancer is diagnosed in the third trimester, radiation may possibly be delayed and adjuvant chemotherapy administered to patients with positive nodes and evidence of metastases, with a lower risk of adverse fetal outcome. Subsequent pregnancies can be considered after 2 to 3 years if no evidence of tumor remains.

GERIATRIC CONSIDERATIONS

Because the incidence of breast cancer increases with age, the preventive measures as described are of utmost importance in this age group.

As the dense breast tissue of youth is replaced with fatty tissue in postmenopausal women, annual mammograms improve diagnostic capability.

The age at which screening should cease largely depends on the patient's functional status and other illnesses. There are no clear guidelines.

PREVENTIVE CONSIDERATIONS

The primary factor in decreasing morbidity and mortality from breast cancer is early detection. In terms of decreased morbidity and mortality, the benefit of annual bilateral mammograms for patients 50 years and older is well established. The benefit of monthly self-breast examination (MSBE) is unclear. However, patient education and vigilance for the signs and symptoms of cancer are certainly important. One tool to increase patient awareness is the MSBE.

Initially, most patients will be unsure of what constitutes normal findings on MSBE. Because "normal" may be dependent on the patient's anatomy, the initial examination should be performed by a competent health care provider, who describes the technique and findings to the patient as the examination progresses. Patients should be encouraged to perform the examination at the same time each month and to report any changes to the provider.

Postmenopausal women desiring hormone replacement therapy (HRT) should receive education on the risk-benefit ratio so that an informed decision can be made. The overall risk of breast cancer in women receiving HRT increases by a factor of 1.023 for each year of use over the risk in women who do not use HRT. After cessation of HRT, the relative increased risk returns to normal within 5 years regardless of the duration of HRT.

PEARLS FOR THE PA

Monthly breast self-examination is important in the early detection of breast tumors and should be taught to all patients.

Mammography performed after the age of 40 may detect early disease.

Because of higher density of breast tissue in younger women, mammography is of limited diagnostic value before the age of 40 years.

Standard of care litigation indicates that patients with a palpable mass on examination should have a biopsy within 2 weeks of discovery of the lesion. Careful follow-up is imperative to ensure prompt evaluation of any suspicious breast mass.

Cervical Cancer

Charles W. Reed, MEd, MPAS, PA-C

DEFINITION

A process of dysplasia leading to metaplasia that results in invasion of the basement membrane of the cervical epithelium.

HISTORY

Symptoms. Vaginal bleeding (postcoital, postmenopausal, irregular), weight loss, pelvic pain, leg edema, leg and back pain.

General. Commonly, the patient has no symptoms until advanced, invasive carcinoma develops. Usually, cervical cancer is found incidentally by an abnormal Papanicolaou (Pap) smear.

Age. Average age at onset of invasive cervical cancer is 35 years; the average age of patients with cervical dysplasia is 25.

Onset. Gradual.

Duration.   May develop over months to years.

Intensity.   The patient may be asymptomatic or may present with significant symptoms.

Aggravating Factors.   Immunosuppression, especially that due to human immunodeficiency virus (HIV) infection.

Alleviating Factors.   Early diagnosis and treatment.

Associated Factors.   Risk is increased in patients with multiple sex partners, history of sexually transmitted diseases (especially human papillomavirus [HPV] infection), early age at first sexual intercourse, and cigarette smoking.

PHYSICAL EXAMINATION

General.   Patient may appear normal or, in advanced stages, appear cachectic.

Extremities.   Observe lower extremities for edema secondary to obstruction.

Gynecologic.   Pap smear will be abnormal. Cervical lesion may be seen on pelvic examination.

Lymphatic.   Evaluate for lymphadenopathy, paying particular attention to the inguinal nodes.

PATHOPHYSIOLOGY

Cervical cancer follows a process of metaplasia and then dysplasia of the epithelium. Infectious cervicitis may contribute substantially to remodeling and repair of the transformation zone. Immunosuppression may also contribute to the development of neoplasia by predisposing the patient to infection by oncogenic viruses and allowing proliferation to escape immune surveillance and other host regulatory mechanisms.

The presence of HPV is an important risk factor for the development of cervical neoplasia. HPV is present in 75% to 100% of cervical cancer specimens and has been estimated as a cause of cervical cancer in 82% to 92% of cases. However, the presence of this virus may not be all that is required for neoplasia. Despite high HPV infection rates in young healthy women, the incidence of cervical cancer is relatively low. This finding would seem to indicate that although HPV is a necessary factor in the development of cervical cancer, it is not the only factor.

DIAGNOSTIC STUDIES

Laboratory

Electrolytes.   Determination of electrolyes is done as a prelude to chemotherapy.

Liver Function Tests.   Values may be elevated with liver metastases.

Complete Blood Count. Elevated white blood cell (WBC) count may be seen in infections.

HIV Testing. As indicated to rule out immunosuppression caused by HIV infection. Especially indicated in persons with multiple or unknown sexual partners.

Radiology
Chest Film. Used to rule out lung metastasis.
Bone scan. Used to rule out bone metastasis.

Other
Colposcopy. As indicated to evaluate level of stromal invasion and any other abnormal areas.

Endocervical Curettage. As indicated to evaluate for neoplastic cells.

Cone Biopsy. For evaluation of the depth of disease.

Intravenous Urography. As indicated to rule out ureteral/urethral compression by the lesion.

DIFFERENTIAL DIAGNOSIS

Traumatic
Postcoital Bleeding. Due to deep penetration or foreign body.

Infectious
Sexually Transmitted Diseases. May cause malodorous discharge or bleeding. Cultures will be positive. Pap smear should be performed.

Metabolic
Hormonal Imbalance. May cause irregular bleeding. Follicle-stimulating hormone, luteinizing hormone, and estradiol levels should be evaluated.

Vascular. Not applicable.
Congenital. Not applicable.
Acquired. Not applicable.

TREATMENT

Once cervical cancer is clinically detected by colposcopy and biopsy, staging should be done according to the system developed by the International Federation of Gynecology and Obstetrics (FIGO) (see Table 11-1).

Indications for surgery and/or irradiation are based on the stage of the cervical cancer.

Low-grade noninvasive lesions are generally treated with cryotherapy, laser ablation, or loop electrosurgical excision procedure (LEEP). These

Table 11–1. FIGO Staging of Carcinoma of the Cervix Uteri

Stage	
0	Preinvasive Carcinoma
	Carcinoma in situ, intraepithelial carcinoma (cases of stage 0 tumors should not be included in any therapeutic statistics)
I	Invasive Carcinoma
	Carcinoma strictly confined to the cervix (extension to the corpus should be disregarded)
	IA: Preclinical carcinomas of the cervix, for example, those diagnosed only by microscopy
	IA1: Minimal microscopically evident stromal invasion
	IA2: Lesions detected microscopically that can be measured; the upper limit of the measurement should not show a depth of invasion of more than 5 mm taken from the base of the epithelium, either surface or glandular, from which it originates, and a second dimension, the horizontal spread, must not exceed 7 mm; larger lesions should be staged as IB
	IB: Lesions of greater dimensions than stage IA2, whether seen clinically or not; preformed space involvement should not alter the staging but should be specifically recorded so as to determine whether it should affect treatment decisions in the future
II	Carcinoma extends beyond the cervix but has not extended onto the wall; the carcinoma involves the vagina, but not the lower third
	IIA: No obvious parametrial involvement
	IIB: Obvious parametrial involvement
III	Carcinoma has extended to the pelvic wall; on rectal examination, there is no cancer-free space between the tumor and the pelvic wall; the tumor involves the lower third of the vagina; all cases with hydronephrosis or nonfunctioning kidney
	IIIA: No extension to the pelvic wall
	IIIB: Extension to the pelvic wall and/or hydronephrosis or nonfunctioning kidney
IV	Carcinoma has extended beyond the true pelvis or has clinically involved the mucosa of the bladder or rectum.
	IVA: Spread of the growth to adjacent organs
	IVB: Spread to distant organs

FIGO, Fédération Internationale de Gynécologie et Obstétrique (International Federation of Gynecology and Obstetrics).

Adapted from Beahrs OH, Henson DE, Hutter RVP, et al: Manual to Staging of Cancer. Philadelphia, JB Lippincott, 1992.

three modalities are of equal efficacy and result in equivalent amounts of tissue destruction.

Invasive stage cancers are generally treated with surgery, radiotherapy, or multimodality approaches.

Radiation therapy methods include teletherapy (external irradiation) and brachytherapy (intracavitary irradiation).

Chemotherapy may be used before radiotherapy to decrease tumor burden or in neoadjuvant fashion as a radiosensitizer. Chemotherapeutic treatment of recurrent cervical cancer is generally palliative in nature.

Eighty percent of cases of recurrent disease are found within 2 years of therapy. Recurrent disease carries a poor prognosis.

PEDIATRIC CONSIDERATIONS

Not applicable to the prepubescent female.

OBSTETRIC CONSIDERATIONS

If the patient wishes to preserve her fertility, she may be treated with cryotherapy, conization, or laser ablation in the case of carcinoma in situ.

In cervical cancer, treatment of carcinoma in situ and cervical dysplasia can be delayed until after delivery as long as these lesions are monitored closely during the pregnancy. Pap smears and colposcopic assessment need to be part of the initial evaluation. However, endocervical curettage should not be performed. A shallow conization can be accomplished with caution if there is evidence of microinvasion of the cancer; bleeding is a complication, even with this conservative approach.

If the cancer is advanced, a radical hysterectomy with pelvic lymphadenectomy is advised in early pregnancy. Alternatively, external irradiation with subsequent fetal death followed by dilatation and curettage and placement of an intracavitary radiation device in the cervix and uterus can also be performed. A hysterotomy performed prior to radiation therapy is the treatment of choice in early second-trimester pregnancies with advanced disease. Treatment can sometimes be delayed in the patient in her late second or third trimester to allow for the fetus to gain more maturity and to increase the likelihood that the fetus will survive an early cesarean section.

In a patient with advanced cervical cancer, overall prognosis will not be affected by a vaginal delivery. Cesarean section is usually advised, however, owing to the possibility that the diseased cervix will fail to dilate or could lacerate with accompanying severe hemorrhage.

GERIATRIC CONSIDERATIONS

There is no empirical evidence indicating a cessation point for screening.

PREVENTIVE CONSIDERATIONS

Avoidance of the sexually transmitted HPV would seem to be an excellent means of preventing cervical cancer.

An effective screening program including public education is a powerful tool in the reduction of morbidity and mortality associated with cervical cancer.

PEARLS FOR THE PA

Early detection by Pap smears is effective if performed correctly.

Pap smears should be performed annually in sexually active women.

Incidental infections discovered during a routine Pap smear can invalidate the results by masking neoplastic changes. If a Pap result indicates an infection, the infection should be treated and the Pap smear repeated.

Colorectal Cancer

Charles W. Reed, MEd, MPAS, PA-C

DEFINITION

Carcinoma that begins as a polypoid adenoma and then invades locally into the colon wall. It subsequently invades the muscularis and proceeds to spread either through the lymphatic system or hematogenously.

HISTORY

Symptoms. Vary according to the anatomic region involved. Early-stage symptoms may include vague abdominal pain (which may be intermittent), flatulence, and minor changes in bowel movements with or without rectal bleeding. Cancers in the left colon usually cause constipation alternating with diarrhea, abdominal pain, nausea, and vomiting. Right-sided lesions produce vague abdominal pain and may be associated with anemia. Rectal lesions may produce a change in bowel movements, a sense of rectal fullness, urgency, bleeding, or tenesmus. Patients can also present with fatigue.

General. Obtain a careful history regarding changes in bowel habits and the presence of melena or bright red blood (hematochezia) in the stools. Melena usually indicates bleeding from the small intestine. Hematochezia usually indicates bleeding from the colon.

Age. Increased risk beginning in the fifth decade and increasing with advancing age. Mean age at presentation is 60 to 65 years.

Onset. Slow and progressive.

Duration. Months to years.

Intensity. Initially mild, but symptoms may progress to intestinal obstruction.

Aggravating Factors. Diet, smoking, low calcium intake, charcoal-prepared foods.

Alleviating Factors. Early diagnosis and treatment.

Associated Factors. Incidence is higher in industrialized regions of the world. A diet rich in fat and charcoal-prepared foods, several genetic polyposis syndromes, inflammatory bowel disease, and a history of pelvic irradiation all have been associated with an increased risk for the development of colorectal cancer. A protective effect has been seen with diets containing cereal fiber, bran, yellow and green vegetables, and calcium-rich foods and with aspirin use.

PHYSICAL EXAMINATION

General. The patient may appear in no acute distress or may be in significant distress if bowel obstruction has developed. A full and complete physical examination is warranted to evaluate for metastatic disease when colorectal cancer is diagnosed.

Gastrointestinal. Perform a digital rectal examination to palpate for tumors. Check for occult blood. Abdominal palpation may reveal masses.

PATHOPHYSIOLOGY

From 90% to 95% of large bowel neoplasms are adenocarcinomas. Mucinoid and signet ring cell tumors are histologic variants of adenocarcinoma. Nonepithelial tumors are very rare.

DIAGNOSTIC STUDIES

Laboratory

Electrolytes. Used as a baseline prior to initiation of therapy and to evaluate for dehydration.

Liver Function Tests. Values may be elevated with metastases; used as a baseline prior to initiation of therapy.

Urinalysis. Used to rule out urinary tract infection.

Complete Blood Count. May reveal anemia; used as a baseline prior to initiation of therapy.

Carcinoembryonic Antigen (CEA) Assay. Normal in nonsmokers: less than 3.0 ng/mL; in smokers: less than 5.0 ng/dL. Elevated with colorectal cancer. Used serially to assess for recurrence.

Radiology
Air Contrast Barium Enema. May show lesions in the colon.

Chest Film. Used to rule out metastatic disease to the lung.

CT Scan of the Abdomen and Pelvis. As indicated to evaluate for mass lesions. Smaller intraluminal masses may be missed.

Other
Colonoscopy. Used for direct visualization, biopsy, or removal of suspected lesions.

DIFFERENTIAL DIAGNOSIS

Traumatic
Foreign Body. May cause rectal bleeding.

Infectious
Colitis. May cause gastrointestinal (GI) bleeding. Will be viewed on anoscopy.

Pseudomembranous Colitis. Positive culture for *Clostridium difficile* and bleeding.

Metabolic
Diverticula. May cause GI bleeding. Diverticula will be seen on barium studies or colonoscopy.

Gastric/Esophageal Varices. Associated with chronic alcohol abuse and prone to bleeding. Upper GI source of the bleeding. May be viewed on esophogastroscopy.

Gastric/Peptic Ulcer. May cause GI bleeding. Patient may have a history of ulcer disease. Viewed on upper GI barium studies or via an endoscopic examination.

Crohn's Disease. May cause GI bleeding. Pain in any abdominal quadrant; can be colicky, with diarrhea or blood. Fever and weight loss may also be present. The hallmark is a chronic history of recurrent symptoms. Patients generally also have nausea/vomiting.

Ulcerative Colitis. Causes GI bleeding and abdominal pain. Patients usually state that their pain occurs immediately after eating a meal, may state that "food passes right through me"; rectal incontinence, several bowel movements a day, fatigue. Fever, nausea or vomiting may also be present.

Anal Fissures/Perirectal Fissures/Abscess. Usually associated with a recent bout of constipation or Crohn's disease.

Vascular

Arteriovenous Malformations. Difficult to detect on routine studies. Biopsies will be negative for tumor.

Hemorrhoids. May be apparent on inspection of the anus. Visualization may require anoscopy.

Mallory-Weiss Tear. Will cause GI bleeding. Can be viewed with the endoscope.

Congenital

Not applicable.

Acquired

Abdominal Surgery. Recent history.

Aortoduodenal Fistula. May be seen following aortic bypass surgery.

TREATMENT

Surgical resection of the involved bowel is the primary mode of therapy, along with adjuvant systemic and local chemotherapy.

PEDIATRIC CONSIDERATIONS

Adenocarcinoma of the colon is rare in the pediatric age group. The transverse colon and rectosigmoid are the two most commonly affected sites. Children are at a greater risk if there is a family history of familial polyposis. Cancer rarely develops before age 15.

OBSTETRIC CONSIDERATIONS

Antineoplastic medications may pose grave risk to the fetus. However, their use is recommended if absolutely needed during pregnancy.

GERIATRIC CONSIDERATIONS

Risk of colorectal cancer increases with age. Amazingly, patients are often reluctant to undergo the screening procedures. Vigilance, knowledgeable enthusiastic counseling, and persistence are critical elements of a beneficial prevention program.

PREVENTIVE CONSIDERATIONS

Prevention

Avoidance of tobacco products reduces risk.

Diets high in fiber and low in fat may inhibit polyp progression to cancer. Daily aspirin may be beneficial in reducing the incidence of colon cancer.

Screening

Periodic screening may allow timely removal of precancerous polyps or of carcinoma in situ prior to metastasis. Screening methods include fecal occult blood testing, double-contrast barium enema, flexible sigmoidoscopy, and colonoscopy.

The National Cancer Institute (NCI), the American College of Surgeons, the American College of Physicians, and the American Cancer Society (ACS) recommend that asymptomatic patients 50 years of age or older undergo a flexible sigmoidoscopic examination every 3 to 5 years.

An annual digital rectal examination with fecal occult blood testing is also recommended for the same age group.

Screening with colonoscopy in patients with a family history of colorectal cancer in a first-degree relative should begin at age 40.

Patients who have a family history of familial adenomatous polyposis (FAP) should be screened for polyps beginning in the early teen years.

Patients with a family history of hereditary nonpolyposis colorectal cancer (HNPCC) syndrome should begin screening examinations by age 20.

PEARLS FOR THE PA

Early detection of localized lesions is the key to improved survival of patients with colorectal cancer.

Digital rectal examination (without sigmoidoscopy) is recommended after age 40 as a screening measure.

Gastric Carcinoma

Charles W. Reed, MEd, MPAS, PA-C

DEFINITION

Primary carcinoma of the stomach, which is mostly (in 95% of cases) adenomatous. It may be of a diffuse or intestinal-type nature.

HISTORY

Symptoms. Gastric carcinoma is often advanced before becoming symptomatic. Symptoms and signs may include anorexia, weakness, early satiety, abdominal pain, weight loss, nausea and vomiting, unremitting "heartburn"/indigestion, anemia, and palpable abdominal mass.

General.   Mortality rates from gastric cancer are lowest in the United States and highest in Costa Rica.

Age.   More common in men older than 50 years of age.

Onset.   Gradual, over months.

Duration.   Progressive if untreated.

Intensity.   Metastatic and fatal if left untreated.

Aggravating Factors.   Delay in diagnosis.

Alleviating Factors.   Appropriate treatment.

Associated Factors.   Smoked, grilled, spicy, or fatty foods in the diet; chronic *Helicobacter pylori* infection with or without chronic gastritis; gastric polyps; African, Asian, and Hispanic American ethnicity; pernicious anemia; achlorhydria (with overuse of histamine H_2 blockers).

PHYSICAL EXAMINATION

General.   Findings on examination may be normal. However, gastric carcinoma spreads via lymphatic and blood vessels; therefore, a thorough examination for lymphadenopathy is required, especially of left axillary and supraclavicular nodes.

Abdomen.   A thorough abdominal examination is critical. Thirty percent of gastric carcinoma patients will have a palpable abdominal mass. The liver is the most common site for metastasis, and hepatomegaly may be noted.

Musculoskeletal.   Bone metastasis is common.

Pulmonary.   Lung metastasis is common.

PATHOPHYSIOLOGY

There are three commonly used classifications based on histology (Lauren), clinical (anatomic), and endoscopic characteristics (Japanese Endoscopic Society [JES]).

DIAGNOSTIC STUDIES

Laboratory

Complete Blood Count and Liver Function Tests.   Important initial baseline studies. Also used to evaluate for anemia or hepatic involvement.

Serum Albumin.   Generally, a decreased serum albumin indicates more advanced disease and is a poor prognostic sign.

Radiology

Abdominal CT.   Useful in determining disease extent but will underestimate extent in about half of all cases. Endoscopic ultrasound examination may be up to 6 times more accurate than CT in staging primary gastric tumors.

Other
Endoscopy. Endoscopy allows for a visual examination of lesions and for the collection of samples for histologic studies.

DIFFERENTIAL DIAGNOSIS

Traumatic. Not applicable.
Infectious. *Helicobacter pylori* and other infections: Differentiated on endoscopy and biopsy.

Metabolic
Gastric Polyps. Various types may be confused with gastric carcinoma, but polyps generally have a low malignant potential.
Peptic Ulcer/Gastroesophageal Reflux Disease (GERD). Differentiated on endoscopy.

Neoplastic
Gastric Lymphoma. Differentiated on endoscopy and biopsy.
Sarcoma. Differentiated on endoscopy and biopsy.
Lipoma. Differentiated on endoscopy and biopsy.
Various Carcinoid Tumors. Differentiated on endoscopy and biopsy.

Vascular
Hemangioma. Differentiated on endoscopy.

Congenital. Not applicable.
Acquired. Gastritis from any cause: Differentiated on endoscopy and biopsy.

TREATMENT

Surgery. Staging is via the tumor-node-metastasis (TNM) system. Treatment and prognosis depend on the degree of tumor extension into the stomach wall, lymph node involvement, and metastasis. The only treatment considered curative is subtotal gastrectomy with wide margins. This necessitates lifelong vitamin B_{12} replacement.
Chemotherapy. Neoadjuvant chemotherapy with 5-fluorouracil (5-FU) in combination with other agents has shown high response rates, but whether response provides survival benefit is not well documented. Adjuvant systemic chemotherapy has not proved beneficial. Intraperitoneal chemotherapy may reduce recurrence at the gastrectomy site. Systemic chemotherapy has proved of minimal benefit in advanced disease.
Radiotherapy. Radiotherapy in combination with chemotherapy with 5-FU may be beneficial in patients with localized, unresectable disease.

PEDIATRIC CONSIDERATIONS

Gastric carcinoma is not a childhood disease

OBSTETRIC CONSIDERATIONS

None specific.

GERIATRIC CONSIDERATIONS

This is the patient population most at risk for gastric carcinoma. Because of the indolent nature of this lesion, high index of suspicion may lead to early diagnosis. Performance status is always an issue affecting prognosis and likely clinical course.

PREVENTIVE CONSIDERATIONS

Avoidance or appropriate management of contributing factors of smoked, grilled, spicy, or fatty foods; chronic *H. pylori* infection with or without chronic gastritis; gastric polyps. It is not currently known if eradicating *H. pylori* during treatment of gastric ulcer has any impact on subsequent development of gastric carcinoma.

PEARLS FOR THE PA

For the prevention and detection of gastric carcinoma, the importance of health care maintenance examinations must be stressed.

A thorough annual comprehensive history and physical examination constitute one of the most important contributions to a patient's health and wellness.

Hodgkin Disease

Charles W. Reed, MEd, MPAS, PA-C

DEFINITION

A malignancy of the lymphatic system that develops in a single lymph node region and then disseminates to distant lymph nodes and extralymphatic organs in the late stages. Also called *Hodgkin lymphoma.*

HISTORY

Symptoms. Painless lymphadenopathy, B symptoms (night sweats, fever, weight loss), early satiety, pruritis. Lymph node pain with alcohol ingestion.

General. Males, in general, have a greater risk of developing the disease.

Age. A bimodal curve is noted. The first peak is during the third decade (ages 20 to 29 years) and the second is after the age of 60.

Onset. Gradual, over months.

Duration. Progressive if left untreated.

Intensity. If untreated, Hodgkin disease is uniformly fatal, usually within 5 years of diagnosis.

Aggravating Factors. Bone marrow involvement, development of B symptoms.

Alleviating Factors. None.

Associated Factors. Higher social class and education level, smaller number of siblings, or abnormal T cell function. Mediastinal involvement.

PHYSICAL EXAMINATION

General. Evaluate for B symptoms (weight loss, fever, and night sweats). Palpate and measure lymph nodes.

Gastrointestinal. Careful evaluation for hepatomegaly and splenomegaly.

Lymphatic. Evaluate for lymphadenopathy by palpating the cervical, supraclavicular, axillary, epitrochlear, and inguinal lymph nodes.

PATHOPHYSIOLOGY

Diagnosis is established by the presence of Reed-Sternberg cells or their equivalent on biopsy of the lymph node. Fibrosis is frequently seen. Hodgkin disease is usually divided into four types according to the characteristic histologic features (the Rye classification): (1) lymphocyte prominent, (2) nodular sclerosis, (3) mixed cellularity, and (4) lymphocytic depletion.

A newer classification from the World Health Organization (WHO) divides Hodgkin lymphoma (HL) into nodular lymphocyte predominance HL and classic HL.

DIAGNOSTIC STUDIES

Laboratory

Complete Blood Count. As indicated to evaluate for anemia, thrombocytopenia, or neutropenia. Eosinophilia can be found in 20% of the patients. Used as a baseline prior to initiation of chemotherapy or radiotherapy.

Liver Function Tests. Used to establish baseline values prior to initiation of chemotherapy or radiotherapy. Also used to assess for liver metastasis.

Erythrocyte Sedimentation Rate. Nonspecific, but may be elevated.

Radiology
Chest Films: Posteroanterior and Lateral Views. As indicated to rule out mediastinal involvement.
CT Scan of the Chest/Abdomen/Pelvis. As indicated to evaluate the extent of mediastinal disease; to evaluate organomegaly and the presence of abdominal nodes.
Bipedal Lymphangiography. Can be useful in detecting early nodal disease missed by CT or MRI.
Bone Scan. In select patients with symptoms suggesting bone involvement.
Gallium Scan. Useful in select patients to evaluate for disease.

Other
Bone Marrow Aspiration and Biopsy. Biopsy/aspiration of bilateral posterior iliac crest to rule out marrow involvement.
Staging Laparotomy. Used only if finding will alter treatment.

DIFFERENTIAL DIAGNOSIS

Traumatic
Hematoma. May affect axillary, supraclavicular, epitrochlear, or inguinal nodes.

Infectious
Cat-Scratch Fever. Usually manifests with a single, enlarged lymph node.
Epstein-Barr Virus Infection. Positive Monospot test, enlarged spleen and tender liver, with fever.
Regional Infection. May cause local lymphadenopathy.

Neoplastic
Non-Hodgkin Lymphoma. May be mistaken for Hodgkin disease. Differentiated on diagnostic testing.

Metabolic. Not applicable.
Vascular. Not applicable.
Congenital. Not applicable.
Acquired. Not applicable.

TREATMENT

Treatment modality and prognosis are largely dependent on the stage of the disease. The *Ann Arbor staging system* was the most often used but has been upgraded to include other important prognostic factors such as mediastinal tumor bulk. The newer system is called the *Cotswolds Staging Classification.* For further information on staging, consult sources in Further Reading at the end of this chapter.

Secondary malignancies may occur after therapy for Hodgkin disease at a rate of 10% to 15%. These malignancies include acute myelogenous leukemia, myelodysplastic syndrome, non-Hodgkin lymphoma, and solid tumors.

PEDIATRIC CONSIDERATIONS

Children who receive radiotherapy to bone may develop growth asymmetry owing to premature epiphyseal closure. Endocrine abnormalities such as hypothyroidism may occur following radiotherapy to the neck. The development of hypothyroidism may occur 11 years or longer after completion of radiotherapy.

OBSTETRIC CONSIDERATIONS

Chemotherapy after the first trimester may be given, but potential risks to the fetus need to be discussed with the mother. Radiotherapy to the abdomen should wait until the postpartum period. Patients' fertility will be affected by the use of combination chemotherapeutic alkylating agents such as cyclophosphamide, chlorambucil, mechlorethamine, and procarbazine.

The most common type of lymphoma that occurs during pregnancy is Hodgkin disease. There are no known adverse affects on maternal or fetal outcome when the mother has Hodgkin disease. However, the use of radiation therapy or chemotherapy can affect the pregnancy. A pelvic shield should be used during the radiation therapy, and chemotherapy is considered relatively safe for use if instituted during the second or third trimester. If therapeutic radiation exposure occurs early in the pregnancy, abortion is recommended.

GERIATRIC CONSIDERATIONS

Awareness of predominance in geriatric population is key to diagnosis.

PREVENTIVE CONSIDERATIONS

None.

PEARLS FOR THE PA

Knowledge of and vigilance for post-treatment malignancies are crucial in the care of survivors of Hodgkin lymphoma.

Early presenting lymphomas may be misdiagnosed as lymphadenopathy due to mononucleosis.

Leukemia

Charles W. Reed, MEd, MPAS, PA-C

DEFINITION

A group of heterogeneous diseases that are similar in spread of neoplastic cells of hematopoietic origin by infiltration of blood, bone marrow, and tissues. Classified as acute lymphocytic leukemia (ALL), acute myelogenous leukemia (AML), chronic lymphocytic leukemia (CLL), or chronic myelogenous leukemia (CML).

HISTORY

Symptoms. Fatigue, anorexia, weight loss, fevers, petechiae, or hemorrhage may be seen in up to 50% of patients at presentation. Bone pain, headache, and lymphadenopathy may be elicited from the patient on further questioning.

General. Rarely asymptomatic except in CML or early-stage CLL.

Age. All ages and both genders are affected. The frequency of leukemia increases with advancing age. ALL typically occurs in childhood, AML in young adults, CML in middle-aged adults, and CLL in the older population.

Onset. Usually a 2- to 3-month prodrome in acute leukemia, with rapid progression. Chronic leukemia may have a slower, asymptomatic period followed by rapidly progressive disease.

Duration. Once clinically apparent, progressive in nature.

Intensity. Severe in association with hemorrhages and infection.

Aggravating Factors. None.

Alleviating Factors. None.

Associated Factors. Radiation and chemical (e.g., benzene) exposure, drugs (e.g., chloramphenicol, phenylbutazone, antineoplastic drugs), viruses (e.g., herpes T cell leukemia virus types I and II [HTLV-I and HTLV-II]), and genetic syndromes (e.g., Down, Klinefelter, and Fanconi syndromes).

PHYSICAL EXAMINATION

General.   The patient may be febrile and/or exhibit pallor or evidence of weight loss.

Cardiovascular.   Evaluate cardiac rate for tachycardia suggesting anemia. Superior vena cava obstruction with facial and upper extremity edema may be present owing to massive adenopathy.

Extremities.   Palpate for bone lesions. Decreased range of motion and tenderness may be present with joint involvement.

Gastrointestinal.   Palpate for hepatosplenomegaly or masses.

Genitourinary.   Palpate testicles for enlargement in males. Inspect for candidal vaginitis in females.

Head, Eyes, Ears, Nose, Throat.   Pallor of mucosal membranes may be seen with anemia. Gingival hyperplasia may be present as a result of infiltration by leukemic cells. Candidal infection may also be seen.

Lymphatic.   Evaluate for lymphadenopathy including all cervical, supraclavicular, axillary, epitrochlear, and inguinal nodes.

Neurologic.   Evaluate for cranial nerve changes, which suggest meningeal involvement by leukemic cells.

Pulmonary.   Ausculate for rales or rhonchi suggesting pneumonia.

Skin.   Reddish purple, raised nodules seen in skin infiltrated with leukemic cells.

PATHOPHYSIOLOGY

Neoplastic infiltration of normal hematopoietic cells and replacement of normal blood constituents with these abnormal cells, resulting in functional pancytopenia and/or thrombocytopenia. Etiology is unknown, but suspected risk factors include radiation, drug, or chemical exposure and genetic aneuploidy.

DIAGNOSTIC STUDIES

Laboratory

Complete Blood Count.   Evaluate for neutropenia, anemia, thrombocytopenia, and extent of peripheral blast cells.

Peripheral Blood Smear.   Will demonstrate an increase of mostly mature or near-mature cells in chronic forms of leukemia and predominance of immature and blast forms in acute leukemia.

Electrolytes.   Used as a baseline prior to chemotherapy.

Liver Function Tests.   Evaluate for hepatic involvement and use as a baseline prior to initiation of chemotherapy.

Uric Acid.   Evaluate for hyperuricemia, which is seen with high blast counts.

Lactate Dehydrogenase (LDH).   Elevated in some leukemias.

Serum Calcium.   Elevated in some leukemias.

Coagulation Profile.   Elevated in patients with certain subtypes of AML, who are at risk for disseminated intravascular coagulation. Decreasing fibrinogen levels and fibrin split products may indicate disseminated intravascular coagulation.

Blood Type and Human Leukocyte Antigen Determination.   As indicated to determine blood type for potential transfusions. Family members should also be tested for potential blood or bone marrow donation.

Radiology
Chest Film.   Used as a baseline prior to initiation of chemotherapy.

Other
Bone Marrow Aspiration and Biopsy.   Evaluate for classification of disease by morphology, cytochemistry, cell membrane markers, cytogenetics, tumor doubling time, immunogloblin, and receptor rearrangement studies, and bcr/abl (in ALL and CML).

Lumbar Puncture.   Used to evaluate for leukemic infiltration. Also used to administer intrathecal chemotherapy.

ECG.   Used as a baseline prior to initiation of chemotherapy.

DIFFERENTIAL DIAGNOSIS

Traumatic
Ecchymosis.   Seen after trauma.

Infectious
Epstein-Barr Virus Infection.   May mimic leukemic process early in the disease with lymphadenopathy and lymphocytosis.

Cytomegalovirus Infection.   May show lymphocytosis.

Metabolic
Not applicable.

Neoplastic
Other Cancers.   May also infiltrate bone marrow. Differentiated on bone marrow aspirate.

Vascular
Not applicable.

Congenital
Genetic Abnormalities: Bloom syndrome, Fanconi congenital pancytopenia, Down syndrome.   Characterized by chromosome aberrations predisposing affected patients to leukemia.

Acquired
Not applicable.

TREATMENT

The chemotherapeutic agent used is dependent on the specific leukemic type. Most regimens include an induction phase followed by postremission chemotherapy.

Acute Lymphoblastic Leukemia

ALL is an acute leukemia affecting mainly the lymphocytic cell lines. Eighty percent of ALL cases occur in children. The peak incidence is between 3 and 4 years of age. Incidence declines after age 9, and ALL is rare after age 40. There is an increased incidence in males.

As with all leukemia, treatment and prognosis depend on presence or absence of cell markers and cytogenetics. A younger patient who presents with a low WBC count, achieves a complete remission (CR) after induction chemotherapy, and who lacks unfavorable cytogenetic aberrations has the best prognosis.

Ninety percent of children with ALL achieve a CR after therapy, and 60% to 70% achieve a cure. Results are less favorable in adults, with a CR rate of 75% and cure rate of 30% to 40%.

In ALL leukemia patients who fail to obtain a remission after induction chemotherapy or who relapse with chemoresistant disease, allogeneic bone marrow transplantation is the only treatment option, resulting in a cure rate of 10% to 20%. Certain patients with unfavorable cell markers or cytogenetic features fare better with allogeneic transplantation after first remission and before the expected relapse occurs.

ALL leukemia is classified on the basis of cell morphology and cell surface markers. Cytogenetics also plays a role in classification, particularly of very early cell types. Less mature cell lines have fewer surface markers and less cellular differentiation and are associated with a worse prognosis.

Acute leukemia is classified within the French-American-British (FAB) system. ALL receives a classification of L1, L2, or L3, depending on the foregoing characteristics. L1 has more differentiation and a better prognosis.

Acute Myelogenous Leukemia

AML is an acute leukemia affecting mainly the myeloid cell lines. In some types of AML, the genetic defect results in a maturation problem, with very early precursor cells affecting maturation of granulocytes, erythrocytes, and/or thrombocytes.

Unlike ALL, AML generally affects adults. The incidence increases with age, with a median of 60 years.

AML is also classified within the FAB system with designations from M0 to M7. M0 through M3 show increasing levels of maturation. M4 and M5 have some monocytic characteristics. M6 demonstrates erythroid differentiation, and M7 is thrombocytic. M3 through M5 also have subtypes.

Chronic Myelogenous Leukemia

CML is characterized by overproduction of myeloid cells. These cells accumulate in the peripheral circulation, resulting in splenomegaly and markedly elevated white blood cell (WBC) counts. Most of the cells will exhibit mature morphologic characteristics. Occasional immature forms may be seen. Due to normal cellular function, patients are generally not immunocompromised as they are in acute leukemia.

Owing to the initial maturity of the cell line, these patients may live for several years with minimal chemotherapy to reduce the WBC count to safe levels. However, eventually the cell line will become unstable and the patient will "blast off" into acute disease. For treatment purposes, the leukemic process then is considered acute.

Chronic Lymphocytic Leukemia

CLL is a chronic B cell disorder characterized by proliferation and accumulation of normal-appearing lymphocytes. The overproduction/accumulation results in splenomegaly and lymphadenopathy. Bone marrow biopsy reveals a predominance of lymphoid cells.

Many patients are asymptomatic and CLL is diagnosed when lymphocytosis is noted in a complete blood count performed for another reason. Autoimmune hemolytic anemia or thrombocytosis may be present.

Massive lymphadenopathy may result in a clinical presentation with obstructive symptoms secondary to compression.

Usually manifests with WBC count of 40 to 150,000/mm^3. May be mistaken for lymphocytosis associated with mononucleosis, cytomegalovirus or other infection. These infections do not generally produce lymphocytosis to this degree.

CLL is incurable with available therapeutic options. Treatment modalities include radiation for bulky adenopathy and chemotherapy including prednisone. Chemotherapy is generally withheld until patients develop progressive symptoms, bone marrow failure, or autoimmune disorders. Efficacy of bone marrow transplantation is still being evaluated.

PEDIATRIC CONSIDERATIONS

ALL in children can mimic many other diseases including brain tumors, nephritis, and carditis. The goal of therapy in childhood ALL is cure. Meningeal and testicular lesions must be considered in this group of patients and are treated with intrathecal chemotherapy and testicular irradiation. Growth potential and secondary sexual development are important long-term considerations in planning therapy and follow-up.

AML is seen in about 20% of children who develop leukemia without specific predilection for age group or gender. Morphology is similar to that in adult AML. Chemotherapy is similar to that recommended for adults. Children have improved survival over adults with this form of disease.

OBSTETRIC CONSIDERATIONS

Acute leukemia has been found to be rapidly fatal in pregnant women, although combination chemotherapy has produced remissions. Chemotherapy should be used despite potential fetal adverse effects. The course of the pregnancy, labor, and delivery is unaltered except for the effect of the leukemia on the general health of the mother.

Chronic leukemia affects pregnancy through the effects of the leukemia on the mother's well-being. Fetal demise correlates with maternal mortality from the leukemia. The disease itself is not adversely affected by the pregnancy. CML is the most common form of chronic leukemia seen in pregnancy. Again, chemotherapy should not be withheld if the disease course is progressing rapidly.

GERIATRIC CONSIDERATIONS

Leukemia is seen in all age groups. Vigilance is important in the elderly. The patient's overall health and performance status are important considerations in therapeutic decisions.

PREVENTIVE CONSIDERATIONS

Avoidance of known contributing factors such as ionizing radiation in doses above 100 Gy and benzene and alkylating agent exposure is important.

PEARLS FOR THE PA

Leukemia is heterogeneous in nature and carries different prognoses depending on the type of disease, patient's age, and other factors.

In childhood leukemia, the goal is cure with chemotherapy and maintenance of near-normal growth and development.

Bone marrow transplantation may offer cure to some groups of patients depending on age and type of disease.

Erythropoietin is contraindicated for anemic patients who have a myeloid leukemia!

Liver Cancer

Charles W. Reed, MEd, MPAS, PA-C

DEFINITION

Hepatocellular carcinoma (HCC) is a common cause of cancer death throughout the world, particularly in Africa and Asia. It is less common in people of Germanic origin.

HISTORY

Symptoms. The most common presenting complaint is right upper quadrant (RUQ) abdominal pain or right shoulder pain from phrenic nerve irritation. Standard neoplastic symptoms of fatigue, anorexia, weight loss, and unexplained fever are present approximately in 30% of cases.

General. Obtain a detailed past history with emphasis on alcohol use, history of hepatitis, medication use, and diabetes.

Age. HCC is rare before the fourth decade of life.

Onset. Months to years.

Duration. The 5-year survival rate for patients with a solitary focus is 45%.

Intensity. Rapidly fatal disease is usually secondary to acute liver failure aggravated by the underlying cirrhosis.

Aggravating Factors. Continued alcohol use.

Alleviating Factors. None.

Associated Factors. Several factors have been implicated as predisposing to HCC. These include hepatitis B virus (HBV) infection, cirrhosis, hepatitis C virus (HCV) infection, aflatoxins, oral contraceptives, anabolic steroids, smoking, alcohol abuse, diabetes, and insulin use.

PHYSICAL EXAMINATION

General. Note any evidence of malnutrition, gynecomastia, cachexia, fever, or jaundice.

Abdomen. Other physical findings in the abdomen may include RUQ tenderness, hepatomegaly, splenomegaly, ascites, or hepatic bruit.

PATHOPHYSIOLOGY

HCC may occur as a solitary lesion (massive), multiple nodules (nodular), or diffuse involvement.

DIAGNOSTIC STUDIES

Laboratory
Liver Function Tests. Levels may or may not be abnormal and offer no real differentiating value. HCC patients with elevated bilirubin and lactate dehydrogenase (LDH) accompanied by a decreased serum albumin often have a poorer prognosis.

Serum α-Fetoprotein (AFP). Elevated in HCC patients but may also be elevated in cirrhosis. Levels are often much higher in HCC. It is also a useful gauge for treatment effectiveness and to follow chronic cirrhosis. Sudden increases in α-FP in patients with cirrhosis may indicate transformation to HCC.

Radiology
Ultrasound Examination. A useful and inexpensive tool in the evaluation of HCC. HCC lesions are usually readily demonstrated on ultrasound studies. CT is superior to ultrasound, and MRI is superior to CT.

Other
Gallium Scans. May be useful in determining whether a liver mass is primary or metastatic. HCC cells take up gallium.

DIFFERENTIAL DIAGNOSIS

Traumatic. Not applicable.

Infectious
Fungal Infection. May appear with intrahepatic nodular densities. Rarely seen in a patient with an intact immune system. The usual culprit is *Aspergillus* spp.

Hepatitis. Differentiated on hepatitis profiles.

Metabolic. Not applicable.

Neoplastic
Liver Cell Adenoma. Although these tumors are often symptomatic, they are rarely malignant and not associated with cirrhosis.

Focal Nodular Hyperplasia (FNH). Nodular tumors without malignant potential. Rarely symptomatic.

Bile Duct Adenoma. Low malignant potential; usually small, single lesions.

Biliary Cystadenoma/Cystadenocarcinoma. Cystic lesions within the biliary system with some malignant potential.

Bile Duct Carcinoma. Less common than HCC, with no relation to cirrhosis.

Vascular. Not applicable.
Congenital. Not applicable.
Acquired. Not applicable.

TREATMENT

Resectable HCC
In most cases, HCC is not resectable. Even when it is resectable, the underlying cirrhosis negatively affects the prognosis. Lobar resection is preferred when possible.

Nonresectable Localized HCC
Localized nonresectable disease can be treated with combination therapy to include external-beam radiation therapy combined with chemotherapy. The chemotherapeutic regimen of choice is doxorubicin with 5-fluorouracil (5-FU). This is occasionally combined with radiolabeled polyclonal antiferritin immunoglobulin conjugate.

Transcatheter arterial embolization (TAE) has also been used in non-resectable localized HCC.

Percutaneous intralesional injection of absolute ethanol has had excellent results in a small group of select patients.

Nonresectable Metastatic HCC
Tamoxifen has been used without much success. Recombinant interferon α-2a has been used in some studies with success. The doses required are associated with significant side effects.

Systemic chemotherapy has a poor response rate in this patient population. When chemotherapy is used, doxorubicin is the agent most often used, as a single agent or in combination.

PEDIATRIC CONSIDERATIONS

None.

OBSTETRIC CONSIDERATIONS

None.

GERIATRIC CONSIDERATIONS

This is the age group most commonly affected. Monitoring serum α-FP in known alcohol abusers may help identify oncologic changes earlier in the disease course. A single, random α-FP assay is probably not beneficial.

PREVENTIVE CONSIDERATIONS

Alpha interferon monotherapy appears to delay or may prevent subsequent development of HCC in patients with either hepatitis B virus (HBV) or hepatitis C virus (HCV) infection. The benefit seems greatest in the HCV patient group.

Moderating alcohol intake would have a positive impact.

PEARLS FOR THE PA

Many patients with hepatocellular carcinoma have vague abdominal discomfort, subjective complaints of fever, and anorexia for up to 2 years before diagnosis.

Never assume a "chronic complainer" deserves no further medical investigation.

Lung Cancer

Charles W. Reed, MEd, MPAS, PA-C

DEFINITION

Carcinoma arising from the endobronchial epithelium, which can lead to metastatic disease.

HISTORY

Symptoms. Rarely asymptomatic. Symptoms are usually related to the location in the tracheobronchial tree. Early, mild pulmonary symptoms include cough and sputum production.

General. Often regional spread of disease to adjacent structures.

Age. Incidence increases with advancing age.

Onset. The latent period prior to clinical disease is prolonged and probably extends over years.

Duration. Relatively rapid course, with non–small cell lung cancers having a slightly more indolent course compared with small cell lung cancer.

Intensity. Once lesion has metastasized, symptoms are rapidly progressive.

Aggravating Factors. Smoking of tobacco products, persistent exposure to pulmonary irritants.

Alleviating Factors. Not applicable.

Associated Factors. Exposure to industrial substances (e.g., arsenic, asbestos, organic compounds), radiation exposure from occupational, medical, and environmental sources. Residential radon exposure may be of increased risk in cigarette smokers. Exposure to second-hand smoke increases the risk in nonsmokers.

PHYSICAL EXAMINATION

General. Observe the patient for evidence of shortness of breath, weight loss, and/or pale appearance suggesting anemia. A full physical examination is performed, paying attention to potential paraneoplastic syndromes from neuroendocrine secretion of hormones from the tumor (e.g., moon facies, buffalo hump, Cushing syndrome).

Cardiovascular. Facial and upper extremity edema may be present with superior vena cava (SVC) syndrome. SVC is a result of blood flow obstruction through the superior vena cava by a pulmonary or mediastial mass. Auscultate and evaluate pulse for arrhythmia. Pulmonary rales may be present with congestive heart failure. Pericardial friction rub may be present with pericardial effusion due to cardiac spread of tumor.

Gastrointestinal. Hepatomegaly may be present with hepatic involvement or right-sided heart failure.

Neurologic. Hoarseness may be present as a result of vocal cord paralysis. Dysphagia may be a complaint, owing to left recurrent laryngeal nerve damage. Phrenic nerve involvement can manifest with cough, dyspnea, and diaphragmatic paralysis. Brachial plexus involvement with arm pain and vasomotor signs. Other neurologic deficits may include symptoms and signs of increased intracranial pressure (papilledema, headache, nausea and vomiting, focal deficits such as hemiparesis or hemisensory loss, dysequilibrium) due to cerebral metastasis. Spinal cord compression due to tumor (direct compression, meningeal or vascular involvement) may manifest with back pain and progressive extremity paralysis.

Ophthalmologic. Horner syndrome (enophthalmos, ptosis, meiosis) may be present owing to interruption of the cervical sympathetic chain from tumor spread.

Pulmonary. Auscultate for decreased breath sounds, rales, or rhonchi, which may suggest atelectasis, pneumonia, or pleural disease. Percuss to evaluate for pleural effusions or masses.

PATHOPHYSIOLOGY

A morphologic chain of events has been linked to squamous cell lung cancer, and a similar sequence is presumed for small cell lung cancer. This sequence involves damage to the tracheobronchial epithelium from a variety of causes including cigarette smoking. The basal epithelial cell proliferates, decreasing the number of ciliated cells. Goblet cells that secrete viscid mucus are thus increased. Prolonged injury allows further disorganization of the epithelial cells, particularly in the basal areas of the mucosa. This process leads to the development of carcinoma.

Eighty-five percent of lung cancers are non–small cell lung cancer, which includes squamous cell, adenocarcinoma, and large cell carcinoma. Therapy in these types of cancers is similar. In 15% of lung cancers, the histologic subtype is small cell carcinoma (oat cell carcinoma), which differs from other lung cancers in natural history, cell biology, and therapeutic response. It is distinct in its rapidly fatal course and propensity for widespread metastases. Small cell lung cancer also exhibits amine precursor uptake and decarboxylation, resulting in hormone secretion and paraneoplastic syndromes such as Cushing syndrome and syndrome of inappropriate antidiuretic hormone secretion (SIADH).

DIAGNOSTIC STUDIES

Laboratory
Complete Blood Count.   Evaluate for anemia and use as a baseline prior to starting chemotherapy.

Chemistry Profile.   Hepatic abnormalities may be seen with metastases. Bone and calcium metabolism may be abnormal owing to bone destruction from metastases. SIADH (hyponatremia) may be present with renal abnormalities.

Radiology
Chest Film.   Evaluate for the presence or extent of pulmonary involvement as well as mediastinal widening suggesting regional spread of disease. Pneumonia may be present.

CT Scan of Chest and Abdomen.   As indicated to evaluate the extent of disease and for selecting radiation ports when planning radiotherapy.

CT/MRI of Brain, Bone, or Liver.   As indicated by the history to evaluate for metastases.

Positron Emission Tomography (PET) Scan.   Used to assess the extent of tumor spread and for staging.

Other
Bone Marrow Aspiration and Biopsy.   This is part of the standard evaluation in SCLC, because of a high incidence of metastases to bone marrow. It is usually not necessary in the evaluation in NSCLC.

ECG.   Used to evaluate for arrhythmias or other abnormalities prior to initiation of medical or surgical therapy.

Pulmonary Function Tests.   Evaluate baseline function prior to surgery or radiotherapy.

Fine Needle Aspiration.   Used to obtain tissue for diagnosis. If diagnosis is not secured, thoracotomy is often necessary.

Bronchoscopy.   Used to evaluate tissue for diagnosis. If diagnosis is not secured, thoracotomy is often necessary.

DIFFERENTIAL DIAGNOSIS

Traumatic
Hematoma.   Following chest trauma. Positive history.

Infectious
Granulomatous Disease. May produce solitary nodules.
Fungal Infections. May manifest with discrete lesions.

Neoplastic
Secondary Tumors. Lymphoma, breast cancer, melanoma, colon cancer, and others may result in lung involvement. These are best differentiated by history of other primary tumors, histology, and presenting symptoms.

Vascular
Pulmonary Embolus. May cause shortness of breath; differentiated on radiographs (ventilation-perfusion scan positive).

Metabolic. Not applicable.
Congenital. Not applicable.
Acquired. Not applicable.

TREATMENT

Treatment is based on the site of disease, the cell type involved, and extent of regional spread or distant metastases, as well as the patient's level of function and underlying medical conditions. Staging is used to evaluate spread of disease in order to select treatments and formulate a prognosis. The site, size, cell type, and anatomic spread of the primary tumor are established. This can be accomplished by clinical, surgical, and pathologic methods throughout the clinical course.

The tumor-node-metastasis (TNM) system is used for staging.

Non–Small Cell Lung Cancers
Surgical resection is the treatment of choice for patients with stage I or II disease. Solitary extrapulmonary masses also require biopsy to determine whether the lesion is metastatic or a benign mass. This distinction is very important to accurate staging and treatment. If the patient is not a surgical candidate, then radiotherapy or chemotherapy may be employed. Stage III disease cannot generally be cured with resection alone. Ongoing clinical trials of adjuvant chemotherapy followed by radiotherapy appear promising, but larger, randomized trials are needed to fully assess long-term survival. Combination chemotherapy does not appear to offer improvement in survival of patients with disseminated disease. Radiotherapy plays a role in offering palliative relief of specific symptoms.

Signs associated with a poor prognosis include but are not limited to loss of greater than 5% of body weight, metastasis, malignant pleural effusion, SVC syndrome, and poor performance status.

Small Cell Lung Cancer
Small cell lung cancer is somewhat sensitive to combination chemotherapy. Although cisplatin and etoposide are often used, new drugs and combina-

tions are evaluated continuously. The average length of survival may be 1 year or more with this therapy, whereas before the advent of combination chemotherapy, the average length of survival was less than 4 months. SCLC has a predilection for brain metastasis. For patients with resectable disease, chemotherapy combined with thoracic radiotherapy and prophylactic cranial irradiation (PCI) has been shown to offer a 5% survival benefit. Palliative radiotherapy may be given in relapsed disease, but chemotherapy does not appear to be beneficial in these cases.

PEDIATRIC CONSIDERATIONS

True carcinoma of the lung is exceedingly rare in childhood. Metastatic lesions, such as Wilms tumor, osteogenic sarcoma, and hepatoblastoma, are the most common forms of pulmonary malignancy in children. Anticipatory guidance given to young children and adolescents should always include serious warnings about the dangers of smoking.

OBSTETRIC CONSIDERATIONS

Antineoplastic medications may pose grave risks to the fetus. However, their use is recommended if absolutely needed during pregnancy.

GERIATRIC CONSIDERATIONS

The risk of lung cancer increases with the amount of "pack years" a patient smokes. Lung cancer often occurs in the geriatric age group.

PREVENTIVE CONSIDERATIONS

Public education about the dangers of smoking is critical. Individual counseling for patients who smoke should be provided, as well as materials and referral to programs the patient needs for success. If possible, procure the aid of family and friends.

PEARLS FOR THE PA

The role of second-hand smoke in the etiology of lung cancer is important to discuss with patients.

Lymphoma

Charles W. Reed, MEd, MPAS, PA-C

DEFINITION

A heterogeneous group of neoplasms whose origin is in the lymphoreticular system.

HISTORY

Symptoms. Usually manifests with asymptomatic lymphadenopathy. Unexplained fevers, night sweats, weight loss, and fatigue (B symptoms) may be present.

General. Commonly, disease has already spread to extranodal sites at the time of diagnosis. Men and women are generally affected equally.

Age. Encompasses all age groups. Several types are more common in children and young adults, but most cases are seen in the 40- to 70-year range.

Onset. In low-grade lymphomas, slow and progressive. In intermediate- and high-grade lymphomas, a more aggressive course is noted, with survival of 12 to 18 months without treatment.

Duration. May have unapparent disease for many years or may have a more aggressive course.

Intensity. Initially asymptomatic or mild.

Aggravating Factors. None known.

Alleviating Factors. None known.

Associated Factors. Patients with congenital or acquired immunodeficiency states have an increased risk for the development of non-Hodgkin lymphoma. This pattern may also be seen in autoimmune disorders following renal, cardiac, and bone marrow transplantation. Environmental exposure has also been implicated.

PHYSICAL EXAMINATION

General. Characteristic B symptoms should be sought (weight loss, fever, fatigue, night sweats).

Gastrointestinal. Size of liver and spleen should be evaluated, as organomegaly may be present.

Head, Eyes, Ears, Nose, Throat. Waldeyer's (lymphatic [tonsillar] tissue that encircles the oropharynx and nasopharynx) ring should be visualized both directly and indirectly.

Lymphatic. Close evaluation of all lymph node areas including size and consistency is important. Include anterior and posterior cervical, supraclavicular, axillary, epitrochlear, retroperitoneal, mesenteric, iliac, inguinal, and femoral nodes.

PATHOPHYSIOLOGY

In low-grade lymphomas, no clear etiologic factor can be identified in a majority of cases. New molecular studies have allowed further characterization of the lineage, clonality, and differentiation stage of lymphomas. The common translocation seen in low-grade lymphomas between chromosomes 14 and 18 (t14;18) places the *bcl-2* oncogene together with the immunoglobulin heavy chain–joining region, resulting in a protein known to inhibit programmed cell death (apoptosis).

In intermediate- and high-grade lymphomas, several immunologic, viral, or environmental factors may be implicated in their pathophysiology. Inherited immune disorders such as Wiskott-Aldrich syndrome and ataxia-telangiectasia carry a greatly increased risk of developing lymphoma. Acquired immunodeficiency also carries an increased risk for the development of lymphoma whether related to human immunodeficiency virus (HIV) infection or iatrogenic immunosuppression such as that seen following organ transplantation. Viruses have been implicated in two human lymphomas: adult T cell lymphoma and Burkitt lymphoma. HTLV-1 has been found to be endemic in some areas, and antibodies to this virus have been found in adult T cell lymphoma. Epstein-Barr virus has been associated with endemic Burkitt lymphoma, especially in Africa. Environmental factors also may play a role in the development of lymphoma, such as radiation exposure, exposure to vinyl chloride, rubber processing, and farming.

DIAGNOSTIC STUDIES

Laboratory
Complete Blood Count. Used to evaluate for anemia and marrow involvement, and as a baseline prior to initiation of chemotherapy or radiotherapy.

Comprehensive Serum Chemistry Profile. Evaluate for hepatic, calcium, or alkaline phosphatase changes as well as for baseline studies. Serum gamma-glutamyltransferase may be elevated in some patients and may be used as a marker of disease.

β_2-Microglobulin. Elevations correlate with tumor burden.

Renal Function Tests. Evaluate for baseline if any metastatic disease is present.

Radiology
Chest Film. Evaluate for intrathoracic disease.

CT Scans. Include chest, abdomen, and pelvis to evaluate for occult disease.

Bipedal Lymphangiography. Can differentiate abnormal lymph nodes not well visualized on CT.

Gastrointestinal Studies. Indicated in patient with Waldeyer's ring disease or when evidence of gastrointestinal disease is present on CT.

Other
Bone Marrow Aspiration and Biopsy. Bilateral evaluations at the time of diagnosis are important. Histology, cytogenetics, immunophenotyping, flow cytometry, DNA analysis, and gene rearrangement studies should be performed.

Lumbar Puncture. Indicated in all patients with lymphoblastic lymphomas and small non–cleaved cell lymphomas as well as in those with neurologic abnormalities.

Pulmonary Function Tests. Evaluate as a baseline prior to beginning chemotherapy or radiotherapy, especially in bleomycin- or doxorubicin-containing regimens.

Liver Biopsy. Indicated only if results would change stage of disease or if there is possibility of hepatic involvement.

Staging Laparotomy. Indicated only in low-grade disease when radiotherapy is the only planned therapy.

DIFFERENTIAL DIAGNOSIS

Traumatic
Hematoma. In nodal site. Usually a history of trauma.

Infectious
Cat-Scratch Fever. Typical finding is solitary enlarged, painful lymph node.

Granulomatous Disease. May manifest with adenopathy and chest abnormalities.

Metabolic. Not applicable.

Neoplastic
Solitary Solid Tumors. May exhibit adenopathy and B symptoms.

Vascular. Not applicable.
Congenital. Not applicable.
Acquired. Not applicable.

TREATMENT

Treatment is dependent on the stage and classification of histologic subtype. Generalizations regarding therapy are difficult owing to the heterogeneous patient population and variables such as stage, histologic subtype, patient age, extent of disease, and underlying medical conditions.

The Ann Arbor system is used for staging both Hodgkin and non-Hodgkin lymphomas; however, owing to the plethora of non-Hodgkin subtypes, the disease course and prognosis are less dependent on stage than on tumor bulk and cytologic subtype.

Low-grade lymphomas, although indolent, cannot be cured with current therapies. Nevertheless, many patients survive 6 to 10 years following diagnosis. In comparison, intermediate-and high-grade lymphomas, although more aggressive, have a potential for cure with combination chemotherapy.

Bone marrow transplantation may be used in selected patients such as those younger than 60 years of age, those who have intermediate- or high-grade lymphomas, and those with a poor prognosis but a partial response to initial therapy. The 60-year age limit is flexible depending on the patient's overall health and functional status. Allogeneic or stem cell transplantation should be considered a last resort. However nonmyeloablative chemotherapy regimens with stem cell support (mini-transplants) are under investigation.

Several monoclonal antibody treatments are also currently under evaluation.

PEDIATRIC CONSIDERATIONS

Toxic effects of radiation therapy and/or chemotherapy in the pediatric population can cause retardation or suppression of bone growth. These treatments also generate significant potential for secondary malignant tumors. Because of the rapid progression of the underlying disease, there is a crucial need for rapid diagnosis and appropriate treatment. Treatment should be administered at a major pediatric treatment facility.

OBSTETRIC CONSIDERATIONS

The most common type of lymphoma that occurs during pregnancy is Hodgkin disease. There are no known adverse affects on maternal or fetal outcome when the mother has Hodgkin disease. However, the use of radiation therapy or chemotherapy can affect the pregnancy. A pelvic shield should be used during radiation therapy, and chemotherapy is considered relatively safe for use if instituted during the second or third trimester. If therapeutic radiation exposure occurs early in the pregnancy, abortion is recommended. (See "Hodgkin Disease" earlier in this chapter.)

GERIATRIC CONSIDERATIONS

Small lymphocytic lymphoma is seen in the elderly.

PREVENTIVE CONSIDERATIONS

None specific.

PEARLS FOR THE PA

Survival rates for patients with lymphoma vary owing to the heterogeneous nature of the disease.

Overall survival rates have improved over the past three decades with newer therapies.

Low-grade lymphoma, although indolent in nature, is not curable with current therapies.

Intermediate-and high-grade lymphomas, although aggressive in nature, respond well to treatment, and cure may be achieved.

Malignant Melanoma

Charles W. Reed, MEd, MPAS, PA-C

DEFINITION

Lesion resulting from the neoplastic transformation of melanocytes that are of neural crest origin.

HISTORY

Symptoms.   Pigmented skin lesions that have changes in color or size, or that begin to itch or bleed spontaneously.

General.   Ascertain a history, occupational or otherwise, of prolonged sunlight or ultraviolet ray (tanning booth) exposure.

Age.   Median age at diagnosis is the mid-40s.

Onset.   Months to years.

Duration.   Slow and progressive growth.

Intensity.   The patient may only notice changes in skin without any other symptoms.

Aggravating Factors.   Overexposure to sunlight, especially intermittent overexposure early in life, is more important than cumulative exposure time.

Alleviating Factors.   Limit exposure to sunlight; early detection improves overall survival.

Associated Factors.   Phenotypic factors associated with melanoma include light skin color; blond or red hair; blue, green, or gray eyes; and family history of melanoma.

PHYSICAL EXAMINATION

General. Evaluate for lymphadenopathy.

Skin. Evaluate all areas of the skin, including palms and soles of feet. Evaluate for changes in nevi. Scales and bleeding lesions are of special concern. Scalloped or notched borders as well as color variegation may be seen. Pigmented lesions of the nail bed, especially of the great toe or thumb, are suspicious for malignant melanoma.

Eyes. Evaluate for presence of choroidal melanoma.

PATHOPHYSIOLOGY

Melanocytes reside in the basal layer of the epidermis and synthesize melanin. Melanin is important in protecting against DNA damage from ultraviolet rays. Neoplastic transformation occurs in these cells, and they are able to produce their own growth factors, with subsequent autonomous growth.

The following four patterns are noted in malignant melanoma:

1. The most common type, occurring in 70% of melanomas, is the superficial spreading pattern. It is usually a flat lesion with pigmented and nonpigmented layers.
2. Nodular melanoma occurs in 15% to 30% of cases. It is usually deeply pigmented (bluish black) and raised. It is most common in men and is more aggressive and fast-growing than the superficial spreading type.
3. Lentigo maligna melanoma is seen in 5% to 10% of melanomas and is usually a facial or neck lesion in older light-skinned patients. It carries a low risk of metastasis.
4. The acral lentiginous type is seen on the palms, soles, and nail beds. It is a rare type, occurring in only 2% to 8% of light-skinned patients with melanoma and in 35% to 60% of dark-skinned patients. Ulceration is commonly observed with this type of melanoma.

DIAGNOSTIC STUDIES

Laboratory
Complete Blood Count. Used as a baseline prior to therapy.
Chemistry Profile. Used as a baseline prior to therapy.

Radiology
CT/MRI. Studies of selected body parts to evaluate for metastasis

Other
Elliptical Excisional Biopsy. At least a 2-mm margin of normal tissue is necessary for diagnostic purposes. Incisional or punch biopsies should be

used only when the anatomic location or lesion so dictates (e.g., facial lesions).

DIFFERENTIAL DIAGNOSIS

Traumatic
Local Trauma. May cause bleeding, bruising, or petechiae. Usually a history of trauma. Will resolve spontaneously.

Infectious
Lesions Associated with an Illness. May be bacterial, such as meningococcal disease in immunocompromised patient, or associated with a viral illness. Lesion subsides with resolution of the illness.

Metabolic
Thyroid Disease, Hypercholesterolemia, Hypertriglyceridemia. May cause macular or lipemic lesions.

Neoplastic
Kaposi Sarcoma, Cutaneous T Cell Lymphomas, Basal Cell Carcinomas. Differentiated on biopsy.

Vascular
Petechiae, Hemangiomata. May bleed. No change in size over time.

Congenital
Café-au-Lait Spots, Hemangiomata. May bleed. No change in size over time.

Acquired
Tattooed Areas. History of tattoo.

TREATMENT

Several staging methods are used, but the American Joint Commitee on Cancer (AJCC) system has grown in popularity because of its simplicity (see Table 11-2).

For excision, the following criteria apply:

Stage IB to early IIA: Excision of 2-mm or thinner lesion with narrow margin (1 cm).

Stage IIA, IIB: Excision of greater than 2-mm-thick lesion with wide margin (3 cm).

The role of elective lymph node dissection at diagnosis is under investigation and controversial at this time. Palpable nodes should be removed.

Traditional chemotherapy as an adjuvant to surgery has not proved to increase survival.

Table 11–2. AJCC Staging System for Melanoma

Stage	Criterion
IA	Localized melanoma <0.75 mm
IB	Localized melanoma 0.76-1.5 mm
IIA	Localized melanoma 1.5-4 mm
IIB	Localized melanoma >4 mm
III	Presence of regional lymph node(s) and/or in transit metastasis
IV	Presence of distant metastasis

AJCC, American Joint Committee on Cancer.

From Pazdur R: Medical Oncology: A Comprehensive Review. New York, PRR Huntington, 1993, with permission.

Interferon-α (IFN-α) has been shown to improve survival but is extremely toxic.

Interleukin-2 (IL-2) occasionally produces a remission and demonstrates a response rate of about 25%. It is extremely toxic and expensive. Both IFN-α and IL-2 are currently under investigation as to efficacy when combined with traditional cytotoxic drugs in a sequential fashion.

PEDIATRIC CONSIDERATIONS

The primary consideration is prevention with the use of sunscreens and limited exposure to sunlight.

OBSTETRIC CONSIDERATIONS

No specific considerations.

GERIATRIC CONSIDERATIONS

No specific considerations.

PREVENTIVE CONSIDERATIONS

Patient education about the potential harmful effects of sun exposure and thorough skin examination should be added to every health care maintenance program. Include explanation of proper use of sunscreens including the meaning of sun protection factor (SPF) numbers. All SPF numbers provide 100% UVA and UVB protection. However, the larger the number, the *longer* the protection lasts.

PEARLS FOR THE PA

Instructing patients about the risk of overexposure to sunlight is an important measure in the prevention of malignant melanoma.

Use of sunscreens should begin in infancy and continue throughout life.

To educate patients about the warning signs of melanoma, use the mnemonic ABCD:

Asymmetry

Border irregularity

Color

Diameter greater than 6 mm

Multiple Myeloma

Charles W. Reed, MEd, MPAS, PA-C

DEFINITION

A malignant proliferation of plasma cells.

HISTORY

Symptoms.   Presentation is variable but may include bone pain, fatigue, renal insufficiency, and infection.

General.   History of radiation exposure or occupational or chemical exposure (to benzenes, formaldehyde) may be elicited from the patient.

Age.   Median age at presentation is 60 years, and incidence increases with advancing age.

Onset.   Unknown, presumed to be over a period of months.

Duration.   Years.

Intensity.   The patient may have no symptoms or may be in severe pain, especially with bone involvement.

Aggravating Factors.   Infections and fractures.

Alleviating Factors.   Early diagnosis and appropriate treatment.

Associated Factors.   A racial difference is seen, with black patients being affected twice as often as whites. A suggestive association between radiation and the development of multiple myeloma is noted. Survivors of atomic bomb blasts had a 60% greater risk of developing the disease. Another potential factor is prolonged benzene exposure. No familial pattern has been established.

PHYSICAL EXAMINATION

General. The patient may appear drowsy or lethargic owing to hyperviscosity of blood. Perform a complete and thorough physical examination. Bones may be tender to palpation. Guarding may be noted on range of motion testing owing to bone pain.

Neurologic. Positive long-tract signs (e.g., Babinski sign, hyperreflexia) may be seen in cord compression. Sensory loss in a "stocking-glove" distribution may be noted with peripheral neuropathy.

PATHOPHYSIOLOGY

It is unclear whether the myeloma process is derived from a stem cell population or a more differentiated plasma cell. Frequent karyotypic abnormalities are seen, although none is specific to myeloma. Various cytokines are produced, which may act as myeloma or osteoclast growth factors. Hypercalcemia is present in up to 20% of patients owing to the production of an osteoclast-activating factor. Patients are at risk for life-threatening bacterial infections as the result of a deficiency of polyclonal immunoglobulins and complement activation defects. There is a monoclonal antibody spike, usually IgG or IgA.

DIAGNOSTIC STUDIES

Laboratory

Complete Blood Count. As indicated to evaluate for anemia and the degree of plasmacytosis. White blood cell (WBC) count elevated with infections.

Renal Function Tests. Elevated blood urea nitrogen (BUN) and creatinine with renal insufficiency.

Creatinine clearance. Used to rule out renal involvement, as a baseline prior to therapy.

Liver Function Tests. Used as a baseline prior to initiation of therapy.

Lactate Dehydrogenase (LDH). Elevated when there is damage to the kidneys, skeletal muscle, liver, heart, spleen, brain, or pancreas. Damage to these organs is associated with decreased survival.

Serum Albumin. Used to correct serum calcium.

Serum Calcium. May be elevated in 20% of patients. Calcium may approach life-threatening levels.

Urine Protein Electrophoresis. Used to evaluate the extent of disease activity.

Immunofixation. As indicated to evaluate the character and quality of monoclonal gammopathies. Can differentiate among polyclonal, monoclonal, and pseudomonoclonal conditions.

β_2-*Microglobulin.* Reflects the extent of disease.

Serum Immunoglobulin Levels. Involved immunoglobulin (either IgG, IgA, IgD, IgE, or kappa or lambda light chains) is elevated, with low levels of uninvolved immunoglobulins.

Radiology
Chest Film. Used to rule out bone disease or underlying pathology.

Complete Skeletal Survey. As indicated to evaluate for bone lesions.

MRI. Evaluation of affected areas for better detail.

Other
Bone Marrow Aspiration. Used to evaluate for plasmacytosis.

DIFFERENTIAL DIAGNOSIS

Traumatic
Solitary Bone Trauma. Usually history of traum to the site.

Infectious
Osteomyelitis. Bone destruction on radiograph, fever, elevated white blood cell count; may have a history of dental procedures, sepsis, or other contributory factor.

Metabolic. Not applicable.

Neoplastic
Metastatic Disease. Due to other causes. A primary lesion will usually be identified.

Vascular
Avascular Necrosis of the Femoral Head. Usually a unilateral and solitary lesion. May have a history of steroid use.

Congenital. Not applicable.

Acquired. Not applicable.

TREATMENT

Treatment includes management of specific complications (e.g., renal failure), radiotherapy to bony lesions, stabilization of humerus or femur fractures with intramedullary rods, and systemic chemotherapy. Prednisone and the alkylating agent melphalan are often used. Use of high-dose, myeloablative melphalan with total body irradiation (TBI) may give higher response rates but at risk of higher toxicity. Autologous stem cell transplantation is required for the myeloablative therapies and carries its own risks. Alpha interferon is being used for maintenance of remissions in select patients, particularly those with IgA paraproteins.

Long-term therapy with vitamin D, calcium, and fluorides may prevent fractures.

PEDIATRIC CONSIDERATIONS

Not applicable to the pediatric age group.

OBSTETRIC CONSIDERATIONS

No specific indications.

GERIATRIC CONSIDERATIONS

This is a disease of the elderly.

PREVENTIVE CONSIDERATIONS

Avoid known contributory factors such as exposure to benzene or prolonged radiation exposure.

PEARLS FOR THE PA

Increased susceptibility to life-threatening infections is a major problem in patients with multiple myeloma, and any infection should be treated aggressively.

Long-term treatment of bone disease with vitamin D, calcium, and fluorides may prevent fractures.

Oropharyngeal Cancer

Charles W. Reed, MEd, MPAS, PA-C

DEFINITION

Heterogeneous group of tumors involving the oropharynx. Natural history and etiology will be unique to each type.

HISTORY

Symptoms. Patient usually notices nonhealing ulcer or change in swallowing or voice character.

General. Obtain a full occupational history including materials that the patient routinely encounters and a social history including tobacco (smoking and spitting tobacco) and alcohol use. Male-to-female ratio is 2:1.

Age. Mean age at onset is 60 years.

Onset. Years.

Duration. Progressive neoplastic change from premalignant to malignant.

Intensity. Pain varies according to the site and extent of lesion.

Aggravating Factors. The primary cause of head and neck cancer is tobacco use.

Alleviating Factors. An inverse relationship between fruit and vegetable intake and head and neck cancer has been noted. Vitamin A and its derivatives decrease susceptibility of patients to develop head and neck cancers.

Associated Factors. Viral contribution to pathogenesis of head and neck cancers has been reported, especially Epstein-Barr virus (EBV), herpes simplex virus (HSV), and human papillomavirus (HPV). Other factors include stimulant use (betel and areca nuts, alcohol) and occupational exposure (nickel, chromium, woodworking, leatherworking, asbestos, and metal processing).

PHYSICAL EXAMINATION

General. The patient usually appears in no acute distress; may sound hoarse or be observed to have difficulty with oral secretions.

Head, Eyes, Ears, Nose, Throat. A complete visual oral inspection is mandated with specific attention paid to the tongue, base of the tongue, floor of mouth, and posterior pharyngeal space, especially the areas in contact with tobacco. Leukoplakia, a localized white film, may be present, suggesting a premalignant state.

Lymphatic. Examine for any lymphadenopathy of the pre-and postauricular, submaxillary, submental, midjugular, and anteroscalene as well as deep cervical and supraclavicular nodes.

PATHOPHYSIOLOGY

Ninety-five percent of head and neck cancers are of the squamous cell type. The remaining 5% include sarcoma, lymphoma, and melanoma. Squamous cell tumors may be categorized as well differentiated, moderately well differentiated, poorly differentiated, and undifferentiated. Oral cavity lesions are usually seen on the lateral and ventral surfaces of the tongue as well as on the floor of the mouth. One-third of these patients have nodal metastases at diagnosis. The oropharyngeal lesions are commonly encountered at the base of the tongue and tonsils and usually appear as advanced disease. Tumors of the pharyngeal spaces are mostly advanced at the time of diagnosis.

The larynx is the most frequent site in head and neck cancers.

Nasopharyngeal tumors are aggressive and usually asymptomatic.

DIAGNOSTIC STUDIES

Laboratory
Complete Blood Count.   Used as a baseline prior to initiation of therapy.
Chemistry Panel.   Used as a baseline prior to initiation of therapy.
EBV Antibody Titers.   As indicated to rule out mononucleosis as a cause for head and neck lymphadenopathy.

Radiology
MRI or CT Scans of the Head, Neck, and Sinuses.   As indicated to rule out cancer or to evaluate the location and extent of the tumor.
Endoscopy, Bronchoscopy and Direct Laryngoscopy.   Performed to stage and evaluate for synchronous malignancies. Synchronous malignancies are present in 10% of cases.
Chest Film.   Used to rule out metastatic spread to the lungs or pneumonia from aspiration.

Other
Pulmonary Function Tests.   Performed in patient scheduled to undergo partial laryngectomy.

DIFFERENTIAL DIAGNOSIS

Traumatic
Intraoral Trauma.   May cause lesions. Usually a history of trauma; will resolve spontaneously.

Infectious
Candidal and Herpetic Infections.   May cause intraoral lesions. Duration, appearance and, recurrence differ.
Otitis Media.   May cause otalgia. Tympanic membrane will be erythematous; condition will usually respond to antibiotic therapy. Note that unilateral serous otitis media is a sign of ear-nose-throat (ENT) cancer.

Metabolic.   Not applicable

Neoplastic
Leukemia, Lymphoma, Melanoma, or Sarcoma.   Will cause lymphadenopathy. Lymphoma may occur in the oropharynx, especially in the posterior pharynx, owing to the presence of lymphoid tissue.

Vascular.   Not applicable.
Congenital.   Not applicable.

Acquired
Mucoceles.   May mimic suspicious intraoral lesions.

TREATMENT

Treatment of any head and neck cancer should be multidisciplinary including surgery (ENT), radiation oncology, medical oncology, and dentistry/oral surgery.

Surgery/External Beam Irradiation/Chemotherapy.   To excise the tumor in situ, perform a wide excision or radical dissection. Adjunctive radiotherapy is used in treating stage III or IV disease. Chemotherapy may be used in some patients to preserve organ function (larynx, tongue, mandible).

Dental Evaluation.   For removal of nonsalvageable teeth prior to radiotherapy.

Nutritional Assessment.   Indicated to maintain good nutritional intake, as well as hydration.

Other.   Presurgery evaluation by maxillofacial prosthodontia for appliance fitting and other considerations.

PEDIATRIC CONSIDERATIONS

Rare in children. Malignant lesions in the oral cavity are most likely to be sarcomas. Mucoepidermoid carcinoma is a malignant tumor of the salivary glands (most frequently the parotids) and is found primarily during the second decade of life.

OBSTETRIC CONSIDERATIONS

No specific indications.

GERIATRIC CONSIDERATIONS

None specific.

PREVENTIVE CONSIDERATIONS

Avoidance of tobacco products and chronic alcohol use would almost eliminate these cancers. Patient education is an important part of any preventive medicine program. "Spit tobacco" or snuff is not a safe alternative to smoking. In fact, the nicotine content of a can of snuff may be equivalent to that in 4 to 6 packs of cigarettes.

PEARLS FOR THE PA

Oropharyngeal cancer is preventable through patient aware-ness, education, and avoidance of carcinogenic substances (tobacco, both smoking and chewing, and alcohol).

Optimal survival is dependent on early identification of the pri-mary site and treatment of any metastases.

Ovarian Cancer

Charles W. Reed, MEd, MPAS, PA-C

DEFINITION

Ovarian cancer is the leading cause of death from gynecologic malignancies. Most cancers are epithelial in origin, accounting for more than 90% of all ovarian malignancies.

HISTORY

Symptoms.   Symptoms are often absent until disease progression with metastases has occurred. When noted, they consist of vague pelvic or abdominal complaints. Most patients at diagnosis have stage III disease.

General.   From 75% to 85% of women have abdominal disease at the time of diagnosis.

Age.   Average age at diagnosis is 55 years, and ovarian cancer is rarely seen before the age of 40.

Onset.   Unknown, but probably months to years.

Duration.   Women with stage IA disease have 5-year survival rates of more than 80%, compared with survival rates of 25% to 30% in those with more advanced disease (stage III or IV).

Intensity.   The patient may be asymptomatic or have only nonspecific complaints of vague pelvic or abdominal discomfort.

Aggravating Factors.   None.

Alleviating Factors.   With every year of oral contraceptive use there is a 10% decreased risk of disease. With each birth there is a decreased risk of 13% to 19%.

Associated Factors.   Residents of industrialized nations and those with a diet high in animal fats have an increased risk of ovarian cancer.

Familial ovarian cancers have been seen in some groups. Women in these groups tend to have bilateral disease and present at an earlier age. The familial factor appears to be an autosomal dominant trait with variable penetration. Women with more than one first-degree relative with ovarian cancer have a 50% chance of also developing the disease. Also, those who carry the *BRCA1* or *BRCA2* gene have a higher incidence.

PHYSICAL EXAMINATION

General.   The patient usually presents in no acute distress.

Gastrointestinal.   Palpate for omental mass.

Gynecologic.   Unilateral or bilateral ovarian enlargement is felt on bimanual examination. Pelvic mass may be palpated.

Pulmonary.   Auscultate for decreased breath sounds or pleural friction rub that may be encountered with a pleural effusion.

PATHOPHYSIOLOGY

Most tumors are of epithelial origin. A small percentage of tumors are of germ cell or stromal cell origin. A number of histologic subtypes are seen in the epithelial group. The serous type is the most frequent (45%), followed by undifferentiated, endometrioid, mucinous, and clear cell. Rare subtypes include Brenner transitional cell type and small cell type.

Ovarian cancer spreads by direct extension or intraperitoneal dissemination, lymphatically, and rarely hematogenously.

DIAGNOSTIC STUDIES

Laboratory

Complete Blood Count.   Used as a baseline prior to initiation of therapy.

Serum Chemistry Profile.   Used as a baseline prior to initiation of therapy.

CA 125 Assay.   Not useful in screening or diagnosis in premenopausal women, but useful in monitoring disease response to therapy. There are too many false-positives for this test to be used as a screening tool.

Radiology

Chest Film.   As indicated to evaluate for metastases.

CT Scans of the Abdomen, Pelvis, and Chest.   As indicated to diagnose a mass lesion and to rule out intraperitoneal, pelvic or pulmonary spread.

Abdominal Ultrasound Examination.   As indicated to evaluate any mass lesions palpated on physical examination.

Other
Barium Enemal/Colonoscopy. Used to evaluate for obstructive lesions.
Laparotomy. For definitive diagnosis and staging.

DIFFERENTIAL DIAGNOSIS

Traumatic
Ovarian Torsion. Usually extremely painful, whereas ovarian cancer is characteristically asymptomatic.

Infectious
Pelvic Inflammatory Disease. Pelvic or abdominal pain and/or vaginal discharge that are usually not present in ovarian cancer.

Metabolic
Ovarian Cyst. May or may not be painful and requires evaluation to distinguish its fluid properties. Usually differentiated on ultrasound examination.

Neoplastic
Cervical Cancer. May be asymptomatic. Noted on Papanicolaou smear.

Vascular
Ovarian Hemorrhage. Associated with moderate to severe pelvic and abdominal pain, whereas patients with ovarian cancer may have only a vague sense of abdominal fullness.

Congenital
Not applicable.

Acquired
Pregnancy. Positive human chorionic gonadotropin (HCG) assay. Pregnancy may be ectopic.

TREATMENT

Primary treatment for stage I disease is surgery, involving a total abdominal hysterectomy with bilateral salpingo-oophorectomy. All other stages of disease require adjunctive chemotherapy in addition to surgery. Radiotherapy is not used as primary treatment but may be used adjunctively in patients with intermediate-risk disease (stage II or III with little postoperative residual disease). Intraperitoneal chemotherapy may be used as consolidation (further therapy given in initial induction doses) in patients who respond to platinum-based regimens. Currently, no ideal salvage therapy is available for recurrent or refractory ovarian cancer.

PEDIATRIC CONSIDERATIONS

A majority of ovarian tumors in children are benign teratomas. Approximately 25% are malignant germ cell tumors. Malignant germ cell tumors are treated by surgery and chemotherapy. Prognosis is generally good.

OBSTETRIC CONSIDERATIONS

The course and prognosis of ovarian cancer are poor overall because of delays in diagnosis owing to lack of symptoms and a dearth of good screening tests for detection. In pregnancy, the same phenomenon of delayed diagnosis is also present. Fortunately, ovarian cancer is fairly rare in pregnancy, and adnexal masses detected during pregnancy are usually not due to malignant processes. Treatment poses grave risks to a successful pregnancy outcome. For epithelial cell tumors, unilateral salpingo-oophorectomy can be carried out if the tumor is confined to one ovary, with delay of the final staging and tumor grading. However, with advanced lesions, particularly in early pregnancy, definitive treatment involving complete hysterectomy, bilateral salpingo-oophorectomy, and tumor debulking must be carried out. If advanced lesions are detected in later pregnancy, treatment options are more flexible.

GERIATRIC CONSIDERATIONS

Annual gynecologic examinations are equally important in postmenopausal women.

PREVENTIVE CONSIDERATIONS

No specific preventive measures exist. However, annual gynecologic examination could detect tumors earlier.

PEARLS FOR THE PA

Ovarian cancer is rarely detected in the early stage.

CA 125 assay is not useful in the screening of asymptomatic patients.

Pancreatic Cancer

Charles W. Reed, MEd, MPAS, PA-C

DEFINITION

A rapidly metastatic primary adenocarcinoma of the pancreas usually associated with an aggressive clinical course and abysmal survival rate.

HISTORY

Symptoms. Most patients are symptomatic at the time of diagnosis. Unfortunately, most patients also have metastatic disease at presentation.

General. Predominant initial symptoms (in descending order of frequency) include abdominal pain, anorexia, weight loss, early satiety, dry mouth, difficulty sleeping, jaundice, fatigue, nausea, depression, indigestion, vomiting, hoarseness, bloating or belching, dyspnea, dizziness, edema, cough, diarrhea, hiccup, and dysphagia.

Age. Rare before the age of 45 years. Peak incidence is between the ages of 65 and 79.

Onset. Onset and progression are usually rapid.

Duration. Less than 20% survival at 1 year after diagnosis and less than 3% at 5 years. Median survival for patients with nonresectable or metastatic disease is 2 to 6 months.

Intensity. Adenocarcinoma, which progresses rapidly, is the most common type.

Aggravating Factors. Delay in presentation or diagnosis.

Alleviating Factors. Early surgical resection if possible.

Associated Factors. Incidence in African Americans is 1.7 times higher than in the remaining U.S. population.

PHYSICAL EXAMINATION

General. Cachexia, anorexia, dyspnea, and weight loss are common findings on initial presentation and often indicate metastatic disease.

Head, Eyes, Ears, Nose, Throat. Scleral jaundice or cervical lymphadenopathy indicates metastasis.

Pulmonary. Tachypnea, dyspnea, hemoptysis, and adventitious breath sounds may be present in pulmonary metastases.

Gastrointestinal. Palpable mass, emesis, fecal incontinence or impaction, ascites, or peritoneal signs may be present.

Musculoskeletal. Pancreatic cancer metastasize to bones in 3% of cases, which may result in focal areas of tenderness or lytic lesions on radiographs. Isolated musculoskeletal presentation would be rare. A polymyositis syndrome has been reported.

Neurologic. Metastasis to the central nervous system is uncommon but, if present, may result in neurologic deficits.

Lymphatic. Supraclavicular lymphadenopathy is most common in metastatic disease.

PATHOPHYSIOLOGY

The etiology of pancreatic adenocarcinoma is unknown. Some factors showing a modest association include cigarette smoking, high-fat diet, partial gastrectomy, diabetes, chronic pancreatitis, and occupational exposure to gasoline, DDT, or benzene products, as well as familial/hereditary pancreatitis.

DIAGNOSTIC STUDIES

Laboratory. There are no specific laboratory analyses used in the diagnosis of pancreatic cancer. Approximately a third of patients will have a serum albumin of less than 3.5 g/dL at the time of presentation. Bilirubin levels may be elevated with liver metastases or direct biliary obstruction from the tumor mass. Elevated serum lipase and amylase are usually noted, but these are also elevated in nononcologic pancreatitis.

Radiology
Abdominal Ultrasound Examination. Ultrasound is noninvasive and inexpensive but is limited by air-containing organs and need for operator experience. It is useful in the early identification of primary pancreatic masses and liver metastasis. It is particularly useful for guided biopsies.

CT. CT is also noninvasive and safe and is much less operator dependent. Both CT and ultrasound examination are limited to detection of tumors greater than 2 cm in diameter. Although CT can detect retroperitoneal masses and lymphadenopathy, it may miss a potentially resectable tumor up to 20% of the time.

MRI. MRI has no advantage over CT in the assessment of pancreatic cancer.

Endoscopic Retrograde Cholangiopancreatography (ERCP). This is the gold standard for evaluating pancreaticobiliary tumors. It allows a more specific look at biliary tree involvement and provides a method for obtaining cells for pathology in some cases.

Other
Percutaneous Fine Needle Aspiration (FNA) Cytology. Cytologic differences between pancreatic tumors may affect treatment decisions and prognosis. FNA provides a safe and reliable means of obtaining that crucial tissue sample. False-negatives may occur when the desired cells are not obtained, but there are no false-positives.

DIFFERENTIAL DIAGNOSIS

Traumatic
Abdominal Trauma.   Can certainly damage the pancreas and result in symptoms of pancreatitis. Onset of symptoms may be delayed. A thorough history and examination will generally identify or eliminate this from the differential diagnosis.

Infectious
Pancreatitis.   May result from infectious seeding of the pancreas. See Metabolic, next.

Metabolic
Pancreatitis.   Acute pancreatitis and exacerbations of chronic pancreatitis are the most difficult to distinguish from pancreatic cancer. Indeed, pancreatic cancer often manifests as acute pancreatitis. There are no specific laboratory analyses reliable for differentiating cancer from pancreatitis. Presence of symptoms such as fatigue, weight loss, night sweats, and low-grade fever for several days or weeks before onset of acute symptoms is more indicative of cancer. Patients presenting with pancreatitis are routinely evaluated with CT to rule out mass or serious complications such as necrotizing pancreatitis. Hypercalcemia, alcohol abuse, hypertriglyceridemia (usually with glyceride concentrations greater than 500 mg/dL), diabetes mellitus, and a variety of drugs may cause pancreatitis.

Vascular
Idiopathic Deep Vein Thrombosis.   May contribute to the development of certain types of pancreatic cancer.

Congenital.   Not applicable.
Acquired.   Not applicable.

TREATMENT

Treatment of pancreatitis is mostly supportive. As with all cancers, pancreatic cancer is staged prior to treatment. The tumor-node-metastasis (TNM) system is used. As research and treatment trials proceed, there are frequent changes to staging criteria.

Surgery
Less than 20% of patients with pancreatic cancer have surgically resectable disease at the time of presentation. The 5-year survival rate for patients with resectable disease is only 3% to 25%. Palliative surgery to relieve obstructive problems secondary to tumor size or location is occasionally an option. However, most patients with these issues generally have advanced disease and a poor performance status, making palliative procedures moot.

Patients with resectable disease often undergo a pancreaticoduodenal resection (Whipple procedure) or a modification.

Adjuvant Therapy
Patients with completely resectable tumor may be treated with adjuvant external-beam radiotherapy (XRT) and 5-fluorouracil (5-FU).

Locally Advanced Disease.   The combination of XRT with 5-FU is also used in this setting. Occasionally, directed intraoperative radiotherapy is used for surgically exposed tumor.

Metastatic Disease.   Chemotherapy with or without XRT is the mainstay. 5-FU or gemcitabine is most often used. Multiagent therapy has not proved more efficacious than single-agent therapy.

PEDIATRIC CONSIDERATIONS

Adenocarcinoma of the pancreas is rare in this age group.

OBSTETRIC CONSIDERATIONS

Chemotherapy and radiation therapy are teratogenic.

GERIATRIC CONSIDERATIONS

Preexisting chronic illnesses may affect treatment decisions and performance status.

PREVENTIVE CONSIDERATIONS

Smoking cessation is strongly recommended. A low-fat, healthy diet and moderation of alcohol use may decrease risk.

PEARLS FOR THE PA

Chronic or nonspecific gastrointestinal complaints in a known ethanol abuser should raise suspicion of pancreatic cancer. Alcohol abusers get cancer too!

Prostate Cancer

Charles W. Reed, MEd, MPAS, PA-C

DEFINITION

A generally slow-growing malignant neoplasm of the adenomatous cells of the prostate gland that can lead to urinary obstruction and metastatic disease.

HISTORY

Symptoms. Rarely symptomatic. May cause symptoms of cystitis, prostatitis, urinary obstruction; in advanced disease, may manifest with bone pain from metastases.

General. Often an incidental finding during rectal examination or transurethral resection of the prostate. When symptomatic, it has commonly already spread beyond the prostate locally or distantly.

Age. Men in their fifth decade make up 10% of cases. Incidence increases by about 10% each decade to the 80s. Mean age at onset is 72.

Onset. Very slow-growing and insidious in most cases; sometimes aggressive and rapidly progressive.

Duration. May have clinically inapparent foci of carcinoma for 50 years.

Intensity. Once metastasized, is rapidly progressive.

Aggravating Factors. Exogenous testosterone.

Alleviating Factors. Orchiectomy in advanced disease.

Associated Factors. African American heritage, family history of prostate cancer, or patient history of bladder outlet syndrome.

PHYSICAL EXAMINATION

General. Shortness of breath, anemia, lymphadenopathy, and weight loss suggest metastatic disease.

Genitourinary. Prostate reveals nodule, asymmetry, and enlargement.

Musculoskeletal. Pathologic fractures and focal neurologic deficits suggest metastasis.

PATHOPHYSIOLOGY

Etiology is unknown. Suspected risk factors include genetic predisposition, hormonal influences, dietary and environmental factors, and infectious agents.

Usually adenocarcinomas appear in the acinar cells in the peripheral zone of the prostate. Biologic aggressiveness is inversely related to its histologic differentiation. Generally, disease progresses at a very slow rate within the prostate and then extends beyond the prostate by local, lymphatic, and hematogenous spread.

DIAGNOSTIC STUDIES

Laboratory
Prostate-Specific Antigen (PSA). Elevated in prostatic carcinoma. However, it may also be elevated in benign prostatic hypertrophy (BPH).
Prostatic Acid Phosphatase. Less reliable indicator of carcinoma in prostate, but increase might indicate metastatic spread.

Radiology
Transrectal Ultrasound Examination. Carcinoma appears as hypoechoic lesions in prostate.
Abdominal/Pelvic CT/MRI. May reveal enlarged lymph nodes indicative of metastasis.
Bone Scan. May indicate metastatic lesions in bone.

Other
Prostate Biopsy. Pathologic confirmation of disease. This information is necessary for grading and prognosis.
Pelvic Lymphadenectomy. Important evidence of lymphatic spread to accurately stage the disease for appropriate treatment.

DIFFERENTIAL DIAGNOSIS

Traumatic. Not applicable.

Infectious
Prostatitis. Will have tender, indurated prostate.

Metabolic. Not applicable.

Neoplastic
Benign Prostatic Hyperplasia. Elevated PSA; gland enlarged but generally smooth and symmetrical. Best differentiated by pathologic examination.

Vascular. Not applicable.
Congenital. Not applicable.
Acquired. Not applicable.

TREATMENT

Treatment is dependent on stage. The tumor-node-metastasis (TNM) staging system is most often used. Disease confined to the prostate is most commonly treated with radical retropubic prevesical prostatectomy or radiation therapy. Disease with local invasion is treated similarly with reduced effectiveness. Disease with distant metastasis is treated with hormonal manipulation using orchiectomy, antiandrogens, luteinizing hormone–releasing hormone (LH-RH) agonists, or estrogens. Chemotherapy may provide some relief in 20% to 30% of symptomatic patients. The use of multiagent chemotherapy has shown no additive benefit when compared with single-agent therapy. Palliative measures are given in advanced disease, including radiation therapy for bone lesions.

PEDIATRIC CONSIDERATIONS

Not applicable to the pediatric age group.

OBSTETRIC CONSIDERATIONS

No considerations.

GERIATRIC CONSIDERATIONS

This is a cancer of the elderly. The patient's age and functional status and presence of comorbid conditions may play a role in treatment.

PREVENTIVE CONSIDERATIONS

Early detection is beneficial in the treatment of prostate cancer. Digital rectal examination should be a part of any health care maintenance program.

The PSA will elevate with age and with BPH. Therefore, PSA assay is not acceptable for screening when used alone.

PEARLS FOR THE PA

Screening for prostate cancer is controversial. The PSA assay may reveal only clinically insignificant disease. Markedly elevated or rapidly increasing PSA levels may be of more clinical significance, but definitive recommendations do not exist.

Digital rectal examinations are recommended for all men older than 50 years of age.

Renal Carcinoma

Charles W. Reed, MEd, MPAS, PA-C

DEFINITION

Primary renal adenocarcinoma accounts for approximately 3% of all adult cancers.

HISTORY

Symptoms. Hematuria, dull flank pain, and weight loss are the most common presenting manifestations. The classic triad of flank pain, flank mass, and hematuria is present in less than 10% of patients.

General. Obtain a history of smoking, family history of renal cancer, von Hippel-Lindau disease, and polycystic kidney disease.

Age. Most commonly seen in the fourth to sixth decades of life.

Onset. Variable.

Duration. Variable.

Intensity. May appear acutely or develop over several years. Without treatment, survival rate after diagnosis is 3% at 5 years.

Aggravating Factors. Smoking.

Alleviating Factors. None specific.

Associated Factors. Smoking, urban living, family history of renal carcinoma, and von Hippel-Lindau disease. Polycystic kidney disease and chronic dialysis may be contributory.

PHYSICAL EXAMINATION

General. Pallor may be suggestive of anemia. Typical B symptoms (night sweats, fever, weight loss), indicate metastatic disease.

Abdomen. Palpable renal mass may be present. A renal mass will be palpable in the flank owing to the retroperitoneal location of the kidney. Costovertebral angle (CVA) tenderness may or may not be present. Metastatic masses may be palpable anywhere in the abdomen.

Lymphatic. Renal carcinoma metastasizes via the lymphatic and circulatory system. A thorough examination for lymphadenopathy is always indicated in the cancer evaluation.

Extremities. Edema in the lower extremities may indicate tumor compression of venous or lymphatic structures.

Musculoskeletal. Bone metastasis is common with renal carcinoma.

Other. The most common sites for metastasis are the lungs, liver, bones, and brain. Renal carcinoma may metastasize to unusual sites such as the fingertips, eyelids, and nose.

PATHOPHYSIOLOGY

Adenocarcinomatous renal tumors have an indolent course and may be present for years before metastasis. They usually are round and have a pseudocapsule composed of thickened stromal and fibrous tissue. Most cases of renal carcinoma (98%) manifest with unilateral involvement. The lesions begin in the proximal tubule and spread from there. Metastatic masses are histologically identical to the primary tumor.

DIAGNOSTIC STUDIES

Laboratory
Urinalysis for protein and blood. Any patient with documented hematuria requires a thorough urologic evaluation.

Complete Blood Count. Elevated red blood cell (RBC) count may indicate an erythropoietin-producing tumor. However, smokers will also have elevated RBC counts. Anemia may be present secondary to urinary blood loss or disruption of erythropoietin production.

Renal Function Tests. Abnormalities suggest more serious disease.

Liver Function Tests. Abnormalities may indicate liver metastasis.

Radiology
Chest Film. May reveal characteristic metastatic tumors resembling multiple large, round (cannonball) lesions. This is a characteristic pattern for renal metastasis.

CT with Ultrasound Examination. The gold standard for evaluation of renal mass.

Intravenous Pyelography. Has been replaced by CT with ultrasound. It is still commonly used as the initial study for the evaluation of hematuria.

Renal Ultrasound Examination. Useful for determining the extent of thrombi when present.

Renal Angiography. Useful in differentiating malignant (vascular) from benign masses, but is invasive, carries risk, and is not generally required.

Other
MRI. Not superior to CT for diagnosis, but can provide a better sense of anatomic relationship prior to surgery.

Percutaneous Fine Needle Aspiration (FNA) Biopsy. FNA biopsy of a renal mass may seed the needle tract or peritoneum.

DIFFERENTIAL DIAGNOSIS

Traumatic
Renal Trauma. May cause hematuria. Differentiated on history.

Infectious
Urinary Tract/Renal Infections. May cause hematuria. Usually associated with leukocytes in urine.

Metabolic
Benign Renal Cysts. May usually be distinguished from carcinoma by ultrasonography.

Neoplastic
Lymphomas and Sarcomas. May begin in the kidney and have the same clinical course as that noted for tumors occurring extrarenally.

Benign Renal Adenomas. May be histologically identical to malignant adenomas. The clinical course with such tumors is difficult to predict when the tumor is less than 3 cm in diameter.

Vascular. Not applicable.
Congenital. Not applicable.
Acquired. Not applicable.

Other
Menses. May result in detection of blood on urinalysis. Repeat urinalysis at a later date as indicated.

TREATMENT

Surgery
Total nephrectomy is the treatment of choice in early disease. When poor renal function exists, nephron-sparing surgery (NSS) is an option.

Regression of metastases has been known to occur after nephrectomy but is rare and not a separate indication for nephrectomy. Early solitary metastases may be resected.

Radiotherapy
Radiotherapy is used palliatively but is not useful in effecting a cure. Radiotherapy and chemotherapy are not used for early disease.

Drug Therapy
High-dose intravenous interleukin-2 (IL-2) may produce response in up to 25% of patients and occasionally a durable remission lasting years. IL-2 therapy carries significant morbidity and mortality and is often administered in an intensive care environment.

Interferon (IFN) may give response rates similar to those obtained with IL-2 and is less toxic, but long-term benefit/durability of response has not yet been determined.

Cytotoxic chemotherapeutic agents are generally ineffective for renal cell carcinoma. Agents for which response has been noted include vinblastine and fluoropyridines.

PEDIATRIC CONSIDERATIONS

Nephroblastoma (Wilms tumor) is generally found in the pediatric population and presents as large bulky masses.

OBSTETRIC CONSIDERATIONS

None specific.

GERIATRIC CONSIDERATIONS

This is also a geriatric cancer. Vigilance is required.

PREVENTIVE CONSIDERATIONS

Cessation of smoking is important.

PEARLS FOR THE PA

Presence of supraclavicular lymphadenopathy with any neoplasm usually indicates that extralymphatic (usually thoracic) metastasis has already occurred.

Sarcomas

Charles W. Reed, MEd, MPAS, PA-C

DEFINITION

Muscle tissue sarcoma is only one of a large category of various primary mesenchymal tumors. Any sarcoma of any nonparenchymal tissue outside the skeleton generally is termed a *soft tissue sarcoma* (STS). For the purpose of this discussion, sarcomas are divdied into two groups: STS and bone sarcoma.

HISTORY

Symptoms.   The most common presenting manifestation is an enlarging, painless swelling on an extremity.

General. Family history is very important with sarcomas, as they are associated with genetic or hereditary factors. Exposure to certain agents or the preexistence of another disease can predispose a patient to certain sarcomas.

Age. All ages are affected. Peak incidence is in childhood and in the fifth decade.

Onset. Onset may be gradual, or the lesion may develop rapidly, depending on the type of sarcoma.

Duration. Course may be indolent or rapidly progressive, depending on tissue type and grade. Sarcomas that metastasize early include rhabdomyosarcoma, synovial sarcoma, and epithelioid sarcoma.

Intensity. May be minimally symptomatic, or symptoms may be acute, especially with tumors that impinge on major blood vessels and nerves.

Aggravating Factors. None specific.

Alleviating Factors. None specific.

Associated Factors. Several sarcomas have been associated with certain agents or diseases:

- Angiosarcoma: exposure to polyvinyl chloride (PVC), thorium dioxide, arsenic, androgens, dioxin
- Fibrosarcoma: radiation (from radiotherapy), Paget disease
- Kaposi sarcoma: cytomegalovirus (CMV), human immunodeficiency virus type 1 (HIV-1) infection
- Leiomyosarcoma: HIV-1 infection in children

PHYSICAL EXAMINATION

General. Until metastasis occurs, characteristic constitutional cancer symptoms may be absent. Sarcomas generally metastasize hematogenously. A comprehensive and thorough soft tissue examination is required.

Pulmonary. Lung metastasis is most common. Thorough search for adventitious sounds and pleural effusion is advised.

Abdomen. Visceral metastases are possible. The retroperitoneum is often a site for metastasis from extremity sarcomas. A thorough abdominal examination is required.

Skin. For subcutaneous tumors, note size, mobility, consistency, fluctuance, and overlying skin color; assess for tenderness and regional lymphadenopathy.

PATHOPHYSIOLOGY

Sarcomas generally behave according to their histologic grade. Low-grade tumors often remain localized and are more likely to be cured surgically. High-grade sarcomas metastasize early and have a much more aggressive course. Sarcomas usually spread along tissue planes, invading local nerves, muscles, and blood vessels as they progress. Owing to this local invasion, presenting symptoms are related to compression of these structures.

Common high-grade sarcomas include rhabdomyosarcoma and osteogenic sarcoma.

Rhabdomyosarcomas arise in the striated muscles. Almost all are of high grade. Embryonal rhabdomyosarcoma is primarily a tumor of infants and children, affecting the head and neck (in 70% of cases) and genitalia (in 15%).

Alveolar rhabdomyosarcoma affects teenagers and may occur in any location.

Pleomorphic rhabdomyosarcoma usually affects adults older than 30 years of age. It is more anaplastic than other rhabdomyosarcomas and more difficult to treat. Five-year survival rate is about 25%.

Osteogenic sarcomas may affect persons of any age but are most common in those in the 10- to 40-year-old age group. Most sarcomas develop in the metaphysis of the long bones, but they may affect any part of the bone. One variety has a predilection for the mandible.

DIAGNOSTIC STUDIES

Laboratory
Serum Alkaline Phosphatase. Usually elevated in osteogenic sarcoma but often not in benign neoplasms of the bones. When it is elevated at the time of diagnosis, it can be used as a tumor marker to evaluate the effectiveness of treatment.

Radiology
Plain Bone Radiographs of Involved Areas. Can be useful in determining the bone involvement from soft tissue sarcomas and is particularly useful with osteogenic sarcoma.

Chest Film. As indicated to evaluate for metastatic lesions.

CT Scan. Best for evaluating retroperitoneal or head and neck tumors. Also required in all sarcoma patients to rule out lung metastasis.

MRI. Comparable to CT in determining tumor extent but often better in obtaining a preoperative evaluation of the tumor's anatomic relationship to other structures.

Bone Scan. May be useful in determining the extent of periosteal reaction.

Other
Open Biopsy. The histologic grade of the sarcoma is key to treatment and prognosis. If the biopsy does not affect subsequent resection, it provides the best sample and allows for an approximation of the anatomical issues involved in the future resection. Because many sarcomas are dense or have osteoid components, fine needle aspiration (FNA) biopsy is generally not the diagnostic procedure of choice. CT-guided biopsies are also performed.

DIFFERENTIAL DIAGNOSIS

Traumatic
Deep Tissue Hematomas. Residual scarring may appear as firm, soft tissue nodules.

Infectious
Trichinosis. Due to *Trichinella spiralis*, a subcutaneous parasite. May manifest with firm nodules in muscle tissue.
Deep Abcesses. May be nodular, but usually do not pose a diagnostic problem.
Tuberculous Processes. In infection due to *Mycobacterium tuberculosis*, subcutaneous nodules may be seen.

Neoplastic
Lipomas. Benign fatty tumors that have no malignant potential.
Soft Tissue Metastasis from Other Primary Cancers. May be mistaken for sarcoma when the primary lesion has not been found. Histology will differentiate.

Vascular
Not applicable.

Congenital
Li-Fraumeni Syndrome, Beckwith-Wiedemann Syndrome, Neurofibromatosis, Familial Retinoblastoma. Syndromes with genetic sarcomatous components.

TREATMENT

Surgery
Surgical removal using wide resection is the treatment of choice for most STSs. The tumor margins must be histologically free of tumor. Wide excision is generally curative for low-grade lesions. Osteosarcoma may require amputation to effect a cure.

Lymph node resection is normally not performed except for angiosarcoma and synovial sarcoma. These tumors tend to metastasize lymphatically.

Radiation Therapy
Radiotherapy is combined with surgical excision for grade 3 and 4 lesions. Chemotherapy may or may not be useful in adults with high-grade tumors.

Chemotherapy
Chemotherapy combined with radiotherapy and excision is standard treatment for pediatric rhabdomyosarcoma. Adjuvant chemotherapy is also the standard of care in the management of all osteosarcomas. Regimens most

often used include mesna, doxorubicin, ifosfamide, and dacarbazine (MAID); cyclophosphamide, vincristine, doxorubicin, and dacarbazine (CyVADTIC); doxorubicin with cisplatin; and ifosfamide with mesna.

PEDIATRIC CONSIDERATIONS

Many STSs present in the pediatric age group. Head and neck sarcomas are more common in the pediatric age group. A thorough well-baby/school physical examination is essential. Embryonal rhabdomyosarcoma is primarily a tumor of infants and children, affecting the head, neck, and genitalia.

OBSTETRIC CONSIDERATIONS

None specific.

GERIATRIC CONSIDERATIONS

Most STSs occur in persons younger than 40 years of age. Bone sarcomas are more common in the geriatric population. Head and neck sarcomas are less common in adults.

PREVENTIVE CONSIDERATIONS

Avoidance of or limiting exposure to certain well-recognized etiologic agents is important:
- For angiosarcoma: PVC, thorium dioxide, arsenic, androgens, dioxin
- For fibrosarcoma: radiation
- For Kaposi sarcoma: CMV, HIV-1
- For leiomyosarcoma: HIV-1 in children

PEARLS FOR THE PA

Multiple types of sarcomas exist. These lesions are generally classified as soft tissue sarcoma or bone sarcoma.

There is a strong familial association for these tumors.

The most common site of metastasis is the lung.

Presenting symptoms are commonly related to compression of adjacent structures (blood vessels, nerves, muscles) as the tumor progresses.

Testicular Cancer

Charles W. Reed, MEd, MPAS, PA-C

DEFINITION

Carcinoma of one or both testes; predominantly of germ cell type in younger age groups and of lymphomatous type in older men.

HISTORY

Symptoms. The most common presenting manifestation is a painless, enlarged testis.

General. Ascertain a history of cryptorchidism in childhood or a family history of reproductive organ cancer.

Age. Usually of germ cell type in patients between 20 and 40 years; lymphomatous type is most common in patients above the age of 60.

Onset. Rapidity of onset depends greatly on the histologic subtype of the tumor. Some patients may present with symptoms similar to those of acute epididymitis.

Duration. Depends on cell type. Seminomas are slower in progression than is embryonal carcinoma or teratoma.

Intensity. Embryonal carcinoma and teratomas grow rapidly, resulting in a large tumor burden.

Aggravating Factors. Failure to perform regular testicular self-examination (TSE) or failure to seek treatment immediately with abnormal findings on TSE.

Alleviating Factors. Underlying bacterial epididymitis will respond to bacterial therapy.

Associated Factors. Cryptorchidism and testicular feminization syndromes increase the risk of testicular cancer.

PHYSICAL EXAMINATION

General. Cardinal cancer symptoms such as weight loss, fatigue, and night sweats may or may not be present. Patients may present for related problems such as gynecomastia, back pain, infertility, or bone pain.

Head, Eyes, Ears, Nose, Throat. Retro-orbital pain or ocular bulging could indicate orbital metastasis.

Chest. Gynecomastia may be present with any tumor that secretes large amounts of human chorionic gonadotropin (HCG).

Lymphatic. A careful examination evaluating for lymphadenopathy is mandatory. Both local and distant lymphatic chains should be examined. Supraclavicular lymphadenopathy indicates thoracic metastasis.

Testicular. A painless swelling of the testicle is the most common finding. Testicular torsion or epididymitis may be an initial finding.

PATHOPHYSIOLOGY

As with most cancers, prognosis and evaluation depend on the histologic subtype of the tumor. There are several histologic subtypes, with four predominating: seminoma, embryonal carcinoma/teratoma, choriocarcinoma, and yolk sac tumors.

Seminoma
A majority of testicular cancers in men older than 30 years of age are seminomatous. Seminomas represent malignant transformation of the spermatocyte. This is the most common form of testicular cancer in men with a history of cryptorchidism. Seminomas tend to be large tumors and metastasize in a predictable manner along the lymphatic chain. The most common sites of visceral metastasis are lung and bone. They may be strictly spermatocytic, anaplastic, or of mixed cell type.

Embryonal Carcinoma/Teratoma
These represent half of all testicular cancers and are most common in 20- to 30-year-old men. They represent malignant transformation of the early cleavage embryo. They are usually bulky and grow aggressively. They metastasize via lymphatics and blood, often to the lung and liver. A majority of patients have metastatic disease at the time of diagnosis.

Choriocarcinoma
Malignant transformation of the chorionic villus results in these uncommon but highly aggressive carcinomas. They are rapidly metastatic.

Yolk Sac Tumors
These are common tumors in children and are generally nonaggressive.

DIAGNOSTIC STUDIES

Laboratory
β-Human Chorionic Gonadatrophin (β-HCG). Tumor marker used for both detection and clinical tracking of testicular cancer. It is present in 100% of choriocarcinomas and in 65% of embryonal carcinomas/teratomas. It is found in only 10% of seminomas.

α-Fetoprotein (α-FP). Tumor marker used for both detection and clinical tracking of testicular cancer. It is rarely found in seminomas or choriocarcinomas but is found in more than 70% of embryonal carcinomas/teratomas.

Alkaline Phosphatase and Lactate Dehydrogenase (LDH). Useful in monitoring for bone metastasis.

Radiology
Metastatic Workup. Including chest film and CT scans as a minimum. Bone scans may be performed when bone metastasis is suspected.

Other
Histologic Examination. Confirmation of tumor cell type(s) is imperative.

DIFFERENTIAL DIAGNOSIS

Traumatic. Not applicable.

Infectious
Epididymitis. Another common condition that rarely may portend an underlying malignancy. Further investigation should be considered if pain or swelling persists after adequate treatment.

Metabolic
Hydrocele. The most common benign condition mistaken for testicular carcinoma. These lesions represent transilluminating fluid collections around the testes. Testicular carcinoma may manifest with a concomitant hydrocele, so thorough evaluation is required, particularly if the hydrocele prevents palpation of the testicle.

Spermatoceles. Cystic transilluminating masses located posterior and superior to the testis.

Neoplastic
Not otherwise applicable.

Vascular
Varicoceles. Engorged veins of the spermatic cord. The classic physical finding is a mass that feels like a "bag of worms." These veins will collapse if the patient is placed in Trendelenburg position.

Congenital
Not applicable.

Acquired
Inguinal Hernia. May appear as a scrotal mass, but generally does not pose a diagnostic dilemma.

TREATMENT

Surgical

Transinguinal orchiectomy is performed in all cases of testicular cancer. It is the definitive treatment for stage A disease. The transinguinal approach is essential to maintain control of the spermatic cord blood supply, preventing hematogenous tumor spread.

Nonsurgical

Nonsurgical treatment of testicular cancer is based on cell type and stage. It generally consists of some combination of bleomycin, etoposide, and cisplatin. Nonresponders may be given high-dose myeloablative chemotherapy followed by autologous bone marrow or peripheral stem cell transplantation.

PEDIATRIC CONSIDERATIONS

Yolk sac tumors are common tumors in children and are generally nonaggressive. A routine testicular screening examination should be part of every school physical.

OBSTETRIC CONSIDERATIONS

Not applicable.

GERIATRIC CONSIDERATIONS

Spermatocytic seminoma is the most common germ cell tumor in older age groups. It may have a bilateral presentation.

PREVENTIVE CONSIDERATIONS

Placement of the undescended testes within the scrotal sac before 6 years of age reduces the risk of testicular carcinoma.

PEARLS FOR THE PA

β-HCG is not present in normal men. Any male patient with a positive HCG assay should be assumed to have testicular cancer until proven otherwise.

Thyroid Cancer

Charles W. Reed, MEd, MPAS, PA-C

DEFINITION

An endocrine malignancy possessing either well-differentiated or anaplastic pathologic subdivision.

HISTORY

Symptoms. Patients may present with an enlarging neck nodule, lymphadenopathy, or voice change. Metastatic disease may produce bone pain or pulmonary symptoms.

General. Ascertain a history of irradiation to the neck during infancy or childhood as well as a family history of thyroid or endocrine tumors.

Age. Rare in children without a history of neck irradiation; incidence increases with advancing age.

Onset. Months to years.

Duration. Well-differentiated tumors may have a long course and highly aggressive tumors a short course.

Intensity. Indolent in papillary tumors; anaplastic tumors are aggressive and rapidly fatal.

Aggravating Factors. None.

Alleviating Factors. None.

Associated Factors. External radiation therapy to the head and neck during childhood as well as high-dose radiation to the head and neck in adults (doses greater than 2000 cGy). Two familial syndromes are associated with follicular thyroid carcinoma: Gardner syndrome and Cowden disease. All patients with inherited multiple endocrine neoplasia type II (MEN-II) present with medullary carcinoma of the thyroid.

PHYSICAL EXAMINATION

General. The patient may exhibit signs of hyperthyroidism or hypothyroidism.

Hypothyroidism. Patients may be obese, may be slow in body movements or have dry skin or alopecia, and invariably complain of fatigue.

Hyperthyroidism. Patients may appear thin and anxious.

Head, Eyes, Ears, Nose, Throat. Thyroid nodule may be present on palpation. Evaluate size, consistency (soft or hard), and fixation to adjacent structures.

Lymphatics. Evaluate for any lymphadenopathy.

PATHOPHYSIOLOGY

Thyroid cancer is subdivided into two main groups; those that are well differentiated and those that are anaplastic.

Well-differentiated tumors include papillary tumors that arise from thyroid follicular cells or follicular cancer. Medullary carcinomas are derived from calcitonin-secreting cells of the thyroid gland and are poorly differentiated. Forty percent of adults with papillary carcinoma will present with regional lymph node metastases. Up to 10% of children with this type of tumor may have lung involvement at the time of diagnosis.

Anaplastic tumors arise from follicular cells. Thyroglobulin is present infrequently in anaplastic carcinomas and not at all in medullary carcinomas. Thyroglobulin immunoreactivity is indicative of follicular epithelial origin.

Hodgkin lymphomas may manifest in the thyroid.

DIAGNOSTIC STUDIES

Laboratory
Complete Blood Count.   Used as a baseline prior to therapy.

Comprehensive Serum Chemistry Profile.   Used as a baseline prior to therapy.

Triiodothyronine (T_3).   May be elevated or decreased.

Thyroxine (T_4).   May be elevated or decreased. Thyroid-binding globulin should be tested when the T_4 is high.

Thyroid-Stimulating Hormone (TSH).   Used as a baseline prior to therapy.

Thyroglobulin Level.   Elevated in destructive lesions of the thyroid.

Antithyroid Antibodies.   High titers seen in Hashimoto disease and lymphadenoid goiter.

Calcitonin Level.   Elevated levels are used to diagnose medullary carcinoma after pentagastrin and/or calcium administration.

Radiology
Ultrasound Examination or Scintigraphy.   May be helpful in some cases, but neither is conclusively diagnostic.

Chest Film.   Obtained in patients with pulmonary symptoms to rule out lung metastases.

Thyroid Scan.   Helpful in identifying hyperfunctional versus nonfunctional lesions. A majority of thyroid nodules (benign or malignant) are hypofunctional and are therefore "cold" on scan.

Other
Fine Needle Aspiration (FNA).   FNA is the single best diagnostic test in the evaluation of thyroid cancer. Many authorities recommend this as the initial diagnostic tool for evaluation of any thyroid nodule.

DIFFERENTIAL DIAGNOSIS

Traumatic. Not applicable.

Infectious
Suppurative Thyroiditis (Bacterial). Usually due to gram-positive organisms. The patient may present acutely ill with severe pain over the gland; associated with fever. Requires appropriate antibiotic therapy and often abscess drainage.

Metabolic
Thyroid Storm. A rare complication that may be seen in patients with Graves disease. Immediate therapy is necessary. It is considered a medical emergency.
Impaired Pituitary or Peripheral Sensitivity to Thyroid Hormone. Rare.
Sick Euthyroid State. Very ill patients may have a normal to low T_4, low T_3, and normal to slightly increased TSH. Their thyroid profile improves as they clinically improve.

Neoplastic
TSH-Secreting Tumor. Very rare cause of hyperthyroidism.

Vascular. Not applicable.
Congenital. Not applicable.
Acquired. Not applicable (see Pathophysiology section).

TREATMENT

Thyroid cancer is staged using the tumor-node-metastasis (TNM) method to determine prognosis and treatment. Surgical excision of the thyroid is the treatment of choice. Surgery is followed by postoperative radioiodine scanning to identify residual or distant foci. Postsurgical treatment with ablative radioactive iodine is often used, but the true efficacy of this therapy is not known. Radioablative iodine therapy has not proved leukemogenic, as was once thought.

Postoperative thyroid replacement and follow-up are necessary. The goal of thyroxine replacement is suppression of the TSH level to normal or below-normal levels, as TSH is known to stimulate most thyroid cancers.

PEDIATRIC CONSIDERATIONS

History of childhood external head or neck radiation should increase the index of suspicion for thyroid cancer. Twenty five percent of symptomatic patients with a positive history may have abnormalities on physical examination or thyroid workup, and up to one-third of these, on aspiration, will have cancer. Up to 10% of children with papillary carcinoma may have lung involvement at the time of diagnosis.

OBSTETRIC CONSIDERATIONS

Antineoplastic medications may pose grave risks to the fetus. However, their use is recommended if absolutely needed during the pregnancy.

GERIATRIC CONSIDERATIONS

Although indiscriminate head and neck irradiation is a thing of the past, some elderly patients may have had this decades ago and should be considered at high risk for the development of thyroid cancer.

PREVENTIVE CONSIDERATIONS

None specific.

PEARLS FOR THE PA

Etiologic factors for hypothyroidism, except for childhood irradiation, are not well understood.

Depression may be the presenting complaint for any condition resulting in hypothyroidism, including neoplasms. Thyroid disease should be considered in any dysphoric or depressed patient.

Uterine Cancer

Charles W. Reed, MEd, MPAS, PA-C

DEFINITION

Primary carcinoma of the endometrium; 90% of uterine cancers are adenocarcinoma.

HISTORY

Symptoms. The most common presenting symptom is abnormal uterine bleeding.

General. Obtain both patient and familial cancer history.

Age. Few cases are diagnosed before the age of 40. Peak incidence is in the sixth and seventh decades.

Onset. Months to years.

Duration. Well-differentiated tumors may have a long course and highly aggressive tumors a short course.

Intensity. Generally indolent in nature.

Aggravating Factors. Continued use of unopposed estrogens and delay in diagnosis. Tamoxifen acts as a mild estrogen and doubles the risk of uterine cancer.

Alleviating Factors. None.

Associated Factors. Anovulatory menstrual cycles, obesity, diabetes, infertility, nulliparity, and hypertension all may be associated with increased risk of endometrial cancer.

PHYSICAL EXAMINATION

General. A general examination to look for common signs of cancer should be performed.

Lymphatic. Thorough and careful examination for lymphadenopathy is critical in any cancer workup.

Abdomen. Large uterine tumors may be palpable on abdominal examination.

Pelvic. Traditional Papanicolaou (Pap) smears have a significantly lower yield in endometrial carcinoma. Endocervical curettage is preferred, and fractional curettage is optimal for an office examination.

Transvaginal ultrasound examination to assess endometrial thickness is under evaluation but seems to yield false-positive results when endometrial thickness is the only criterion evaluated.

PATHOPHYSIOLOGY

Two main cell types predominate: adenocarcinoma (accounting for 90% of these cancers) and adenosquamous (10%). Unopposed estrogen causes changes in the endometrium ranging from hyperplasia to invasive carcinoma. Tumors generally spread via direct extension. Primary site of visceral metastasis is the lung. Staging is done using the 1971 International Federation of Gynecology and Oncology (FIGO) system. This system is based on results from endometrial curettage, hysteroscopy, cystoscopy, proctoscopy, and chest/bone radiographs.

DIAGNOSTIC STUDIES

Laboratory
Histology. Curettage as described. Peritoneal washings containing cancer cells may indicate retrograde sloughing of tumor cells via the fallopian tubes.

Radiology
Transvaginal Ultrasound Examination. Assessment of endometrial thickness is under evaluation but seems to yield false-positive results when endometrial thickness is the only criterion evaluated.
Radiographs of Chest and Bones. For metastasis.
CT. If visceral metastasis is suspected.

DIFFERENTIAL DIAGNOSIS

Traumatic. Not applicable.
Infectious. Not applicable.
Metabolic. Not applicable.

Neoplastic
Uterine Fibroid Tumors. Benign, but may be quite large and palpable on examination.

Vascular. Not applicable.
Congenital. Not applicable.
Acquired. Not applicable.

TREATMENT

Any cause of abnormal uterine bleeding requires full and complete evaluation to rule out uterine cancer. As with most cancers, treatment is dependent on stage. Hyperplasia and low-stage well-differentiated lesions may respond to high-dose progestin hormones. This may actually be curative. However, if hyperplasia persists after progestin therapy or if the patient's performance status is adequate for surgery, total abdominal hysterectomy with bilateral salpingo-oophorectomy (TAH/BSO) is the treatment of choice.

Radiotherapy (RT) may be combined with surgery. The standard has been to use RT preoperatively. However, this approach may be detrimental to accurate staging, so postoperative RT is becoming more popular.

Chemotherapy has limited use in the treatment of uterine cancer. It is recommended in the treatment of papillary serous or clear cell carcinoma. The most commonly used agents are carboplatin and paclitaxel.

PEDIATRIC CONSIDERATIONS

None.

OBSTETRIC CONSIDERATIONS

Uterine cancer is rare during the childbearing years.

GERIATRIC CONSIDERATIONS

Peak incidence occurs in the geriatric age group, so index of suspicion should be high.

PREVENTIVE CONSIDERATIONS

Use of unopposed estrogen in postmenopausal women should be avoided. This prohibition also applies to anovulatory women with endometrial hyperplasia.

PEARLS FOR THE PA

Any postmenopausal woman developing uterine bleeding greater than 1 year after cessation of menses should be assumed to have uterine cancer until proven otherwise.

Further Reading

Casciato D: Manual of Clinical Oncology, 4th ed. Philadelphia, Lippincott Williams & Wilkins, 2000

Chu E, DeVita V: Physician's Cancer Chemotherapy Drug Manual 2001. Boston, Jones & Bartlett, 2001.

Fischer D, Knobf M, Durivage H (eds): The Cancer Chemotherapy Handbook, 5th ed. St. Louis, Mosby–Year Book, 1997.

Lee G, Foerster J, Luken J, et al (eds): Wintrobe's Clinical Hematology, 10th ed. Philadelphia, Lippincott Williams & Wilkins, 1999.

Slamon D, Leland-Jones B, Shak S, Fuchs H: Use of chemotherapy plus a monoclonal antibody against HER2 for metastatic breast cancer that overexpresses HER2. N Engl J Med 344: 783-792, 2001.

Stoller J, Ahmad M, Longworth D: The Cleveland Clinic Intensive Review of Internal Medicine, 2nd ed. Philadelphia, Lippincott Williams & Wilkins, 2000.

Woods M: Hematology/Oncology Secrets, 2nd ed. Philadelphia, Hanley & Belfus, 1999.

The work on which this chapter is based was supported in part by grants CA 18029, CA 18221, CA 15407, CA 09645, and HL 36444 from the National Institutes of Health, DHHS.

OPHTHALMOLOGY

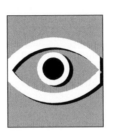

12

Cataract

George L. White, Jr., PhD, MSPH, PA-C

DEFINITION

Any opacity of the normally clear crystalline lens is termed a *cataract*. Cataracts may be congenital, traumatic, iatrogenic, or physiologic with aging.

HISTORY

Symptoms. Gradual, progressive, painless, unremitting blurriness of vision experienced unilaterally or bilaterally at *all* distances. The world appears as if viewed from behind a waterfall—hence the name "cataract."

General. Difficulty seeing in settings with increased reflected or direct bright light, especially the lights of incoming traffic at night. Difficulty with night driving in general may be the earliest manifestation. Halos may be seen (without pain) around bright objects (e.g., street lamps). Full review of systems including trauma history is important to rule out contributing factors.

Age. All patients will develop some degree of cataract by age 60 years. Congenital cataracts do occur and must be recognized and the patient referred promptly to salvage vision. One of the remnants of the fetal hyaloid system, the Mittendorf dot, may appear as a small cataract but very rarely alters vision.

Onset. Physiologic cataracts develop over months to years, congenital cataracts are present at birth, traumatic cataracts may develop rapidly within days to weeks, and iatrogenic cataracts (e.g., steroid-induced) usually develop over many months.

Duration. In the absence of injury and underlying disease, formation is relentlessly progressive; symptoms are not intermittent.

Intensity. Initially may be asymptomatic for months to several years, but later can range from very mild to visually incapacitating.

Aggravating Factors. Glare and low-light conditions may make vision especially difficult. Trouble with night driving often prompts a request for evaluation.

Alleviating Factors. Surgical replacement of the natural lens with an artificial lens. Corrective eyeglasses or contact lenses may help when vision is only slightly impaired.

Associated Factors. Smoking, ultraviolet light exposure, metabolic disorders, certain dermatologic conditions, long-term steroid use (topical or systemic), chlorpromazine, and amiodarone all are potential contributing factors.

PHYSICAL EXAMINATION

General. A full physical examination needs to be performed with special attention paid to the endocrine and dermatologic systems.

Ophthalmologic.   Decreased visual acuity in one or both eyes. Cataract is most easily detected through a dilated pupil from a distance of 20 to 30 cm using the +4 to +5 lens diopter (black) of the ophthalmoscope. During direct ophthalmoscopic examination, a small cataract will appear as a black spot against the red reflex, when viewed while the patient looks straight ahead. Funduscopic examination may be difficult or impossible owing to opacity of the lens. The cornea and anterior chamber of the eye are not involved with cataract.

PATHOPHYSIOLOGY

The lens contains a subcapsular epithelium, subepithelium, nutrient-rich fluid that bathes the lens, and lamellar fibers that lie in the subepithelium. Over time or with certain irritants, edema, necrosis, and general disruption of the orderly stratification of the lamellar fibers develop, resulting in lens opacification. Metabolic disease further disrupts the lens fluid. The exact cause of the opacification is unknown, but lifetime exposure to ultraviolet light has been implicated.

DIAGNOSTIC STUDIES

Laboratory
Chemistry Profile.   May show elevated glucose with diabetes mellitus or hypercalcemia/hypocalcemia.

Radiology
Not applicable.

Other
Not applicable.

DIFFERENTIAL DIAGNOSIS

Traumatic
Blunt Trauma.   May cause slow or rapid development of a cataract, usually over months to years.
Trauma with Penetration of the Lens Capsule.   Causes rapid cataract formation.
Thermal, Electrical, and Radiation Injuries.   Can also lead to cataract formation.

Infectious
Uveitis/Intraocular Infection.   May develop cataract from inflammation, steroid use, or both.

Metabolic
Acute Glaucoma. May cause *painful* halos around bright objects.
Diabetes Mellitus. May be associated with development of cataract earlier than in the general population.
Hypocalcemia and Dystrophia. May lead to cataract formation.

Neoplastic
Metastatic Tumors (Rarely Affecting Lens). May be seen in other ocular structures.

Vascular. Not applicable, as the lens is avascular.

Congenital
Congenital Remnants. May be seen in the vitreous or retina (Bergmeister papilla, Mittendorf dot), but do not involve the lens.
Congenital Lens Opacities. May be seen at birth or develop within 3 months after birth.

Acquired
High-Dose, Chronic Steroid Use and Chronic Exposure to Ultraviolet Light. May predispose to cataract formation.

TREATMENT

Elective surgical repair is the only treatment. Surgical removal is indicated if visual impairment interferes with quality of life and eyeglasses can no longer satisfactorily improve vision. The cataract is removed and a clear acrylic or silicone foldable lens is substituted.

PEDIATRIC CONSIDERATIONS

The three most commonly accepted factors predisposing to the development of congenital cataracts are prenatal pelvic irradiation; prenatal infections, primarily the TORCH group (toxoplasma, rubella, cytomegalovirus, herpes simplex or herpes zoster); and maternal use of certain medications (corticosteroids, sulfonamides, and chlorpromazine). Various inborn errors of metabolism have been implicated, as cataracts are common in Down syndrome patients (developing after the onset of puberty) and in those with galactosemia. Cataracts in newborns with galactosemia are reversible with early treatment.

Removal of congenital or acquired cataracts may be indicated in early childhood to prevent development of amblyopia. An ophthalmologist should be consulted.

OBSTETRIC CONSIDERATIONS

No specific indications.

GERIATRIC CONSIDERATIONS

All patients will develop some degree of cataract by age 60 years. Cataract may be the cause of difficulty with night driving

PREVENTIVE CONSIDERATIONS

Routine use of protective eyewear will reduce the chance of ocular injury with subsequent cataract formation. Smoking cessation should be encouraged in all patients. Limit ultraviolet light exposure and/or use polarized sunglasses. Optimal control of metabolic disorders (e.g., diabetes mellitus) is recommended. Patients in whom long-term steroid use (topical or systemic) is required should be screened for cataract formation.

PEARLS FOR THE PA

Cataracts cause painless, unremitting blurriness of vision, unilateral or bilateral, at all distances.

Trouble with night driving often leads to evaluation.

All persons will develop some degree of cataract by age 60.

Conjunctivitis

George L. White, Jr., PhD, MSPH, PA-C

DEFINITION

Inflammation and erythema involving the outer covering of the eye due to infection, allergic reaction, or toxic exposure. The most common ophthalmologic condition seen by the primary health care provider. Although a minor concern in the industrialized world, chlamydial conjunctivitis, if left untreated, causes corneal scarring and is the major cause of blindness worldwide.

HISTORY

Symptoms. Infectious conjunctivitis is characterized by progressive redness and discharge. Usually begins unilaterally and becomes bilateral. Allergic conjunctivitis is associated with nasal discharge, sneezing, scratchy throat, or local reaction only from eye drops or facial cream. Chemical conjunctivitis is related to chemical exposure and manifests with conjunctival injection and swelling. Contact lenses that have become soiled or contaminated are often implicated. Contact lenses should be removed and not worn until the conjunctivitis is resolved.

General. Infectious conjunctivitis is usually associated with an upper respiratory infection, which may be concurrent with or precede the eye infection. Allergic conjunctivitis may be seasonal or related to an otherwise nontoxic ocular exposure. Chemical conjunctivitis will have an association with a noxious chemical exposure.

Extreme pain, photophobia, and visual loss are *not* consistent with primary care conjunctivitis, and the patient should be referred for immediate ophthalmologic consultation.

Age. Any, but most cases occur in school-aged children.

Onset. Most cases are fairly rapid in onset (over 12 to 48 hours), but with some causes (e.g., *Chlamydia* infection), can exhibit a gradual onset over many weeks.

Duration. Days to years, depending on appropriate diagnosis and treatment.

Intensity. Ranges from a very mild "gritty" discomfort to severe pain, depending on the cause and the patient's tolerance (marked pain suggests corneal involvement).

Aggravating Factors. Mechanical irritation of the eye and coexisting disease (e.g., allergy, diabetes mellitus).

Alleviating Factors. Cool water rinse.

Associated Factors. Poor hygiene, seasonal hay fever, close contact with affected persons, especially in day care centers, schools, shelters, or jails.

PHYSICAL EXAMINATION

General. The patient may be in acute or mild discomfort, depending on the cause. Preauricular lymph node enlargement may be present and is commonly associated with viral conjunctivitis.

Ophthalmologic. Visual acuity is not affected unless the cornea is involved. Palpebral and bulbar conjunctival inflammation is a classic sign. Hypertrophy of the lymphoid follicles may be seen as shiny red swellings in the lower fornix. Enlarged conjunctival papillae may also be seen on the everted upper and lower lids.

PATHOPHYSIOLOGY

The conjunctiva is the clear outer covering of the eye and therefore comes into contact with more microorganisms than any other mucous membrane. It is highly vascularized and has a high proportion of mucus-producing cells. As there is no closed cavity or space, infections (bacterial and viral) are generally self-limited owing to a profuse polymorphonuclear response and to intrinsic cleansing mechanisms of the eye. Tears themselves are antibacterial, and the eyelids are mechanical cleansers of the external eye. Allergens cause a mast cell histamine release, which provokes an extreme inflammatory response in the highly vascular tissue. Chemical irritants are directly toxic to the conjunctival tissue, and the extent of damage or irritation is related to the type of chemical.

DIAGNOSTIC STUDIES

Laboratory
Culture and Sensitivity Testing/Gram Stain/Viral Transport Medium. As indicated to identify a bacterial or viral agent; performed prior to instituting antibiotic therapy. Not necessary in "routine" conjunctivitis.

Radiology
Not applicable.

Other
Fluorescein Stain. Should be done in patients complaining of a foreign body sensation or poor vision to rule out corneal involvement.

Schirmer Test/Rose Bengal Stain. Used to rule out dry eye in selected patients.

Gram and Wright Stains. Stains of conjunctival scrapings may be helpful when allergic etiology is suspected.

Skin Testing for Potential Allergens. May be helpful as a preventive measure in persons with seasonal or chronic allergic conjunctivitis.

Intraocular Pressure Measurement. If acute glaucoma or iritis is suspected.

DIFFERENTIAL DIAGNOSIS

Traumatic
Foreign Body/Corneal Abrasion. Fluorescein stain reveals the abrasion or foreign body.

Infectious
Iritis. Extreme photophobia, generalized periocular ache, erythema radiating from the corneoscleral junction ("ciliary flush") that is usually unilateral, pupillary asymmetry, mobile pupil, decreased vision that improves with blinking, intraocular pressure slightly decreased or markedly increased compared with the contralateral eye; cornea is clear and does not stain.

Metabolic
Acute Glaucoma. Pupil is mid-dilated and fixed, cornea is "steamy," conjunctiva is erythematous, pain is excruciating. Visual acuity is markedly diminished, intraocular pressure is markedly elevated unilaterally, and cornea does not stain.

Neoplastic. Not applicable.
Vascular. Not applicable.
Congenital. Not applicable.
Acquired. Not applicable.

TREATMENT

Infectious
- Topical antibiotic
    Trimethoprim sulfate and polymyxin B sulfate (Polytrim) oph-
    thalmic solution four to six times daily for 7 to 10 days
- Topical steroids: Not usually recommended owing to potential side
  effects. Viral conjunctivitis will not respond to antibiotic therapy.

Allergic
- Topical vasoconstrictor
    Vasocon-A ophthalmic solution 2 to 3 times daily as required.
- Antihistamine
    Oral: Diphenhydramine 50 mg every 4 hours as required
    Topical: Nedocromil sodium (Alocril) ophthalmic solution, 1 or 2
        drops in each eye twice a day
- Topical steroids: For resistant cases and only with ophthalmologic
  supervision.

Chemical
Remove contact lenses if worn. Copious amounts of water irrigation immediately following the event, regardless of the suspected substance. Once the
patient has arrived in the medical setting, irrigation is again instituted, and
ophthalmologic consultation is immediately obtained.

PEDIATRIC CONSIDERATIONS

Prevention includes careful handwashing and use of individual towels,
washcloths, and eye drops.

Newborn
Topical ophthalmic prophylaxis at birth with 0.5% erythromycin or 1%
silver nitrate. Conjunctivitis in the newborn, however, is often caused by a
secondary inflammation resulting from the use of silver nitrate. Passage
through a birth canal colonized or infected by *Neisseria gonorrhoeae,
Chlamydia trachomatis,* group B streptococci, or herpes simplex virus type 2
may result in newborn conjunctivitis. Other bacteria, most commonly
Staphylococcus aureus, are usually acquired after birth.

Inflammation secondary to silver nitrate usually develops within 6 to 12 hours after instillation. Therefore, conjunctivitis appearing after 48 hours should be evaluated for infectious cause. The incubation period for conjunctivitis due to *N. gonorrhoeae* is 2 to 5 days, and for *C. trachomatis,* 5 to 14 days.

General Pediatrics

Conjunctivitis is common in childhood and may be infectious or noninfectious. Conjunctivitides are often associated with systemic viral infections such as the childhood exanthems (particularly measles) and may be associated with Kawasaki disease and mucocutaneous diseases such as erythema multiforme and Stevens-Johnson syndrome.

OBSTETRIC CONSIDERATIONS

Cesarean section is indicated for an active herpes simplex infection of the birth canal.

GERIATRIC CONSIDERATIONS

Extreme pain, photophobia, and visual loss are *not* consistent with conjunctivitis, and the patient should be referred for prompt ophthalmologic consultation.

Conjunctival erythema, pain, mid-dilated pupil, "steamy" cornea, decreased visual acuity, and elevated intraocular pressure are symptoms of acute glaucoma rather than primary conjuctivitis.

PREVENTIVE CONSIDERATIONS

Infectious (Bacterial and Viral)

Avoid direct contact with infected persons or their personal items (e.g., towels, blankets, visual equipment such as glasses, binoculars, microscopes). Wash hands with soap and water; do not rub eyes.

Allergic

Avoid contact with known allergens (e.g., scented face lotion, mascara, eyeliner). Keep sleeping environment free from allergens, especially bed linen. Because allergens adhere to hair and skin, it is important to shower before going to bed. Learn to avoid hand-to-eye contact as much as possible. Wash hands with soap and water before touching eyes or contact lenses. Avoid windy or dusty environments. Rinse eyes with cool water and pat dry.

PEARLS FOR THE PA

Conjunctivitis is the most common ophthalmologic condition seen by the primary health care provider.

Contact lenses should be removed and not worn until the conjunctivitis is completely resolved.

Etiology is infectious, allergic, or chemical.

Extreme pain, photophobia, and visual loss are not consistent with conjunctivitis and should prompt ophthalmologic consultation.

Glaucoma

George L. White, Jr., PhD, MSPH, PA-C

DEFINITION

An abnormal increase in intraocular pressure, occurring chronically or acutely, that causes impaired vision.

HISTORY

Symptoms.   *Chronic* glaucoma is usually asymptomatic and painless until visual loss is profound and causes diminished-field (tunnel) vision.

Acute glaucoma causes sudden, usually unilateral pain, blurring, and loss of peripheral vision, followed by a loss of central vision, incandescent light halos, and headaches. Associated with a fixed pupil.

General.   *Chronic* glaucoma may be suspected in middle-aged patients who require frequent changes in refractive prescriptions, complain of seeing halos around lights, are increasingly bothered by mild headaches, and report decreased visual acuity at night.

Acute glaucoma is characterized by sudden unexplained unilateral eye pain with a loss of vision. A full review of systems is required to rule out contributing systemic diseases. Ask the patient about prolonged use of steroids and any prior ocular surgery, especially cataract surgery.

Age
Chronic.   After age 30.
Acute.   Typically affects one eye and occurs at any age.

Onset
Chronic.   Gradual and surreptitious.

Acute. Occurs suddenly with pain and often loss of vision.

Duration
Chronic. Usually progressive and unremitting if untreated.
Acute. Lasts until attack is treated or spontaneously resolves.

Intensity
Chronic. Initially imperceptible, progressing (without treatment) to significant loss of vision or blindness.
Acute. Pain usually subsides after treatment, but each subsequent episode may further impair visual acuity.

Aggravating Factors. Definite aggravating factors include diabetes mellitus, family history, and myopia. Suggested factors include hypertension, thyroid disease, excessive water intake, tobacco abuse, excessive use of coffee, fatigue, and emotional upset.

Alleviating Factors. Probably none. Decreased use of tobacco and caffeine as well as cessation of steroid therapy in selected patients may be possibly beneficial.

Associated Factors. Risk for developing glaucoma is 4 to 5 times greater in blacks than in whites.

PHYSICAL EXAMINATION

General
Chronic. Findings on physical examination may be unremarkable.
Acute. The patient usually complains of eye pain.

Ophthalmologic
Chronic. The external eye may appear normal. Visual acuity may or may not be affected. The earliest finding on funduscopic examination is an increased cup-to-disc ratio with asymmetry on comparison between the eyes. Visual field abnormalities to confrontation will be present only in very late, profound cases. A Marcus Gunn pupil (afferent pupillary defect) may be present.
Acute. Pupil is mid-dilated and immobile. Cornea has a "steamy" appearance. Conjunctiva is chromatic, erythematous, or injected. Visual acuity is severely affected. Funduscopic examination reveals excavated cupping of the optic disc, shallowness of the anterior chamber, and possible aqueous turbidity. Intraocular tension is increased and visual field defects are common.

PATHOPHYSIOLOGY

The ciliary body produces aqueous humor at the normal rate, but uptake of this fluid is impeded by obstructions or narrowing within the canal of

Schlemm. Intraocular pressure develops and compresses the lens, vitreous body, and optic disc, causing irreversible damage to the head of the optic nerve and consequent visual impairment. Acute episodes of glaucoma tend to be associated with shallow anterior chambers (acute angle glaucoma). Chronic glaucoma is characterized by a normal-appearing anterior chamber that is incompetent in its uptake of aqueous humor (open angle glaucoma).

DIAGNOSTIC STUDIES

Laboratory
Serum Glucose.   As indicated to rule out diabetes mellitus.
Thyroid Profile.   As indicated to rule out thyroid disease.

Radiology
Not applicable.

Other
Tonometry.   Used to measure intraocular pressure.

DIFFERENTIAL DIAGNOSIS

Traumatic
Ocular Trauma.   Positive history of trauma. Requires tonometry as well as careful ophthalmologic examination of the anterior compartment for the presence of blood or other pathologic process that may block the canal of Schlemm.

Infectious
Conjunctivitis and Uveitis.   In acute glaucoma, the injected vessels are more numerous near the corneoscleral limbus, whereas conjunctival vascularization tends to occur peripherally on the sclera.

Metabolic
Diabetes Mellitus.   Elevated serum glucose. Contributes to glaucoma formation (chronic).
Thyroid Disease.   Abnormal thyroid function profile. Contributes to glaucoma formation (chronic).
Hypertension.   Elevated blood pressure measurement. Contributes to glaucoma formation (chronic).
Leukemia, Sickle Cell Disease, Rheumatoid Arthritis, Atopic Disorders. Require the use of steroids and should arouse clinical suspicion for related glaucoma.

Neoplastic
Malignant Melanoma of the Ciliary Body and Choroid.   Seen on MRI scan. Rare.

Vascular
Idiopathic Conjunctival Vascularization. Absence of funduscopic cavitation and undermining of the optic discs.

Congenital
Congenital Glaucoma. Rare. Presence of photophobia, tearing, corneal edema, corneal haziness, and protrusion of the eye (buphthalmos, or "ox eye").

Acquired
Long-Term Steroid Use, Ocular (Especially Cataract) Surgery. Known to contribute to glaucoma formation.
Medications. Steroids, amphetamines, chlorpromazine. Can result in elevation of intraocular pressure.

TREATMENT

Chronic. Ophthalmologic referral is recommended.
Acute. Immediate ophthalmologic referral. Once pressure is normalized, laser iridotomy is indicated to prevent recurrence.

Medical Therapy
- Topical medications
     Pilocarpine (0.5% or 2%) 1 or 2 drops three to six times a day (use weaker preparation first)
     Timolol maleate (0.25% to 0.5%) 1 or 2 drops added to the pilocarpine regimen as required
     Betaxolol HCl (0.5%) 1 drop daily
- Systemic medications
     Carbonic anhydrase inhibitors
     Dichlorphenamide 50-200 mg/day OR
     Acetazolamide 125-250 mg three to four times a day
     Other
     Mannitol (20%) 500 mL by slow intravenous drip

Surgical Intervention
Laser Trabeculoplasty or Iridotomy. For refractory cases.

PEDIATRIC CONSIDERATIONS

Glaucoma is very rare in children but should be a consideration in the Apgar evaluation and in cases of prolonged conjunctivitis or with other refractory eye symptoms.

OBSTETRIC CONSIDERATIONS

No specific indications.

GERIATRIC CONSIDERATIONS

Glaucoma is typically a disorder affecting older persons.

PREVENTIVE CONSIDERATIONS

Optimal control of metabolic conditions (e.g., diabetes mellitus) is essential. Possible contributing factors that may be modified by behavioral change and medical treament include hypertension, thyroid disease, excessive water intake, tobacco abuse, excessive use of coffee, fatigue, and emotional upset. Protective eyewear is recommended during participation in any activity that may cause ocular injury. Screening for glaucoma is recommended in persons requiring long-term steroids.

PEARLS FOR THE PA

Tonometry is the single most useful diagnostic tool for identifying glaucoma.

Chronic glaucoma tends to be bilateral and insidious in onset. The anatomy of the anterior chamber may appear normal (open angle).

Acute glaucoma is usually associated with intense, unilateral eye pain, increased conjunctival vascularity, and shallow (closed angle) anterior chamber.

Acute glaucoma requires prompt diagnosis and treatment, as visual acuity is rapidly and often permanently lost in the untreated patient.

Ocular Hemorrhage

George L. White, Jr., PhD, MSPH, PA-C

DEFINITION

Bleeding into any of the intraocular structures. There are four major types: subconjunctival hemorrhage, anterior chamber hemorrhage (traumatic hyphema), and vitreous and retinal hemorrhages.

HISTORY

Symptoms. Ocular hemorrhages are almost always painless. Subconjuctival hemorrhages are identified as deep red, flat, and well-circumscribed lesions outlined against the white sclera. Anterior chamber hemorrhages (traumatic hyphemas) do not usually affect vision, are half-moon shaped, and do not tend to form a solid clot. Vitreous hemorrhages generally cause decreased vision in the affected eye. Retinal hemorrhages are associated with impaired vision and visual field defects.

General. The patient may have a history of direct trauma to the eye or of minor trauma such as sneezing, or may have a systemic condition such as diabetes mellitus, hypertension, or a blood dyscrasia.

Age. Usually unrelated to the occurrence of ocular hemorrhage.

Onset. Anterior chamber and vitreous hemorrhages are acute, typically following head or eye trauma. Subconjunctival hemorrhages occur spontaneously or after barely perceptible trauma such as sneezing. Retinal hemorrhages are acute and may follow trauma but are more commonly associated with systemic conditions.

Duration. Subconjunctival hemorrhages clear up in about 1 to 2 weeks. Anterior chamber and vitreous hemorrhages generally resolve over varying amounts of time, years in some cases. Retinal hemorrhages usually clear up but may leave areas of retinal scarring, which may impair vision.

Intensity. Most hemorrhages in the eye are relatively painless.

Aggravating Factors. The use of aspirin and anticoagulation medications, physical activities involving transient straining, and hypertensive episodes.

Alleviating Factors. Time for spontaneous resolution or surgery in selected cases to preserve vision.

Associated Factors. Use of anticoagulants, systemic diseases such as diabetes mellitus, hypertension, or blood dyscrasias.

PHYSICAL EXAMINATION

General
A full physical examination including blood pressure measurement needs to be performed to rule out systemic disease.

Ophthalmologic
Visual acuity should be measured and documented in all cases.

Subconjunctival hemorrhages are flat and deep red in color outlined against a white sclera.

Anterior chamber hemorrhages typically have a settled layer of blood between the cornea and the iris and resemble a half-moon. The blood does not tend to clot but settles to the bottom of the anterior chamber and remains horizontal despite changes in body position.

Vitreous hemorrhages, on ophthalmologic examination, produce diffusely scattered dots or lines that may appear black in the early stages of the bleed, changing to lighter colors later. View of the retina is obscured on funduscopic examination.

Retinal bleeding produces flame-shaped markings on the innermost surface of the retina and round ("dot and blot") lesions in the deeper layers.

PATHOPHYSIOLOGY

Ocular hemorrhages are often related to direct trauma to the head or orbit but may be associated with congenital and retinal vascular abnormalities, atherosclerotic disease, and retinal vein occlusion from such conditions as sickle cell anemia.

The vitreous is an avascular structure. As age advances, the vitreous becomes less viscous and may come loose from the retina. Any tear in the retina or other ocular structures may allow blood into the vitreous.

Retinal hemorrhage may result from tears due to trauma (stretches that deform the eye), age (retina becomes brittle), and loss of vitreous viscosity (allows the retina to bulge).

Anterior chamber hemorrhage may cause glaucoma or scarring of the iris, which may result in visual dysfunction.

Subconjunctival hemorrhages are rarely associated with underlying pathology and are self-limiting.

DIAGNOSTIC STUDIES

Laboratory
Serum Glucose.　As indicated to rule out diabetes mellitus.
Coagulation Screen.　As indicated to rule out blood dyscrasias.

Radiology
Skull Radiographs, CT/MRI Scan of the Orbits or Head.　As indicated to evaluate trauma.

Other
Visual Field Testing.　Used to evaluate for visual field deficits.

DIFFERENTIAL DIAGNOSIS

Traumatic
Penetrating Trauma to the Globe.　Small objects may penetrate the globe even with apparently innocuous trauma. Conjuctiva may be bloody or bulge (bloody chemosis). Injury is a primary cause of serious ocular hemorrhages within the interior compartments of the eye.

Infectious
Vitreous Infection.　Hemorrhagic artifacts may be confused with tissue and white blood cell inclusions or with bacteria that aggregate in clusters

within the vitreous body. These artifacts tend to develop surreptitiously, whereas ocular bleeding is sudden.

Metabolic
Retinal Aberrations/Floaters/Refractive Defects Associated with Aging. Generally differentiated from vitreous bleeding by being structurally larger and less diffuse.

Neoplastic
Leukemia. Produces retinal hemorrhages with white centers (Roth spots).

Vascular
Chronic Hypertension. Damage and occlusions of the fundic vasculature, resulting in ischemia and destruction of portions of the retina.

Congenital
Telangiectasia/Sickle Cell Anemia. Can produce varyious types of ocular hemorrhage.

Acquired. Not applicable.

TREATMENT

Subconjunctival Hemorrhage
No treatment.

Anterior Chamber and Vitreous Hemorrhages
Surgical drainage is indicated with intraocular pressures in excess of 50 mm Hg, persistently high pressures (for longer than 5 to 7 days), or hemorrhagic staining of the cornea.

Retinal Hemorrhage
Treatment of the underlying condition. Surgery is indicated when retinal separation has occurred.

PEDIATRIC CONSIDERATIONS

Subconjunctival and intraocular hemorrhages are relatively common in traumatic deliveries but almost always clear without sequelae.

In the examination of the newborn, a finding of conjunctival and retinal hemorrhages by themselves is not significant; the bleeding usually is thought to result from a sudden increase in intrathoracic pressure during passage of the chest through the birth canal. Retinal hemorrhages resulting from violent shaking of infants and children who have been physically abused are well documented. Often, no direct signs of trauma to the eye, periocular region, or head are obvious in these cases.

OBSTETRIC CONSIDERATIONS

No specific indications.

GERIATRIC CONSIDERATIONS

Patients requiring aspirin or anticoagulation medications and those with hypertension or atherosclerotic disease are at higher risk for ocular hemorrhage.

With advancing age, the vitreous becomes less viscous and may come loose from the retina. The retina becomes more brittle. Any tear in the retina or other ocular structures may allow blood into the vitreous.

PREVENTIVE CONSIDERATIONS

Appropriate protective eyewear is the most effective preventive measure against ocular hemorrhage. Optimal control of systemic conditions (e.g., diabetes mellitus, hypertension) is recommended.

PEARLS FOR THE PA

Subconjuctival hemorrhages are characterized by blood outlined against the white of the sclera.

Anterior chamber hemorrhages are usually painless (aside from the precipitating trauma) and may or may not interfere with vision.

Vitreous hemorrhages are painless and often cause decreased vision in the affected eye.

Retinal hemorrhages are painless and associated with impaired visual acuity, visual field deficits, and the appearance of sudden new floaters.

Anterior chamber and vitreous hemorrhages necessitate immediate referral of the patient for ophthalmologic care.

Avoid the use of aspirin for analgesia.

Prompt ophthalmologic referral is prudent for all intraocular hemorrhages except conjunctival bleeding.

Optic Neuritis

George L. White, Jr., PhD, MSPH, PA-C

DEFINITION

An inflammatory, demyelinating, and degenerative condition associated with the optic nerve.

HISTORY

Symptoms. About three-fourths of the cases of optic neuritis involve unilateral visual changes including blurring of vision, blind spot (scotoma), impaired color vision, and poor depth perception. Eye pain with movement occurs in a majority of cases and frequently precedes the onset of visual changes.

General. Patienta may have a history of viral or bacterial infection involving the eye, systemic conditions, multiple sclerosis (MS), autoimmune disorders, demyelinating disease, environmental exposure, alcohol abuse, or long-term steroid use.

Age. Unilateral disease is most common in the 30- to 50-year age group. Pediatric optic neuritis, although rare, is generally bilateral.

Onset. There is often a dull prodromal pain in one eye several days prior to visual changes. Visual changes, sometimes progressing to blindness, may occur rapidly, after about 12 hours in some cases.

Duration. Typically a progressive loss of vision over a 5-day period. Recovery may take 1 to 2 weeks to several months.

Intensity. Ocular pain is present in about two-thirds of cases. The pain may be a generalized, dull, periorbital ache or a sharp pain.

Aggravating Factors. Pain may be exacerbated by eye movement or pressure to the globe.

Alleviating Factors. None.

Associated Factors. Women, especially those in their 30s, are more likely to develop optic neuritis than men. There is a high correlation with multiple sclerosis (MS) (almost half of the patients who present with optic neuritis have a history of MS or go on to develop the disease within a few years), systemic lupus erythematosus, syphilis, meningitis, and autoimmune encephalitis.

PHYSICAL EXAMINATION

General. A full physical examination is performed, with attention given to the neurologic component to rule out contributing systemic disease.

Ophthalmologic. Often a decreased pupillary light reflex in the affected eye. Visual acuity should be measured and documented and visual field defects identified. Funduscopic examination may reveal papilledema and splinter hemorrhages of the optic disc, along with varying degrees of retinal edema and hyperemia.

PATHOPHYSIOLOGY

The etiology of optic neuritis is obscure. The condition is associated with inflammation of the optic nerve, often with demyelination.

DIAGNOSTIC STUDIES

Laboratory
Complete Blood Count. Elevated white blood cell count with infections; decreased hemoglobin and hematocrit with anemias.
Serologic Studies. As indicated to rule out syphilis, mononucleosis, and the rickettsial diseases.
Chemistry Profile. Elevated serum glucose with diabetes mellitus, decreased serum iron with deficiency states.
Thyroid Function Studies. As indicated to rule out hyperthyroidism/ hypothyroidism.

Radiology
Skull Radiographs/MRI Scan of the Orbits and Brain (with and without Contrast). As indicated to evaluate for MS or tumors.

Other
Lumbar Puncture. As indicated to rule out meningitis, neurosyphilis, and MS.

DIFFERENTIAL DIAGNOSIS

Traumatic
Hysterical Vision Loss after Head Trauma. Normal examination.

Infectious
Chickenpox, Malaria, Pertussis. May manifest with papilledema.

Metabolic
Diabetes mellitus, Addison disease, Hyperthyroidism. May mimic signs and symptoms of optic neuritis; differentiated on laboratory testing.
Pseudotumor Cerebri. Papilledema associated with elevated intracranial pressure and, occasionally, an abducens nerve palsy.

Neoplastic
Intracranial Neoplasms.   May exhibit papilledema; positive MRI scan.

Vascular
Malignant Hypertension, Iron Deficiency Anemia, Leukemia.   Similar funduscopic signs; differentiated on laboratory testing.

Congenital
Not applicable.

Acquired
Alcohol Abuse, Chronic Lead Ingestion, Chronic Use of Corticosteroids, Pregnancy, Systemic Effects of Bee Stings.   All have resulted in optic neuritis and related ophthalmic findings.

TREATMENT

Pulsed, intravenous steroids have been shown to be effective. This should be done under the direct supervision of a neuro-ophthalmologist.

PEDIATRIC CONSIDERATIONS

Optic neuritis is very rare in children, but it should be considered when there is a high index of suspicion for lead ingestion. When pediatric optic neuritis occurs, it is generally bilateral.

OBSTETRIC CONSIDERATIONS

No specific indications.

GERIATRIC CONSIDERATIONS

No specific indications.

PREVENTIVE CONSIDERATIONS

Avoidance of alcohol abuse is important. Safe sex practices should be encouraged to prevent contributing factors such as syphilis. Optic neuritis may be the initial symptom of multiple sclerosis, so full neurologic evaluation should be performed to appropriately diagnose and treat patients.

PEARLS FOR THE PA

There is about a 50% correlation between optic neuritis and the presence of MS.

Prompt identification and treatment of optic neuritis are important in preventing permanent visual damage.

The typical patient with optic neuritis is a woman in her early 30s.

Papilledema is an indication for immediate ophthalmologic and neurologic referral.

Retinal Detachment

George L. White, Jr., PhD, MSPH, PA-C

DEFINITION

Separation of the retina from the underlying choroid.

HISTORY

Symptoms. Shower of flashing lights associated with eye movements and new floaters may be appreciated initially. Progresses to a painless visual field loss that spreads from the periphery to the center of the visual field.

General. Often described as a curtain-like defect of the visual field. History of previous ocular surgery and family history of retinal detachment and systemic disease should be ascertained.

Age. In the absence of blunt trauma, detachment occurs most often in persons older than 60 years.

Onset. May be sudden or gradual.

Duration. Progresses relentlessly to blindness, if neglected over hours to days.

Intensity. Varying degrees of visual loss that can be permanent if left untreated.

Aggravating Factors. Continued activity after the detachment has occurred. The patient should lie flat.

Alleviating Factors. Retinal surgery, using protective eyewear when appropriate.

Associated Factors. High myopia, family history of retinal detachment, previous ocular surgery, blunt trauma, intraocular tumors, ocular inflammatory disease, and renal failure.

PHYSICAL EXAMINATION

General. The patient will ordinarily be in no acute distress.

Ophthalmologic. When examined through a dilated pupil, the detachment appears grayish blue and may extend or "balloon" anteriorly into the vitreous humor. The vessels appear darker than those viewed on an attached retina. There is a loss of the red light reflex on viewing the affected area. A Marcus Gunn pupil (afferent pupillary defect) may be present. Confrontation may reveal a visual field deficit.

PATHOPHYSIOLOGY

The detachment is that of the sensory retina (rods and cones) separating from the underlying pigmented epithelium, allowing fluid accumulation between the two. The majority of detachments are associated with retinal holes created by vitreous traction.

DIAGNOSTIC STUDIES

Laboratory. Not applicable.
Radiology. Not applicable.
Other. Not applicable.

DIFFERENTIAL DIAGNOSIS

Metabolic
Migraine Aura. Shimmering, flashing lights with geometric borders, seen with the eyes open or closed, not related to head motion and spontaneous resolution.

Neoplastic
Leukemia. Produces retinal hemorrhages with white centers (Roth spots).

Vascular
Vitreous Hemorrhage. On ophthalmologic examination, presence of diffusely scattered dots or lines that may appear black in the early stages of the bleeding, changing to lighter colors later. View of the retina is obscured on funduscopic examination.
Chronic Hypertension. Damage and occlusions of the fundal vasculature, resulting in ischemia and destruction of portions of the retina.

Traumatic. Not applicable.
Infectious. Not applicable.
Congenital. Not applicable.

TREATMENT

On diagnosis, the patient should be placed on NPO status. Immediate ophthalmologic referral is made for surgical reattachment of the retina.

PEDIATRIC CONSIDERATIONS

Detachment of the retina in children usually is associated with severe ocular trauma, high myopia, or other ocular abnormalities or disease processes such as retinopathy of prematurity, persistent hyperplastic primary vitreous, Coat disease, retinoblastoma, toxocariasis, and certain optic nerve head anomalies. Retinal detachment also is a feature of Pierre Robin syndrome and a number of other systemic syndromes.

A child with retinal detachment may complain of progressively more severe blurred vision and may present with signs of secondary strabismus and/or nystagmus, or leukokoria (white pupillary reflex).

OBSTETRIC CONSIDERATIONS

No specific indications.

GERIATRIC CONSIDERATIONS

In the absence of blunt trauma, detachment occurs most often in persons older than 60 years of age.

PREVENTIVE CONSIDERATIONS

Protective eyewear is recommended. Immediate referral of suspected cases is recommended to prevent visual loss.

PEARLS FOR THE PA

Retinal detachment is often described as a curtain-like defect of the visual field.

The condition progresses relentlessly to blindness, if neglected over hours to days.

Immediate ophthalmologic referral is indicated.

Further Reading

Apple DJ, Rabb MF: Ocular Pathology, 5th ed. St. Louis, Mosby, 1998.

Behrman RE, Kliegman RM, Jenson HB, et al: Nelson Textbook of Pediatrics, 17th ed. Philadelphia, Saunders, 2003.

Hay WW Jr, Hayward AR, Levin MJ, et al (eds): Current Pediatric Diagnosis and Treatment, 16th ed. East Norwalk, CT, McGraw-Hill/Appleton & Lange, 2002.

Newell FW, Patel, S: Ophthalmology: Principles and Concepts, 8th ed. St. Louis, Mosby, 1996.

Rakel RE (ed): Textbook of Family Practice, 6th ed. Philadelphia, WB Saunders, 2002.

OTORHINOLARYNGOLOGY

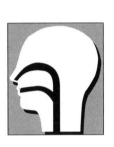

13

Benign Paroxysmal Positional Vertigo

Debra S. Munsell, MPAS, PA-C

DEFINITION

Benign paroxysmal positional vertigo (BPPV): A disorder characterized by recurring episodes of objective (measurable) vertigo with or without nausea and vomiting, lasting from seconds to minutes, associated with changes in head or body position.

HISTORY

Symptoms.   Severe vertigo occurring with rapid changes in head or body position. Vertigo may be described as a swimming or rocking sensation. Symptoms are reported to be of sudden onset, lasting seconds only. Usually occurs when rising from bed or lying down. There is no associated hearing change, tinnitus, or aural fullness.

General.   No specific etiologic factor has been documented; the patient may have a history of a closed head injury or recent infection or otologic surgery. Certain drugs may produce vertigo, but not a positional vertigo. This condition should not be confused with postural hypotension.

Age.   Mean age at onset in the fourth to fifth decades of life, but cases in persons from 11 to 84 years of age have been reported. Incidence increases with age.

Onset.   Immediate after changes in body or head position.

Duration.   Vertiginous periods last seconds, rarely over a minute.

Intensity.   Severe, can be transiently disabling.

Aggravating Factors.   Rapid changes in head or body position (e.g., lying down, looking up, bending, rolling over in bed).

Alleviating Factors.   Rest and slow head and body movements.

Associated Factors.   Alcohol ingestion, concurrent inner ear infections, pharmacologic agents.

PHYSICAL EXAMINATION

General.   The patient, if unaffected at the time of examination, will appear normal.

Head, Eyes, Ears, Nose, Throat.   Usually normal. The presence of hearing loss indicates a separate underlying process. Dix-Hallpike maneuver is often positive (i.e., elicits a classic rotatory nystagmus with a fast component). The response usually fatigues with repeated maneuvers, diagnostic of BPPV.

Neurologic.   A complete neurologic examination including cranial nerve testing should be performed to rule out mass lesions or other neurologic syndromes associated with vertigo.

PATHOPHYSIOLOGY

Lodging of free-floating degenerated otoliths in the posterior semicircular canal is reported as the responsible mechanism. These particles stimulate the neuroepithelium of the semicircular canal, producing the symptoms.

DIAGNOSTIC STUDIES

Laboratory. None.
Radiology. Not useful unless mass lesion needs to be ruled out.

Other
Audiogram. Usually normal findings or, if abnormal, commensurate with age group.
Electronystagmography (ENG). Usually normal findings. May be positive when the Dix-Hallpike maneuver is performed with electrode monitoring. A positive result on Dix-Hallpike is diagnostic of BPPV.

DIFFERENTIAL DIAGNOSIS

Traumatic
Labyrinthine Concussion. History of trauma.

Infectious
Vestibular Neuronitis/Labyrinthitis. Often associated with vertigo, nausea, and vomiting.

Metabolic
Meniere Disease. Classic triad of episodic vertigo, decreased hearing, and tinnitus. Patient usually has nausea and vomiting.

Neoplastic
Acoustic Neuroma. Hearing loss and tinnitus and possibly dizziness with positive findings on CT/MRI.

Vascular
Basilar Artery Insufficiency. Vertigo associated with gait imbalance and possible vital sign and visual changes.

Congenital. Not applicable.
Acquired. Not applicable.

TREATMENT

Treatment is geared toward reducing symptoms.

Vestibular rehabilitation using vestibular exercises, administered by a vestibular therapist, may increase tolerance of the vertigo. Vestibular rehabilitation is the treatment of choice.

Suppression of vestibular function with medications is ineffective and may delay recovery.

The canalith repositioning procedure described by Epley is effective.

Surgical interventions include singular neurectomy, vestibular neurectomy, and posterior semicircular canal occlusion. Surgical risks include sensorineural hearing loss.

PEDIATRIC CONSIDERATIONS

Brief attacks of vertigo (BPPV) may occur in young children, often prior to the third year. The attacks are sudden and associated with ataxia. Horizontal nystagmus may be identified during the attacks. The youngster appears pale and frightened, and nausea and vomiting may occur. The attacks vary in duration and frequency. There is no lethargy or drowsiness noted following the episode. These children are often susceptible to motion sickness, and some will develop migraine headaches later in life. Findings on neurologic evaluation are normal, and medications are usually unnecessary.

OBSTETRIC CONSIDERATIONS

Vestibular suppressants are generally ineffective; vestibular rehabilitation should be utilized.

GERIATRIC CONSIDERATIONS

Elderly patients should be cautioned to avoid activities that could result in injury should an episode occur. These may include climbing, reaching, and driving.

Caution should be used in prescribing sedating medication for patients with BPPV, as this may compound the problem when an attack occurs.

PREVENTIVE CONSIDERATIONS

None.

PEARLS FOR THE PA

BPPV can usually be diagnosed from the history.

Symptoms are precipitated by rapid changes in head or body position in the absence of other otologic symptoms.

Cerumen Impaction

Debra Munsell, MPAS, PA-C

DEFINITION

Obstruction of the external auditory canal by excessive earwax, which may incorporate hair or epithelial debris.

HISTORY

Symptoms.   Hearing loss is the most common complaint, but patients may complain of aural fullness, plugging, itchy external auditory canal, or sensitivity.

General.   Inquire about any history of attempts to clean the ear canal. A history of traumatic tympanic membrane perforation or prior ear surgery needs to be ascertained. Patients who have undergone external beam radiotherapy involving the external auditory canal must be examined carefully, preferably using the otologic microscope.

Age.   Any.

Onset.   Gradual with the buildup of cerumen.

Duration.   As long as the impaction remains.

Intensity.   Mild, unless sensitivity or secondary infection develops.

Aggravating Factors.   Prior history of ionizing radiation to region of the external auditory canal, and insertion of foreign bodies into the canal.

Alleviating Factors.   Removal of the impaction.

Associated Factors.   Use of foreign bodies in the external auditory canal.

PHYSICAL EXAMINATION

General.   The patient is usually in no apparent distress.

Head, Eyes, Ears, Nose, Throat.   Otoscopic examination reveals impaction obstructing the view of the tympanic membrane.

PATHOPHYSIOLOGY

Excess accumulation of cerumen produced by the cerumen glands of the external auditory canal, squamous epithelium, and external auditory canal hair combine to form a plug, which becomes impacted.

DIAGNOSTIC STUDIES

Laboratory.   None.
Radiology.   None.
Other.   None.

DIFFERENTIAL DIAGNOSIS

Traumatic
Foreign Body.   Seen on otoscopic examination.

Infectious
Otitis Externa.   Pain on manipulation of auricle; reddened external auditory canal.

Metabolic
Skin Diseases (e.g., Psoriasis).   May produce squamous epithelial plugs.

Neoplastic
Tumors Impinging on the External Auditory Canal.   Seen on otoscopic examination.

Vascular
Vascular Tumors (e.g., Glomus Tumor).   Can affect the middle ear.

Congenital
Canal Atresia.   Absence of external auditory canal.

Acquired
Radiation-Induced.   Prior history of external beam radiotherapy involving the external auditory canal.

TREATMENT

Removal can be accomplished by irrigation (contraindicated in patients with a history of tympanic membrane perforation) with tepid water or curettage under direct otoscopic vision.

Ceruminolytic agents may be required (e.g., Debrox or Cerumenex drops). In persistent cases, otology consultation may be indicated.

Microscopic otologic evaluation with careful cleaning of the canal performed by a knowledgeable clinician must be provided for the patient with a prior radiation history. Trauma to the delicate tissues of the irradiated canal can lead to devastating consequences such as osteoradionecrosis of the canal and associated bone structures as well as serious infections.

PEDIATRIC CONSIDERATIONS

Removal of cerumen can be accomplished with the use of an otoscope with a surgical head and a wire loop or cerumen curette. Care must be taken in the pediatric patient to provide an appropriate and adequate level of restraint to avoid injury. Cerumen may also be removed by gentle irrigation of the ear canal with warm water using an irrigation syringe or dental irrigation device (set at low pressure). Softening the cerumen first with the instillation of hydrogen peroxide (3% solution) may facilitate removal. A perforated tympanic membrane or in-place ventilation tube is a contraindication to any form of irrigation. History of allergic response to ceruminolytics should be ruled out prior to use.

OBSTETRIC CONSIDERATIONS

No specific indications.

GERIATRIC CONSIDERATIONS

Patients should be admonished to change positions slowly after cerumen removal, to avoid a vertiginous episode.

PREVENTIVE CONSIDERATIONS

None.

PEARLS FOR THE PA

The diagnosis of ceruminal impaction is usually apparent on otoscopic examination.

Inquiry should be made about history of tympanic perforations, previous ear surgery, or history of external beam irradiation prior to irrigation procedures or instillation of cerumen-softening agents.

Eustachian Tube Dysfunction

Debra Munsell, MPAS, PA-C

DEFINITION

Abnormal eustachian tube function associated with symptoms referable to the ear, but not involving a middle ear effusion.

HISTORY

Symptoms. The most common complaints are otalgia, vertigo, tinnitus, aural fullness, and plugging. May also be associated with autophony (hearing one's own voice) and abnormal speech.

General. A recent history of an upper respiratory infection, environmental allergies, or surgery is common. Patients may mention that after swallowing, they experience canal fullness or plugging, decreased hearing, and autophony. Eustachian tube dysfunction can be caused by an obstruction or by an unusual degree of patency, in which case the tube is referred to as a *patulous* eustachian tube. A history of recent rapid weight loss, pregnancy, or neuromuscular disease may be elicited.

Age. Any.

Onset. Usually immediate, but can be gradual.

Duration. Acute to chronic.

Intensity. Varies. May become painful if infection develops.

Aggravating Factors. Environmental allergies, upper respiratory infection, recent rapid weight loss, pregnancy, neuromuscular disease.

Alleviating Factors. Appropriate therapy.

Associated Factors. Coexisting infections, recent nasopharyngeal surgery, recent barotrauma, craniofacial deformities.

PHYSICAL EXAMINATION

General. The patient usually is in no acute distress.

Head, Eyes, Ears, Nose, Throat. Eustachian tube dysfunction associated with obstruction may yield signs of middle ear negative pressure and a retracted tympanic membrane (TM). Erythema of the TM may be present after recent barotrauma. Physical signs of a patulous eustachian tube may include movement of the TM synchronous with speaking and respiration.

PATHOPHYSIOLOGY

Eustachian tube dysfunction may be acute or chronic, and involve obstruction or a patulous tube. It may be the result of inefficient or ineffective function of the tensor veli palatini muscle. Acute conditions are usually associated with an infectious or a neoplastic process such as an acute upper airway infection or tumor mass. Chronic dysfunction may be the result of allergies, neuromuscular disorders, or craniofacial deformities or may be entirely idiopathic in nature.

DIAGNOSTIC STUDIES

Laboratory
Allergen Testing. May be considered if allergic etiology suspected.

Radiology
CT/MRI of the Head/Inner Ear. May show a mass lesion.

Other
Audiogram.   Nondiagnostic.
Tympanometry.   Will usually show negative middle ear pressures.

DIFFERENTIAL DIAGNOSIS

Traumatic
Head Injury.   History of concussion or basilar skull fracture.
Concussive Injury to the Ear Canal.   Commonly seen with hand slaps to the pinna.
Barotrauma.   Associated with rapid changes in atmospheric pressure.

Infectious
Upper Respiratory Infection.   History of cough, congestion, and erythema of oropharynx.

Metabolic
Otosclerosis.   Differentiated on otoscopic examination.

Neoplastic
Nasopharyngeal or Vascular Tumor.   Positive biopsy findings, progressive growth, positive findings on CT/MRI.

Vascular
Not applicable.

Congenital
Congenital Stapes Fixation.   Characterized by otosclerosis that develops after birth.
Craniofacial Deformities.   Associated with cleft anomalies.

Acquired
Post–Head/Neck Irradiation.   History of radiation therapy with ports that involve the eustachian tube.
Rapid Weight Loss, Pregnancy.   Positive history.

TREATMENT

Non-Patulous Pathology

Pharmacologic Management
- Antihistamines: either over-the-counter preparations such as diphenhydramine or prescriptive preparations (e.g., loratadine, cetirizine), if allergies are suspected
- Decongestants: over-the-counter preparations such as pseudoephedrine

- Immunotherapy for allergic symptoms
- Steroids: oral prednisone or intranasal steroids beneficial in some patients

Surgical Correction

Tympanotomy with or without insertion of polyethylene tube.

Patulous Eustachian Tube

Abnormally patent eustachian tube is not treated in the same manner. Decongestants and antihistamines may aggravate the condition. Most cases are self-limited, and attempts at surgical correction have been met with mixed results. Re-gaining the weight previously lost may be helpful. Surgical obstruction of the eustachian tube has been performed to relieve symptoms of a patulous tube.

PEDIATRIC CONSIDERATIONS

In the young child, the eustachian tube is shorter, more compliant, and more horizontally placed than in older children or adults. The increased frequency of upper respiratory tract infections in the young child adversely affects the function of the eustachian tube and predisposes the child to middle ear effusion. This dysfunction prevents middle ear secretions from draining and creates negative pressure within the middle ear space. The negative pressure predisposes the child to aspiration of bacteria from nasopharyngeal secretions, which frequently results in otitis media.

OBSTETRIC CONSIDERATIONS

Abnormally patent eustachian tube is sometimes seen in pregnant patients.

Decongestants, which can be used in eustachian tube dysfunction, are considered relatively safe to use during pregnancy if clearly indicated. However, studies have demonstrated some possible connections between maternal decongestant use and increased risk of clubfoot and inguinal hernia.

GERIATRIC CONSIDERATIONS

As with all geriatric patients, care should be given when prescribing sedating medications.

PREVENTIVE CONSIDERATIONS

None.

PEARLS FOR THE PA

Most cases of eustacian tube dysfunction are self-limiting.

Commonly associated with upper respiratory infections.

The patient with an abnormally patent eustachian tube may have similar symptoms, but treatment with decongestants and antihistamines may aggravate the symptoms.

Labyrinthitis

Sue M. Enns, MHS, PA-C

DEFINITION

An acute inflammation of the labyrinth (internal ear) either of viral or bacterial etiology, often causing disabling vertigo, nausea, and vomiting.

HISTORY

Symptoms. Patients typically experience acute onset of continuous, severe vertigo with hearing loss, nausea and vomiting, and occasional tinnitus. The diagnosis of labyrinthitis is usually made clinically on the basis of the classic findings on history and physical examination.

General. May have a recent history of an upper respiratory infection.

Age. Any, but more common in adults.

Onset. Acute.

Duration. Symptoms gradually resolve over a period of 7 to 10 days. Some patients may experience dysequilibrium for weeks to months. Hearing may return to normal or remain permanently impaired in the affected ear.

Intensity. Vertigo is usually moderate to severe. The most severely affected patients may require hospitalization for parenteral fluids and medications to control nausea and vomiting.

Aggravating Factors. Physical activity, especially rapid movements of the head and neck.

Alleviating Factors. Bed rest and sedation.

Associated Factors. Upper respiratory infection.

PHYSICAL EXAMINATION

General. Patients may appear quite ill or dehydrated secondary to the vertigo, nausea, and vomiting.

Head, Eyes, Ears, Nose, Throat. Otolaryngologic examination findings are usually negative. Horizontal nystagmus is almost always present.

Neurologic. Ataxia may be present. Full examination with attention given to the cranial nerves and cerebellar function is mandatory to rule out primary neurologic disease.

PATHOPHYSIOLOGY

Acute inflammation of the labyrinth (inner ear). The exact cause is unknown, although it frequently follows an upper respiratory infection. Rarely, bacterial infection is the cause.

DIAGNOSTIC STUDIES

Diagnostic studies are not routinely needed, as the diagnosis is made clinically.

Laboratory
Electrolytes and Urine Specific Gravity. As indicated to evaluate for dehydration in patients with severe nausea and vomiting.

Radiology. Not generally indicated.

Other
Audiogram/Electronystagmography (ENG). Not generally indicated unless further investigation is indicated based on unusual presentation or neurologic abnormalities.

DIFFERENTIAL DIAGNOSIS

Traumatic
Head Injury. History of injury. May be associated with labrynthine concussion and may cause dizziness. Symptoms gradually resolve over several days but may be prolonged over several months.

Infectious
Central Nervous System Infection (e.g., Meningitis/Encephalitis). Fever and neurologic signs and symptoms are typically present; positive findings on examination of cerebrospinal fluid (CSF) in meningitis.

Vestibular Neuronitis. Due to inflammation of the vestibular nerve. Symptoms essentially the same except for the absence of hearing loss and tinnitus.

Tertiary Syphilis. Positive result on Venereal Disease Research Laboratory (VDRL) test.

Metabolic
Meniere Disease. Classic combination of episodic vertigo, fluctuating hearing loss, tinnitus, and aural fullness. Usually with nausea and vomiting. Episodes typically last only for hours as opposed to several days.

Diabetes Mellitus. Diabetics are at risk for autonomic neuropathy resulting in dizziness or lightheadedness.

Multiple Sclerosis (MS). Patients may suffer from episodic vertigo and chronic imbalance. Other neurologic signs may be present. In rare cases, the presentation of MS is an acute attack of vertigo.

Neoplastic
Intracranial Tumors. Positive CT/MRI. Tumors can cause vertigo from increasing intracranial pressure or from direct effect on the vestibular nerve. Symptoms become progressively worse.

Acoustic Neuroma. A benign tumor involving the eighth cranial nerve. Progressive, unilateral hearing loss is the most common symptom; however, it may manifest with continuous, progressive dysequilibrium.

Vascular
Vertebrobasilar Artery Insufficiency. Dysequilibrium as a result of a transient reduction in blood flow to the brainstem. May be triggered by changes in posture or extension of the neck.

Cerebrovascular Disease. Transient ischemic attacks (TIAs) may result in dysequilibrium for a variable length of time. Stroke may also manifest with dizziness or dysequilibrium. Other neurologic deficits will typically be present.

Acquired
Benign Paroxysmal Positional Vertigo. Vertigo associated with rapid head movements and lasting only a few seconds to minutes. Symptoms are fatigable.

History of Ototoxic Medication (e.g., Aminoglycosides). May result in dizziness secondary to peripheral end-organ damage. Patients usually report progressive unsteadiness.

Congenital. Not applicable.

TREATMENT

- Antihistamines
  Meclizine 25-50 mg PO every 6 to 8 hours
  Dimenhydrinate 50-100 mg PO/IM/IV every 4-6 hours; maximum 400 mg/day
  Diphenhydramine 25-50 mg PO/IM/IV every 6 hours; maximum 100 mg/dose; 400 mg/day

- Anticholinergics
  Scopolamine patch 1.5 mg/patch
- Antiemetics
  Prochlorperazine 5-10 mg PO/IM or 25 mg rectally every 6-8 hours
  or 25 mg rectally every 12 hours
  Promethazine 12.5-25 mg PO/IM or rectally every 4 to 6 hours

PEDIATRIC CONSIDERATIONS

Labyrinthitis is rare in children. Treat the same as adults with pediatric medication doses.

OBSTETRIC CONSIDERATIONS

Meclizine can be used for symptomatic relief. Prochlorperazine should be avoided because of serious fetal effects such as jaundice, protracted extrapyramidal signs, hyperreflexia, and hyporeflexia. Scopolamine should be used only if clearly indicated.

GERIATRIC CONSIDERATIONS

Elderly patients with residual postional vertigo following labyrinthitis should be cautioned to avoid activities that may involve quick head movements inducing dizziness, possibly resulting in injury (e.g., standing on ladders, changing light bulbs).

Medications (e.g., antihistamines) that potentially cause drowsiness and resulting unsteadiness should be used with caution in the elderly.

Prescribe anticholinergic medications with caution in the elderly patient, who may be more likely to have prostatic hypertrophy, hypertension, or glaucoma.

Closely monitor the elderly patient with severe nausea and vomiting for dehydration and electrolyte disturbance.

The incidence of cerebral hypoperfusion as a cause of dizziness increases with advancing age, and this possibility should always be considered in the differential diagnosis.

PREVENTIVE CONSIDERATIONS

None.

PEARLS FOR THE PA

Acute labyrinthitis is often associated with a precipitating upper respiratory infection or central nervous system infection.

Diagnosis is dependent on ruling out disorders causing similar symptoms.

Meniere Disease

Sue M. Enns, MHS, PA-C

DEFINITION

Is thought to be due to excessive endolymphatic fluid in the cochlea, semicircular canals, or both. Typically, the disease occurs unilaterally, although bilateral disease may be present.

HISTORY

Symptoms.   The hallmark of this disorder is the combination of fluctuating, low-frequency sensorineuronal hearing loss, tinnitus (usually a low roaring noise), vertigo, nausea, and aural fullness. In many cases the vertigo is severe, resulting in nausea and vomiting. These symptoms may or may not occur simultaneously, so a thorough history is important.

General.   The patient should be asked if the symptoms are positional or if there are any subjective signs of cranial nerve abnormalities (e.g., diplopia, facial numbness/weakness, dysphagia, dysarthria).

Age.   Any, but most frequently onset is between 30 and 50 years of age. Rarely noted for the first time in older persons. Both genders affected equally.

Onset.   Usually develops gradually, with a sensation of aural fullness, plugging, pressure, and tinnitus, followed in rapid progression by vertigo, nausea, and vomiting.

Duration.   Episodes can last from several minutes to several hours. Episode frequency may vary from days to weeks, months to years.

Intensity.   Mild to disabling; may require hospitalization for rehydration.

Aggravating Factors.   High-sodium diet, caffeine/alcohol ingestion, smoking, and lifestyle stress are thought to increase the frequency of episodes.

Alleviating Factors.   Bed rest and sedation.

Associated Factors.   None.

PHYSICAL EXAMINATION

General.   During asymptomatic periods, the patient will appear normal. During an episode, the patient may appear quite ill and be unwilling to move. Nausea and vomiting usually accompany severe vertigo.

Head, Eyes, Ears, Nose, Throat.   Usually normal. Lateral gaze nystagmus may be present.

Neurologic.   Usually normal. Full examination with attention given to the cranial nerves and cerebellar function is mandatory to rule out primary neurologic disease.

PATHOPHYSIOLOGY

The precise mechanism is unknown. Etiologic possibilities include distention of the endolymphatic spaces. The endolymphatic sac, which is thought to be responsible for excretion of endolymphatic fluid, is felt to be the primary source of the condition. Two conditions known to affect the endolymphatic sac are syphilis and head trauma.

DIAGNOSTIC STUDIES

Laboratory

Chemistry Profile, Complete Blood Count, and Serologic Tests.   As indicated to rule out underlying or concurrent illness.

Radiology

CT/MRI of the Head, with and without Contrast.   As indicated to rule out cerebellopontine angle lesions (e.g., acoustic neuroma, plaques of multiple sclerosis).

Other

Electronystagmography (ENG).   Evaluate for the presence of hypoactive/hyperactive labyrinth function.

Posturography.   An elaborate test to check for central nervous system integration of muscles, eyes, and the vestibular apparatus.

Audiologic Reflexes and Reflex Decay.   Audiometric test to check for retrocochlear nerve function.

Brainstem Auditory Evoked Response.   Used to measure the conduction of the vestibulocochlear nerves.

DIFFERENTIAL DIAGNOSIS

Traumatic

Head Injury.   If causing labyrinthine concussion, may result in dizziness. Symptoms gradually resolve over several days but may be prolonged for months.

Infectious

Labyrinthitis. Acute vertigo with nausea and vomiting. Hearing loss and tinnitus are also noted. Vertigo lasts for several days, then resolves.

Vestibular Neuronitis. Symptoms similar to those of labyrinthitis; however, hearing loss and tinnitus are absent.

Neurosyphilis. Syphilis is one known cause of endolymphatic hydrops.

Metabolic

Hyperthyroidism/Hypothyroidism. Abnormal results on thyroid function tests.

Benign Paroxysmal Positional Vertigo (BPPV). Vertigo is brought on by head movement.

Multiple Sclerosis. Episodic neurologic complaints in the past, positive MRI for demyelinating disease, or positive findings on cerebrospinal fluid (CSF) studies for multiple sclerosis.

Neoplastic

Acoustic Neuroma. A benign lesion involving cranial nerve VIII. Symptoms include nonepisodic, progressive hearing loss and tinnitus.

Cerebellar Tumors or Disease. Ataxia and incoordination, positive result on Romberg test (worsening of symptoms on movement with eyes closed).

Vascular

Vertebrobasilar Artery Insufficiency. Dysequilibrium or unsteadiness occurring as a result of a transient reduction in blood flow to the brain. May be triggered by changes in posture or extension of the neck.

Congenital

Not applicable.

Acquired

Acute Toxic Labyrinthitis. History of ototoxic medication use.

TREATMENT

The goal of therapy is to prevent or reduce the frequency of the episodes and preserve hearing.

A low-sodium diet (less than 2 g daily) supplemented by a diuretic (e.g., hydrochlorothiazide 50-100 mg daily) is effective to control symptoms for many patients.

Treatment of acute vertigo usually requires medications to suppress the vestibular system and to alleviate the accompanying nausea and vomiting. The drug classes commonly used are:

- Antihistamines
  Meclizine 25-50 mg PO every 6 to 8 hours
  Dimenhydrinate 50-100 mg PO/IM/IV every 4-6 hours; maximum 400 mg/day

> Diphenhydramine 25-50 mg PO/IM/IV every 4 to 6 hours; maximum 100 mg/dose, 400 mg/day
- Anticholinergics
  Scopolamine 1.5 mg patch, place behind ear; may replace every 3 days
- Antiemetics
  Prochlorperazine 5-10 mg PO/IM every 6-8 hours; 25 mg rectally every 12 hours
  Promethazine 12.5-25 mg PO/IM or rectally every 4 to 6 hours

For severe cases or when conservative management has failed, surgical decompression of the endolymphatic sac may be indicated.

PEDIATRIC CONSIDERATIONS

Meniere disease is rare in children. Exhaustive search for cause of any symptoms is mandatory.

OBSTETRIC CONSIDERATIONS

No specific indications.

GERIATRIC CONSIDERATIONS

Medications (e.g., antihistamines) that cause drowsiness and resulting unsteadiness should be used with caution in the elderly.

Prescribe anticholinergic medications with caution in the elderly patient, who may be more likely to have prostatic hypertrophy, hypertension, or glaucoma.

The incidence of cerebral hypoperfusion as a cause of dizziness increases with advancing age, and this possibility should always be considered in the differential diagnosis.

PREVENTIVE CONSIDERATIONS

Follow dietary guidelines for low-sodium diet and avoidance of caffeine.

PEARLS FOR THE PA

Meniere disease is a diagnosis of exclusion.

Characterized by a classic constellation of four symptoms: episodic hearing loss, tinnitus, vertigo, and aural fullness.

Nasal Polyps

Sue M. Enns, MHS, PA-C

DEFINITION

Benign, pale or translucent edematous masses found in the nasal fossae, originating in the maxillary or ethmoid sinuses. They occur as a result of chronic edema of the nasal mucosa with susequent prolapse of nasal and sinus mucosa into the nasal cavity.

HISTORY

Symptoms.   Nasal obstruction and pressure, rhinorrhea, anosmia.

General.   Usually the result of chronic mucosal edema in the nose and sinuses. Many patients have a history of allergic rhinitis. A symptom triad involving nasal polyps, asthma, and aspirin sensitivity may also be encountered.

Age.   Children to adults.

Onset.   Gradual, months to years.

Duration.   Slow, will continue to grow and may recur if removed.

Intensity.   Initially asymptomatic, but later cause nasal obstruction and pressure.

Aggravating Factors.   Vasomotor or allergic rhinitis.

Alleviating Factors.   Surgical removal.

Associated Factors.   Aspirin sensitivity, nonallergic asthma, chronic sinusitis, and cystic fibrosis.

PHYSICAL EXAMINATION

General.   The patient may appear normal or may sound congested.

Head, Eyes, Ears, Nose, Throat.   Smooth, pale, pear-shaped masses that appear singly or in clusters in the nasal fossae; easily movable, nontender. May be unilateral or bilateral.

PATHOPHYSIOLOGY

Edema of the sinus submucosa can form irregular folds within the sinus and result in polyp formation. The exact etiology of the polyp development is poorly understood.

DIAGNOSTIC STUDIES

Laboratory

Usually not necessary, but increased eosinophils are commonly seen on nasal smear.

Radiology

Sinus Radiographs.   Soft tissue density that may totally opacify a sinus. Will not erode or destroy the sinus wall as would be seen with a malignancy. With long-standing nasal obstruction, changes such as spreading of the nasal bones with widening of the bridge of the nose may be seen.

Other

Not applicable.

DIFFERENTIAL DIAGNOSIS

Traumatic.   Not applicable.
Infectious.   Not applicable.
Metabolic.   Not applicable.

Neoplastic

Malignant Tumors of the Paranasal Sinuses, Nasal Fossa or Septum. May resemble polyps.

Squamous Cell Carcinoma.   The most common malignancy. Associated with nasal mass, facial swelling and pain, epistaxis, and palate swelling. The patient may present with a nonhealing lesion in the nasal vestibule or anterior portion of the septum.

Inverted Papilloma.   Unilateral tumor arising from the lateral wall of the nose that may bleed intermittently; may occur with nasal polyps or malignant nasal tumors. Patients present with nasal obstruction, epistaxis, and/or rhinorrhea.

Squamous Papilloma.   Benign wart-like tumor that occurs on the anterior nasal septum or lateral wall of the nose and may cause nasal obstruction or hemorrhage. May also involve the sinuses.

Vascular

Juvenile Angiofibroma.   Benign tumor found in teenage boys that can cause massive bleeding; may also arise from the lateral wall of the nose. Manifests with epistaxis, nasal obstruction, and occasionally, deformity of the cheek.

Congenital

Cystic Fibrosis.   Children with cystic fibrosis may have recurrent nasal polyps that can deform the nasal bones.

Acquired

Not applicable.

TREATMENT

Initial treatment with topical nasal steroids may be effective for small polyps. Surgical removal may be necessary when medical management is unsuccessful. After removal, topical beclomethasone spray used twice a day may decrease the incidence of recurrence and must be used indefinitely.

If allergies are the primary cause of polyp formation, desensitization, decongestants, and antihistamines help decrease the incidence of recurrence.

PEDIATRIC CONSIDERATIONS

Nasal polyps develop in 25% of children with cystic fibrosis. Every child with nasal polyps, even in the absence of typical respiratory and digestive symptoms, should be tested for cystic fibrosis. Nasal polyps in children are also associated with chronic allergic rhinitis, chronic sinusitis, and asthma. Children may often present with the complaint of persistent mouth breathing and/or hyponasal phonation.

OBSTETRIC CONSIDERATIONS

No specific indications.

GERIATRIC CONSIDERATIONS

None.

PREVENTIVE CONSIDERATIONS

None.

PEARLS FOR THE PA

If epistaxis is present, along with nasal obstruction, the causative disorder is probably not nasal polyps, and further investigation is warranted.

Patients with nasal polyps and asthma should be advised to avoid aspirin.

Cystic fibrosis should always be considered in a patient with nasal polyps.

Otitis Externa

Sue M. Enns, MHS, PA-C

DEFINITION

Inflammation of the external auditory canal commonly caused by a bacterial infection. Also known as *swimmer's ear*.

HISTORY

Symptoms. Itching of the ear canal, intense pain, tenderness, swelling, drainage; hearing loss may occur secondary to obstruction.

General. The usual presentation includes maceration of the external canal caused by retained water from swimming or showering or by minor trauma from attempting to clean the external ear canal. This causes maceration of the canal skin, which gives favorable conditions for bacterial growth.

Age. Early childhood to advanced age.

Onset. Rapid, with progressive pain and purulent drainage.

Duration. Several days to weeks; may be a recurrent problem (several times a year).

Intensity. Minor itching to severe pain.

Aggravating Factors. Water exposure, local trauma, insertion of foreign objects into the ear (e.g., cotton swabs, fingernails, hearing aids, ear plugs).

Alleviating Factors. Maintaining clean, dry conditions in ear canals.

Associated Factors. Eczema, psoriasis, seborrhea, diabetes mellitus, and untreated acute suppurative otitis media with perforation.

PHYSICAL EXAMINATION

General. Patients frequently present in mild distress with ear pain and possibly fever.

Head, Eyes, Ears, Nose, Throat. Tenderness over the tragus and pain with movement of the auricle; watery to purulent drainage, erythema and swelling of the external auditory canal. Enlarged cervical nodes may be present. If swelling is sufficient to occlude the external canal, the patient may complain of aural fullness, and a conductive hearing loss may be present.

Neurologic. Necrotizing or malignant otitis externa is a life-threatening extension of the infection into the mastoid or temporal bone leading to severe headache or other neurologic abnormalities.

PATHOPHYSIOLOGY

The most common etiologic agents are *Pseudomonas aeruginosa* and *Staphylococcus aureus*. Fungal overgrowth is responsible for a small number of cases.

DIAGNOSTIC STUDIES

Laboratory
Culture and Sensitivity Testing of Purulent Drainage. For organism identification and antibiotic sensitivity studies.

Serum Glucose. In patients with recurrent problems or in elderly persons with first severe episode.

Radiology
CT of Head in Suspected Malignant Otitis Externa. Indicated to rule out bone involvement of the external auditory canal and base of the skull; may have acute osteomyelitis of the temporal bone.

Other
Audiologic Testing. After removing debris from the canal, a screening hearing evaluation should be performed.

DIFFERENTIAL DIAGNOSIS

Traumatic/Infectious/Metabolic
Not applicable.

Neoplastic
Ear Malignancies. Most involve the auricle and are rarely associated with otitis externa. Primary complaint is otorrhea with pain that is intense and out of proportion to clinical findings.

Congenital
Not applicable.

Acquired
Irritant or Allergic Contact Dermatitis. Contact dermatitis may involve the pinna as well as the external canal. Common agents causing allergic reactions are topical anti-infectives and anesthetics.

Eczematoid Otitis Externa. Usually caused by topical antibiotics, allergies to chemicals or metals used around the ear, atopic reaction caused by ingested or inhaled substances, or contact of the ear canal with middle ear drainage.

Seborrheic Otitis Externa. Common condition, associated with seborrheic dermatitis of other areas, especially the scalp.

TREATMENT

Inspection and cleaning and drying of the ear canal are necessary. Gentle suctioning of the debris through an otoscope helps dry and clear the canal and permits visualization of the tympanic membrane to look for perforation or middle ear pathology. Flushing the canal with water is not recommended, particularly if tympanic membrane cannot be visualized.

Topical antibiotic therapy is routinely indicated. Numerous antibiotic preparations are available (e.g., neomycin, polymyxin, aminoglycosides, quinolones) both with and without steroids to reduce inflammation. Two percent acetic acid solution (V̄oSol) can also be very effective in mild cases.

Oral antibiotics are not indicated unless the patient has significant fever (temperature greater than 101° F) or adenopathy or appears septic.

Special attention must be given to the diabetic or other immunocompromised patient, who is at risk for developing malignant otitis externa, a severe, potentially life-threatening form of diffuse otitis externa. These patients require close monitoring and referral to an otologist for management with parenteral antibiotics if infection is severe or does not improve.

Future infections may be prevented by the use of ear molds or by instillation of a few drops of dilute alcohol or an acetic acid solution after bathing or swimming. The external canal may also be dried using a hair dryer on a low setting.

PEDIATRIC CONSIDERATIONS

Excessive wetness, dryness, and trauma are three conditions that may predispose the skin of the ear canal to infection. In children, rule out foreign bodies, trauma, and referred pain from other sites in the head or neck. Children who swim frequently and are susceptible to recurrences of otitis externa may prevent infection by instillation of dilute alcohol or acetic acid immediately following swimming or bathing.

OBSTETRIC CONSIDERATIONS

No specific indications.

GERIATRIC CONSIDERATIONS

The patient should avoid wearing hearing aids until the infection has completely cleared.

PREVENTIVE CONSIDERATIONS

Patients should be advised not to attempt self-cleaning of the ears with cotton swabs or other objects. Patients with recurrent problems should be advised to keep the ear canal dry by using a hair dryer on low setting after bathing, showering, or swimming. A tight-fitting cap or molded ear plugs are recommended for swimming.

Otitis Media

Debra S. Munsell, MPAS, PA-C

DEFINITION

Inflammation of the middle ear caused by pathogens from the nasopharynx secondary to eustachian tube dysfunction. Can occur after rapid pressure changes (barotrauma).

HISTORY

Symptoms.   Otalgia, fever, enlarged, tender cervical lymph nodes, and hearing loss; irritability in young children.

General.   Patient may have a history of persistent middle ear fluid or recurrent ear infections. Young children are usually irritable, have difficulty sleeping, and pull at the affected ear.

Age.   Any, but most common in children younger than 5 years of age.

Onset.   Acute, can progress to chronic.

Duration.   Usually 2 weeks. Becomes a chronic problem if not treated; may also recur after symptoms of upper respiratory infection.

Intensity.   Mild to severe pain.

Aggravating Factors.   Infections of the nose and throat. Rapid pressure changes.

Alleviating Factors.   Antibiotic treatment.

Associated Factors.   Serous otitis media, upper respiratory infections including viral infections.

PHYSICAL EXAMINATION

General. Patients generally present with fever, children may be crying and pulling at their ears.

Head, Eyes, Ears, Nose, Throat. Normal external canal unless tympanic membrane has been perforated and purulent drainage is present.

Tympanic Membrane. Erythematous, bulging, and unresponsive to pneumatic testing. Possible purulent effusion or otorrhea from tympanic membrane perforation, loss of bony landmarks in late stages.

Neck. Enlarged, tender cervical nodes may be present.

PATHOPHYSIOLOGY

Streptococcus pneumoniae, Haemophilus influenzae, and *Moraxella catarrhalis* are the most common etiologic agents. Other possible pathogens include viruses, *Streptococcus pyogenes*, and *Staphylococcus aureus*.

DIAGNOSTIC STUDIES

Laboratory

Culture and Sensitivity Testing. If purulent drainage is present, for appropriate antibiotic treatment. Tympanocentesis may be required to appropriately treat patients who are immunocompromised.

Radiology
Not applicable.

Other
Audiologic Testing. Mild conductive hearing loss with a negative pressure in the middle ear noted on tympanometry.

DIFFERENTIAL DIAGNOSIS

Traumatic
Rupture of the Tympanic Membrane. Can give infectious organisms an entrance into the middle ear. Positive traumatic history.

Infectious
Viral Otitis Media. Slight thickening of tympanic membrane without marked hyperemia.

Bullous Myringitis. Bleb or vesicle present on tympanic membrane; associated with a viral infection, but may have a secondary bacterial infection.

Chronic Otitis Media. Persistent middle ear effusion or painless drainage noted in the ear canal from the middle ear. Cholesteatoma may be present.

Metabolic
Not applicable.

Neoplastic
Malignancies Involving the Middle Ear. Rare. When present, associated with intense pain due to invasion of the bone; bleeding from the auditory canal may be present. External auditory canal may be occluded by tumor or debris.

Vascular
Not applicable.

Congenital
Acute Otitis Media. May be associated with sepsis, pneumonia, and meningitis in the newborn.

Acquired
Serous Otitis Media. Sterile fluid in the middle ear with air fluid level or bubbles often noted; caused by eustachian tube dysfunction, barotrauma.

TREATMENT

Ten-day course of antibiotics constitutes definitive therapy. First-line agents include amoxicillin and amoxicillin-clavulanate. Penicillin-allergic patients may be given trimethoprim-sulfamethoxazole.

Oral pain medicine can be given as needed.

Auralgan otic drops may be used every 1 to 2 hours (if no perforation is present) to relieve pain.

If drainage is present, keep water out of ear canal.

Referral to ear-nose-throat (ENT) physician is indicated if patient is not significantly improved in the first 2 or 3 days.

PEDIATRIC CONSIDERATIONS

Infants and young children (ages 4 months to 2 years) are at highest risk. Children who develop otitis media in the first year of life have an increased risk of chronic disease. The high-risk populations include children with cleft palate and other craniofacial anomalies, children with Down syndrome, Alaskan natives, and Native Americans. Incidence of otitis media is highest in the winter months.

The child with frequent bouts of recurrent otitis media may benefit from a prophylactic dose of antibiotics (a daily dose of amoxicillin or sulfonamides). Myringotomy and ventilating tubes should be reserved for patients who suffer recurrences despite antimicrobial prophylaxis or in whom, because of allergy to penicillin or sulfonamides, chemoprophylaxis is not desirable.

Children who have chronic otitis media with effusion (duration longer than 3 months) lack the clinical manifestations of acute infection. They do not have pain or fever but often have decreased auditory acuity. Although most of these effusions resolve spontaneously, referral and treatment may be indicated, especially for the child with bilateral chronic effusions with marked hearing loss.

OBSTETRIC CONSIDERATIONS

Sulfonamides, erythromycin, and ciprofloxacin should be used with caution. Tetracycline is contraindicated.

GERIATRIC CONSIDERATIONS

Otitis media in the adult is uncommon. An elderly patient presenting with signs or symptoms of otitis media should be referred to an ENT physician for further evaluation for neoplastic disease.

PREVENTIVE CONSIDERATIONS

Avoidance of risk factors may help prevent recurrence of otitis media in children. Tobacco smoke exposure should be limited, as well as attendance at day care facilities Pneumoccal and influenza vaccines may prevent some recurrences.

PEARLS FOR THE PA

Pain should resolve soon after antibiotic therapy begins.

Nose and nasopharynx should be carefully evaluated for causative factors such as adenoid hypertrophy or throat infection.

Follow-up evaluation of the hearing is mandatory.

Pharyngitis

Debra S. Munsell, MPAS, PA-C

DEFINITION

Inflammation of the pharynx, usually viral in origin. Cannot be diagnosed by clinical examination alone.

HISTORY

Symptoms. Pharyngeal pain, fever, odynophagia, malaise, cough, lymphadenopathy. Headache, abdominal pain, and vomiting are commonly seen in streptococcal disease, whereas accompanying symptoms of upper respiratory infection are more indicative of a viral etiology.

General. Associated with the common cold.

Age. Children to adults.

Onset. Gradual.

Duration. Usual course is 7 to 10 days; can be chronic.

Intensity. Mild to moderate discomfort.

Aggravating Factors. Tobacco use; chemical abuse with alcohol and mouthwashes.

Alleviating Factors. Throat lozenges, discontinuing tobacco or exposure to chemical irritants, vocal rest, adequate hydration.

Associated Factors. Respiratory infections. Untreated streptococcal infection may lead to acute rheumatic fever, otitis media, lymphadenitis, peritonsillar abcess, or acute glomerulonephritis.

PHYSICAL EXAMINATION

General. Patients may present with sore throat, malaise, pain with swallowing, and occasionally fever. Nasal congestion and discharge may be present.

Head, Eyes, Ears, Nose, Throat. Normal to mild erythema and mildly injected posterior pharyngeal wall, dry mucosa, lymphoid hyperplasia on the posterior pharyngeal wall.

Neck. Possible mild adenopathy.

PATHOPHYSIOLOGY

Causative viral organisms include coxsackievirus, adenovirus, enterovirus, herpes simplex virus, Epstein-Barr virus, rubella virus, influenza virus, and other viruses. Bacterial infections can occur with beta-hemolytic group A streptococci, pneumococci, or staphylococci.

DIAGNOSTIC STUDIES

Laboratory

Rapid Streptococcal Antigen Test. Should be done as soon as possible. In suspected cases, a throat culture to rule out beta-hemolytic group A streptococcal infection should be done. Testing for infectious mononucleosis should be done if clinically indicated.

Complete Blood Count with Differential. If patient is febrile. Elevated white blood cell count with bacterial infections.

Monospot Test. As indicated to rule out infectious mononucleosis.

Radiology. Not applicable.
Other. Not applicable.

DIFFERENTIAL DIAGNOSIS

Traumatic
Foreign Body (e.g., Swallowing a Fish Bone). Usually scratches the throat, and patient swallows the object.

Infectious
Streptococcal Pharyngitis. Associated with severe pain, fever, and cervical adenopathy.
Acute Tonsillitis. Swollen erythematous tonsils present. Exudate with purulent material may be present on the tonsils or crypts.
Infectious Mononucleosis. Associated with lymphadenopathy, lymphocytosis with atypical lymphocytes on the peripheral smear, splenomegaly, hepatomegaly, and petechiae of the soft palate.
Gonococcal Pharyngitis. History of sexual activity involving oral-genital contact. May be asymptomatic or have throat pain and usually has a bright red pharynx with superficial ulcerations and yellow exudate. Confirmed by pharyngeal Gram stain and culture.

Metabolic
Not applicable.

Neoplastic
Squamous Cell Carcinoma. Ulcerative or submucosal mass that may manifest with referred otalgia. A history of tobacco use and alcohol abuse should warrant a comprehensive head and neck examination by an otolaryngologist.

Vascular. Not applicable.
Congenital. Not applicable.
Acquired. Not applicable.

TREATMENT

Viral infections may be treated conservatively. Bed rest, fluids, saline gargles, analgesics such as acetaminophen, and decongestants (if postnasal drainage is present) are usually sufficient.

Discontinue tobacco, alcohol, and mouthwash use if they are an irritant to the throat.

Streptococcal pharyngitis should be treated with a 10-day course of oral penicillin V potassium or an intramuscular injection of penicillin G benzathine. Erythromycin should be used for patients with a penicillin allergy.

Otherwise, treat with an antibiotic effective against beta-lactamase–producing organisms (amoxicillin-clavulanate, erythromycin, or cephalosporin). In the case of a patient or family member with repeated frequent streptococcal infections or when a family member has a history of rheumatic fever or glomerulonephritis, further attempts at treating the "carrier" may be indicated (a 10-day course of clindamycin). Other considerations in recurrent infection include daily penicillin prophylaxis during winter months and referral for tonsillectomy.

PEDIATRIC CONSIDERATIONS

Viral infections account for about 90% of cases of childhood pharyingitis. The most common etiologic agents include rhinovirus, coronavirus, coxsackieviruses, echoviruses, adenovirus, enteroviruses, Epstein-Barr virus, cytomegalovirus, and herpes simplex virus.

Generally, the treatment of acute viral pharyngitis is symptomatic. Fluids or sucking on lozenges or hard candy will help by keeping the mouth moist. Older children may gargle with salt water solution or antacid solution (e.g., Mylanta). Acetaminophen is sometimes helpful, whereas antibiotics are contraindicated.

OBSTETRIC CONSIDERATIONS

Sulfonamides, erythromycin, and ciprofloxacin should be used with caution. Tetracycline is contraindicated.

GERIATRIC CONSIDERATIONS

Dental appliances may be foreign body sources of sore throat in the elderly. Hydration and electrolyte issues can occur rapidly if the patient is not receiving adequate oral intake.

PREVENTIVE CONSIDERATIONS

Proper hand washing technique can help prevent spread of viral and bacterial organisms.

PEARLS FOR THE PA

Culture throat to rule out beta-hemolytic group A streptococcal infection.

Physical examination findings may be unremarkable.

Rhinitis

Sue M. Enns, MHS, PA-C

DEFINITION

Inflammation of the nasal mucous membranes causing edema, nasal obstruction, and rhinorrhea.

HISTORY

Symptoms. Sneezing, rhinorrhea, nasal obstruction, itchy nose and eyes.
General. Self-limiting or chronic problem depending on the cause.
Age. Typically in the first two decades of life, with prevalence decreasing with age. Atrophic rhinitis is a condition affecting the middle-aged to elderly.
Onset. Acute.
Duration. Few days to chronic or recurrent condition.
Intensity. Mild to severe obstruction.
Aggravating Factors. Allergens, excessive use of topical nasal decongestants, inhaled irritants, nasal obstruction, environmental pollution, cigarette smoke.
Alleviating Factors. Allergy desensitization, avoidance of irritants, discontinuance of topical decongestants, surgery.
Associated Factors. Nasal infections, nasal polyps, hypothyroidism, pregnancy, oral contraceptives, recurrent upper respiratory infections and/or sinusitis.

PHYSICAL EXAMINATION

General. Patients are usually afebrile unless acute viral or bacterial infection is present.

Head, Eyes, Ears, Nose, Throat
Nose. Swollen boggy turbinates; may be pale or erythematous. Thin watery to purulent nasal secretions will be present.
Eyes. Lacrimation or injected conjunctivae.
Mouth. Dry mucosa secondary to mouth breathing.
Oropharynx. Postnasal drainage.

PATHOPHYSIOLOGY

Rhinitis is typically classified as infectious, allergic, vasomotor (nonallergic), or mixed. Rhinitis caused by infection is almost always caused by viruses. Many different serologic types of rhinoviruses and adenoviruses are implicated in the development of rhinitis. Allergic rhinitis is a common condition caused by the inhalation of allergens to which the patient has become sensitized. Vasomotor rhinitis is a chronic condition for which the etiology is unclear. It is thought to result from reaction to inhaled irritants and/or weather changes.

DIAGNOSTIC STUDIES

Laboratory
Serum Immunoglobulin E (IgE). Used to assist in the confirmation of allergic rhinitis. Elevated levels are indicative of an allergic state, but a normal level does not rule out allergy.

Nasal smears. An elevated eosinophil count may be present in allergic rhinitis or nonallergic rhinitis with eosinophilia syndrome (NARES).

Allergy Skin Testing. If indicated by history.

Complete Blood Count. Eosinophilia in the peripheral smear may indicate allergy.

Thyroid Function Studies. As indicated to evaluate for hypothyroidism.

Radiology
Sinus Radiographs. Chronic sinusitis may also cause nasal congestion and purulent drainage.

Other
Not applicable.

DIFFERENTIAL DIAGNOSIS

Traumatic
Facial Fracture. May have a cerebrospinal (CSF) rhinorrhea with basal skull fracture. CSF is typically clear and rhinorrhea is profuse, especially with positional changes. CSF may be differentiated from nasal drainage by the presence of glucose.

Infectious
Not applicable

Metabolic
Hypothyroidism. Manifests with chronic nasal obstruction that resolves with correction of the hypothyroidism.

Neoplastic
Neoplasms. Tumors of the nasal cavity and nasopharynx are rare. Unilateral nasal obstruction, epistaxis, and pain are the most common presenting symptoms. Patients presenting with persistent or unilateral symptoms (adults) should be referred for further evaluation.

Congenital
Wegener Granulomatosis and Sarcoidosis. May manifest with nasal congestion, obstruction, and rhinorrhea.

Acquired
Rhinitis Medicamentosa. Prolonged, excessive use of topical nasal preparations produces a rebound phenomenon of severe nasal congestion.

Hormonal Rhinitis. Nasal congestion is a common complaint during pregnancy. This is due to vascular engorgement and increased estrogen levels. A similar effect may be seen in patients taking oral contraceptives.

Mechanical Obstruction by Deviated Nasal Septum, Foreign Body. May cause unilateral nasal congestion and inflammation.

TREATMENT

Treatment is determined by the specific cause of the rhinitis and may include medications, surgery, avoidance of known irritants, and allergy desensitization.

Allergic Rhinitis
Best treated with allergen avoidance.

Pharmacotherapy includes numerous over-the-counter antihistamines such as chlorpheniramine or brompheniramine. Prescription antihistamines include fexofenadine and loratadine. The prescription preparations tend to be less sedating but are more expensive.

Use of intranasal topical corticosteroids is a mainstay of treatment. Several preparations are available including beclamethasone, fluticasone, and mometasone.

Oral steroids can be extremely effective in very severe allergic rhinitis if used infrequently. A regimen of an initial dose of 40 mg prednisone and then gradually decreasing doses over the next 10 days is usually sufficient. Patients with severe symptoms should be referred to an allergist.

Vasomotor Rhinitis
Treated with avoidance of tobacco smoke, rapid changes in temperature or humidity, and chemical irritants.

Pseudoephedrine every 4 to 6 hours may provide some relief. A combination antihistamine-decongestant may provide some nonspecific drying effect, but an antihistamine alone is not effective.

Viral Rhinitis (Common Cold)
Supportive measures including decongestants (pseudoephedrine 30-60 mg every 4 to 6 hours as needed) and acetaminophen or ibuprofen for fever and muscle aches are generally effective. Antibiotics are not indicated unless there is evidence of secondary infection.

Hormonal Rhinitis
Topical corticosteroid may be safely used twice a day for 1 to 2 weeks at a time, during pregnancy, to relieve the congestion of hormonal rhinitis, as there are minimal systemic effects.

Rhinitis Medicamentosa
Topical decongestants must be discontinued. This will trigger significant nasal congestion for 1 to 2 weeks. Intranasal corticosteroids may be a useful adjunctive therapy. Severe cases may require a short tapered course of oral corticosteroid.

PEDIATRIC CONSIDERATIONS

If the purulent discharge is foul-smelling or unilateral, or recurs after adequate treatment, the possibility of foreign body must be considered.

Many infants in the first 2 months experience frequent periods of stuffy nose with a clear discharge. Young infants (younger than 4 months) are often obligate nasal breathers and may commonly present with nasal congestion and subsequent difficulty breathing that is worsened during feeding. Instillation of normal saline nose drops followed by gentle suction with a bulb syringe will usually relieve the symptoms. Differential diagnosis in the infant should include congenital syphilis, hypothyroidism, choanal atresia, and cow's milk allergy.

OBSTETRIC CONSIDERATIONS

Decongestants are considered relatively safe to use during pregnancy if clearly indicated. However, studies have demonstrated some possible connection between decongestant use and increased risk of clubfoot and inguinal hernia in the fetus.

GERIATRIC CONSIDERATIONS

Medications (e.g., antihistamines) that potentially cause drowsiness and resulting unsteadiness should be used with caution in elderly patients.

PREVENTIVE CONSIDERATIONS

Environmental control measures and avoidance of allergen exposure can greatly reduce symptoms of allergic rhinitis in susceptible patients. Smoking cessation should be advised and environmental exposure to cigarette smoke should be avoided. Parents of children with allergic rhinitis should not smoke at home or around the child.

PEARLS FOR THE PA

Antibiotics are not indicated in the treatment of viral rhinitis. Purulent drainage in the first week of a "cold" is a component of viral rhinitis.

Consider desensitization therapy in patients who cannot avoid allergens or in whom the condition is not controlled by medication alone.

Adult patients who have persistent unilateral nasal obstruction, epistaxis, and/or pain should be referred for further evaluation.

Foreign body should be considered in children presenting with persistent, unilateral, foul-smelling nasal discharge.

Sinusitis

Sue M. Enns, MHS, PA-C

DEFINITION

Inflammation of the paranasal sinuses secondary to nasal congestion from a viral, bacterial, or fungal infection and/or an allergic reaction.

HISTORY

Symptoms.   Common symptoms include facial or dental pain, headache, nasal congestion, purulent rhinorrhea, postnasal drainage, and cough. Fever, fatigue, and sore throat are less common.

General.   Sinusitis is usually preceded by an upper respiratory infection. Typically, the patient's symptoms begin to resolve but then worsen again.

Age.   Small children to the elderly.

Onset   Acute.

Duration.   Seven days to a chronic condition with acute exacerbations.

Intensity.   Mild facial pain to severe headaches.

Aggravating Factors.   Rhinitis, nasal polyps, cigarette smoking, adenoid hypertrophy, cleft palate, immunodeficiency, nasal septal deviation, barotrauma.

Alleviating Factors.   Nasal saline irrigation or steam inhaler.

Associated Factors.   Nasal polyps, rhinitis, deviated nasal septum, adenoid hypertrophy, dental caries or abscesses. Debilitating conditions such as uncontrolled diabetes, malignancies, malnutrition, chronic steroid therapy, cystic fibrosis.

PHYSICAL EXAMINATION

General.   Fever is uncommon.

Head, Eyes, Ears, Nose, Throat
Nose.   Swollen, inflamed nasal mucosa and turbinates, obstructing secretions or polyps, blood-tinged or purulent nasal drainage.
Sinuses.   Tenderness to palpation and percussion of the soft tissues overlying the sinus. Transillumination of the maxillary and frontal sinuses may be reduced.
Oropharynx.   Purulent drainage on the posterior pharyngeal wall.
Neck.   Cervical lymphadenopathy is uncommon.

Neurologic.   Occasional loss of sense of smell.

PATHOPHYSIOLOGY

A majority of cases of acute sinusitis occur following upper respiratory infection. Obstruction of the sinus ostia by inflammation and edema or other anatomic abnormality leads to impaired drainage and subsequent infection. Common causative organisms in adults and children include *Streptococcus pneumoniae, Haemophilus influenzae,* and *Moraxella catarrhalis. Staphylococcus aureus* and other anaerobic bacteria may predominate in chronic cases. Fungi may be encountered in the immunocompromised patient.

DIAGNOSTIC STUDIES

Laboratory
Cultures.   Although not routinely used because of expense and invasiveness, culture of specimen obtained by sinus puncture provides definitive diagnosis.

Radiology
Sinus Radiograph with Waters View.   Routine radiographs are not indicated in the diagnosis of uncomplicated sinusitis. They may be helpful in patients with atypical symptoms or recurrent disease. Findings of an air-fluid level, sinus opacity, or mucosal thickening are indicative of sinusitis. Radiographs are not routinely indicated in children, especially those younger than 6 years of age.

CT of Sinuses/Head. Sinus CT is not indicated for routine management. In the patient with chronic or recurrent disease, CT may be helpful in obtaining a detailed view of the sinus anatomy and mucosal surfaces.

Other
Not applicable.

DIFFERENTIAL DIAGNOSIS

Traumatic.   Not applicable.
Infectious.   Not applicable.
Metabolic.   Not applicable.

Neoplastic
Squamous Cell Carcinoma.   Most common malignant tumor of the paranasal sinuses. When present, it is usually found in maxillary sinuses. Destruction of bone will be noted on plain films and CT scan. Persistent, unilateral purulent drainage, epistaxis, and pain are typical presenting symptoms.

Vascular
Wegener Granulomatosis (Necrotizing Granulomatous Vasculitis).   A majority of patients have involvement of the nose and sinuses. Friable mucosa and blood-stained crusting may be clues for further investigation.

Congenital
Cystic Fibrosis.   Patients tend to have chronic or recurrent cough. These patients are predisposed to upper respiratory infection secondary to impaired mucociliary function and chronic colonization of the respiratory tract.

Acquired.   Not applicable.

TREATMENT

Symptoms in two-thirds of patients with uncomplicated disease will resolve without treatment. Antibiotics are the mainstay of treatment to reduce symptom severity and length of illness.

Current clinical guidelines recommend amoxicillin or trimethoprim-sulfamethoxazole as the antibiotics of first choice. If the patient is allergic to these medications, a cephalosporin, macrolide, or quinolone should be used. Antibiotic treatment should be continued until the patient has been well and asymptomatic for 7 days (usual course of treatment is 10 to 14 days)

Topical or oral decongestants may be recommended for adjunctive therapy to improve symptoms of drainage. These include oral pseudoephedrine

(30-60 mg every 4 to 6 hours, with a maximum daily dose of 240 mg). Topical decongestants such as oxymetazoline (0.5%) may be used (1 or 2 sprays in each nostril every 6 to 8 hours) for up to 3 days only.

If the patient fails to respond to usual therapy or the infection recurs, the patient should be evaluated for underlying anatomic anomalies or risk factors, including immunodeficiency. Consider referral in these cases.

PEDIATRIC CONSIDERATIONS

Maxillary and ethmoid sinuses and the sphenoid sinus are present by age 3. The frontal sinuses are usually not present until the age of 8. Symptoms of sinusitis in small children are less specific than in adults and may include persistent nasal drainage, nasal congestion, cough, and feeding difficulties. Routine radiographic studies or CT scans are not indicated unless the patient is refractory to therapy, has unusual symptoms (e.g., unilateral facial or periorbital swelling), or if surgical therapy is being considered.

Complications of paranasal sinusitis include preseptal periorbital cellulitis, orbital cellulitis or abscess (manifested by decreased extraocular movements, proptosis, edema, altered visual acuity), epidural or subdural empyema, brain abscess, osteitis of the frontal bone (Pott puffy tumor), dural sinus thrombosis, and meningitis. Maxillary sinusitis may result in buccal cellulitis. Any of these complications should be treated with drainage and broad-spectrum parenteral antibiotics.

OBSTETRIC CONSIDERATIONS

Sulfonamides, erythromycin, and ciprofloxacin should be used with caution. Tetracycline is contraindicated.

GERIATRIC CONSIDERATIONS

Medications (e.g., antihistamines) that potentially cause drowsiness and resulting unsteadiness should be used with caution in elderly patients.

PREVENTIVE CONSIDERATIONS

Avoid medications such as antihistamines (unless the patient has a documented inhalant allergy), which dry the mucosa and secretions of the upper respiratory tract, resulting in decreased mucociliary clearance. Patients with chronic sinusitis should be advised and counseled regarding smoking cessation.

```
┌─────────────────────────────────────────────────────────────┐
│                    PEARLS FOR THE PA                          │
│  ─────────────────────────────────────────────────────────   │
│  Antibiotic treatment should be continued for at least 7 days │
│  after the patient is asymptomatic (feels well).             │
│                                                               │
│  Amoxicillin and trimethoprim-sulfamethoxazole are considered │
│  first-line agents in routine cases.                         │
│                                                               │
│  Routine radiographs are not indicated in the management of   │
│  uncomplicated sinusitis.                                     │
└─────────────────────────────────────────────────────────────┘
```

Tonsillitis

Debra S. Munsell, MPAS, PA-C

DEFINITION

Inflammation of the tonsillar tissue, most usually of the palatine tonsils. May be caused by viral or bacterial agents.

HISTORY

Symptoms. Severe pain in the throat, dysphagia, fever, chills, general malaise, referred ear pain, and sometimes headaches. Also reported are fullness in the throat, referred otalgia, altered speech, and limb and back pains.

General. A disease of childhood, with peak around 5 to 6 years of age.

Age. Small children to adults.

Onset. Abrupt.

Duration. Appropriate antibiotic treatment should control bacterial infections within 48 hours. Viral infections last up to 10 days. May have recurrent episodes as a child. Chronic tonsillitis sometimes seen in teenagers and adults; this is usually a polymicrobial disorder.

Intensity. Moderate to severe pain with dysphagia.

Aggravating Factors. Concurrent upper respiratory infections.

Alleviating Factors. Antibiotics if appropriate, warm saline gargles, analgesics, bed rest, and antipyretics.

Associated Factors. Adenotonsillar hypertrophy.

PHYSICAL EXAMINATION

General. Fever, nasal-sounding voice, generalized malaise, odynophagia.

Head, Eyes, Ears, Nose, Throat. Tender cervical adenopathy.

Oropharynx. Swollen, erythematous tonsils, possibly with gray to white exudate. In adults with chronic tonsillitis, the tonsils may be small and pink. The tongue may be dry.

PATHOPHYSIOLOGY

Usually caused by beta-hemolytic group A streptococci; may be secondary to group C beta-hemolytic streptococci, *Mycoplasma pneumoniae*, *Chlamydia* spp., *Neisseria gonorrhoeae*, or viral infections.

DIAGNOSTIC STUDIES

Laboratory
Rapid Streptococcal Antigen Test. If appropriate. May yield false-negative results. In high-risk seasons or populations, combination with throat culture is appropriate.
Throat Culture. Used to detect beta-hemolytic group A streptococci. A negative throat culture does not always rule out a streptococcal infection, and the patient should be treated according to severity of symptoms.
Complete Blood Count with Differential. As indicated to look for leukocytosis and elevated polymorphonuclear count.
Monospot Test. If the throat culture is negative, indicated to rule out infectious mononucleosis.
Radiology. Not applicable.
Other. Not applicable.

DIFFERENTIAL DIAGNOSIS

Traumatic. Not applicable.

Infectious
Viral Tonsillitis. Similar to acute bacterial tonsillitis, but usually afebrile with less severe symptoms. Negative results of throat culture and Monospot test. Need symptomatic treatment with no antibiotics. Resolves in 3 to 10 days.
Infectious Mononucleosis. Usually includes lymphadenopathy, petechiae of the soft palate, splenomegaly, hepatomegaly, lymphocytosis with atypical lymphocytes in the peripheral smear, and positive result of Monospot test. Antibiotics are needed if patient has a secondary bacterial infection.
Peritonsillar Abscess. Complication of tonsillitis with unilateral peritonsillar pain and swelling of the anterior pillar and soft palate. There will be marked bulging of the tonsil into the oropharynx. May occur when patient is already on antibiotics.

Metabolic

Not applicable.

Neoplastic

Squamous Cell Carcinoma of the Tonsils.   May manifest with sore throat and pain radiating to the ear on the same side. A high index of suspicion must be held if the patient is long-term tobacco and alcohol user. Lesions may be ulcerative or submucosal and often have a foul, distinct odor. The patient may complain of unilateral otalgia only.

Leukemia.   May be associated with swollen, necrotic tissue of the tonsils and palate, fever, and oral ulcerations.

Vascular.   Not applicable.

Congenital.   Not applicable.

Acquired.   Not applicable.

TREATMENT

Beta-hemolytic group A streptococcal infections requires 250 mg of penicillin three times a day for 10 days or 500 mg three times a day (or equivalent doses of erythromycin in the penicillin-sensitive patient). These are recent recommendations from the American Heart Association. Oral and intramuscular routes of administration are equally effective.

Viral infections require only symptomatic treatment with warm saline gargles, bed rest, and analgesics.

Tonsillectomy should be considered if the patient has repeated infections that have failed medical treatment, airway obstruction, or peritonsillar abscess. Obstructive sleep apnea secondary to hyperplasia is also an indication for tonsillectomy in patients diagnosed with chronic tonsillitis.

If malignancy is suspected, a biopsy of the tonsil should be performed, or the patient should be referred to an otolaryngologist.

PEDIATRIC CONSIDERATIONS

Most hypertrophied tonsils seen in the school-aged child are actually normal in size. Failure to note that tonsils are relatively larger in children than in later years will lead to inappropriate concern for and overdiagnosis of tonsillitis.

Parents often wrongly attribute frequent upper respiratory infections and other problems such as chronic mouth breathing, recurrent purulent or serous otitis media, and recurrent or chronic sinusitis to chronic tonsillitis. Tonsillectomy and adenoidectomy, however, do not decrease the incidence of these problems in children.

OBSTETRIC CONSIDERATIONS

Sulfonamides, erythromycin, and ciprofloxacin should be used with caution. Tetracycline is contraindicated.

GERIATRIC CONSIDERATIONS

Maintain a high index of suspicion for malignancy in elderly populations. If no response to antibiotic treatment is seen with one course of antibiotic therapy, consult an otolaryngologist.

PREVENTIVE CONSIDERATIONS

None.

PEARLS FOR THE PA

Culture for beta-hemolytic group A streptococci and treat for 10 days if present.

Refer to ENT physician if the patient has repeated infections.

Further Reading

Alper CM, Myers EN, Eibling DE: Decision Making in Ear, Nose, and Throat Disorders. Philadelphia, WB Saunders, 2001.

Cummings CW, Fredrickson JM, Harker LA, et al (eds): Otolaryngology—Head and Neck Surgery, 3rd ed. St. Louis, Mosby–Year Book, 1998.

Fairbanks DNR: Pocket Guide to Antimicrobial Therapy in Otolaryngology—Head and Neck Surgery, 10th ed. Alexandria, VA, American Academy of Otolaryngology—Head and Neck Surgery, 2001.

Woodson GE: Ear, Nose, and Throat Disorders in Primary Care. Philadelphia, WB Saunders, 2001.

PSYCHIATRY

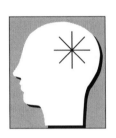

14

Adjustment Disorders

James B. Labus, PA-C

DEFINITION

Adjustment disorder is an acute, short-term pathologic response to a known acute or chronic psychosocial stressor. The stress causes a disturbance of mood, particularly depression and anxiety, sufficiently severe to cause impairment in function.

HISTORY

Symptoms. The maladjustment may be manifested by emotional problems (e.g., depression, anxiety), or by behavior (e.g., withdrawal, "acting out"). Symptoms occur within 3 months of the event.

General. Manifestations include abusive alcohol/drug use, legal problems, reckless driving, and various risk-taking behaviors. It is important to define the precipitating stressor (e.g., divorce, job loss), previous experience with similar stressors, and the likelihood of continuation of the stressor.

Age. Physical manifestations are more common in children and in elderly persons. Reaction to the stressor differs with emotional and chronologic age.

Onset. The presentation may vary widely. The timing of clinical symptoms may not parallel the occurrence of the stressor. Maladaptive responses may be delayed, to up to 3 months later (e.g., psychoactive substance abuse, conflicts, isolation, school/job problems).

Duration. Maladjustment persisting no longer than 6 months, although continuation of the stress may increase the duration of symptoms.

Intensity. Moderate to severe; may require psychiatric hospitalization. People vary significantly in their response to stress.

Aggravating Factors. Related to previous level of functioning and success in dealing with life stressors. Continuation of stressor.

Alleviating Factors. Early intervention, psychotherapy, and removal or escape from stressor.

Associated Factors. The existence of comorbid conditions, such as a personality disorder or an organic mental disorder, may significantly influence the formation and duration of the adjustment disorder. Secondary gain may increase the duration of symptoms.

PHYSICAL EXAMINATION

General. A full physical examination with emphasis on the neurologic system is warranted to rule out coexisting physical disorders.

Psychiatric. Psychomotor agitation, impaired concentration, and anxiety may be present. Symptoms of depression and/or anxiety may be manifest.

PATHOPHYSIOLOGY

Although adjustment disorders have a clear precipitating stressor, the reason why a person reacts with a particular intensity or for a particular duration is unknown. Different schools of thought in psychiatry account for this range of reactive variance according to their philosophical reference. Thus, the existence and extent of the adjustment disorder may be considered a result of biologic/constitutional determinants, environmental/developmental factors, or child rearing.

DIAGNOSTIC STUDIES

Adjustment disorders can be characterized by specific features that determine their particular subtype. The disorder types are as follows:
- With depressed mood
- With anxious mood
- With mixed emotional features (depression/anxiety)
- With disturbance of conduct
- With mixed disturbance of emotions and conduct
- Not otherwise specified

Diagnostic Criteria
Adjustment disorders are precipitated by many life problems such as divorce, financial stresses, death, illness, or relocation. Features common to all types of maladjustment include the following:
- Clearly identifiable stressor
- Onset within 3 months of the occurrence of stressor
- A maladaptive response to the stressor
- Impairment of occupational, school, or social activities; impairment of relationships
- Symptomatic reaction beyond normal expectations
- Maladaptive reaction not longer than 6 months
- Disturbance not related to a characteristic pattern of overreaction
- Not attributable to another mental disorder

DIFFERENTIAL DIAGNOSIS

Because the diagnosis of an adjustment disorder is based on clinical experience and judgment, it is important to distinguish characteristic types from other diagnostically identifiable conditions or mental disorders that may be associated with similar symptoms.

Bereavement.   Self-limited and normal process occurring after the death or loss of a loved one. May cause temporary symptoms of psychosis and/or general anxiety.

Post-Traumatic Stress Disorder (PTSD).   Occurs as a result of significant stress that is not a usual component of normal human experience and is expected to cause a response in an otherwise normal person.

Major Depression. May cause symptoms suggestive of an adjustment disorder, but symptoms may be prolonged and/or not directly associated with an identifiable stressor.

Developmental and Learning Delays. Differentiated on neuropsychologic testing; symptoms may be worsened by stressors.

TREATMENT

Psychotherapy, behavioral or insight-oriented, is indicated to promote healthy readjustment, to decrease the intensity and duration of the problem, and to prevent recurrence.

The use of psychopharmacologic therapy is dependent on the severity and duration of symptoms. The use of antidepressant, antianxiety, or even antipsychotic medication follows the guidelines for use of such agents in related primary disorders. Medications are used only briefly and are not used without adjunctive psychologic therapy.

Therapy is directed at assisting the patient to work through current trauma and to develop strategies for dealing with similar traumas in the future. Supportive group and family therapy seems to be an effective treatment.

Patients usually return to baseline function within 3 months, provided that the stressor is not ongoing.

PEDIATRIC CONSIDERATIONS

Adjustment disorders in childhood and adolescence often involve either "acting out" behaviors (anger, outbursts, oppositional stance, disturbances of conduct) or, conversely, avoidant behaviors (psychosomatic illness, school phobia, excessive dependency). Decreased school performance, impaired relationships, and overreactivity may be the first signs of an adjustment problem. Patients may go on to develop mood disorders or substance abuse problems.

OBSTETRIC CONSIDERATIONS

Pregnancy is a stressor for most women. Concerns about pain on delivery, fetal development, and physical changes after delivery are apt to cause transient psychologic changes. Education about the delivery process can lessen the stress and prevent untoward reaction to the stress. Screening for potential mental disorders should be performed to effectively address potential problems in the antepartum or postpartum period.

GERIATRIC CONSIDERATIONS

Acute or subacute changes in the mental functioning of the geriatric patient require investigation to rule out a primary medical condition or medication side effect. Retirement, death of loved ones, job loss, financial changes, and medical illness all are more frequently encountered in the elderly population. Individual methods of dealing with life stressors are also more established.

PREVENTIVE CONSIDERATIONS

Patients should be supported in maintaining a realistic attitude with expectation of inevitable stressors in life and should be educated in developing defense mechanisms to deal with the stressors. Effective treatment involves strategies in coping with future stressors.

PEARLS FOR THE PA

Adjustment disorders are important to recognize as maladjustment behavior due to a clear stressor.

Although adjustment disorders are not exacerbations of preexisting psychopathology, psychotherapy is still the treatment of choice.

Anxiety Disorders

Pamela A. Van Bevern, MPAS, PA-C

DEFINITION

A group of mental disorders that includes panic disorder, generalized anxiety disorder, phobias (specific and social), obsessive-compulsive disorder (OCD), and post-traumatic stress disorder (PTSD). Anxiety is the predominant symptom in all of these conditions.

HISTORY

Symptoms. Anxiety disorders involve an acute and intense psychologic and physiologic response to environmental stimuli. These responses may involve motor tension, autonomic hyperactivity, apprehensive expectations, and hypervigilance. Motor tension may be identified by trembling or twitching, inability to relax, and increased startle response. Autonomic hyperactivity may be manifested by dry mouth, tachycardia, paresthesias, diarrhea, nausea, and hyperventilation. Consequently, patients may experience difficulty in concentration, insomnia, and irritability or impatience.

The intensity and duration of these symptoms may vary, ranging from limited panic episodes to a more generalized, persistent anxiety. Phobic and panic disorders are characterized by their brief episodic nature, whereas generalized anxiety disorder and OCD are more chronic. PTSD is marked by recurrent, painful, intrusive recollections of a traumatic event including dreams, flashbacks, and nightmares. Patients with OCD are consumed with performing rituals or compulsions that are so frequent or complex that they interfere with normal functioning.

General. Anxiety and depression frequently occur together, which can complicate the clinical picture. This co-depression is generally less debilitating than depression occurring alone. It is not uncommon for patients with severe anxiety to develop alcohol or drug dependence.

Age. Although most of the anxiety disorders tend to occur in adolescence and early adulthood, they can begin at any time in life.

Onset. Panic disorder is characterized by abrupt onset without warning or any associated external factors, whereas specific phobias are often attributed to a particular frightening episode experienced as a child or young adult. The remainder of these disorders tend to develop more gradually and become more complex over time.

Duration. Generalized anxiety involves symptoms that persist for longer than 6 months and are present on a continual basis. Conversely, panic attacks may last for only a few minutes. Anxiety disorders tend to persist indefinitely unless identified and treated appropriately.

Intensity. The degree of severity associated with anxiety disorders may range from extremely mild, such as with some of the specific phobias, to extreme and incapacitating. Patients with severe anxiety may become so agoraphobic that they are unable to leave the home. If left untreated, many of these disorders may often affect patients' social and recreational activities.

Aggravating Factors. Specific phobias are directly related to certain activities or conditions (flying, heights) or to insects or animals. Social phobias involve circumstances in which patients are subjected to scrutiny (e.g., performing or speaking in public). Panic attacks are generally provoked by repeated exposure to the setting or activity that precipitated the attacks (e.g., stores, concerts, driving). PTSD is attributable to a specific traumatic event that was experienced or even witnessed directly by the affected person.

Alleviating Factors. Prompt recognition and diagnosis are key. Cognitive behavior therapy and patient education help to reduce the fear of isolation and to dismiss patients' fears that they are "going crazy." Medications such as selective serotonin reuptake inhibitors (SSRIs) and anxiolytics are often very beneficial in alleviating symptoms and decreasing the severity of the condition.

Associated Factors. The occurrence of depression is common to most anxiety disorders and may lead to suicide attempts or self-medication with alcohol or other illicit drugs. Psychosocially, patients may find it difficult to maintain relationships, jobs, and finances.

PHYSICAL EXAMINATION

General. It is very common for a patient with an anxiety disorder to present to the emergency room with hyperventilation, dyspnea, tachycardia, palpitations, and numbness in the hands or around the lips. The patient may also complain of nausea, diarrhea, or a lump in the throat. These symptoms require a complete physical examination, as an anxiety disorder may coexist with other medical illness.

Patients may exhibit signs of restlessness and agitation. Vital signs may reveal tachycardia and increased blood pressure and respirations.

Neuropsychiatric.   The neurologic evaluation may be remarkable for tremors, hyperreflexia, or autonomic symptoms (e.g., diaphoresis, dry mouth). The patient may complain of hot and cold flashes or areas of numbness, with loss of sensation in the hands, lips, or feet. The gait will be normal, but the patient may complain of dizziness, vertigo, or unsteadiness. The mental status examination in all anxiety disorders will show decreased concentration but in PTSD will also reveal impaired memory. Mental function will be affected by apprehensive expectations including worries, fears, ruminations, obsessions, and rituals, all with the intent to relieve the anxious mood.

Neck.   A complete thyroid examination is warranted. The presence of a thyroid bruit may indicate hyperthyroidism, causing the anxiety.

Cardiovascular.   Assess for rate and regularity of rhythm. Unifocal premature ventricular contractions (PVCs) are common in anxiety disorders. A systolic click may indicate mitral valve prolapse.

Pulmonary.   Auscultate for expiratory wheezes or decreased breath sounds that may indicate asthma or pulmonary embolus (which may be associated with anxiety due to hypoxia).

Neurologic.   Assess for postural tremors, hyperreflexia, decreased sensation, or gait disturbances.

Mental Status.   Mini Mental Status Examination is necessary to determine mood symptoms or psychotic symptoms that are uncharacteristic of anxiety disorders

PATHOPHYSIOLOGY

The etiology of anxiety disorders includes biologic abnormalities and behavioral factors. Many patients have autonomic nervous systems that exhibit increased sympathetic tone and do not adapt as well to external stimuli. The areas of the brain known to be affected in patients with these disorders include the limbic system, prefrontal cortex, noradrenergic neurons of the locus ceruleus, and serotonergic neurons of the median raphe nucleus. Behavioral considerations include counterproductive thinking that leads to maladaptive behaviors.

DIAGNOSTIC STUDIES

Laboratory
Thyroid Panel, Complete Blood Count, Serum Chemistry.   Performed to rule out physical ailments causing the anxious behavior.

Toxicology Screen.   As indicated to rule out substance abuse.

Radiology.   Not applicable.

Other
ECG.   As indicated to rule out a cardiac condition causing the anxious behavior.
Pulse Oximetry.   As indicated to rule out hypoxia causing the anxious behavior

Diagnostic Criteria
Diagnostic criteria are specified in the *Diagnostic and Statistical Manual of Mental Disorders*, 4th edition (DSM-IV):

Generalized anxiety disorder: Excessive worry and anxiety for 6 months about a number of events. This is accompanied by three additional symptoms including but not limited to restlessness, becoming easily fatigued, and increased muscle tension. The focus of the worry is not associated with features of other anxiety disorders.

OCD: Recurrent obsessions or compulsions that are severe enough to be time-consuming and lead to significant impairment in daily living.

PTSD: Development of symptoms following exposure to traumatic stressor. These may develop acutely (within 3 months) or be delayed as long as 6 months following the event.

Panic disorder: Recurrent and unexpected attacks of intense fear or discomfort in which at least four physiologic symptoms occur. At least one of the attacks has been followed by persistent fear of another attack, worry about the implications of the attack, and a resultant behavioral change as a result of the attacks.

Specific phobias: Marked and persistent fear that is unwarranted and illogical and provoked by the presence or anticipation of exposure to a certain object or situation.

Social phobia: A fear of situations in which the person is placed where he or she will be observed by others and subject to the possibility of embarrassment.

DIFFERENTIAL DIAGNOSIS

Establishing the differential diagnosis in anxiety may be difficult because anxiety may be the consequence of a medical illness such as in the cardiac patient. Anxiety may also occur concomitantly with other medical conditions; therefore, careful evaluation of the patient is required. It cannot be assumed that physical symptoms are simply secondary to an anxiety disorder.

Traumatic/Infectious.   Not applicable.

Metabolic
Hyperthyroidism.   Will have abnormal thyroid function studies.

Neoplastic.   Not applicable.

Vascular

Mitral Valve Prolapse. Systolic murmur and click may be present. Echocardiogram is diagnostic.

Arrhythmias. Irregular pulse will be present. ECG and/or Holter monitoring may be warranted.

Congenital. Not applicable.

Acquired

Drug Side Effects/Withdrawal. Cocaine, amphetamines, caffeine, cannabis, beta agonists have been implicated.

TREATMENT

Because of the prevalence of anxiety disorders, primary caregivers are vital in recognizing the signs and symptoms to ensure prompt diagnosis. Treatment strategies should involve immediate referral for cognitive behavior therapy and/or pharmacotherapy. The importance of supportive counseling should be stressed and patients urged to become as educated as possible with regard to prevalence, treatment options, and the availability of local support groups.

Supportive counseling requires time, understanding, compassion, and empathy, which provides reassurance to the patient and emphasizes the importance of psychologic treatment. Follow-up is necessary in order to maintain rapport and further emphasize that the patient will work in conjunction with the psychotherapist to facilitate recovery.

Pharmacotherapy

The SSRIs provide effective first-line treatment for panic disorder, OCD, social phobias, and PTSD. Paroxetine has been approved for panic disorder, social phobia, OCD, and PTSD. As a rule, it is best to start at the lower dosages, as patients with these disorders tend to be quite sensitive to medications in general. Adjunctive treatment with low-dose benzodiazepines may be offered for the initial 2 to 4 weeks of therapy until the therapeutic range of the SSRI has been achieved. It is also important to instruct patients to have these medications available when break-through symptoms do occur, because of the rapid onset of action that they provide. With any benzodiazepine, the possibility of sedation, memory impairment, or abuse is a concern. It is important for patients on benzodiazepines or SSRIs to avoid quick discontinuation of these drugs as withdrawal symptoms can be very severe. Patients with social anxiety disorder may benefit from low-dose beta blockers as well.

Generalized anxiety disorder may be treated with benzodiazepines such as low-dose diazepam or lorazepam. Dependence on these medications is a concern, and the chronic nature of this disorder has led many clinicians to prescribe SSRIs initially. Buspirone is very useful in patients who have a history of alcohol or drug dependence owing to its nonaddictive nature.

Venlafaxine, a mixed serotonin and norepinephrine reuptake inhibitor, has also been approved for use in generalized anxiety disorder.

PEDIATRIC CONSIDERATIONS

Anxiety and fear are a part of the experience of childhood and can be on a continuum of normal development. Anxiety can be pathologic in childhood if (1) it occurs at a time that is not synchronous with normal development, (2) if the discomfort and distress interfere with the child's ability to participate in age-appropriate social and academic activities, and (3) if it is characterized by inflexibility that limits adaptive behavior. Some anxiety disorders have their onset in childhood. Animal phobias begin in childhood, severe performance anxiety in late childhood, and social phobia in adolescence. Children may have PTSD following significant stressors including physical or sexual abuse, witnessing violence, or diect experience of war or natural disasters.

Current treatment is administration of high-potency benzodiazepines (alprazolam and clonazepam) and tricyclic antidepressants.

OBSTETRIC CONSIDERATIONS

Many patients experience situational anxiety with pregnancy, often in the last trimester. Patient education and counseling usually suffice for management of the anxiety. Anxiolytics should be avoided if at all possible during pregnancy. The long-term influence of benzodiazepines can lead to withdrawal symptoms in the newborn. There is also an increased incidence of congenital malformations with minor tranquilizer use. Diazepam has been associated with a greater possibility of cleft palate. Sustained diazepam or administration of a large single diazepam dose can cause "floppy infant syndrome" (hypotonia, difficulty in suckling, and hypothermia).

GERIATRIC CONSIDERATIONS

It is unusual for adults to suddenly develop anxiety disorders during the geriatric years. Acute or subacute changes in the mental functioning of the geriatric patient require investigation to rule out a primary medical condition or medication side effect. Long-term effects of medications or substances (e.g., alcohol) may cause mental changes later in life.

Hypoxia can manifest as acute anxiety. A pulse oximeter should be available for use as a screening tool.

PREVENTIVE CONSIDERATIONS

Early recognition of phobias is necessary to prevent the disorder from significantly affecting the patient's social life. Appropriate medication and psychologic therapy can allow the patient to lead a more fulfilling life.

PEARLS FOR THE PA

Use benzodiazepines, but monitor for abuse or sale. Watch for symptoms of mild depression exacerbated by the medication.

Benzodiazepine maintenance is effective therapy for chronic disorders.

Discontinuation of benzodiazepines requires careful monitoring for discontinuation syndrome, seizures, or rebound.

SSRI medications provide a constructive alternative to the pharmacologic regimen.

Complete history and physical examination affords accurate diagnosis and appropriate referral to avoid problems later in treatment (e.g., other psychiatric or medical illness).

Monitor carefully for other substance abuse and withdrawal symptoms.

Remember, regularly scheduled office visits, supportive counseling, and physician assistant availability can do more for treatment than medications.

Attention-Deficit Hyperactivity Disorder

James B. Labus, PA-C

DEFINITION

Attention-deficit hyperactivity disorder (ADHD): Persistent hyperactivity and/or inattention that is age inappropriate. The hyperactivity/inattention must be present in at least two settings (work, school, home, social). The level of dysfunction is usually different between the settings. Symptoms must be present before the age of 7 years.

HISTORY

Symptoms.   Symptoms must interfere with normal, age-related function; must be present for at least 6 months; and must include excessive motor activity and/or inattention. Other related symptoms include impulsive behavior, poor attention span, distractibility, misbehavior, emotional lability, and/or irritability.

General. Behavior that leads to evaluation includes the inability to complete a task, inability to be unattended, inability to control emotions, and lack of impulse control. Obtain a history of the patient's home life, school or work functioning, and social interactions. The condition may lead to criticism, school difficulty, legal trouble, and risk-taking behavior of the affected child. Diagnosis should only be made by professionals with experience in treating ADHD and not by laypersons or school personnel.

Age. Symptoms must have been present before the age of 7 years (although not necessarily diagnosed). Boys are affected (or diagnosed as a result of behavior difficulty) more than girls.

Onset. Symptoms may not be recognized and diagnosis may be delayed until the child enters a structured environment.

Duration. Symptoms must be present for a minimum of 6 months before a diagnosis can be made. Most children "grow out" of symptoms by adolescence or adulthood. Hyperactivity is usually the first symptom to resolve, with distractibility the last.

Intensity. Symptoms can significantly affect school, work, or social situations.

Aggravating Factors. Non-diagnosis, coexisting learning disabilities, ridicule or reinforcement from peers.

Alleviating Factors. The presence of emotional support. Comprehensive treatment plan that involves all affected settings.

Associated Factors. Siblings are often affected by ADHD. School performance may suffer. Other mood disorders (e.g., depression) may coexist. Twenty-five percent of biologic parents are affected by ADHD, and there is a higher incidence of substance abuse and other psychiatric disorders. The patient may also have learning disability or uncoordination.

PHYSICAL EXAMINATION

General. A comprehensive examination is performed with emphasis on the neurologic system to rule out primary neurologic or medical illnesses contributing to the behavior.

Psychiatric. Affect and thought content should be normal. No evidence of psychosis should be present. Depression and/or anxiety may be revealed. The diagnosis of ADHD is made clinically on the basis of history and symptoms; degree of effect on school, home, work, and social activities; and consideration of age-appropriate nature of the behavior.

PATHOPHYSIOLOGY

The origin of ADHD is probably multifactorial. Genetic and environmental factors and exposures have been suggested as contributing factors. The genetic theory is supported by an increased incidence in monozygotic twins and in siblings and parents of affected persons. Furthermore, neurochemical pharmacologic manipulation seems to benefit the condition, suggesting a physical cause.

Environmental causes such as life changes, stress, anxiety, or lack of supportive home life may contribute to symptoms of ADHD.

Exposures to maternal infections have also been implicated.

DIAGNOSTIC STUDIES

Laboratory. None specific.

Radiology
MRI/CT of Brain. As indicated to rule out structural intracranial lesion.
Positron Emission Tomography (PET) Scan. May be used in selected cases for support of the diagnosis.

Other
Electroencephalography (EEG): Sleep and Awake. Performed to rule out absence seizures as a cause of the inattention.
Cognitive Testing. May reveal impulsive behavior.
Intelligence/Psychoeducational Testing. Testing in mathematics, reading, spelling, and writing, as indicated to rule out coexisting learning disorder.
Vision and Hearing Tests. Should be performed to rule out a physical cause of the inattention/hyperactivity.

DIFFERENTIAL DIAGNOSIS

Traumatic
Brain Injury. History of injury. Usually does not exhibit the hyperactivity and inattention symptoms.

Infectious. Not applicable.

Metabolic
Absence Seizure. A generalized seizure disorder that causes brief loss of consciousness. May be misdiagnosed as inattention. Differentiated on EEG.

Neoplastic
Brain Tumor. Any focal neurologic deficit or symptoms suggesting increased intracranial pressure requires full evaluation including MRI with and without contrast.

Vascular. Not applicable.

Congenital
Prenatal Factors. Exposure to toxins, maternal infections, prematurity have been associated with the development of ADHD.

Age-Appropriate Behavior. May be difficult to differentiate in the very young child (younger than 3 years). This should be the first consideration in the differential diagnosis, rather than ADHD.

Depression. Usually results in lower activity rather than hyperactivity. May coexist with ADHD.

Manic-Depressive Disorder (Bipolar Disorder). Increases and decreases in severity instead of the relatively constant features of ADHD.

Learning Disorder. May coexist with ADHD. May be a cause of the behavior issues alone.

Acquired. Not applicable

TREATMENT

Pharmacotherapy should be used only in combination with psychotherapy and/or behavior therapy. Parents as well as children should undergo counseling in order to provide a coordinated and long-term approach to the problem. Coordination of and involvement in the process by the school system are also helpful. Identification and appropriate treatment of coexisting learning disorders are indicated.

Behavior therapy is useful to redirect the disruptive deeds into productive activities.

Stimulant medication includes:
- Methylphenidate (Ritalin)
- Pemoline (Cylert)
- Dextroamphetamine (Dexedrine)

Antidepressants, antipsychotics, and selective serotonin reuptake inhibitors (SSRIs) have been used for primary treatment when stimulants are contraindicated or not effective.

Medications should be prescribed by health care professionals with experience treating ADHD and as a part of a comprehensive treatment program.

PEDIATRIC CONSIDERATIONS

According to the *Diagnostic and Statistical Manual of Mental Disorders*, 4th edition (DSM-IV), symptoms must be present before the age of 7. This is a pediatric condition.

OBSTETRIC CONSIDERATIONS

Not applicable.

GERIATRIC CONSIDERATIONS

Not applicable.

PREVENTIVE CONSIDERATIONS

Appropriate recognition and treatment. Identification of coexisting learning disabilities and mood disorders and appropriate treatment.

PEARLS FOR THE PA

Diagnosis of ADHD should be performed by those with experience and not by schools or lay people.

Symptoms of ADHD must have been present before age 7, be persistent, involve at least two settings, and interfere with normal function.

Behaviors must be age inappropriate.

Eating Disorders

R. Ellen Davis-Hall, PhD, PA-C

DEFINITION

There are two major types of eating disorders:

Anorexia nervosa: An eating disorder characterized by a disturbed sense of body image, an intense fear of gaining weight, and significant self-imposed dietary restrictions and weight loss.

Bulimia nervosa: Characterized by uncontrolled, compulsive overeating over a short period of time, terminated by physical discomfort and feelings of guilt and depression, followed by induced vomiting and/or abuse of laxatives or diuretics or other artificial means of purging.

HISTORY

Symptoms

Symptoms are as listed in the *Diagnostic and Statistical Manual of Mental Disorders*, 4th edition (DSM-IV).

Anorexia Nervosa.   The patient has an intense fear of gaining weight, a disturbance in self-perception of body image, weight loss to less than 85% of the body weight expected, and in females, absence of at least three consecutive menstrual cycles.

Bulimia nervosa. There is a feeling of lack of control over recurrent binge eating, with regular engagement in purging activity (self-induced vomiting, diuretic, laxative, or ipecac use, strict dieting or fasting, or vigorous exercise) to prevent weight gain; there must be a minimum average of two binge episodes a week for at least 3 months; history must also convey the patient's overconcern with body shape and weight.

General

Although these are distinct disorders, the features of bulimia and anorexia tend to overlap.

Anorexia. Patients with anorexia nervosa have a large part of their lives focused on food, have elaborate diets (including vegetarianism), sometimes becoming recipe collectors, and cook large meals for others. They also tend to have an intense interest in exercise, demonstrate high academic achievements, come from families with high-achievement orientation, and be perfectionistic. Anorexia is considered to be more common in the higher socioeconomic groups. Somatic complaints such as epigastric complaints are common; patients may have a decreased interest in sex, complain of cold intolerance, have chronic constipation. Much more common in females than in males.

Bulimia. Bulimic patient's history may reveal precipitating factors such as adolescent life events. The patient may privately consume huge amounts of food and then induce vomiting by placing the fingers down the throat; later, the patient may be able to vomit at will. History may also reveal episodes of stealing, or shoplifting food items. Bulimics are more sexually active than anorexics; a history of amenorrhea is rare. The disease is observed to be more common in higher socioeconomic classes; families may be unaware of binging but may notice that food bills are increasing or that high-calorie foods disappear; frequently, the parents of the bulimic patient are obese. Much more common in females than in males.

Age

Anorexia. Adolescence or young adulthood.
Bulimia. Adolescence through the 30s.

Onset

Anorexia. Onset in early teen years is most common.
Bulimia. Initial behaviors usually begin in the late teens through the early 20s. Childhood obesity may precede bulimia with onset in adolescence or adulthood.

Duration

Anorexia. Symptoms are usually manifested between 10 and 30 years of age; the duration of the actual disorder depends on the timing of diagnosis and intervention.
Bulimia. The disease is chronic over many years until diagnosis is made and intervention is taken.

Intensity
Anorexia. May be from mild to life-threatening, or fatal.

Bulimia. Rarely incapacitating unless there is very frequent binging and purging; for this reason it is more difficult to diagnose than anorexia. There may be periods of normal eating between binge and purge cycles. Cardiac arrhythmias and sudden death, as well as esophageal tears and gastric ruptures from vomiting, may be life-threatening.

Aggravating Factors
Anorexia. The outcome of this disease is worse if there is parental conflict, a comorbid personality disorder, older age at onset, or coexisting bulimia.

Bulimia. Morbidity of the disease may increase if esophageal tears occur, and as the frequency of the binging and purging cycles increases.

Alleviating Factors
Anorexia. Usually none until a medical intervention is made.

Bulimia. The fact that weight may remain stable, and may not be grossly abnormal, masks the seriousness of the disorder; there is some improvement in bulimia with antidepressant therapy.

Associated Factors
Anorexia. There may be an associated major depression, substance abuse, anxiety disorder, obsessive-compulsive disorder, or a personality disorder.

Bulimia. Careful family history may reveal obesity in other family members; in addition, adolescent obesity in the patient may predispose to bulimia in adulthood. As with anorexia, depression may be a concurrent problem in the bulimic. These patients may also have a predisposition to chemical dependency.

PHYSICAL EXAMINATION

General
Anorexia. Weight will be 15% below usual weight; the patient will appear emaciated despite the patient's verbalization of concern with overweight.

Bulimia. Weakness or lethargy may be noted (secondary to electrolyte disturbance); weight may be in the normal range, or patient may be mildly over- or underweight.

Cardiovascular
Anorexia. Bradycardia, hypotension, edema.

Head, Eyes, Ears, Nose, Throat
Bulimia. Dental erosion and caries may be obvious; parotid gland enlargement or throat inflammation may be present.

Skin
Anorexia. Check for signs of hypothermia, purplish cast to the hands, petechiae, dry skin, hair loss, and lanuginous hair development.

Bulimia. Scratches and/or calluses may be seen on the back of the hand (from repeated placing of the fingers down the throat); poor turgor may reflect dehydration.

PATHOPHYSIOLOGY

Anorexia

Attempts have been made to explain this disorder with genetic, biologic, psychologic, and social theories. Anorexia tends to run in families. Neurotransmitter theories have been suggested.

Bulimia

Disorders of the hypothalamic-pituitary axis have been theorized; hormonal levels, however, are normal. The neurotransmitter theories cite findings of reduced norepinephrine activity and turnover.

DIAGNOSTIC STUDIES

Expected/possible changes are as given in DSM-IV.

Laboratory

Serum Electrolytes
Anorexia/Bulimia. Important to assess initially and periodically during treatment to evaluate for any changes.

Thyroid Function Studies
Anorexia. May reveal a low triiodothyronine (T_3).

Hormone Levels
Anorexia. Low LH and FSH levels, elevated growth hormone and plasma cortisol levels.

Complete Blood Count
Anorexia. Leukopenia may be present.

Serum Chemistry
Anorexia. May reveal elevated transaminases and serum cholesterol.

Bulimia. Hypocalcemia, hypokalemia; serum transaminase levels may be elevated; fatty degeneration of the liver may develop; elevated serum amylases may be present.

Radiology. Not applicable.

Other

ECG
Anorexia. Sinus bradycardia may occur as well as arrhythmias secondary to electrolyte abnormalities.
Bulimia. Cardiac arrhythmias may occur secondary to electrolyte disturbances.

DIFFERENTIAL DIAGNOSIS

Anorexia
Other psychiatric disorders such as major depression, schizophrenia, obsessive-compulsive disorder, and somatization disorders must be ruled out. A careful history should also rule out bulimia.

Bulimia
Other psychiatric disorders such as major depression and schizophrenia must be ruled out; a personality disorder, such as borderline personality, may coexist.

TREATMENT

Anorexia
Referral to a practitioner or center specializing in eating disorders for medical management, behavior modification, and individualized therapy; management is multidisciplinary and may be on an inpatient or outpatient basis. Certain medications may be helpful including cyproheptadine hydrochloride, phenothiazines, and benzodiazepines. Evaluate patients for and treat concurrent problems. Family therapy may be indicated if the patient is still living at home or has close family contact.

Bulimia
Referral to a practitioner or center specializing in eating disorders for medical management, behavioral modification, and individualized therapy. Ensure metabolic balance is achieved by ongoing monitoring of electrolytes. Tricyclic antidepressants, monoamine oxidase (MAO) inhibitors, trazodone, and fluoxetine have been shown to improve bulimia. Family therapy may be indicated if the patient is still living at home.

PEDIATRIC CONSIDERATIONS

Eating disorders of childhood include failure to thrive, obesity, rumination disorder (rare), pica (rare but more common in developmentally delayed or neglected children), anorexia nervosa, and bulimia.

Failure to thrive may be either organic or nonorganic. In nonorganic failure to thrive, disorders in the parent-child interaction are common. Treatment is focused on restoration of adequate calories and nutrition, optimizing feeding behavior, and improving parent-child interactions.

Anorexia nervosa rarely occurs before puberty and rarely affects males. When it does occur before menarche, the effects may be devastating including prolonged delay of puberty or menarche and serious impairment of growth in stature and breast development. In premenarchal forms, weight loss may not occur; rather, failure to gain weight in accordance with developmental expectations may be noted.

OBSTETRIC CONSIDERATIONS

Pregnancy is unusual owing to the amenorrhea that results from the loss of body fat in anorexia nervosa. Careful monitoring of nutritional intake should be performed in bulimic patients.

GERIATRIC CONSIDERATIONS

Not applicable.

PREVENTIVE CONSIDERATIONS

Recognition, vigilance by professionals who regularly encounter adolescents, and education and treatment are imperative to prevent health risks. Education of students, teachers, counselors, church workers, and so on can assist in identifying youth at risk.

PEARLS FOR THE PA

Anorexic and bulimic patients can be very manipulative, critical, and secretive and commonly lie about food intake.

Patients have a strong denial system and are resistant to treatment.

Being firm about behavioral guidelines and encouraging the family members to do the same are important.

Mood Disorders

R. Ellen Davis-Hall, PhD, PA-C

DEFINITION

Classified as either depression or bipolar disorder:

Depression: A condition characterized by a depressed mood or loss of interest or pleasure in usually enjoyable activities and associated symptoms.

Bipolar disorder: A condition characterized by one or more manic episodes and usually accompanied by one or more major depressive episodes. The manic period is distinctly abnormal, with persistent elevated, expansive, or irritable mood, sufficiently severe to cause marked impairment in occupational or social functioning.

HISTORY

Symptoms

Symptoms are as listed in the *Diagnostic and Statistical Manual of Mental Disorders*, 4th edition (DSM-IV).

Depression. Depressed mood, diminished interest or pleasure in all (or almost all) activities most of the time, significant unintentional weight loss or weight gain, insomnia or hypersomnia, psychomotor agitation or retardation, fatigue or loss of energy, feelings of worthlessness or inappropriate guilt, diminished ability to think, concentrate, or make decisions, and recurrent thoughts of death or suicide. A careful past history may reveal prior episodes of depression; family history is important. Past treatments for the patient's depression and the success of these treatments should also be recorded.

Bipolar Disorder. Depressive symptoms and also manic symptoms including inflated self-esteem or grandiosity, decreased need for sleep, increased talkativeness or subjective experience of pressure to talk, flight of ideas or subjective experience that thoughts are racing, distractibility, increase in goal-directed activity or psychomotor agitation, excessive involvement in pleasurable activities that have a high potential for painful consequences.

General

Depression. Patient may present with depressed mood as a chief complaint, but be unaware of the depression; may be brought in by concerned others who have noted withdrawal from usual activities of prior interest; women are more commonly affected than men.

Bipolar Disorder. The patient may have a contagious euphoria and have little insight into his/her behavior; family members may be the first to recognize the abnormality and inappropriateness of the behavior; euphoria may change to irritability if patient's activities are impeded or inhibited. The incidence is equal in males and females and among races. Bipolar disorder is considered an inheritable disorder; because of mania, history is unreliable.

Age
Depression. Early childhood through old age.
Bipolar Disorder. Adolescence through old age.

Onset
Depression. Approximately half of the patients have their initial episode after age 40 years. Progression is usually insidious.

Bipolar Disorder. Usually starts with depression; the initial manic episode usually occurs prior to 50 years of age, with a mean onset in the 30s; the symptoms may have a rapid or insidious onset, developing over a few hours to a few weeks.

Duration
Depression. Untreated episodes may last 6 to 13 months; a treated episode may last 3 months.

Bipolar Disorder. An untreated manic episode may last for approximately 3 months.

Intensity
Depression. Outward manifestations of symptoms (affect) may include severe agitation or profound psychomotor retardation, so that the patient cannot initiate activities; inward manifestations (mood), if severe, can lead to suicide.

Bipolar Disorder. There can be significant social consequences from the impulsiveness and impaired judgment that are often present; at times patients may be assaultive, threatening, or psychotic, and require physical restraints or intramuscular tranquilizers.

Aggravating Factors
Depression. Significant life events are sometimes implicated in onset of symptoms. Chronic medical illnesses may exist concurrently. Isolated living conditions as well as certain medications are also known factors in depression. Chemical dependency may predispose to depression.

Bipolar Disorder. As the patient's age increases and the disease progresses, there may be more frequent episodes of mania that last longer. Coexisting dysthymia, active chemical dependency, and anxiety increase the risk of recurrence.

Alleviating Factors
Depression. Caution should be given that patients may present with a single or clustering of physical symptoms only (masked depression); treating these somatic complaints may seem temporarily effective, but may only serve to distract the health care provider from the real cause of the complaints.

Bipolar Disorder. Early and appropriate psychiatric or medical intervention.

Associated Factors
Depression. Increase in somatic complaints (especially gastrointestinal symptoms including constipation or dry mouth) and a decrease in sex drive are common.
Bipolar Disorder. See under Aggravating Factors.

PHYSICAL EXAMINATION

General
Depression. A complete physical examination is necessary because depression may coexist with serious medical problems. Weight change, more commonly a loss, may be prominent. Agitation or psychomotor retardation may be obvious. Patient may have an unkempt appearance.
Bipolar Disorder. Patients are excited and talkative; flight of ideas may be prominent. May be euphoric or irritable, emotionally labile.

Neuropsychiatric
Depression. Findings on Mental Status Examination including memory may be abnormal, but secondary to an inability to concentrate; delusions may also be detected; thought processes may reflect a negative view of the world.
Bipolar Disorder. Orientation and memory are intact. Impaired judgment is prominent. There will be little insight into the disease. Thought process may reflect grandiosity.

PATHOPHYSIOLOGY

Etiologic theories include biologic (including genetic) and psychosocial hypotheses. Biologically, norepinephrine and serotonin are the two neurotransmitters most strongly implicated; it is unclear whether these neurotransmitter abnormalities are the result of depression or result in depression. Both unipolar and bipolar forms of depression run in families, but the evidence for heritability is stronger for bipolar disorder.

DIAGNOSTIC STUDIES

Laboratory
Bipolar Disorder. Prior to drug treatment with lithium, certain laboratory screening should be performed including thyroid studies, urinalysis, electrolytes with blood urea nitrogen (BUN) and creatinine, and complete blood count, to rule out concurrent or contributing disorders.

Radiology
CT/MRI scan of brain as indicated to evaluate for lesion causing symptoms.

Other

Objective Rating Scales
Depression.   The Zung or Hamilton Depression Rating Scale may be helpful in confirming the diagnosis.

Diagnostic Criteria

Diagnostic criteria are specified by DSM-IV.

Depression.   At least five of the nine symptoms listed under Symptoms earlier must be present during the same 2-week period; at least one of the symptoms must be depressed mood or loss of interest or pleasure in usually pleasurable activities.

Bipolar Disorder.   The patient must have an elevated, expansive, or irritable mood lasting at least one weekend sufficient to cause marked occupational or social functioning and at least three of the seven symptoms listed under Symptoms.

DIFFERENTIAL DIAGNOSIS

Traumatic

Head Injury.   May be remote history and decreased intellectual capacity or neurologic deficit.

Infectious

Depression
Viral Pneumonia.   Especially in the elderly. Chest film will show infiltrate.

Mononucleosis.   Especially in the adolescent. Positive Monospot test, lymphadenopathy.

Depression/Bipolar Disorder
Acquired Immunodeficiency Syndrome (AIDS).   If patient is in the high-risk group for this disease.

Metabolic

Depression
Parkinson Disease.   Tremors present, cogwheel rigidity on passive range of motion of the extremities, slow shuffling gait, masked facies.

Dementia.   Patients are unaware of their condition.

Depression/Bipolar Disorder
Epilepsy.   History of seizures.

Thyroid Abnormalities.   If weight problems are prominent. Positive thyroid profile.

Adrenal Abnormalities (Addison Disease).   Weakness, fatigue, lethargy, hyperpigmentation, electrolyte abnormalities, weight loss, dehydration. Decreased 24-hour urinary free cortisol.

Bipolar Disorder
Migraines.   History of recurrent unilateral headaches, may have visual scotoma or positive family history.

Multiple Sclerosis.   History of waxing and waning focal neurologic signs. Positive MRI or cerebrospinal fluid examination.

Menstrual Abnormalities.   History specifically relating mood alterations to menstrual cycles.

Systemic Lupus Erythematosus.   Fever, weight loss, skin and oral lesions, multiple organ system involvement. Patient may have a positive antinuclear antibody assay, and a further workup with anti–native DNA may be diagnostic.

Uremia.   Multiplicity of physical findings, elevated BUN and creatinine suggesting renal failure.

Neoplastic

Depression
Brain Tumors.   Positive CT/MRI. May have symptoms of increased intracranial pressure.

Malignancies: Notably Pancreatic, Gastrointestinal.   May manifest with depression and few other symptoms. Positive CT of abdomen.

Vascular

Depression/Bipolar Disorder
Stroke.   Positive CT/MRI of brain. May have carotid bruit, cardiac arrhythmia, or murmur.

Congenital
Not applicable.

Acquired

Depression
Drug Side Effects.   May be the etiology of the depression, and discontinuance of drug is the primary treatment (e.g., analgesics, antibacterials, antineoplastics, antiparkinsonians, antiepileptics, antipsychotics, hypnotics, sedatives, antihypertensives, or cardiac drugs).

Bipolar Disorder
Drug Side Effects.   Captopril, cimetidine, cocaine, corticosteroids, hallucinogens, hydralazine, levodopa have been implicated.

Vitamin Deficiencies.   History of poor nutrition (in the elderly) or a malabsorption syndrome.

TREATMENT

Depression
Hospitalize if patient is suicidal or if there is severe psychomotor retardation that impairs ability for self-care.

Tricyclic antidepressants and monoamine oxidase (MAO) inhibitors are the mainstays of therapy (see Table 14-1). Newer drugs now available, such as the second-generation antidepressants, are probably no more efficacious but may have fewer side effects. As a rule, agitated depressed patients should be treated with a sedating antidepressant, and those with psychomotor retardation should be treated with a nonsedating drug.

Electroconvulsant therapy is the most effective treatment for depression but is usually reserved for the most severe cases or for depression resistant to drug therapy, or for cases in which a rapid therapeutic response is particularly desirable. Electroconvulsant therapy is considered safer for cardiac patients than certain antidepressants.

Referral for psychotherapy.

Bipolar Disorder

Psychiatric consultation/referral. Hospitalization is indicated if full manic syndrome is present; hypomania may be managed on an outpatient basis in some cases.

After laboratory evaluation, lithium may be started; antipsychotics may also be required (under a psychiatrist's supervision); this drug should be continued for 4 to 6 months, with frequent serum lithium levels assessed.

Psychotherapy may be helpful, especially to increase drug compliance.

Electroconvulsant therapy has been used in treatment of mania.

Table 14–1. Medical Therapy for Depression Daily Drug Dose*

First-Generation Antidepressants	
Tricyclic Derivatives	
Amitriptyline (Elavil, etc.)	50-150 mg
Desipramine hydrochloride (Norpramin)	100-300 mg
Doxepin hydrochloride (Sinequan, etc.)	25-300 mg
Imipramine hydrochloride (Tofranil, etc.)	75-200 mg
Nortriptyline (Pamelor)	100-300 mg
MAO Inhibitors	
Phenelzine sulfate (Nardil)	45-90 mg
Tranylcypromine sulfate (Parnate)	30-60 mg
Second-Generation Antidepressants	
Tricyclic Derivatives	
Trimipramine maleate (Surmontil)	75-200 mg
Other	
Bupropion (Wellbutrin)	200-300 mg
Citalopram (Celexa)	20-60 mg
Escitalopram (Lexapro)	10-20 mg
Fluoxetine (Prozac)	10-40 mg
Trazodone (Desyrel)	100-600 mg
Venlafaxine (Effexor)	37.5-225 mg

*Daily oral therapeutic dose.
MAO, monoamine oxidase.

PEDIATRIC CONSIDERATIONS

Depression

The diagnosis of depression in childhood can be difficult. Children may be limited in their capacity to recognize and articulate features of depression. Children referred to mental health centers commonly are diagnosed with depression, but there is considerable overlap with other conditions (anxiety, attention-deficit disorder, conduct disorder, drug use, anorexia nervosa, and school refusal). Physical symptoms such as recurrent abdominal pain or headaches may be the initial presentation of depressive disorders. Children with depression are at increased risk for subsequent episodes of depression.

Medication use in treatment for childhood depression has not been very promising. Tricyclic antidepressants can be used for significant depression unresponsive to other interventions. Because cardiovascular side effects have been reported, albeit rarely, caution should be utilized. There have been reports of sudden death in children receiving tricyclic antidepressants in therapeutic ranges. Patients need regular electrocardiogram, pulse, and blood pressure monitoring. Because tricyclic antidepressants are lethal in overdose, parents should administer the medication and care should be exercised so that siblings do not accidentally ingest the medication.

Bipolar Disorder

Bipolar disorder can appear prior to adolescence. Superficially, children with hyperactivity disorder may seem hypomanic. However, in bipolar illness there is a more pronounced mood shift, activity is more goal-oriented, and there may be accompanying delusions or hallucinations. In older children, grandiosity and paranoia are common, whereas irritability and emotional lability are more often present in younger children. Family history is important because bipolar illness seems to have a substantial genetic component.

Treatment may include use of neuroleptics for acute mania and lithium for bipolar depression. Appropriate laboratory studies should be performed before initiation of lithium therapy. Tricyclics and MAO inhibitors may cause hypomanic reactions in susceptible patients.

OBSTETRIC CONSIDERATIONS

Most antidepressant medications are category C (adverse affects have been demonstrated by animal studies; no well-controlled human studies are available) and should be used only if the benefits of their use clearly justify the risk of adverse effects in the fetus.

GERIATRIC CONSIDERATIONS

Depression. About 50% of patients have initial symptoms after age 40. Changes in lifestyle that accompany aging can lead to significant depression.

Bipolar Disorder. As the patient's age increases and the disease progresses, there may be more frequent episodes of mania that last longer.

PREVENTIVE CONSIDERATIONS

Vigilance, recognition, and appropriate treatment are indicated for both depression and bipolar disorder. These conditions are treatable. Lessening the "mental illness" stigma by inquiring and providing the patient the opportunity to discuss mental health issues, even in a routine visit, will assist in the identification and treatment of these conditions.

PEARLS FOR THE PA

Depression
If a patient makes you feel depressed, then depression is probably the primary diagnosis.

If a particular antidepressant drug has worked successfully in the past for the patient or a family member, it will probably work well again.

As a patient's depression improves with treatment, remain vigilant for suicidal ideation, as sometimes seemingly significant improvement can precede a suicide attempt.

Inquiry must always be made into thoughts of suicide.

Bipolar Disorder
Use diuretics with caution in a patient on lithium, as serum levels will be affected.

Supervise prescription compliance carefully during the manic phase; the depressive phase carries a risk for suicide attempt by overdosing.

Personality Disorders

James B. Labus, PA-C

DEFINITION

Personality disorder: A fixed, maladaptive behavioral and emotional approach to the personal and social challenges of life (personality), reflecting the "character." A personality disorder occurs when the behavior deviates from what is considered culturally normal, is maladaptive, and causes a functional impairment and/or emotional distress.

HISTORY

Symptoms. People with personality disorders may be egosyntonic to the degree that their personality structure and preferred psychologic defenses shield them from the consequences of their dysfunction. Patients may have impaired insight (or denial) regarding their condition. Generally, they do not require psychiatric hospitalization other than for a concurrent or superimposed problem (such as psychoactive substance abuse or acute anxiety).

General. Antisocial, paranoid, and obsessive-compulsive disorders are more common in men. Borderline, dependent, and especially histrionic personality disorders are more common in women.

The repertoire of behaviors underlying a personality disorder lead to problems in legal, occupational, and interpersonal areas. Depending on the specific disorder, the person may experience distress from divorce, arrest, job loss, alcohol/psychoactive substance abuse, or other social conflict.

Age. Specific dysfunctional personality traits or styles may be evident from adolescence or early adult life.

Onset. Although symptoms may be present from an early age, the diagnosis is usually not made until age 18 years or older.

Duration. There is generally a lifelong pattern of conflict and dysfunction.

Intensity. Discord and dysfunction range from moderate to severe.

Aggravating Factors. These patients are quite difficult to treat, as they generally do not experience anxiety directly as a result of the maladaptive behaviors.

Alleviating Factors. Support groups for substance abuse may be of benefit.

Associated Factors. Many defense mechanisms, particularly projection and blaming, are used by persons with a personality disorder to resist therapeutic change. Work and social life are affected by the disorder. Substance abuse, depression, and mild brain damage may be associated with personality disorder.

PHYSICAL EXAMINATION

General. The physical examination usually does not provide diagnostic information, other than through complications manifest in the Mental Status Examination.

Psychiatric. Depending on the specific personality disorder, affective intensity and inappropriateness may be present (e.g., borderline, histrionic). Psychomotor changes associated with anxiety or depression may be observable (e.g., in dependent or obsessive-compulsive styles).

PATHOPHYSIOLOGY

Specific dysfunctional personality traits or styles may be evident from adolescence or early adulthood. Personality disorders are generally thought to be a learned response to developmental and environmental forces. As such, they represent patterns of behavior characteristic of most of adult life. Well-defined types of personality disorders are recognized (see Table 14-2).

Etiologic factors in the formation of a personality disorder may include genetic (more common in families) as well as psychodynamic and learned components. The prevalence of personality disorders in the community is thought to be 10% of the population.

DIAGNOSTIC STUDIES

The diagnosis of a personality disorder is based on the patient's history and on clinical assessment. Laboratory abnormalities may be associated but are not diagnostic.

Laboratory
Testosterone/17-Estradiol/Estrone. May be elevated.
Dexamethasone Suppression Test. May be abnormal.
Serotonin. May be low.

Table 14–2. Classification of Personality Disorders

Personality Type	Features
Antisocial	Fails to respect social norms
Avoidant	Timid, reticent, easily embarrassed, sensitive, "inferiority complex"
Borderline	Intense and unstable moods and relations
Dependent	Submissive, needy, subordinate
Narcissistic	Grandiose, hypersensitive, sense of entitlement
Obsessive-compulsive	Perfectionistic, inflexible
Paranoid	Expects harm, questions loyalty, distrustful, blames others for paranoia
Schizoid	Lifelong indifference to social relationships, "eccentric"
Schizotypal	Peculiar ideas, appearance, behavior, and communication
Not otherwise specified	
Passive-aggressive	Procrastination, ineffectual
Depressive	Pessimism, long-term unhappiness
Sadomasochistic	One or the other component may predominate, or both may be present; *sadism*: causing physical or psychologic pain in others, *masochism*: inflicting physical or emotional pain on the self

Radiology
MRI/CT of the Brain.   As indicated (if there is an acute personality change, poor impulse control, and/or no history of a mental disorder) to rule out mass lesion.

Other
Electroencephalography (EEG).   May reveal changes; more common with antisocial and borderline personality disorders.
Minnesota Multiphasic Personality Inventory (MMPI) and Projective Testing.   May be helpful in some cases to assist with diagnosis.

DIFFERENTIAL DIAGNOSIS

Traumatic
Brain Injury.   Mild head injury is associated with the development of personality disorder.

Infectious
Encephalitis.   May have a positive history.
Neurosyphilis.   Positive result of Venereal Disease Research Laboratory (VDRL) test.
Acquired Immunodeficiency Syndrome (AIDS).   Positive human immunodeficiency virus (HIV) assay; may have cerebral lesions on CT/MRI.

Metabolic
Dementia.   Global disorientation, decline in intellectual function; usually seen in the elderly.
Seizure Disorder.   Differentiated on careful history and positive EEG.

Neoplastic
Cerebral Lesion.   Identified on CT/MRI of brain.

Vascular
Not applicable.

Congenital
Not applicable.

Acquired
Anabolic Steroids.   Can cause both personality and behavioral changes. Steroids are used to increase muscle mass, increase athletic performance; may cause " 'roid rage."

TREATMENT

Persons with personality disorders are notoriously resistant to therapy owing to the deeply ingrained nature of the problem. Interventions are aimed at behavioral restructuring. Patients benefit from clearly defining behavioral boundaries and consequences for actions. Psychotherapy, behavior therapy, and cognitive behavior therapy all may be beneficial. Group therapy may be beneficial in all cases except those involving a paranoid personality disorder.

Medications are typically reserved to treat associated conditions such as anxiety or depression rather than the primary condition.

Self-help groups such as Alcoholics Anonymous (AA) are very helpful to those persons who have psychoactive substance abuse problems.

PEDIATRIC CONSIDERATIONS

Personality disorders are, by definition, diagnoses of adult behavior and dysfunction. Certain patterns characteristic of a personality disorder may be recognizable in childhood and adolescence such as identity disorder (precursor of borderline personality disorder) or conduct disorder (harbinger of antisocial personality disorder).

OBSTETRIC CONSIDERATIONS

Careful screening and appropriate psychotherapeutic intervention are indicated.

GERIATRIC CONSIDERATIONS

Personality disorders are usually evident early in adult life. Acute or subacute changes in the mental functioning of the geriatric patient require investigation to rule out a primary medical condition or medication side effect. Long-term effects of medications or substances of abuse (e.g., alcohol) may cause mental changes later if life.

PREVENTIVE CONSIDERATIONS

Recognition and awareness are paramount in identification and effective treatment for personality disorders. Patients should be counseled regarding abuse of alcohol or other substances.

PEARLS FOR THE PA

The personality disorders tend to provoke strong reactions and countertransference in the clinician.

Be aware of the potential for associated substance abuse.

Treatment success may come slowly and require strong intervention to break through the "character armor."

Psychotic Disorders

James B. Labus, PA-C

DEFINITION

Psychosis is, literally, a loss of contact with "reality" in the context, structure, and expectations of social life. Hallmark features of these disorders are delusions or hallucinations and a distortion of cognitive functions, particularly in content and process of thought.

Schizophrenia is a type of psychosis that lasts for at least 6 months and includes at least 1 month of active symptoms. Symptom complex must include two or more of the following: delusions, hallucinations, disorganized speech, disorganized behavior, or catatonic behavior.

HISTORY

Symptoms. The first 6 months constitutes the *active phase*, which includes psychotic, or "positive," symptoms including delusions, hallucinations, flat affect, and illogical thinking. The active phase is usually followed by a *residual phase*, including such "negative" symptoms as social isolation, poor hygiene, odd behavior, speech, and thought, and lack of interests or initiative. With respect to the course of disease, schizophrenia may be classified as follows:

- Subchronic
- Chronic
- Subchronic with acute exacerbation
- Chronic with acute exacerbation
- Remission
- Unspecified

General. Schizophrenia tends to be an illness characterized by periods of relapse and recovery. Patients may or may not perceive their behavior as unusual. There may be limited insight into the condition. Schizophrenia has an equal male and female distribution and affects about 1% of the population. It is important to determine educational level when taking the history.

Age. Schizophrenia appears in adolescence or early adulthood. In males, peak age range is 15 to 25 years; in females, 25 to 35.

Onset. Chronic, characterized by periods of relapse and recovery.

Duration. Usually lifelong.

Intensity. Patients may be able to function marginally in society or may be incapacitated and require long-term hospitalization.

Aggravating Factors. Variations from daily routine. Significant environmental stressors may exacerbate or cause symptoms.

Alleviating Factors. Appropriate medication, strict adherence to a daily routine.

Associated Factors. Positive family history of similar disorders. There is a generally increased mortality and increased incidence of suicide, depression and anxiety, substance abuse, homelessness, and complex partial epilepsy.

PHYSICAL EXAMINATION

General. There are no diagnostic physical findings in psychosis. Impairment of fine motor activity may be seen.

Eyes. May have difficulty tracking a moving object. Increased blink or tic may be apparent.

Psychiatric

Affect. The range, intensity, and content of the patient's emotional state all are significantly altered. The affect is usually flat, with a paucity of expression. Patients may laugh inappropriately, seeming to respond to internal mental stimuli, or relate in a bland, monotonous fashion.

Perception. Hallucinations, involving any of the senses but particularly auditory, are a prominent feature of the illness. Patients frequently experience "voices," often critical or persecutory in nature.

Thought Form. Loose associations between thoughts. Speech and thinking may be random, disconnected, and very idiosyncratic.

Thought Content. Delusions (fixed false beliefs) indicate major disturbance. The delusions are often religious or somatic in nature and are often systematized. Patients may feel that people are talking about them, or conversely, that they can control others or broadcast their thoughts. See Table 14-3 for list of types of delusions.

PATHOPHYSIOLOGY

Many hypotheses have been presented for the cause of schizophrenia: genetic, viral, hormonal, family dynamics, anatomic, and biochemical.

Table 14–3. Types of Delusions	
Erotomanic	Belief that someone of higher status is in love with the person
Grandiose	Inflated sense of self-worth, power, or knowledge
Jealous	Centered on unfaithfulness of a sexual partner
Persecutory	Perceptions of being mistreated
Somatic	Perceptions of having a physical defect or disease
Unspecified	No prominent theme, do not fit any other category

Currently there is no cure for schizophrenia or noninduced psychosis, as there is no specifically identified etiology.

It is postulated that there is a "premorbid personality," and that specific environmental stressors trigger the psychotic episodes.

See Table 14-4 for a classification of psychotic disorders.

DIAGNOSTIC STUDIES

The diagnosis of psychotic disorders is made on clinical grounds. Laboratory and radiographic data are of little use except to rule out physical illness appearing as psychosis.

Laboratory
Complete Blood Count with Differential and Blood Cultures.   Performed if septicemia is suspected of causing psychosis.

Thyroid Function Studies.   Performed to rule out hyper- or hypothyroidism as a cause of the psychologic symptoms.

Radiology
MRI.   As indicated to rule out mass lesion causing symptoms.

Other
Neuropsychiatric Testing, Intelligence Testing, Projective (e.g., Rorschach), Personality Tests.   Used as indicated to assist with diagnosis.

Electroencephalography (EEG).   May show changes with psychosis or may reveal seizure disorder.

DIFFERENTIAL DIAGNOSIS

See Table 14-5 for differential diagnosis of schizophrenia-like symptoms.

TREATMENT

The first consideration is whether the patient requires hospitalization. Criteria for hospitalization include the following:
- Danger to self or others (suicidal/homicidal)
- Inability to maintain activities of daily living
- Grossly inappropriate behavior
- For diagnostic purposes
- For stabilization of medical conditions

A primary treatment focus is the use of antipsychotic medications. Appropriate referral should be made to a psychiatric facility so that appropriate medical therapy and psychotherapy can commence.

Equally important is building a bridge between the patient's needs and the support systems available in the community. Patient and family education,

Table 14–4. Classification of Psychotic Disorders

Disorder	Features
Schizophrenic type	
Paranoid	Preoccupation with a specific theme, usually persecutory in nature within a delusional system
Catatonic	Characterized by significant motor symptoms including rigidity, posturing, and/or mutism; may cause self-injury or exhibit violence to others.
Disorganized	Marked incoherence and disorganized behavior
Undifferentiated residual type	Prominent delusions, hallucinations, and bizarre behavior
	Symptoms persist but do not include all active symptoms
Delusional (paranoid) type	Delusions are primary symptom; other symptoms of schizophrenia (disorganized speech/behavior, catatonia/flat or inappropriate affect) may be absent
Other psychoses	
Delusional disorder	Differentiated from delusional schizophrenia by plausibility of delusions (e.g., there is some basis in reality for beliefs)
Brief psychotic episode	Psychotic response to a significant stressor without a prodrome, lasting at least 1 day but less than 1 month
Schizophreniform disorder	Psychotic episode lasting at least 1 month but less than 6 months
Schizoaffective disorder	A mood disorder existing concurrently with schizophrenia-type symptoms
Substance-induced psychotic disorder	Symptoms are associated with intoxication or withdrawal; features are hallucinations and impaired grasp on reality
Atypical psychosis	A variety of psychotic symptoms exist that do not meet the criteria for any other nonorganic psychosis
Shared psychotic disorder	Symptoms of psychosis developing in a person in close relationship to the primary psychotic person
Postpsychotic depressive disorder	Occurs during the residual phase of schizophrenia and includes symptoms of a major depressive disorder
Simple deteriorative disorder (Simple schizophrenia)	Progressive social withdrawal consistent with deficit symptoms of schizophrenia
Culture-bound psychotic disorder	Seen only in certain cultures; may be psychosis with strong societal influences.

Table 14–5. Differential Diagnosis of Schizophrenia-Like
Symptoms

Medical and Neurologic

Substance-induced—amphetamine, hallucinogens, belladonna alkaloids, alcohol
   hallucinosis, barbiturate withdrawal, cocaine, phencyclidine (PCP)
Epilepsy—especially temporal lobe epilepsy
Neoplasm, cerebrovascular disease, or trauma—especially frontal or limbic
Other conditions
   Acquired immunodeficiency syndrome
   Acute intermittent porphyria
   Vitamin B$_{12}$ deficiency
   Carbon monoxide poisoning
   Cerebral lipoidosis
   Creutzfeldt-Jakob disease
   Fabry disease
   Fahr disease
   Hallervorden-Spatz disease
   Heavy metal poisoning
   Herpes encephalitis
   Homocystinuria
   Huntington disease
   Metachromatic leukodystrophy
   Neurosyphilis
   Normal-pressure hydrocephalus
   Pellagra
   Systemic lupus erythematosus
   Wernicke-Korsakoff syndrome
   Wilson disease

Psychiatric

Atypical psychosis
Autistic disorder
Brief psychotic disorder
Delusional disorder
Factitious disorder with predominantly psychologic signs and symptoms
Malingering
Mood disorders
Normal adolescence
Obsessive-compulsive disorder
Personality disorders—schizotypal, schizoid, borderline, paranoid
Schizoaffective disorder
Schizophrenia
Schizophreniform disorder

as well as behavioral (social skills) therapy and individual and group therapy, contributes to the integration of the patient into a productive social life.

Compliance must be addressed. The patient may have no insight into the condition or, even with insight, may deny the condition exists. Regular follow-up or hospitalization is needed.

PEDIATRIC CONSIDERATIONS

Psychotic disorders are generally not childhood illnesses and are very rare before the age of 10 years. A pediatric presentation of psychosis would indicate evaluation for a neuropsychiatric developmental disorder such as autism, or a workup for an atypical psychosis related to conditions such as post-traumatic stress disorder (PTSD) or toxicity. Schizophrenia and manic-depressive illness may have their onset in adolescence.

OBSTETRIC CONSIDERATIONS

Postpartum psychosis manifests in the new mother with depression, delusions, cognitive defects, mood disturbances, occasional hallucinations, and thoughts of doing harm to the infant or herself. The incidence is 1 to 2:1000 births. There appears to be a close relation with mood disorders. Symptoms usually occur 2 to 8 weeks post partum. Medical treatment consists of antidepressants, lithium, and antipsychotics. The mother should not breastfeed when receiving these medications. Psychotherapy is also instituted. Other physical causes for symptoms, including hypothyroidism, Cushing disease, analgesic effect, toxemia, and cerebral neoplasm, should be investigated. Postpartum psychosis must be differentiated from "postpartum blues," which affects about 50% of mothers who have recently given birth.

GERIATRIC CONSIDERATIONS

It is rare to diagnose a psychotic disorder after the age of 50 years. Acute or subacute changes in the mental functioning of the geriatric patient require investigation to rule out a primary medical condition or medication side effect. Long-term effects of medications or substances (e.g., alcohol) may cause mental changes later in life.

PREVENTIVE CONSIDERATIONS

Recognition and appropriate treatment are necessary for optimal function. Society must not stigmatize mental illness.

PEARLS FOR THE PA

During psychotic states, there is an elevated risk for suicide.

Schizophrenia is a chronic, debilitating illness characterized by exacerbations and relative remissions.

It may be difficult to establish a therapeutic relationship with the psychotic patient.

Somatoform/Dissociative Disorders

R. Ellen Davis-Hall, PhD, PA-C

DEFINITION

Somatoform/dissociative disorders include the following disorders as specified in the *Diagnostic and Statistical Manual of Mental Disorders*, 4th edition (DSM-IV):.

Conversion disorder: A disorder characterized by a loss of or alteration in physical functioning suggesting a physical disorder but in fact resulting from a psychologic conflict.

Hypochondriasis: A preoccupation with the fear of acquiring or the belief that one has a serious disease, based on the person's interpretation of physical signs and symptoms as illness.

Somatization disorder: A disorder characterized by multiple somatic complaints (the eight symptoms from the DSM-IV criteria list) when no organic pathology can be found; these symptoms must not have occurred during a panic attack and must have caused the patient to take medication (other than over-the-counter medication), see a physician, or alter lifestyle.

Somatoform pain disorder: A preoccupation with severe and prolonged pain lasting at least 6 months, for which there is no organic explanation; or when there is organic pathology, the subjective pain impairment is in excess of what would be expected from the physical findings.

Psychogenic amnesia: The sudden inability to recall important personal information, beyond forgetfulness, in the absence of underlying brain disease, and not due to multiple personality disorder or organic mental disorder.

Psychogenic fugue: A rare amnesia state with associated unexpected travel from usual home or work settings, often with the assumption of a new identity. Owing to its rarity, it is not considered further in this section.

Multiple personality disorder: This disorder represents the existence within the person of two or more distinct personalities or personality states, each with its own pattern of perceiving and relating to the environment and the self; at least two of these personalities take full control of the person's behavior.

Depersonalization disorder: A disorder characterized by feeling detached from one's body or mental processes or feeling as if in a dream.

HISTORY

Symptoms

Conversion Disorder. Paresthesias or anesthesias are common, especially involving the extremities, including hemianesthesia from the waist downward. Sensory impairment may include the classic stocking and glove pattern rather than a dermatomal distribution. Other sensory or motor disturbance including paralysis and visual, speech, or hearing loss may occur.

Hypochondriasis. Patients classically have varied symptoms from multiple systems and body area. Chest pain and gastrointestinal symptoms are common. The most pervasive symptom of the disease is the persistence of the belief despite normal evaluations.

Somatization Disorder. The DSM-IV requires eight symptoms from the following list. The italicized items may be used for screening purposes; the presence of two or more is considered significant. Symptoms are often vague, inconsistent, or bizarre.

Each of the following criteria must be met:

Four pain symptoms: A history of pain related to at least four different sites or functions (e.g., head, abdomen, back, joints, extremities, chest, rectum, during menstruation, during sexual intercourse, during urination).

Two gastrointestinal symptoms: A history of at least two gastrointestinal symptoms other than pain (e.g., nausea, bloating, vomiting other than during pregnancy, diarrhea, intolerance of several different foods).

One sexual symptom: A history of at least one sexual or reproductive symptom other than pain (e.g., sexual indifference, erectile or ejaculatory dysfunction, irregular menses, excessive menstrual bleeding, vomiting throughout pregnancy).

One pseudoneurologic symptom: A history of at least one symptom or deficit suggesting a neurologic condition not limited to pain (conversion symptoms such as impaired coordination or balance, paralysis or localized weakness, difficulty swallowing or lump in throat, aphonia, urinary retention, hallucinations, loss of touch or pain sensation, double vision, blindness, deafness, seizures; dissociative symptoms such as amnesia; loss of consciousness other than fainting).

Somatoform Pain Disorder. Some of the more common pain presentations include neck, low back, and pelvic pain and headache. The pain may stem from a specific injury or may be documented as neuropathic, or no pathology is demonstrable.

Psychogenic Amnesia. Sudden memory loss, including of identity, confusion, and disorientation.

Multiple Personality Disorder. It may be easily observable that, at different times, personalities may be quite different (even opposite); the patient will not admit awareness of this; the patient's belief that he or she is "possessed" may be a symptom.

Depersonalization Disorder. Subjective reports may be elicited of existing outside the body, perhaps watching oneself. There may be a feeling of difference or separateness relative to the environment.

General

Conversion Disorder. Review of systems is often strongly positive. To fit this diagnosis, the symptoms cannot follow a culturally sanctioned response pattern, nor can they be explained by a physical disorder. The patient has no insight into the psychologic nature of the symptoms; there is no definable gender predominance, although one common symptom, globus hystericus, is more common in women.

Hypochondriasis. Patients may be "doctor shoppers," seeking multiple evaluations for specific symptoms, or to have someone confirm their beliefs of having a specific disease (e.g., cancer); this quest for a diagnosis frequently results in unnecessary surgery. Patients may also undergo many unnecessary treatments and receive many prescription drugs. Requesting and reviewing past medical records may save both time and money. The disorder is equally common in men and women.

Somatization Disorder. Patients may "doctor shop" and have a history of multiple treatments without cure. Women may have a history of early life gynecologic surgery and multiple other surgical procedures; a history may be elicited of growing up in a low-functioning family with multiple addictions and abuses, and/or marrying either an addict or an enabler. There may be a family history of a relative with similar somatizing behaviors; this pattern becomes deeply ingrained in lifestyle. It is more common in women.

Somatoform Pain Disorder. Pain syndromes, particularly involving low back pain, is one of the most common medical complaints; the resultant disability is very costly to both society and the affected person, financially and otherwise. The patient may have an extensive history of both medical and surgical treatments, as well as analgesic use; "doctor shopping" frequently occurs. A history of pain unresponsive to analgesic use suggests psychogenic pain; the patient may be excessively preoccupied with the pain and its presence as a solitary event.

Psychogenic Amnesia. History may reveal a precipitating traumatic event; more common in women, although war experiences commonly involve men.

Multiple Personality Disorder. Existence of up to ten personalities is not uncommon; multiple prior psychiatric diagnoses are common. Some personalities may be aware of hearing voices, or of other personalities; these personalities may have proper names. More common in women.

Depersonalization Disorder. This is very common in its mild form; it is only a problem when severe and causes life stress; although equally common in men and women, the most severe form may be more common in women.

Age

Conversion Disorder/Somatization Disorder. May appear at any age, although it may be somewhat more common in teenage and young adult years.

Hypochondriasis. May occur at any age, peaking in the mid-40s.

Somatoform Pain Disorder. Throughout adulthood.

Psychogenic Amnesia/Depersonalization Disorder. Occurs in adolescence and young adulthood primarily.

Multiple Personality Disorder. Most common in childhood through young adulthood.

Onset

Conversion Disorder. Often the symptoms can be traced to a precipitating life event, and the symptoms may be modeled after a prior actual experience or one to which the patient has had some exposure.

Hypochondriasis. Usually between age 20 and 30 years; it may follow a period of actual health threat, persisting beyond competent reassurances of good health.

Somatization Disorder/Depersonalization Disorder. Usually before age 30.

Somatoform Pain Disorder. Peak onset is in the 30s and 40s.

Psychogenic Amnesia. Very sudden.

Multiple Personality Disorder. Usually in childhood or adolescence.

Duration

Conversion Disorder. Usually short, may be single or multiple episodes.

Hypochondriasis/Somatization Disorder. Should be considered a chronic illness with cyclic improvements and exacerbations.

Somatoform Pain Disorder. Chronic.

Psychogenic Amnesia. From several minutes to several days, the majority of the episodes lasting less than 1 week with spontaneous recovery.

Multiple Personality Disorder. Chronic; over time the switching of personalities decreases.

Depersonalization Disorder. Chronic course, with cyclic improvements and exacerbations; lasts from minutes to several days with spontaneous resolution.

Intensity

Conversion Disorder. The impairment suffered by the patient may be mild or very prominent depending on the symptoms; perceived paralysis, blindness, or deafness may significantly impair functioning.

Hypochondriasis. Symptoms may worsen at times of acute problems and may be medical, psychiatric, or social in origin, with significant social and occupational impairment.

Somatization Disorder. Symptoms may worsen during times of excess stress; patients are rarely without symptoms.

Somatoform Pain Disorder. Although intensity is variable after mid-adulthood, pain threshold seems to lower with increasing age. Pain is frequently incapacitating, and an invalid role is assumed.

Psychogenic Amnesia. Memory loss is complete for identifying information; if affected person is alone and without identifying information, can have a significant life impact; impairment is most usually minimal and temporary.

Multiple Personality Disorder. Dramatic changes may be observed, with a wide range of physical and emotional responses including anger and violence; the amount of the impairment may be based on the relationship between various personalities.

Depersonalization Disorder. Symptoms may be very mild to disabling.

Aggravating Factors

Conversion Disorder. Attempts to talk the patient out of the symptoms, pointing out that they are imaginary, or (conversely) giving excess attention to the symptoms may exacerbate the symptoms. The amount of primary or secondary gain can also affect the intensity or duration of the symptoms.

Hypochondriasis/Somatization Disorder. Concurrent (perhaps untreated) psychiatric disorders.

Somatoform Pain Disorder/Depersonalization Disorder. Symptoms may be aggravated or precipitated by personal and social stresses such as relationship discord.

Psychogenic Amnesia. None.

Multiple Personality Disorder. Severe child abuse, including sexual abuse, has been observed as a related history; stressful psychosocial conflicts may trigger the personality switches.

Alleviating Factors

Conversion Disorder/Hypochondriasis/Somatoform Pain Disorder. None except addressing the psychologic issues.

Somatization Disorder. If symptoms are acute and secondary to anxiety disorder or major depression, treatment of the primary disorder will bring relief.

Psychogenic Amnesia/Depersonalization Disorder. Resolves spontaneously.

Multiple Personality Disorder. Unknown.

Associated Factors

Conversion Disorder. On occasion, "la belle indifférence" may be seen (the patient may appear indifferent to what would to most be considered a major health change); conversion symptoms may also be seen as a part of the clinical picture of depression or schizophrenia.

Hypochondriasis. These patients may be almost compulsively well organized in documenting the symptoms, citing or directing you to specific medical texts, articles, and so forth. They may be people who isolate themselves and whose major social activities are health care interactions.

Somatization Disorder. These patients often have personality disorders (including histrionic and antisocial personalities), major psychosocial problems, and addictive tendencies, as well as anxiety and/or depressed mood. They may be predisposed by their disease to substance abuse.

Somatoform Pain Disorder. Depression and addictions, as well as other associated psychiatric disorders, may coexist with this disorder.

Psychogenic Amnesia. The episode is often preceded by an overwhelming event or life-threatening natural disaster; there may also be a finding of relative indifference toward the memory disturbance.

Multiple Personality Disorder. May also be diagnosed with other disorders including somatization disorder, borderline personality, and depression. Suicide attempts/ideation, self-violence, and substance abuse may be concurrent.

Depersonalization Disorder. Anxiety, hyperventilation, other psychiatric disorders including schizophrenia and depression.

PHYSICAL EXAMINATION

General

Conversion Disorder. No abnormal physical findings are observed that could explain the patient's complaints.

Hypochondriasis. Complete physical examination is mandatory. Findings may be completely normal or a variant of normal; findings related to past surgical procedures may also be prominent. Symptoms of anxiety may be present.

Somatization Disorder. Complete examination is mandatory initially, and a systems examination repeated as new symptoms arise. Findings will often be minimal.

Somatoform Pain Disorder. A complete physical examination is indicated with specific attention given to the site of the pain.

Psychogenic Amnesia/Depersonalization Disorder. Usually negative findings.

Multiple Personality Disorder. Although it may take an extended period of observation, the change in personalities may be observed suddenly. Voice may change, as well as personality type, age, or gender; mood may be variable, ranging from anger to passivity. May be highly sexual or inhibited.

Neuropsychiatric

Conversion Disorder. A complete neurologic examination may support the complaints while lacking diagnostic potential. In cases of paralysis, the subjective complaints voiced by the patient are inconsistent with neural pathways; reflexes will be normal; gait, tremor, or other abnormal movements that are part of the present illness may worsen when the patient is examined.

Hypochondriasis. Neurologic examination and Mental Status Examination normal.

Somatization Disorder/Depersonalization Disorder.   Reality testing is intact.

Somatoform Pain Disorder.   The patient's subjective descriptions may be inconsistent with known neurologic sensory patterns.

Psychogenic Amnesia.   Signs of head injury should be sought. Mental Status Examination will help determine whether amnesia is localized, generalized, or selective.

Multiple Personality Disorder.   Normal findings on Mental Status Examination. May demonstrate periods of apparent amnesia.

PATHOPHYSIOLOGY

Conversion Disorder

Multidimensional etiologic aspects to the disease process (biologic, psychologic, and cultural factors). A stressful circumstance or event appears to trigger a psychologic conflict, with the resultant physical "conversion."

Hypochondriasis

Psychodynamic in origin, but with sociocultural aspects as well; repressed anger, guilt, may be prominent parts of the process.

Somatization Disorder

Psychodynamic in origin, but with sociocultural aspects, including growing up in a chaotic or otherwise dysfunctional family.

Somatoform Pain Disorder

There are multiple psychologic aspects to pain; it may be a learned behavior. In our society, often this provides a strong secondary gain (relatives, employers, the legal system); pain also has strong manipulation capability.

Psychogenic Amnesia

Usually thought to be secondary to intense emotions such as fear or conflict; may also have a component of primary or secondary gain.

Multiple Personality Disorder

Current theories observe that multiple personality disorder has a similarity to self-hypnosis, citing it as a response to severe trauma/abuse; different personalities are formed to handle the abuse. Some authorities consider etiologic mechanisms of this disorder to be similar to those of post-traumatic stress disorder (PTSD).

Depersonalization Disorder

There may be an organic component such as endocrine disease, epilepsy, or brain tumor; there may also be a relationship with other psychiatric disorders (schizophrenia, depression, anxiety, sensory deprivation, or emotional trauma); iatrogenic causes, including drugs, must be considered. Also may be considered as a post-traumatic stress response.

DIAGNOSTIC STUDIES

Laboratory

Hypochondriasis/Somatization Disorder/Somatoform Pain Disorder. If the diagnosis is uncertain, a cost-effective, stepwise approach to ordering tests to evaluate the specific complaint is recommended. Careful review of prior tests performed can save both time and money. Likewise, it is important to consider the patient's epidemiologic risk for the targeted disorder, including family history; costly or invasive laboratory procedures are warranted primarily when there are objective (rather than subjective) findings of disease.

Psychogenic Amnesia. Screening laboratory tests, including blood chemistry, glucose, complete blood count, and toxicology studies may be advisable because the patient cannot offer a medical history.

Multiple Personality Disorder. Minimal usefulness.

Depersonalization Disorder. Screening tests may rule out organic disorders.

Radiology
CT/MRI Scan of the Brain. As indicated to evaluate for organic disease.

Skull Films/CT Scan of Head
Psychogenic Amnesia. If any findings of head injury.

Other
Electroencephalogram (EEG). If seizure disorder is suspected.

Personality Inventories
Multiple Personality Disorder. If administered at different times to different personalities, results may be quite variable.

DIFFERENTIAL DIAGNOSIS

Conversion Disorder

Organic disease as defined by the system involved in the chief complaint, including multisystem diseases (e.g., multiple sclerosis, systemic lupus erythematosus). Other organic diseases that may be present include myopathies, polymyositis, and brain tumors. Acquired conditions such as malingering also need to be considered. Psychiatric disorders that may contribute include schizophrenia and factitious disorders.

Hypochondriasis

Even known hypochondriacs can suffer from organic disease. Therefore, new symptoms require a reasonable evaluation for a definable disorder, especially when symptoms cross several organ systems (i.e., endocrine, dermatologic, rheumatic, or neurologic). A contributing physical ailment such as organic brain syndrome needs to be considered. Acquired conditions such as malingering, depression, anxiety, and panic disorder also need to be considered. Psychiatric disorders that may contribute include Munchausen syndrome and schizophrenia.

Somatization Disorders
Rule out physical disorders with multisystem manifestations (i.e., endocrine, rheumatic, and so forth). Other psychiatric disorders such as schizophrenia or panic attacks may be present.

Somatoform Pain Disorder
Pathologic pain (which is more likely than psychogenic pain to respond to analgesics) is the primary consideration in the differential diagnosis. Psychiatric disorders such as depression may mimic this disorder or may be concurrent. Other psychiatric diagnoses to consider are schizophrenia, somatization disorder, hypochondriasis, and drug and/or alcohol addiction. Acquired conditions such as malingering also need to be considered.

Psychogenic Amnesia
Traumatic and neoplastic conditions such as head injury (postconcussion amnesia) and brain tumor (with symptoms of increased intracranial pressure) may manifest with amnesia. Other organic causes of amnesia include organic brain syndrome, dementia, and seizure disorder. Acquired conditions such as alcoholic blackout or psychoactive substance intoxication and malingering need to be included in the differential diagnosis.

Multiple Personality Disorder
The primary organic condition that may present as multiple personality disorder is seizure. Other psychiatric disorders, including schizophrenia, depression, and borderline personality (may be concurrent diagnosis), need to be differentiated from other dissociative disorders (e.g., fugue, amnesia). Acquired conditions such as malingering also need to be considered.

Depersonalization Disorder
Organic disease such as endocrinopathies, epilepsy, brain tumors, and migraine all may present as depersonalization disorder. Other psychiatric disorders such as schizophrenia, depression, anxiety disorders, and addictions need to be considered.

TREATMENT

Conversion Disorder
After thorough medical evaluation without findings indicative of organic disease, the patient should be reassured that there is no physical problem. Referral should be made for psychologic management (psychotherapy, anxiolytics if indicated, and/or hypnotherapy).

Hypochondriasis

Identify and treat any identifiable organic disorder. Reassure the patient that past and present tests indicate no disease. Schedule regular, periodic follow-up visits to reassure the patient of your commitment to ongoing evaluation and support. Drugs are useful only in treating an actual organic condition, or if depression or anxiety is a concurrent diagnosis. Referral for psychiatric treatment may be resisted; it may, however, be acceptable to the patient if therapy will include education, group support, and stress reduction. Once the pattern is established (duration of 6 months or more for DSM-IV diagnosis), resolution or "cure" may occur but is unlikely.

Somatization Disorder

Identify and treat any organic disorders. Offer reassurance and supportive treatment. Schedule regular follow-up visits for ongoing evaluation. Referral for psychiatric treatment may be of benefit to educate the patient about how to cope with prominent symptoms. Drug use should be minimized.

Somatoform Pain Disorder

Avoid use of analgesics or antianxiety agents in these patients, as they will be of little help. Antidepressants are frequently of benefit, whether by treating an underlying depression or through an analgesic effect. Referral for hypnotism or biofeedback may be of some benefit, as well as transcutaneous nerve stimulation in the case of neck or back pain. Nerve block may offer temporary relief but is not curative. Referral to a tertiary care center for a chronic pain program may be beneficial in its multidisciplinary approach including individual and group therapy and patient education.

Psychogenic Amnesia

Careful observation alone may result in spontaneous recovery. Referral to a psychiatrist for hypnosis or intravenous barbiturate use may allow recall. Although spontaneous recovery is the usual course, psychiatric therapy is advised to help the patient process the event.

Multiple Personality Disorder

Psychiatric referral for long-term therapy—depending on approach, either to integrate the personalities or to promote placement of a dominant healthy personality in charge. Hypnotherapy may be helpful. Medications are of little use unless an additional disorder (i.e., major depression) coexists.

Depersonalization Disorder

Treat any organic disorder such as migraine. Refer to psychiatrist for possible hypnotherapy if it is disruptive to life and relationships.

Benzodiazepines are of some use if anxiety is concurrent, and antidepressants if major depression is concurrent; no drug therapy is of help in the pure form of depersonalization.

PEDIATRIC CONSIDERATIONS

Conversion symptoms in childhood often occur after significant psychologic stress. In younger children, the symptoms are usually limited to gait problems or seizures.

Care should be utilized in the evaluation of a child with multiple somatic complaints without apparent organic etiology. A nonjudgmental approach is essential. The initial workup often sets the tone for future perceptions and interactions. The family should be informed that a comprehensive evaluation of the symptoms will include both psychologic and physical components. A thorough history should include both medical and psychologic aspects, especially attending to recent stressors. The possibility of an evolving organic illness should not be dismissed. Once a strong psychologic component is suspected in the presence of a normal physical examination, the primary care provider must try to avoid the temptation toward further diagnostic evaluations, which may reinforce the concept of illness.

OBSTETRIC CONSIDERATIONS

Careful screening and appropriate psychiatric referral are indicated.

GERIATRIC CONSIDERATIONS

Acute or subacute changes in the mental functioning of the geriatric patient require investigation to rule out a primary medical condition or medication side effect. Long-term effects of medications or substances (e.g., alcohol) may cause mental changes later in life.

PREVENTIVE CONSIDERATIONS

It is important to identify stress and dysfunction in the home and with social interaction. Be aware that sexual abuse may present with conversion disorder. Query the patient in a non-accusatory fashion to evaluate for the potential of secondary gain. Awareness of somatoform disorders, referral, and treatment are key secondary preventive measures.

PEARLS FOR THE PA

Conversion Disorder
Establishment of an empathetic, supportive relationship with the patient will be therapeutic.

It is important to remember that these patients have no insight into the psychologic nature of their physical problems.

Continued

PEARLS FOR THE PA—cont'd

Hypochondriasis
Remember that the patient is truly suffering; trying to minimize or trivialize reported symptoms may only make the patient feel worse.

It may be necessary to set limits on time spent with the patient; inquire at each visit about the patient's expectations of what you can do.

Offer ongoing support and return visits as frequently as agreed necessary by practitioner and patient.

Somatization Disorder
Remember that pain is a prominent symptom of this disorder and that the pain is very real to the patient.

Use medications cautiously, as patients are not always reliable with their use.

Attempt to minimize the number of practitioners involved in the patient's care; consistency is important.

Be honest about your inability to take away all their symptoms, but provide assurance that you will work with the patient in management of the disorder.

Somatoform Pain Disorder
Keep in mind the common association of addiction in these patients, and the limited benefit of analgesics in psychogenic pain.

Always document because of the frequency of a litigation component to these medical problems.

Remember that most complications of this disease are iatrogenic.

Psychogenic Amnesia
Prompt return of memory is indicative of a psychogenic cause.

A lasting episode may require continued medical workup.

Multiple Personality Disorder
Care should be taken to avoid the overuse of medications, as polypharmacy may complicate the clinical situation.

Depersonalization Disorder
Be supportive and patient.

Further Reading

American Psychiatric Association: Diagnostic and Statistical Manual of Mental Disorders, 4th ed. Washington, DC, American Psychiatric Association, 1994.

Cunningham FG, MacDonald PC, Gant NF, et al (eds): Williams Obstetrics, 19th ed. East Norwalk, CT, Appleton & Lange, 1993.

Dunnihoo DR: Fundamentals of Gynecology and Obstetrics, 2nd ed. Philadelphia, JB Lippincott, 1992.

Kaplan HI, Sadock BJ (eds): Synopsis of Psychiatry, Behavioral Sciences/Clinical Psychiatry, 8th ed. Baltimore, Williams & Wilkins, 1997.

Karboski JA: Medication selection for pregnant women. Physician Assist 15:59, 1991.

Labus JB, Lauber AA: Patient Education and Preventive Medicine. Philadelphia, WB Saunders, 2001.

Lewis M: Child and Adolescent Psychiatry: A Comprehensive Textbook. Baltimore, Williams & Wilkins, 1991.

Murphy, JL (ed): Physician Assistant's Prescribing Reference, Fall 2003. New York, Prescribing Reference Inc., 2003.

Rutter M, Taylor E, Hersov L: Child and Adolescent Psychiatry, Modern Approaches, 3rd ed. London, Blackwell Scientific Publications, 1994.

Steiner JF: Anxiety: An update on pharmacologic therapy. J Am Acad Physician Assist 4:421, 1991.

Widmer R: Anxiety and depression in women. Physician Assist 12:168, 1988.

Web Sites

American Academy of Child and Adolescent Psychiatry: http://www.aacap.org

American Psychiatric Association: http://www.psych.org/public_info/adhdfactsheet42401.pdf

American Academy of Child and Adolescent Psychiatry: http://www.aacap.org/press%5Freleases/1999/june24ad.htm

PULMONOLOGY

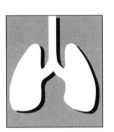

15

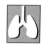

Acute Hypoxemic Respiratory Failure

Judith E. Colver, MMS, PA-C

DEFINITION

Acute hypoxemic respiratory failure (AHRF) arises from the acute collapse or filling of the alveoli, resulting in a ventilation-perfusion mismatch. This leads to further problems with gas exchange, fluid accumulation (interstitial or alveolar), and decreased lung compliance. If uncorrected, the process leads to tissue hypoxia, respiratory distress, respiratory arrest, and death.

AHRF may be categorized as diffuse or focal. *Diffuse* AHRF is due to an increase in fluid in the lungs, as from edema or hemorrhage, whereas *focal* AHRF is usually due to acute processes such as pneumonia or lung contusion. The origin of pulmonary edema may be either cardiogenic, from increased pressure, or pulmonary, from increased permeability or low pressure. The most common pulmonary cause of reduced-pressure edema is acute respiratory distress syndrome (ARDS). A less severe form of ARDS is now recognized and often termed *acute lung injury* (ALI).

HISTORY

Symptoms. Dyspnea.
General. Usually has history of injury to the lungs.
Age. Any.
Onset. Rapid following injury.
Duration. Short term. Mortality rate from respiratory failure alone is 20%; with associated additional organ system failure, mortality rate approaches 70%.
Intensity. Life-threatening.
Aggravating Factors. Precipitating factors include trauma (embolic phenomenon or lung contusion) aspiration (gastric contents, near drowning, hydrocarbons), inhalation (smoke, corrosive chemicals), sepsis, shock, reexpansion following thoracic surgery, or multiple blood transfusions.
Alleviating Factors. Aggressive treatment of underlying cause.
Associated Factors. Metabolic conditions (e.g., uremia, diabetic ketoacidosis), pneumonia (viral, bacterial, tuberculosis, fungal, *Pneumocystis carinii*), drugs (heroin, methadone, propoxyphene, barbiturates, colchicine, aspirin, hydrochlorothiazide), eclampsia, ascent to high altitude, brain injury, collogen vascular disease, immunocompromised state.

PHYSICAL EXAMINATION

General. Patient often appears anxious. Hypotension (with sepsis), hyperthermia (temperature greater than 38° C, or 100.4° F) or hypothermia (less than 36° C, or 96.8° F, especially with near drowning).

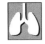

Cardiovascular.   Tachycardia. Auscultate for S_3, S_4, or gallop suggestive of cardiogenic etiology.

Extremities.   Edema of lower extremities suggests cardiogenic etiology.

Head, Eyes, Ears, Nose, Throat.   Funduscopic examination to evaluate for papilledema; evaluate for jugular venous distention and adenopathy.

Gastrointestinal.   Abdomen may be tender to palpation with pancreatitis or spontaneous bacterial peritonitis.

Genitourinary.   Renal failure may predispose to or follow AHRF.

Neurologic.   Alteration in mental status may indicate underlying metabolic abnormality, drug ingestion, or neurogenic etiology.

Pulmonary.   Dyspnea and tachypnea with respiratory rate greater than 30 breaths/minute; evaluate for use of accessory muscles. Auscultate for diffuse crackles and/or focal findings.

Skin.   May be cyanotic.

PATHOPHYSIOLOGY

Cardiogenic pulmonary edema occurs with increases in left ventricular end-diastolic pressure or, less commonly, with increases in left atrial pressure as in mitral valve abnormalities. It also is seen in acute volume overload (with exogenous fluid administration, in renal failure, or with translocation of fluid to central compartment).

Edema from pulmonary mechanisms (as in ARDS) is due to injury to the microcirculation of the lungs with resultant extravasation of fluid and protein into the interstitium. Early manifestations are rapid fluid accumulation followed by hyaline membrane formation in the alveoli and frequently necrosis. Possible sequelae on healing include extensive fibrosis and pulmonary hypertension.

Severe hypoxemia results as a result of ventilation-perfusion mismatch, and there is decreased pulmonary compliance.

DIAGNOSTIC STUDIES

Laboratory

Arterial Blood Gas Analysis.   Usually severe hypoxemia (Pao_2 less than 50 mm Hg) with a normal to decreased $Paco_2$ (less than 35 mm Hg). Increased alveolar-arterial (A–a) gradient (normal less than 10 mm Hg).

Complete Blood Count.   May show leukocytosis if infection is present.

Amylase/Lipase.   Elevated in pancreatitis.

Blood Urea Nitrogen (BUN)/Creatinine.   Elevated in renal failure.

Toxicology Screen.   If drug overdose/involvement is suspected.

Blood Cultures.   As indicated to rule out sepsis.

Radiology

Chest Film.   Diffuse (usually bilateral), generalized interstitial infiltrate(s). Predominantly clear bases.

Other
Swan-Ganz Catheter. Pulmonary capillary wedge pressure (PCWP) of less than 18 mm Hg usually indicates ARDS, whereas a value of 20 mm Hg or more usually indicates a cardiogenic etiology for pulmonary edema.

DIFFERENTIAL DIAGNOSIS

AHRF and ARDS are radiologic and physiologic responses to underlying disorders resulting in increased fluid in the lungs, ventilation-perfusion mismatch, and decreased lung compliance. The strict concept of differential diagnosis does not apply.

TREATMENT

Supportive measures, with aggressive pursuit of underlying pathology, constitute the mainstay of treatment. Endotracheal intubation and mechanical ventilation are often required.

Positive end-expiratory pressure (PEEP) may improve oxygenation but has not been shown to alter the course of the disease process.

Medications to effect diuresis and/or translocate fluids from the central to peripheral compartment may help. Furosemide may help reduce preload. Ionotropic support may be required, as well as afterload reduction, especially when there is a cardiogenic etiology.

Surfactant may be helpful in some patients. Inhaled nitric oxide (iNO) may be of benefit.

Steroids may be used if there is an inflammatory component. Steroids should be avoided in patients with sepsis or acute myocardial infarction, but there is some support for prophylactic use of these agents following aspiration.

Packed red blood cells may be required to keep the hematocrit above 25% and to maintain oxygenation to the tissues.

Parenteral nutritional support is often required to maintain adequate intravascular volume and oncotic pressure.

PEDIATRIC CONSIDERATIONS

AHRF may occur at any age. Neonatal causes include prematurity and congenital malformations of the lungs, heart, and thoracic vasculature.

OBSTETRIC CONSIDERATIONS

Sepsis and aspiration are the leading causes of ARDS in pregnancy. Eclampsia and amniotic fluid embolism may also predispose a patient to AHRF.

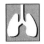

GERIATRIC CONSIDERATIONS

Geriatric patients generally have less compliant lung tissue and are therefore at higher risk for developing AHRF. Geriatric patients also have a higher incidence of heart failure, which may predispose them to developing AHRF.

PREVENTIVE CONSIDERATIONS

In most cases, AHRF is preceded by direct insult to the lung. Prevention may be possible through aggressive/expectant treatment following traumatic injury (lung contusion), inhalation injury, aspiration of gastric contents or near drowning, in sepsis or shock, or following lung surgery or multiple blood transfusions. Early identification and treatment of thrombophlebitis may prevent pulmonary embolism, another cause of AHRF.

PEARLS FOR THE PA

Search for the underlying etiology. Could be metabolic cause that produces insult to lung and subsequent problems. Not always precipitated by hypoxemia.

Treatment is supportive while correcting underlying problem.

PCWP may help to distinguish underlying pathology.

Asthma
Judith E. Colver, MMS, PA-C

DEFINITION

Asthma is a largely reversible, chronic obstructive pulmonary disease characterized by inflammation, airway hyperresponsiveness and reversible narrowing, and increased secretions. There is an associated accumulation of cells in the airways that contributes to changes in airway structure and function.

HISTORY

Symptoms. Dyspnea and anxiety, often accompanied by coughing, wheezing, chest tightness, and/or shortness of breath.

General. Allergic component may be familial. Increasing incidence among urban dwellers and in low-socioeconomic-level groups may be due in part to environmental causes.

Age. May occur at any age. Childhood asthma often abates with adolescence. Adult onset often due to late-onset atopy or sensitization in workplace, but condition may also arise as recurrence of childhood asthma.

Onset. Symptoms are often of abrupt onset, especially in hypersensitivity reaction. Onset may be gradual, over hours to days.

Duration. Acute episodes with frequent remissions are common.

Intensity. Mild to life-threatening and fatal.

Aggravating Factors. Allergens (dust mites, animal dander, molds, pollens), exercise, viral infections, medications (aspirin and other nonsteroidal anti-inflammatory drugs [NSAIDs], beta blockers, angiotensin-converting enzyme [ACE] inhibitors, and others), sulfites (in multiple foods—e.g., dried fruits, red wine, pickles), gastroesophageal reflux disease (GERD), and stress may cause acute exacerbations. Occupational irritants may cause or intensify symptoms. Symptoms often worsen at night.

Alleviating Factors. Appropriate therapy, if used early in an attack, may minimize symptoms. Daily use of leukotriene modifiers and/or inhaled anti-inflammatory drugs (steroids, cromolyn or nedocromil) may reduce the severity and frequency of exacerbations.

Associated Factors. Most often associated with low birth weight, atopy, allergic rhinitis, and GERD.

PHYSICAL EXAMINATION

Findings often normal between acute episodes.

General. Tachypnea, often with audible wheezing. Patients may use accessory muscles of respiration, sit forward, and breathe through pursed lips.

Cardiovascular. Tachycardia and pulsus paradoxus (decrease of greater than 20 mm Hg in systolic blood pressure with inspiration) common in acute attacks.

Extremities. Cyanosis is late finding in severe attacks. Clubbing suggests an etiology other than asthma.

Head, Eyes, Ears, Nose, Throat. Nasal polyps common. Chronic allergic rhinitis/sinusitis often present.

Gastrointestinal. GERD may cause or exacerbate acute attacks.

Pulmonary. Chest hyperresonant to percussion. Auscultation reveals wheezing. Decreased breath sounds with prolonged expiratory phase constitutes late and often ominous finding.

Skin. Cyanosis in severe attacks. Atopic dermatitis or eczema common.

PATHOPHYSIOLOGY

Cell-derived mediators influence inflammation and airway muscle tone and stimulate mucus production. Airway hyperresponsiveness is characterized

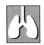

by contraction of smooth muscle and ultimately proliferation of tissue. Airflow is further compromised by edema and the secretion of mucus. In most cases, the process is reversible. When there is irreversible airflow limitation, it is usually caused by increased airway wall thickness, fibrosis, remodeling of the airway wall, and/or obstruction of the lumen by exudates or mucus plugs.

DIAGNOSTIC STUDIES

Findings may be normal between acute exacerbations.

Laboratory
Arterial Blood Gas Analysis. Usually normal until late, when hypoxia and then hypercapnea occur. Hypercapnea often heralds respiratory failure.

Complete Blood Count. May show eosinophilia.

Serum Protein Electrophoresis. Often shows an increase in serum immunoglobulin E (IgE).

Sputum Examination. May contain eosinophils, Curschmann spirals (bronchiolar casts of mucus and cells), or Charcot-Leyden crystals (crystallized eosinophil proteins).

Nasal Swabs. May see eosinophils.

Radiology
Chest Film. Hyperinflation of lungs during acute exacerbations. Occasionally may see complications of disease such as pneumothorax or pneumomediastinum.

Other
Pulmonary Function Tests. Decreased airflow rates in acute exacerbations, including reduced peak expiratory flow rate (PEFR), reduced forced expiratory volume in 1 second (FEV_1), and decreased forced vital capacity (FVC). Reversibility may be demonstrated by inhalation of $beta_2$ agonist. Bronchial provocation (metacholine or histamine challenge) may be useful in cases in which diagnosis remains uncertain.

Skin Tests. May be helpful in identifying allergens.

ECG. Usually normal. May see tachycardia, right bundle branch block, right axis deviation, increased voltage of P wave in leads II, III, and aVF.

DIFFERENTIAL DIAGNOSIS

Traumatic
Pneumothorax. Usually acute onset of dyspnea and evidence on chest film.

Foreign Body Inhalation. May be associated with stridor acutely or with chronic pulmonary infections if long-standing. Forced expiratory films may demonstrate hyperinflation in affected lung segment.

Infectious
Bronchospastic Bronchitis. May mimic asthma, but is not recurrent and less responsive acutely to beta agonists.

Neoplastic
Bronchogenic Cancer. Mass may be seen on chest film or CT scan of chest. If the mass is intraluminal or juxtaluminal, may be identified on bronchoscopy.

Vascular
Pulmonary Embolism. Acute onset of dyspnea with chest pain. May have associated lower extremity pain/edema with deep vein thrombosis.

Congestive Heart Failure. Echocardiogram will differentiate asthma from cardiogenic wheezing.

Acquired
Chronic Obstructive Pulmonary Disease (COPD). Less evidence of reversibility with beta agonists. Pulmonary function tests may show persistent obstructive changes between exacerbations.

GERD. Upper gastrointestinal radiographs or endoscopy helpful in differentiation.

Vocal Cord Dysfunction. Factitious, somatoform disorder associated with breath holding and resultant hypercarbia with normal Pao_2 levels.

Panic/Anxiety. Difficulty breathing is commonly noted on inspiration rather than expiration.

Metabolic. Not applicable.
Congenital. Not applicable.

TREATMENT

The key to therapy is maintenance of adequate oxygenation. Pulse oximetry is helpful in the outpatient setting. Pulse oximeter readings of 90% to 92% Sao_2 correspond roughly to a Pao_2 of 60 mm Hg.

- Beta agonists: Mainstay of bronchodilator treatment. Action is through stimulation of the beta-adrenergic receptors, which leads to the relaxation of constricted smooth airway muscle. Patients should be cautioned to seek medical help if they require more than the prescribed daily dosage.

    Albuterol (Ventolin, Proventil) 0.083% solution for nebulizer or 2.5 mg (0.5 mL of 0.5% solution diluted to 3.0 mL with normal saline) up to 10 mg three or four times a day; metered dose inhaler 90 µg/inhalation—2 inhalations every 4 to 6 hours, maximum 16 to 20 inhalations daily. Acute exacerbations: 2.5-5 mg by nebulizer every 20 minutes for three doses, then 2.5-10 mg by nebulizer every 1 to 4 hours or 10-15 mg/hour by continuous nebulizer.

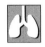

Albuterol extended release tablets (Volmax, Vospire ER) 2 mg and 4 mg tablets, 4-8 mg every 12 hours; maximum 32 mg/day. *Not for treatment of acute attacks.*

Formoterol (Foradil) 12 µg capsules for inhalation with device—1 inhalation twice daily. Long-acting beta agonist, not for treatment of acute attacks.

Pirbuterol (Maxair) metered dose inhaler 200 µg/inhalation—1-2 inhalations every 4 to 6 hours, maximum 12 inhalations daily.

Metaproterenol (Alupent) metered dose inhaler 0.65 mg/inhalation—2-3 inhalations every 3 to 4 hours, maximum 12 inhalations daily.

Salmeterol (Serevent) metered dose inhaler 21 µg/inhalation—2 inhalations twice daily. Long-acting beta agonist, not for treatment of acute attacks.

Terbutaline (Brethine) 2.5-5 mg tablets three times daily at 6-hour intervals; *age 12-15 years*: 2.5 mg three times a day at 6-hour intervals; also available in injectable form 0.25 mg given subcutaneously, repeat in 15 to 30 minutes, maximum 0.5 mg every 4 hours.

- Anticholinergics

Atropine 0.025 mg/kg diluted with 3-5 mL normal saline by nebulizer every 6 to 8 hours.

Ipratropium (Atrovent) nebulizer solution 500 µg/2.5 mL three or four times a day; metered dose inhaler 18 µg/inhalation—2 inhalations four times a day, maximum 12 inhalations daily.

- Methylxanthines: Various products for intravenous/oral administration. *Note*: May cause toxicity. Monitor serum levels. Symptoms of toxicity include nausea, vomiting, flushing, and tachycardia.

Aminophylline OR theophylline: *initial (loading) dose*: 5-6 mg/kg IV over 20 minutes; *maintenance*: 0.5-0.9 mg/kg/hour. Therapeutic range is 10-20 µg/mL, oral form 300-600 mg twice daily, titrate to reach therapeutic range.

- Systemic steroids: Reserved for moderate/severe exacerbations, usually given as a 3- to 14-day course, occasionally on low-dose maintenance. Some forms available for intravenous/intramuscular administration acutely. Usually convert to oral therapy as soon as symptoms are controlled or patient tolerates. Taper dose if using for more than 5 consecutive days.

Prednisone 10-50 mg/day

Methylprednisolone (Medrol, Solu-Medrol) 1-2 mg/kg every 4 to 6 hours IV or IM

Hydrocortisone (Solu-Cortef) for status asthmaticus: Start 1-2 mg/kg every 6 hours IV or IM for 24 hours, then 0.5-1.0 mg/kg per day.

- Anti-inflammatory medications: Not for treatment of acute attack.

Cromoglycates: Not for treatment of acute attack.

Cromolyn (Intal) nebulizer solution 20 mg/2 mL four times a day, metered dose inhaler 0.8 mg/inhalation—2 inhalations four times a day

Nedocromil (Tilade) metered dose inhaler 1.75 mg/inhalation—2 inhalations two or three times a day

Inhaled steroids: Not for treatment of acute attack.

Beclomethasone (QVAR) metered dose inhaler 40 µg or 80 µg/inhalation—2 inhalations twice daily, maximum 320 µg per day

Budesonide (Pulmicort) metered dose inhaler 200 µg/inhalation—1-4 inhalations twice daily, maximum of 4 inhalations twice daily

Flunisolide (AeroBid) metered dose inhaler 250 µg/inhalation—2 inhalations twice daily, maximum 8 inhalations daily

Fluticasone (Flovent) metered dose inhaler with 44 µg, 110 µg, or 220 µg/inhalation—2 inhalations twice daily

Triamcinolone (Azmacort) metered dose inhaler 100 µg/inhalation—2 to 4 inhalations twice daily, maximum 16 inhalations daily

- Other anti-inflammatory agents: Not for treatment of acute attack.

Nedocromil sodium (Tilade) metered dose inhaler 1.75 mg/inhalation—2 inhalations 4 times daily

Systemic gold and oral methotrexate: Experimental medications that have been used in patients with severe asthma who require long-term suppression.

- Leukotriene inhibitors: Not for treatment of acute attack.

Montelukast (Singulair) 10 mg tablet at bedtime; *age 2 to 5 years*: 4 mg chewable; *age 6 to 14*: 5 mg chewable

Zafirlukast (Accolate) 20 mg tablet twice daily 1 hour before or 2 hours after meals; *age 7 to 11 years*: 10 mg tablet twice daily; not recommended for children younger than 7

- Lipoxygenase inhibitors: Not for treatment of acute attack.

Zileuton (Zyflo) 600 mg tablet four times a day; need to monitor liver function

- Combination products: Not for treatment of acute attack.

Albuterol/ipratropium (Combivent) metered dose inhaler 18/90 µg/inhalation—2 inhalations four times a day, maximum 12 inhalations daily

Salmeterol/fluticasone (Advair) metered dose inhaler 50/100 µg, 50/250 µg, or 50/500 µg formulation—1 inhalation twice daily

Table 15-1 presents the recommended stepwise approach to the management of asthma.

PEDIATRIC CONSIDERATIONS

Asthma is the leading cause of chronic illness in childhood and is the most frequent cause of pediatric emergency room visits, hospital admissions, and

Table 15–1. Stepwise Approach for Managing Asthma in Adults and Children Older than 5 Years of Age: Treatment

Classify Severity: Clinical Features Before Treatment or Adequate Control			Medications Required to Maintain Long-Term Control
	Symptoms: Day/Night	PEF or FEV$_1$/PEF Variability	Daily Medications
Step 4 **Severe persistent**	Continual/ Frequent	≤60%/ >30%	**Preferred treatment:** • High-dose inhaled corticosteroids AND • Long-acting inhaled beta$_2$ agonists *If needed*, add: • Corticosteroid tablets or syrup long term (2 mg/kg/day, generally do not exceed 60 mg/day) (make repeat attempts to reduce systemic corticosteroids and maintain control with high-dose inhaled corticosteroids)
Step 3 **Moderate persistent**	Daily/ >1 night/week	>60-<80%/ >30%	**Preferred treatment:** • Low- to medium-dose inhaled corticosteroids AND • Long-acting inhaled beta$_2$ agonists **Alternative treatment:** • Increase inhaled corticosteroids within medium-dose range OR • Low- to medium-dose inhaled corticosteroids PLUS either leukotriene modifier or theophylline *If needed* (particularly in patients with recurring severe exacerbations): **Preferred treatment:** • Increase inhaled corticosteroids within medium-dose range PLUS long-acting inhaled beta$_2$ agonists **Alternative treatment:** • Increase inhaled corticosteroids within medium-dose range PLUS either leukotriene modifier or theophylline

Continued

Table 15–1. Stepwise Approach for Managing Asthma in Adults and Children Older than 5 Years of Age: Treatment—cont'd

Classify Severity: Clinical Features Before Treatment or Adequate Control			Medications Required to Maintain Long-Term Control
	Symptoms: Day/Night	PEF or FEV$_1$/PEF Variability	Daily Medications
Step 2 **Mild persistent**	>2×/week but >1×/day/ >2 nights/month	≥80%/ 20-30%	**Preferred treatment:** • Low-dose inhaled corticosteroids **Alternative treatment** (listed alphabetically): cromolyn, leukotriene modifier, nedocromil, OR sustained-release theophylline to serum concentration of 5-15 μg/mL
Step 1 **Mild intermittent**	≤2 days/week/ ≤2 nights/month	≥80%/ <20%	**No daily medication needed** Severe exacerbations may occur, separated by long periods of normal lung function and no symptoms. A course of systemic corticosteroids is recommended.

Quick Relief
All patients
• Short-acting bronchodilator: 2-4 puffs of short-acting inhaled beta$_2$ agonist as needed for symptoms.
• Intensity of treatment will depend on severity of exacerbation; up to 3 treatments at 20-minute intervals or a single nebulizer treatment as needed. Course of systemic corticosteroids may be needed.
• Use of short-acting beta$_2$ agonists >2 times a week in intermittent asthma (daily, or increasing use in persistent asthma) may indicate the need to initiate (increase) long-term control therapy.

⇓ **Step down**

Review treatment every 1 to 6 months; a gradual stepwise reduction in treatment may be possible.

⇑ **Step up**

If control is not maintained, consider step up. First, review patient medication technique, adherence, and environmental control.

Note
- The stepwise approach is meant to assist, not replace, the clinical decision making required to meet individual patient needs.
- Classify severity; assign patient to most severe step in which any feature occurs (PEF is % of personal best; FEV$_1$ is % predicted).
- Gain control as quickly as possible (consider a short course of systemic corticosteroids); then step down to the least medication necessary to maintain control.
- Provide education on self-management and controlling environmental factors that make asthma worse (e.g., allergens and irritants).
- Refer to an asthma specialist if there are difficulties controlling asthma or if step 4 care is required. Referral may be considered if step 3 is required.

Goals of Therapy: Asthma Control

Minimal or no chronic symptoms day or night.

Minimal or no exacerbations.

No limitations on activities; no school or work missed.

Maintain (near) normal pulmonary function.

Minimal use of short-acting inhaled beta$_2$ agonist (<1×/day, <1 canister/month).

Minimal or no adverse effects from medications.

FEV$_1$, forced expiratory volume in 1 minute; PEF, peak expiratory flow.

school absenteeism. Fifty percent of childhood asthmatics will experience remission by age 20 years; however, there is a growing number of recurrences in adults with a history of childhood asthma.

History is important to the diagnosis. Airway patency decreases at night. Thus, children often have nocturnal exacerbations, manifested by a tight nonproductive cough. Wheezing is not always present, but a history of recurrent cough (especially nocturnal or exercise-induced) or vomiting copious amounts of mucus following a spasm of coughing is suggestive of asthma. Abdominal pain may be present in younger children owing to accessory muscle use. Vomiting may be present and often provides temporary relief of symptoms. Some children will also have a low-grade temperature.

Children may assume a tripod position and may breathe through pursed lips. Infants may exhibit nasal flaring and grunting. Hyperexpansion of the chest and resultant chest deformity may be seen in children with chronic asthma.

Wheezing prior to 3 months of age suggests pulmonary malformations, cardiac or gastrointestinal abnormalities, or cystic fibrosis. In children younger than 3 years, bronchiolitis due to respiratory syncytial virus infection is a common cause of wheezing. Other causes of airway obstruction include foreign bodies in the airway or esophagus, immunodeficiency, and other rare conditions.

Identification and avoidance of allergens, reduction of inflammation, and bronchodilatation are the mainstays of treatment. Children can use metered dose inhalers (MDIs) with the addition of a spacer (AeroChamber or InspirEase) as early as age 2 years. By age 3 or 4, many can perform peak flow maneuvers, which provide some guidance for treatment.

Infants and young children with intermittent and mild symptoms can be treated with oral beta-adrenergic agonists such as albuterol (0.1-0.2 mg/kg/dose given three times daily, maximum 12 mg/day). Aerosolized nebulizers are indicated and effective in children with moderate symptoms, or those too young to use an MDI. Montelukast may be used prophylactically in children 2 years of age or older. Cromolyn is especially useful in preventing exercise-induced asthma in children age 2 or older. Steroid bursts may be used acutely at 1-2 mg/kg/24 hours with severe exacerbations. Inhaled steroids (fluticasone may be used from age 4 years, triamcinolone from age 6, and beclomethasone from age 8) may be helpful in obtaining daily control. However, some studies suggest that regular use of inhaled steroids may cause growth retardation.

OBSTETRIC CONSIDERATIONS

Asthma may be exacerbated, remain unchanged, or remit during pregnancy. Approximately 33% of pregnant asthmatic women will experience worsening of their condition. Roughly 40% of pregnant asthmatics require hospitalization owing to exacerbation of their asthma during pregnancy. The clinical course may be predicted by symptom presentation during the first trimester. Most patients will respond similarly in subsequent pregnancies. If

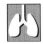

a pregnant asthmatic experiences an exacerbation of symptoms, the possibility of pulmonary embolism should be considered.

The ultimate goal of the treatment of asthma in pregnancy is to maintain adequate oxygenation. Routine management is essentially unchanged during pregnancy except for corticosteroid use. Corticosteroids have been implicated in fetal growth retardation. Therefore, steroids should be used only after careful consideration of the potential fetal risk versus the maternal benefit. Beclomethasone is the most frequently studied steroid in pregnancy and has not been implicated in fetal malformations. All inhaled steroids are considered class C drugs in pregnancy. Maintenance of hydration is essential in the management of the pregnant asthmatic. Asthma is usually inactive during the labor period. However, if systemic steroids are required in the 4 weeks prior to the onset of labor, hydrocortisone (100 mg every 8 hours IV) should be given through 24 hours after delivery to prevent adrenal crisis.

Caution is advised in the use of prostaglandin $F_{2\alpha}$ for control of postpartum hemorrhage, as its use may precipitate an asthmatic attack.

GERIATRIC CONSIDERATIONS

Contrary to the belief that new-onset asthma does not occur in the geriatric population, there is growing evidence that asthma may commonly manifest after age 65. Asthma deaths rise dramatically with advancing age. Elderly patients with new-onset wheezing or nocturnal cough should be evaluated for GERD. Patients with COPD may have a reversible bronchospastic component to their disease that is often treatable as for asthma.

Geriatric patients often respond better to anticholinergic medications for bronchodilatation, in part because beta-adrenergics may stimulate arrhythmias. However, ipatropium has been associated with the precipitation of acute angle closure glaucoma in the elderly population. Consider the use of spacers (AeroChamber or InspirEase) when prescribing metered dose inhalers, as hand-eye coordination decreases with age. Cromoglycates are generally not used in the geriatric population. Elderly patients are at increased risk of developing life-threatening toxicity with the use of methylxanthines.

PREVENTIVE CONSIDERATIONS

Treatment of asthma is largely preventive. Use of long-acting beta agonists, methylxanthines, cromoglycates, leukotriene inhibitors, and inhaled steroids is considered preventive therapy, and one or more of these agents should be used on a daily basis.

Patients with an allergic component to their asthma may benefit from allergen desensitization. Avoidance of known triggers such as pollution, cold weather, exercise, sulfite-containing foods, and aspirin-containing drugs may lessen the frequency of attacks. Patients with gastroesophageal reflux disease (GERD) should receive histamine H_2 blockers (cimetidine, ranitidine, famotidine) or proton pump inhibitors (lansoprazole, omeprazole, rabeprazole, pantoprazole) as indicated to reduce exacerbations.

PEARLS FOR THE PA

Strongly consider hospitalization if pulse oximetry shows Sao$_2$ (oxygen saturation) of 92% or less in acute asthma attack.

Acute attacks are best treated with beta agonists, anticholinergics, and methylxanthines. Steroid onset of action is delayed, but steroids may speed resolution of airflow obstruction and reduce relapse.

Bronchitis

Judith E. Colver, MMS, PA-C

DEFINITION

Inflammation of the large airways of the lower respiratory tract. Acute bronchitis is due to viral or bacterial infection. Bronchitis is considered chronic when the patient exhibits hypersecretion of mucus and cough in 3 or more months of two consecutive years.

HISTORY

Symptoms. Cough, sputum production, often wheezing. May have substernal chest discomfort or burning, and mild dyspnea.

General. Low-grade fever; may have antecedent viral upper respiratory illness or history of smoking or other tobacco abuse.

Age. Affects all ages. Chronic form seen in older adults, usually the result of smoking tobacco.

Onset. Insidious over 1 to 2 days.

Duration. Depending on etiology, cough may persist for up to 6 weeks.

Intensity. Usually mild and self-limited. In children, may lead to persistent airway hyperreactivity and asthma.

Aggravating Factors. Tobacco smoke, inhalation irritants, underlying pulmonary pathology.

Alleviating Factors. Rest, fluids, avoidance of irritants.

Associated Factors. Frequently associated with tobacco smoking and may follow acute upper respiratory illness.

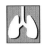

PHYSICAL EXAMINATION

General. Rarely ill-appearing; frequent cough.
Cardiovascular. May have mild tachycardia, especially if febrile.
Head, Eyes, Ears, Nose, Throat. Evidence of resolving upper respiratory infection (URI) such as serous otitis, recent otitis media, sinusitis, rhinorrhea, pharyngitis, and/or cervical adenopathy.
Pulmonary. Diffuse adventitious sounds (crackles, rhonchi, wheezes) that often clear with coughing. Bronchitis is the most common etiology for hemoptysis.

PATHOPHYSIOLOGY

Microorganisms are aspirated from a previously colonized oropharynx. Pulmonary macrophages may produce mediators that draw leukocytes to the area. Inflammation and overproduction of sputum ensue. Cough reflex removes sputum and debris from the lower airways. Viruses cause 40% of infections. *Haemophilus influenzae*, pneumococci, and *Mycoplasma* account for another 10%. Recently, *Moraxella* and *Chlamydia* have been implicated.

DIAGNOSTIC STUDIES

Laboratory
Complete Blood Count. May show leukocytosis if bronchitis is of bacterial origin.
Arterial Blood Gas Analysis. May show hypoxia if infection is severe.
Sputum Culture. Generally not helpful in the outpatient setting.

Radiology
Chest Film. Usually normal.

Other
Pulmonary Function Tests. Usually normal values.

DIFFERENTIAL DIAGNOSIS

Infectious
Bronchiolitis. Infection of the smaller airways, more common in the first year of life.
Bronchiectasis. History of recurrent lower respiratory infections, hemoptysis and clubbing of digits if long term.

Neoplastic
Primary or Metastatic Pulmonary Neoplasm in Early Stages. Mass may be noted on chest film or chest CT scan.

Vascular

Congestive Heart Failure. Occasionally mainfests as chronic cough. Echocardiogram will reveal cardiogenic etiology.

Acquired

Chronic Cough from Angiotensin-Converting Enzyme (ACE) Inhibitors. Careful history and resolution on withdrawal of offending agent.

Traumatic. Not applicable.
Metabolic. Not applicable.
Congenital. Not applicable.

TREATMENT

Treatment is largely supportive. Antibiotics do little to affect the course of the disease in otherwise healthy patients. However, patients with chronic pulmonary problems (including chronic bronchitis with an acute overlay) may benefit from antibiotics, especially if clinical manifestations include increased sputum volume, increased sputum purulence, or increased dyspnea.

- Antibiotics
  Augmentin 500 mg three times a day OR
  Macrolides: azithromycin 500 mg day 1, then 250 mg daily for 4 days, OR clarithromycin 500 mg twice daily OR
  Doxycycline 100 mg twice daily OR
  Fluoroquinolones: ciprofloxacin 500 mg twice daily, levofloxacin 500 mg daily, OR gatifloxacin 400 mg daily. A 10-day course is usually effective.

Amoxicillin, erythromycin, and trimethoprim-sulfamethoxazole are no longer reliable choices.

Increased oral fluids, antipyretics, and cough suppressants are generally effective. Smoking cessation should be addressed.

- Cough suppressants
  Benzonatate 100-200 mg three times a day OR dextromethorphan 10-15 mg (often with guiafenesin) every 4 to 6 hours as needed

Maintain hydration to reduce mucus plugging. Humidified air may provide some relief. Inhaled bronchodilators may reduce wheezing if present.

PEDIATRIC CONSIDERATIONS

Acute bronchitis is rarely an isolated disease in childhood. Instead, bronchitis frequently occurs in concert or following associated upper or lower respiratory infection. Shortly after a viral URI, the child develops a nonproductive cough. Occasionally the child will have post-tussive emesis, usually of phlegm loosened by the coughing.

Physical findings differ with age of the child and stage of the illness. Treatment is largely supportive. Children with repeated episodes of acute

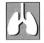

bronchitis should be evaluated for abnormalities of the respiratory tract including foreign body aspiration, allergic rhinitis, and sinusitis, and for cystic fibrosis.

OBSTETRIC CONSIDERATIONS

Treatment is largely supportive. When antibiotics are indicated, avoid fluoroquinolones, tetracyclines, and erythromycin.

GERIATRIC CONSIDERATIONS

Although acute bronchitis is a disease of all ages, chronic bronchitis is more common in the geriatric population.

PREVENTIVE CONSIDERATIONS

Tobacco use is the single most important factor in the development of chronic bronchitis. Smoking cessation should be encouraged in all patients. Patients with chronic bronchitis who have an increase in sputum production or change in sputum color should be considered for antibiotic therapy.

PEARLS FOR THE PA

Bronchitis is the most common cause of hemoptysis.

Most causes of acute bronchitis are viral. Reserve the use of antibiotics for severe infections or acute-on-chronic infections.

Smoking cessation should be encouraged.

Chronic Obstructive Pulmonary Disease

Judith E. Colver, MMS, PA-C

DEFINITION

Chronic obstructive pulmonary disease (COPD) is the leading pulmonary cause of morbidity and mortality in the 21st century. COPD has two major components: emphysema and chronic bronchitis.

Emphysema is an anatomic alteration of the lung characterized by enlargement of the air spaces and destruction of alveolar walls. Patients are known as "pink puffers."

Chronic bronchitis is a chronic inflammatory process involving the major airways and is characterized by hypersecretion of mucus and cough in 3 or more months of two consecutive years. Patients are often referred to as "blue bloaters" because of chronic hypoxia and resultant cyanosis.

HISTORY

Symptoms. Dyspnea and weight loss are common with emphysema; chronic productive cough, with chronic bronchitis.

General. History of tobacco abuse in most cases. Exacerbations occur following exposure to pulmonary irritants or after upper respiratory infections.

Age. Emphysema usually becomes symptomatic after age 50, although familial form (due to lack of α_1-antitrypsin) may be symptomatic by mid 30s. Chronic cough with bronchitis often starts in the mid to late 30s.

Onset. Gradual over years; however once symptomatic, patients usually remain symptomatic.

Duration. Progressive.

Intensity. High morbidity and mortality rates. COPD is the second leading cause of disability and fourth most common cause of death in adults in the United States.

Aggravating Factors. Antecedent respiratory infection, respiratory irritants, environmental pollution.

Alleviating Factors. Smoking cessation has shown some benefit, particularly in chronic bronchitis.

Associated Factors. Familial deficiency of α_1-antitrypsin, tobacco abuse.

PHYSICAL EXAMINATION

General. As dyspnea progresses, patients may sit forward and lean on elbows or hands, use accessory muscles of respiration, and breathe through pursed lips. Emphysema patients are usually thin (may be cachectic), often with ruddy complexion, barrel chest, and dyspnea. Chronic bronchitis patients, on the other hand, are often obese and cyanotic, but generally less dyspneic until late in the disease course. Fever may be present if there is a superimposed acute infection.

Cardiovascular. Often mild tachycardia. Jugular venous distention indicates accompanying right-sided heart failure. Palpation of the precordium may reveal displaced point of maximal intensity (PMI) and/or right ventricular heave suggestive of right-sided heart enlargement and pulmonary hypertension. Auscultation frequently reveals S_3, murmur of tricuspid insufficiency, and/or loud pulmonary component of the second heart sound.

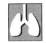

Extremities. Pitting pedal edema that fails to subside with leg elevation is indicative of right-sided heart failure. Digital clubbing is not normally seen and should prompt evaluation for other pulmonary comorbid conditions.

Gastrointestinal. Liver enlargement and ascites when right-sided heart failure is present.

Genitourinary. Inguinal hernias common in emphysema patients.

Pulmonary. Tachypnea (respiratory rate greater than 18 breaths/minute). Emphysematous patients will have increased chest anteroposterior diameter and hyperresonance to percussion. Decreased breath sounds are common with prolonged expiratory phase. Heart sounds may be muffled or displaced to midline owing to hyperinflation of lungs. Patients with chronic bronchitis may have rhonchi from increased secretions. Either may have wheezing or crackles.

Skin. Pink to ruddy in emphysema; cyanotic in chronic bronchitis.

PATHOPHYSIOLOGY

Cigarette smokers develop a chronic inflammatory reaction and often edema in the bronchioles. Macrophages infiltrate the area and the process progresses to fibrosis or actual obliteration of the airways by smooth muscle hyperplasia. Goblet cell metaplasia and resulting increase in secretions further obstruct the airways. With emphysema there is actual destruction of the acinus. Ultimately, COPD leads to hypoxia, pulmonary hypertension, and cor pulmonale (right-sided heart failure).

DIAGNOSTIC STUDIES

Laboratory
Complete Blood Count. Polycythemia and thrombocytosis in advanced stages.

Arterial Blood Gas Analysis. Hypoxemia (Pao_2 less than 55 mm Hg) as disease progresses; worse with acute exacerbations.

Emphysema. Normal to decreased Pao_2 (55-60 mm Hg); normal to mild decrease in $Paco_2$ (30-40 mm Hg).

Chronic Bronchitis. Markedly decreased Pao_2 (less than 55 mm Hg); increased $Paco_2$ (greater than 45 mm Hg). This patient group often is referred to as the "50-50 club" because the Pao_2 and $Paco_2$ values approximate 50.

Serum α_1-Antitrypsin. Absent or decreased in familial emphysema.

Radiology
Chest Film. Loss of vascular markings, hyperinflation, flattened hemidiaphragms, and increased anteroposterior diameter. May show evidence of right ventricular enlargement (cor pulmonale).

Other

Pulmonary Function Tests. Decreased forced vital capacity (FVC), forced expiratory volume in 1 minute (FEV_1), and FEV_1/FVC ratio. In emphysema, total lung capacity (TLC) is increased, FRC is increased, and there is a decreased diffusion capacity.

DIFFERENTIAL DIAGNOSIS

Traumatic

Pneumothorax. Usually history of acute onset of dyspnea and/or chest pain. Patients with emphysema may experience spontaneous rupture of a large bleb, causing a pneumothorax.

Infectious

Bronchiectasis. Recurrent history of pneumonia, hemoptysis, and digital clubbing.

Neoplastic

Primary or Metastatic Lung Tumor. May have dyspnea, hemoptysis, chest pain; mass may be seen on chest film or chest CT scan.

Vascular

Pulmonary Embolism. Usually acute onset dyspnea and chest pain. May have associated leg/calf pain from deep vein thrombosis.

Metabolic. Not applicable.
Congenital. Not applicable.
Acquired. Not applicable.

TREATMENT

Smoking cessation should be encouraged. Patients who continue to smoke have the greatest deterioration of pulmonary function over time. Treatment is largely symptomatic.

Bronchodilators play an important part in the treatment of many patients with COPD and can provide considerable symptomatic relief.

- Beta agonists: Mainstay of bronchodilator therapy.
    Albuterol (Ventolin, Proventil) 0.083% nebulizer solution or 2.5 mg (0.5 mL of 0.5% solution diluted to 3.0 mL with normal saline) up to 10 mg three to four times a day; metered dose inhaler 90 µg /inhalation—2 inhalations every 4 to 6 hours, maximum 16 to 20 inhalations daily
    Formoterol (Foradil) 12 µg capsules for inhalation with device—1 inhalation twice daily. Long-acting beta agonist, not for treatment of acute exacerbations

Pirbuterol (Maxair) metered dose inhaler 200 µg /inhalation—1-2 inhalations every 4 to 6 hours, maximum 12 inhalations daily

Metaproterenol (Alupent) metered dose inhaler 0.65 mg/inhalation—2 or 3 inhalations every 3 to 4 hours, maximum 12 inhalations daily

Salmeterol (Serevent) metered dose inhaler 21 µg/inhalation—2 inhalations twice daily. Long-acting beta agonist, not for treatment of acute exacerbations

Terbutaline (Brethine) 2.5-5 mg tablets three times daily at 6-hour intervals

- Anticholinergics: May be more effective than (and/or synergistic with) beta agonists in COPD; have the added benefit of reducing secretions.

Atropine 0.025 mg/kg diluted with 3-5 mL normal saline by nebulizer every 6 to 8 hours

Ipratropium (Atrovent) nebulizer solution 500 µg 2.5 mL three or four times a day; metered dose inhaler 18 µg/inhalation—2 inhalations four times a day, maximum 12 inhalations daily

- Methylxanthines: Various products for intravenous or oral administration. *Caution*: Numerous drug interactions. *Note*: May cause toxicity; monitor serum levels. Symptoms of toxicity include nausea, vomiting, flushing, tachycardia, and mental status changes.

Aminophylline OR theophylline: *initial (loading) dose*: 5-6 mg/kg IV over 20 minutes; *maintenance*: 0.5-0.9 mg/kg/hour. Therapeutic range is 5-15 µg/mL; oral form 200-600 mg twice daily, titrate to reach therapeutic range.

- Anti-inflammatory medications: Useful in the routine management of COPD.

Inhaled steroids

Beclomethasone (QVAR) metered dose inhaler 40 µg or 80 µg/inhalation—2 inhalations three or four times a day, maximum 320 µg per day

Budesonide (Pulmicort) metered dose inhaler 200 µg/inhalation—1 to 4 inhalations twice daily, maximum of 4 inhalations twice daily

Flunisolide (AeroBid) metered dose inhaler 250 µg/inhalation—2 inhalations twice daily, maximum 8 inhalations daily

Fluticasone (Flovent) metered dose inhaler with 44 µg, 110 µg, or 220 µg/inhalation—2 inhalations twice daily

Triamcinolone (Azmacort) metered dose inhaler 100 µg/inhalation—2 to 4 inhalations twice daily, maximum 16 inhalations daily

Cromoglycates: generally ineffective in COPD

Oral steroids: frequently used in acute exacerbations

Methylprednisolone 125 mg IV every 6 hours

Hydrocortisone 2 mg/kg IV bolus, then 0.5 mg/kg/hour IV

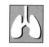

Prednisone 40-100 mg/day, taper dose once controlled. May ultimately be able to taper patient to an inhaled steroid.

Chest physiotherapy may be beneficial in mobilizing and clearing secretions.

Antibiotics are generally not needed but may be helpful with overlying acute exacerbations heralded by increase in sputum quantity, sputum purulence, or dyspnea.

Administration of supplemental O_2 to patients with significant hypoxia may reduce somnolence and significantly improve quality of life. Patients usually respond to even small amounts of supplemental oxygen. A low flow rate (1-2 liters/minute) via nasal cannula is usually effective and well tolerated. Some patients only require supplementation at night, when airway resistance is lessened. Goal is to shift the Pao_2 into a range greater than 60 to 65 mm Hg.

α_1-Antitrypsin replacement therapy is appropriate when deficiency has been determined.

Pulmonary rehabilitation may help increase exercise tolerance and the patient's sense of well-being. Nutrition status should be maximized.

Mechanical ventilation is generally reserved for those patients with acute respiratory failure. Noninvasive forms should be considered (nasal cannula, continuous positive-pressure mask).

Lung volume reduction for emphysematous patients may be of benefit. Lung transplantation may be appropriate in some patients.

PEDIATRIC CONSIDERATIONS

Not applicable to pediatric patients.

OBSTETRIC CONSIDERATIONS

Generally not applicable to obstetric patients. When needed, use of steroids should be weighed against the potential risk to the fetus.

GERIATRIC CONSIDERATIONS

COPD is largely a disease of the geriatric population and is the leading cause of pulmonary morbidity and mortality in the United States.

PREVENTIVE CONSIDERATIONS

Tobacco use is the single most important factor in the development of COPD. Smoking cessation should be encouraged in all patients. Pneumococcal vaccination and annual influenza vaccination is indicated for all patients with COPD.

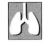

PEARLS FOR THE PA

Primary prevention of COPD through smoking cessation is crucial.

Administration of pneumonia vaccine (single vaccination, booster should be considered if 5 years have elapsed since vaccination and patient is older than 65) and annual influenza vaccination are indicated as preventive measures in patients with COPD.

Interstitial Lung Disease

Judith E. Colver, MMS, PA-C

DEFINITION

Interstitial lung disease is a term used to describe a number of disorders that have in common an inflammatory-fibrotic infiltration of the alveolar walls. Interstitial fibrosis follows injury to the alveolar-capillary membranes. In many of these diseases, collagen accumulates within the airway lumina, further compromising the ability of gas exchange. Over 100 entities are known, all of which produce disease processes similar in clinical manifestations, radiographic findings, and physiologic features. The most common of these etiologic disorders include rheumatologic diseases (scleroderma, polymyositis, systemic lupus erythematosus, rheumatoid arthritis, and ankylosing spondylitis), drug-induced changes (from numerous antibiotics, antiarrhythmics, anti-inflammatories, anticonvulsants, narcotics, and others), primary diseases (sarcoid, amyloidosis, neurofibromatosis, pulmonary neoplasm/lymphoma), occupational/environmental diseases (silicosis, asbestosis, talc pneumoconiosis, siderosis), hypersensitivity pneumonitis (bird breeder's lung, farmer's lung), and idiopathic causes (acute interstitial pneumonitis, bronchiolitis obliterans organizing pneumonia, autoimmune pulmonary fibrosis, and idiopathic pulmonary fibrosis).

HISTORY

Symptoms.   Dyspnea on exertion is the most common presenting symptom, usually associated with cough. Eventually most patients will have dyspnea, tachypnea, and cyanosis. Substernal or pleuritic chest pain is also common. Hemoptysis is common with some causative disorders.

General.   Fever may accompany hypersensitivity pneumonitis or drug-induced pneumonitis. Joint pain or inflammation may herald a rheumatologic disease.

Age. Any, depending on the etiology. Becomes more frequent with advancing age.

Onset. Subacute onset is seen with hypersensitivity pneumonitis and bronchiolitis obliterans organizing pneumonia. Slowly progressive with sarcoidosis, pneumoconiosis, rheumatologic diseases, and idiopathic pulmonary fibrosis. Acute with infection, hypersensitivity pneumonitis, drug reactions, and toxic ingestions.

Duration. Usually slow and progressive, occasionally rapid deterioration.

Intensity. Frequent relapses and remissions are common. Exacerbations usually worsen with the length of the disease.

Aggravating Factors. Tobacco abuse, exposure to environmental or occupational dusts/toxins.

Alleviating Factors. None.

Associated Factors. In malignant conditions, patients are often immunosuppressed.

PHYSICAL EXAMINATION

General. Tachypnea is common. Fever, chills may be present.

Cardiovascular. Accentuation of pulmonary component of S_2 may be heard with pulmonary hypertension.

Extremities. Clubbing is frequently seen; cyanosis is a late finding. Joint inflammation/effusion may be present in rheumatic diseases.

Head, Eyes, Ears, Nose, Throat. Coexisting iritis/uveiitis and/or keratitis sicca is common finding with rheumatic diseases and sarcoid. Cervical adenopathy may be present in sarcoid or with lymphoma/malignancy. Jugular venous distention (JVD) may be present if heart failure is present.

Gastrointestinal. Dysphagia and reduced intestinal motility in scleroderma. Hepatosplenomegaly may be present.

Genitourinary. Glomerulonephritis and nephrotic sydrome may occur, especially with rheumatologic diseases.

Neurologic. Organic brain syndrome may accompany rheumatologic diseases. Depression is common.

Pulmonary. Bibasilar inspiratory crackles are common. Breath sounds may be normal or accentuated.

Skin. Rashes (i.e., malar in systemic lupus, erythema nodosum) may accompany rheumatologic diseases. Cyanosis is a late finding.

PATHOPHYSIOLOGY

Alveolar spaces bring inspired air into close proximity with the pulmonary capillaries. Surrounding these air-exchange units is the interstitium of the lung. This area is a potential space where inflammatory cells and fluid can accumulate. In early stages, inflammation is usually localized to the alveoli. Later in the disease, derangement of the noncellular supporting structures causes fibrosis and distortion of the lung tissue. Some diseases also have associated granuloma formation and/or sclerosis that affect the lungs as well as other organ systems.

DIAGNOSTIC STUDIES

Laboratory
Erythrocyte Sedimentation Rate.   Elevated in 90% of cases with acute exacerbation, but rarely exceeds 100 mm/hour.

Serologic Tests for Rheumatologic Diseases.   May be helpful, but generally are neither sensitive nor specific.

Immunoglobulins.   Elevated in 40% of cases.

Complement.   Often reduced in acute exacerbations.

Complete Blood Count.   Often shows a mild anemia of chronic disease that is indistinguishable from iron deficiency anemia. Eosinophilia is present in some syndromes.

Arterial Blood Gas Analysis.   Low Pao_2, low $Paco_2$, and elevated alveolar-arterial (A–a) oxygen gradient.

Radiology
Chest Film.   Diffuse "ground glass" or honeycomb appearance of the lungs, worsening with progression of the disease. Prominent hilar adenopathy in most cases. Nodules may be seen with primary malignancy or metastatic disease.

Conventional CT.   May miss up to 10% of cases. High-resolution computed tomography (HRCT) is preferred.

Other
Pulmonary Function Tests.   Will show a restrictive pattern and, in advanced disease, a reduced total lung capacity (TLC), vital capacity (VC), forced residual capacity (FRC), and residual volume (RV). Evidence of obstruction is usually minimal as evidenced by a normal forced expiratory volume in 1 minute to forced vital capacity (FEV_1/FVC) ratio.

Bronchoalveolar Lavage (BAL).   May assist with histologic diagnosis and staging of disease. Also may provide diagnosis of eosinophilic lung disease. If findings are inconclusive, transbronchial biopsy should be considered, followed by open lung biopsy if needed to establish the diagnosis.

DIFFERENTIAL DIAGNOSIS

Infectious
Chronic Pneumonia.   Presence of effusion or infiltrates on chest film; productive cough.

Neoplastic
Bronchogenic Cancer/Pulmonary Metastatic Disease.   Mass seen on chest film or HRCT scan.

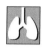

Vascular

Recurrent Pulmonary Emboli.   Definitive diagnosis made by pulmonary angiogram. Ventilation-perfusion (V/Q) scan may be helpful. Chest film may reveal evidence of pulmonary infarction.

Congestive Heart Failure.   Echocardiogram is helpful in differentiating cardiac from pulmonary etiology of disease. Chest film may show cardiomegaly.

Acquired

Chronic Obstructive Pulmonary Disease (COPD).   Classically a history of productive cough. Pulmonary function tests reveal an obstructive pattern.

Other

Pleural Effusion.   Chest film shows blunting of costophrenic angle and/or fluid in the plural space.

Traumatic/Metabolic/Congenital

Not applicable.

TREATMENT

Treatment is largely supportive. The central goal of treatment is to maintain adequate oxygenation.

- Supplemental oxygen therapy: Titrate to keep oxygen saturation greater than 90%.
- Corticosteroids: Prednisone 1 mg/kg/day may be given.
- Cytotoxic agents: Azathioprine/cyclophosphamide may be useful in patients who are resistant to corticosteroids. Penicillamine is often more effective in patients with rheumatologic diseases.

Remove environmental/occupational irritants, or remove the patient from further exposure. Encourage smoking cessation. Prophylactic use of pneumococcal and influenza vaccines is encouraged. Lung transplantation may be indicated in some patients.

PEDIATRIC CONSIDERATIONS

Interstitial lung fibrosis is predominantly a disease of lung immaturity in the premature infant (born at less than 32 weeks of gestation). It is characterized by insidious onset of dyspnea, tachycardia, and cyanosis, usually in the first month of life. Viral infections, meconium aspiration, and hyperoxygenation all have been implicated. Symptoms increase over a 2- to 6-week period and may include spontaneous pneumothorax, oxygen dependence (for up to several months), and progressive respiratory and right-sided heart failure. Infants who survive are at increased risk for development of lower respiratory infections during the first year of life. Treatment is largely supportive, and mechanical ventilation is often indicated.

Older children may develop interstitial lung disease following infection or aspiration, or as the result of underlying cardiac disease or pulmonary vascular disease. Onset of symptoms is usually gradual. Children frequently present with a dry cough or dyspnea. As the disease progresses, they often exhibit tachypnea, tachycardia, use of accessory muscles, cyanosis, digital clubbing, and weight loss.

Auscultation reveals fine crackles, especially at the lung bases. Breath sounds may be diminished. Chest radiographic appearance is variable, with normal findings in up to 15% of cases. In the remainder of cases, a diffuse or perihilar interstitial infiltrate is commonly seen. Peribronchial cuffing, hilar adenopathy, and nodular infiltrates also may be noted. Pulmonary function tests often indicate a restrictive pattern, with decreased lung volume and compliance. Diagnostic evaluation includes BAL or lung biopsy. Treatment is directed at the primary disorder, and prognosis varies according to specific impairment and severity. Lung transplantaion is indicated in some children.

OBSTETRIC CONSIDERATIONS

Pregnant women with interstitial lung disease are considered high-risk patients. Steroids should be used with caution. The pregnancy is generally not at risk as long as pulmonary function is not compromised. Serial pulmonary function testing should be considered to monitor the disease process during pregnancy.

GERIATRIC CONSIDERATIONS

Up to one-third of all patients with idiopathic pulmonary fibrosis (IPF) do not exhibit symptoms of the disease until after age 65 years. The incidence of idiopathic drug reactions causing IPF increases with age.

PREVENTIVE CONSIDERATIONS

All patients with interstitial lung disease should receive pneumococcal vaccination and annual influenza vaccination.

Prevention is key with the pneumoconioses. Use of a respirator by persons who work with or around asbestos, talc, silica, iron filings, or other substances known to induce interstitial lung disease is imperative in the prevention of the disease.

Smoking cessation is imperative.

PEARLS FOR THE PA

Carefully evaluate occupational, travel, and environmental history in patients with interstitial lung disease.

Pleural Effusion

Judith E. Colver, MMS, PA-C

DEFINITION

Pleural effusion is the accumulation of free fluid in the pleural space. Fluid accumulates when the rate of fluid formation exceeds the rate of removal by the pulmonary lymphatic system. Effusions may be transudative or exudative.

Transudative effusions are due to decreased colloidal pressure and a transfer of fluid into the pleural space from the vascular or peritoneal space. Transudates are seen in pulmonary embolism, myxedema, congestive heart failure (CHF), nephrotic syndrome, pericardial disease, and cirrhosis/ascites.

Exudative effusions arise within the pleura and reflect increased pleural capillary permeability or interference with thoracic lymphatic drainage. Exudates are seen with acute infections (bacterial, viral, fungal, or parasitic), infarction of the lung tissue (often following pulmonary embolism), pancreatitis, neoplasms and rheumatic diseases.

HISTORY

Symptom. Dyspnea, cough, orthopnea, paroxysmal nocturnal dyspnea. Pain may or may not be present and if present may be localized or pleuritic in nature.

General. The medical history may help in identifying the underlying causative disorder (e.g., congestive heart failure, liver disease).

Age. All ages, but incidence increases with advancing age.

Onset. Usually gradual but may be abrupt.

Duration. Usually short-term if treated.

Intensity. Mild to debilitating, depending on the underlying causative disorder.

Aggravating Factors. Preexisting medical conditions and noncompliance with treatment.

Alleviating Factors. Therapeutic thoracentesis may reduce dyspnea while appropriate therapy for underlying disorder is instituted.

Associated Factors. Underlying illness that leads to general physical deterioration.

PHYSICAL EXAMINATION

General. Fever if infectious etiology.

Cardiovascular. Tachycardia is common. Gallop rhythm may be present if CHF is the etiologic disorder. Cardiac friction rub may be heard in pericarditis.

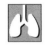

Extremities.   Pedal edema may be present in CHF.

Head, Eyes, Ears, Nose, Throat.   Jugular venous distention may be noted if CHF is present

Gastrointestinal.   Hepatomegaly and/or ascites with cirrhosis. In hepatic failure, the liver may be normal or shrunken in size.

Genitourinary.   Proteinuria if uremia or nephrotic syndrome is present. Rarely, patients with urinary obstruction will have an effusion.

Pulmonary.   Tachypnea is present. Decreased tactile fremitus, dullness to percussion, diminished or absent breath sounds over the area of the effusion are common. Decreased chest expansion and egophony may be present immediately above the level of the effusion.

Skin.   Edema may be noted with CHF or nephrotic syndrome

PATHOPHYSIOLOGY

Pleural effusions occur with CHF as the result of the reduced clearance of pulmonary interstitial fluid across a leaky mesothelium. With CHF, it is common to have bilateral effusions. Effusions occur in cirrhosis/ascites with a translocation of ascitic fluid across the diaphragm due to increased abdominal pressure. With cirrhosis, the effusion is usually right-sided. The incidence of effusion in nephrotic syndrome is 30%, and the effusion appears to be the result of decreased plasma oncotic pressure due to hypoproteinemia in association with increased hydrostatic pressure secondary to sodium retention and the resultant hypervolemic state. In the presence of nephrotic syndrome, the effusions most often are bilateral. The mechanism responsible for the presence of effusion in pericardial disease is not clear; however, often the effusion is only left-sided.

Parapneumonic effusions are the result of an acute infection. Initially there is inflammation and increased interstitial fluid, which leaks into the pleural space. The infective agent then invades the pleural fluid (resulting in the condition known as empyema), and fibrin is deposited. Loculation may occur with the formation of limiting membrane(s). Finally, fibroblasts grow into the exudates, producing an inelastic membrane also known as a *pleural peel*. This peel may encase the entire lung and render it virtually functionless.

DIAGNOSTIC STUDIES

Laboratory
Pleural Fluid Evaluation.   Often diagnostic. Transudates generally are clear and demonstrate low specific gravity (<less than 1.016), absence of clot formation, low protein (less than 3 g/dL), glucose equal to serum level, and a low lactate dehydrogenase (LDH). Exudates are turbid or cloudy and demonstrate high specific gravity (>1.016), presence of clot formation, higher protein level (greater than 3 g/dL), glucose lower than serum level, and high LDH (greater than two-thirds of the upper normal level for serum). Leukocyte

count will be elevated in parapneumonic effusions. Gram stain and cultures (for aerobic, anerobic, and acid-fast organisms) should be performed. Malignant cells may be seen on cytology with associated neoplasm.

Arterial Blood Gas Analysis. Values remain nearly normal or may show hypoxemia.

Complete Blood Count. Will show a leukocytosis with infectious etiology.

Serum Protein, Glucose, and LDH. Should be performed to compare with pleural fluid values.

Rheumatoid Factor/Antinuclear Antibody (ANA) Assay, Serum Amylase, Lung Function Tests, Chemistry Panel, Thyroid Studies (TSH,T_3,T_4), BUN and/or Creatinine. May be indicated depending on the underlying pathology.

Radiology
Chest Film. The earliest radiographic manifestation of a pleural effusion is blunting of the posterior costophrenic angle. As fluid increases, the lateral costophrenic angle is blunted. Free fluid may layer out on lateral decubitus film and is said to be loculated when it does not change with position of the patient. Cardiomegaly is often present with CHF.

Ultrasound Examination. May be helpful in differentiating pleural fluid from solid tissue.

Chest CT. Generally valuable in differentiating pleural from parenchymal disease.

Other
Purified Protein Derivative (PPD). Indicated if tuberculosis is suspected.

DIFFERENTIAL DIAGNOSIS

Traumatic
Hemothorax. Blood (not fluid) accumulates in the pleural space.

Infectious
Empyema. Pus accumulates in the pleural space. Fungal "balls" may be seen in the fluid and elsewhere in the thorax with fungal infection.

Metabolic
Chylothorax. Lipid effusion due to obstruction of lymphatic drainage.

Neoplastic
Primary or Metastatic Cancer. May cause a bloody effusion.

Acquired
Following Liver Transplantation. Effusions are common. Although they may be bilateral, the effusion is almost always worse on the right side. Effusions are also common following cardiac injury or coronary bypass surgery.

Vascular/Congenital
Not applicable.

TREATMENT

Treatment of the underlying pathology is key in obtaining resolution of the effusion.

With parapneumonic effusions, antibiotic choice should be guided by Gram stain and culture of sputum, blood, and pleural fluid. Thoracentesis is both diagnostic and therapeutic. Chest tube insertion and drainage may be required in the treatment of empyema. Thoracoscopy with lysis of adhesions should be considered in patients who have inadequate drainage at 24 hours following tube thoracostomy. Open thoracotomy with decortication is reserved for those patients in whom tube thoracostomy with drainage or thoracoscopy with lysis fails.

Intrapleural thrombolytic agents should be considered in complicated parapneumonic effusions to reduce loculations and the formation of pleural peel. Streptokinase 250,000 units or urokinase 100,000 units diluted in 30-60 mL of normal saline is administered via chest tube; the tube is clamped for 1 to 2 hours after drug administration. May be repeated daily up to 14 days.

Lung resection may be required in fungal infections.

Prednisone may be required in the treatment of rheumatic effusions, especially lupus-induced effusions.

PEDIATRIC CONSIDERATIONS

The most common cause of pleural effusion in children is a parapneumonic effusion secondary to bacterial pneumonia. Plural effusions may also be seen in children with heart failure, metastatic thoracic malignancy, tuberculosis, rheumatic fever, aspiration pneumonitis, uremia, pancreatitis, Still disease (juvenile rheumatoid arthritis), and subdiaphragmatic abscess.

OBSTETRIC CONSIDERATIONS

Pleural effusions that compromise oxygenation of are special concern during pregnancy. Treatment is aimed at maintaining proper oxygenation and correcting the underlying abnormality.

Obstetric patients with HELLP (*h*emolysis, *e*levated *l*iver enzymes, *l*ow *p*latelets) syndrome (up to 12% of patients with severe preeclampsia or eclampsia) are at increased risk for development of a pleural effusion. Thoracentesis may be required for diagnosis and may be therapeutic if oxygenation is poor. Extreme caution must be used because hemorrhage is a major concern. These patients are best managed at a tertiary care facility.

GERIATRIC CONSIDERATIONS

The incidence of CHF increases with age, and CHF is one of the leading causes of pleural effusion. Half of all lung cancers occur in patients age 65 years and older, with the peak incidence at age 75. Pleural effusions should be carefully evaluated to rule out an underlying neoplasm.

PREVENTIVE CONSIDERATIONS

Aggressive treatment of underlying conditions may decrease the incidence of pleural effusion. Smoking cessation should be encouraged in all patients, as tobacco use increases the risk of lung cancer and hence pleural effusion.

PEARLS FOR THE PA

Chest film and thoracentesis are the keys to diagnosis.

Pleurisy

Judith E. Colver, MMS, PA-C

DEFINITION

Chest pain that worsens with chest wall movement. Most commonly associated with inflammation of the parietal pleura. May be due to any of various causes including infection, trauma, inflammation, and neoplasm.

HISTORY

Symptoms.   Sharp pain that is worsened by movement of the chest wall, especially with deep inspiration, coughing, or sneezing. May lead to the sensation of dyspnea.

General.   History of similar chest pain is helpful. Recent or concurrent bronchitis is the most common etiology.

Age.   Any.

Onset.   Gradual to abrupt, depending on etiology.

Duration.   Short to long term, depending on etiology.

Intensity.   May be incapacitating.

Aggravating Factors.   Sudden movement of the thorax or deep inspiration.

Alleviating Factors.   Shallow respirations and lack of movement.
Associated Factors.   Infection, trauma, inflammation, and neoplasm.

PHYSICAL EXAMINATION

General.   Shallow respirations with splinting.

Cardiovascular.   May have mild tachycardia. Cardiac friction rub if pericarditis is present.

Pulmonary.   Tachypnea with shallow respirations. May hear a friction rub with respiration (often is intermittent). Unless trauma is involved, chest wall is usually not tender with palpation.

Skin.   Examine for vesicular rash on hemithorax if herpes zoster is suspected.

PATHOPHYSIOLOGY

The visceral pleura is not innervated by pain sensors, but inflammatory processes in the periphery of the visceral pleura may extend and involve the parietal pleura. The parietal pleura is innervated by adjacent intercostal nerves; thus, pain is often localized to the cutaneous distributions of the involved nerves. Because the diaphragm is innervated by the phrenic nerve, inflammation of the parietal pleura that lies in the central region of the diaphragm may be associated with pain referred to the shoulder or neck on the ipsilateral side.

DIAGNOSTIC STUDIES

Laboratory

Complete Blood Count.   May show leukocytosis if bacterial infection is present.

Erythrocyte Sedimentation Rate.   Usually elevated with inflammatory or metastatic process.

Radiology

Chest Film.   Chest film is usually normal but may be helpful in underlying pneumonia or neoplasm or in cases of acute trauma. Occasionally will show a diffuse haziness at the pleural surface or a dense, sharply demarcated shadow, which is diagnostic.

Spiral CT of the Chest.   In some institutions, CT is replacing ventilation-perfusion (V/Q) scan as study to rule out pulmonary embolism.

Other

V/Q Scan.   Helpful in ruling out pulmonary embolism.

DIFFERENTIAL DIAGNOSIS

Traumatic
Chest Wall Trauma. May mainfest as pleuritic pain. Patient will exhibit pain with light palpation, and chest film may reveal fracture or hemothorax/pneumothorax.

Infectious
Pneumonia. Infiltrative process seen on chest film.

Pericarditis. Pericardial friction rub, may be associated with jugular venous distention (JVD), reduced heart sounds. Pain is limited to the precordial area; is often worsened by turning and relieved by sitting up and leaning forward.

Herpes Zoster. Pain may precede rash, usually more constant. Vesicular rash in dermatomal distribution confined to one hemithorax.

Metabolic
Uremia. Elevated creatinine and blood urea nitrogen (BUN). Patients may have pleuritic pain secondary to the underlying uremia.

Neoplastic
Primary Lung Neoplasm/Metastatic Disease. Chest film and/or chest CT will help identify mass.

Vascular
Pulmonary Embolism. Acute onset of dyspnea with chest pain. May have lower extremity deep vein phlebitis. V/Q scan or spiral (helical) chest CT will assist with diagnosis.

Acquired
Acute Rib Trauma/Fracture. May mainfest as pleuritic chest pain.

Other
Multiple Rheumatologic Diseases. May have a component of pleuritic chest pain.

Congenital
Not applicable.

TREATMENT

Treat the underlying cause if known. Pleurisy associated with acute illness is usually self-limiting and lasts days to weeks.

Pain can usually be controlled with nonsteroidal anti-inflammatory drugs (NSAIDs) such as ibuprofen 800 mg three times a day or naproxen 500 mg twice a day. Occasionally, narcotic medication is required; a combination agent such as acetaminophen/codeine 300/30 or acetaminophen/ hydrocodone 500/5, 1 or 2 tablets every 4 to 6 hours, can be given as needed for pain.

Cough suppressants are indicated if cough is present. Dextromethorphan/guaifenesin, 30/600 1 or 2 tablets every 12 hours, or benzonatate 200 mg three times daily can be given.

PEDIATRIC CONSIDERATIONS

No specific pediatric considerations.

OBSTETRIC CONSIDERATIONS

The extent of pulmonary compromise is commensurate with the magnitude of effect on the pregnancy.

GERIATRIC CONSIDERATIONS

Herpes zoster in elderly persons may appear as pleuritic chest pain, even before the vesicular rash occurs.

PREVENTIVE CONSIDERATIONS

Generally, there are no preventive considerations in the development of pleurisy.

PEARLS FOR THE PA

If the appearance on chest film is normal, diagnosis should be directed to ruling out pulmonary embolism, herpes zoster, or inflammation associated with rheumatic disease.

If patient has pleurisy and associated pneumonia with effusion, screen for tuberculosis.

Pneumonia

Judith E. Colver, MMS, PA-C

DEFINITION

Pneumonia is characterized by inflammation of the lung parenchyma secondary to the presence of an infectious agent, usually with an associated exudative fluid accumulation in the alveoli (consolidation). It is the most common cause of infection-related mortality and the sixth leading cause of death in the United States. Debilitated patients and those who are very young (less than 1 year of age) or are older than 60 years are at increased risk. Treatment is often empirical depending on the infectious agent. Causative agents and means of bacterial spread are listed in Table 15-2.

HISTORY

Symptoms.   Cough, sputum production, dyspnea, and fever all are hallmarks of acute pneumonia.

General
Fever with or without chills, general malaise.

In the form of pneumonia termed *chronic pneumonia*, constitutional symptoms including fever, chills, and malaise often are present early in the course but may disappear with chronicity. Anorexia and weight loss are common.

Any patient in a debilitated state with new or changing pulmonary symptoms such as cough, sputum production, hemoptysis, chest pain (often pleuritic), or dyspnea deserves careful evaluation. Chest film may or may not be helpful, and often CT of the chest is required. On physical examination, wheezing is common, and sputum production is often too scant for usual Gram stain and culture. Treatment is directed at the underlying pathogen, and empirical treatment is NOT recommended. The most common etiologic disorders include tuberculosis, human immunodeficiency virus (HIV) infection, and alcoholism with aspiration.

Age
Any, more prominent in the very young and elderly.
  In infants: Viral etiology is most common.
  In young adults: *Mycoplasma pneumoniae* is the most common pathogen.
  In adults: *Streptococcus pneumoniae* is most frequent cause.

Onset
Typical Pneumonia.   Abrupt, with high fever (temperature greater than 38.3° C [101° F]), chills, and purulent sputum production.

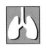

Table 15–2. Common Pathogens in Pneumonia

Type of Pneumonia	Agent	Pathogen	Signs/Symptoms/Circumstances
Nosocomial	Bacterial	*Staphylococcus aureus*	Hematogenous spread
		Gram-negatives	Leukopenia, hypotension
Community-acquired			
Typical	Bacterial	*Streptococcus pneumoniae*	Rusty sputum, high WBC count
		Haemophilus influenzae	URI, nausea, vomiting
Atypical	Mycoplasmal	*Mycoplasma pneumoniae*	Headache, dry cough
	Chlamydial	*Chlamydia trachomatis*	ST, hoarseness, dry cough
	Viral	Influenza virus, adenovirus	Rhinitis, pharyngitis, cough

ST, sore throat; URI, upper respiratory infection; WBC, white blood cell.

Atypical Pneumonia. Insidious onset with fever, headache, hacking cough, and scant sputum.

Duration. Usually 1 to 2 weeks.
Intensity. Mild to life-threatening.
Aggravating Factors. Aspiration of gastric fluids, preexisting infection, comorbid disease (congestive heart failure, diabetes mellitus, HIV infection).
Alleviating Factors. Appropriate therapeutics and symptomatic treatment.

Associated Factors

Alcoholism. Increased risk for infection due to *Klebsiella, S. pneumoniae*, or *Haemophilus influenzae*. increased risk of aspiration.

Aspiration. Altered mental status, intoxication, intubation, seizure, stroke all increase risk of aspiration. Increased risk for infection by gram-negative organisms and anerobes.

Chronic Obstructive Pulmonary Disease (COPD)/Smoking. Increased risk for infection due to *S. pneumoniae, H. influenzae, Legionella, Moraxella*, and *Chlamydia.*

Cystic Fibrosis. Increased risk for infection due to *Pseudomonas* and *Staphylococcus aureus.*

Diabetes. Increased risk for *S. aureus, Klebsiella, Mycobacterium tuberculosis* infection.

Immunocompromised States. *Pneumocystis carinii* pneumonia (PCP), infection due to cytomegalovirus, *Mycobacterium avium* complex (MAC), *Legionella*, gram-negative organisms, or fungi.

Intravenous Drug Abuse. Increased risk for *S. aureus* infection.

Nosocomial Infections. Members of family Enterobacteriaceae, *Pseudomonas aeruginosa*, and *S. aureus* are the most common prominent pathogens. *S. aureus* is often resistant to methicillin (methicillin-resistant *S. aureus* = MRSA) or to both vancomycin and methicillin (VRMRSA).

Post–Viral Bronchitis. Increased risk for infection due to *S. pneumoniae*, rarely *S. aureus.*

PHYSICAL EXAMINATION

General. Fever is usually present and may be intermittent or sustained. Hypotension warrants close observation and further investigation.

Cardiovascular. Tachycardia is common, and heart rate commonly increases by 10 beats for each degree Celsius above normal. A relative bradycardia (lower than expected for the magnitude of fever) should suggest viral infection, mycoplasmal infection, chlamydial infection, tularemia, or infection with *Legionella* spp.

Extremities. Presence of clubbing (pulmonary) or edema (cardiac) may indicate an underlying comorbid condition that could compromise treatment.

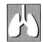

Head, Eyes, Ears, Nose, Throat.   May note findings of residual upper respiratory infection. Bullous myringitis suggests a mycoplasmal etiology.

Neurologic.   Altered mental status suggests hypoxemia, which should be aggressively addressed.

Pulmonary.   Tachypnea and accessory muscle use are ominous findings. Splinting (or an inspiratory lag on the side of the lesion) is suggestive of bacterial pneumonia. Tactile fremitus is usually increased over the area of consolidation. Adventitious breath sounds (especially crackles) with petriloloquy, bronchophony, and egophony are common overlying the involved region of the lung. Pleural friction rubs may be present intermittently.

Skin.   Cyanosis suggests severe respiratory compromise.

PATHOPHYSIOLOGY

Pneumonia develops when host defenses are insufficient to meet the level of infectious agent presented to the lungs. Bacterial challenges occur with aspiration of contaminated oropharyngeal secretions, inhalation of microorganisms, or hematogenous spread of bacteria from extrapulmonary infections, and occasionally by direct extension into the lungs. Host defenses include the upper airway anatomy, cough reflex, mucociliary clearance, phagocytosis by polymorphonuclear neutrophils (leukocytes) (PMNs) along with alveolar macrophages, and immune response at both the cellular and humoral levels.

DIAGNOSTIC STUDIES

Laboratory

Complete Blood Count.   White blood cells (WBCs) are generally increased in bacterial pneumonia, normal in atypical pneumonia, and decreased in viral pneumonia.

Arterial Blood Gas Analysis.   Variable.

Sputum Gram Stain and Cultures.   Mainstay of identification of pathogenic organisms, but with frequent false positives (normal flora) and false negatives. Sample is adequate for use if there are greater than 25 PMNs and fewer than 10 epithelial cells per low-power field.

Other Cultures.   Samples should be collected before the initiation of antibiotic therapy whenever possible. Two sets of blood cultures (for aerobic and anaerobic organisms) should be obtained from two different sites. Culture pleural fluid if applicable.

Acid-Fast Stain for Mycobacteria.   Modified acid-fast stain for *Nocardia*. Potassium hydroxide (KOH) preparation for identification of fungi. Methenamine silver sputum stain for *Pneumocystis carinii*.

Serology: Antigen/Antibody Assays.   May establish a diagnosis of infection with *Streptococcus pneumoniae*, *Haemophilus influenzae*, *Pseudomonas*,

P. carinii, *Mycoplasma*, *Legionella*, influenza virus, respiratory syncytial virus (RSV), and *Chlamydia*.

Polymerase Chain Reaction (PCR) Assay. Available for *Legionella*, *Mycoplama pneumoniae*, *Chlamydia pneumoniae*, cytomegalovirus, and *P. carinii*.

Radiology
Chest Film. Helpful to rule out associated pneumothorax, pleural effusion, empyema, or abscess. Findings are highly variable depending on organism and host defenses (see Table 15-3).

Other
Skin Tests. May help in diagnosis of tuberculosis or coccidioidomycosis.
Bronchoscopy, Bronchoalveolar Lavage (BAL), or Transtracheal Aspiration. May be needed to obtain adequate sputum specimen in critically ill patients with pneumonic processes refractory to therapy.
Open Lung Biopsy. Reserved for those patients in whom empirical therapy has failed and less invasive diagnostic procedures have been exhausted.

DIFFERENTIAL DIAGNOSIS

Infectious
Tuberculosis. Differentiated by demonstration of acid-fast bacilli in sputum and positive purified protein derivative (PPD) skin test.
Lung Abscess. Cavitary lesion on chest film or chest CT scan.
Inhalation Anthrax. Prodrome—influenza-like illness. High fever, hypotension, and hemoptysis may be present. Chest film shows widened mediastinum; peripheral blood smear with gram-positive bacilli. Prophylaxis constitutes most effective approach to management.
Numerous Pneumoconioses. Environmental and occupational history may help to identify/differentiate.

Neoplastic
Primary or Metastatic Lung Neoplasms. A mass is usually seen on chest film or chest CT scan.

Vascular
Congestive Heart Failure. Echocardiogram is diagnostic. Patient usually afebrile and may have pedal edema.

Acquired
Hypersensitivity Pneumonitis. Classically differentiated by dyspnea with nonproductive cough.

Traumatic. Not applicable.
Metabolic. Not applicable.
Congenital. Not applicable.

Table 15–3. Common Radiographic Pathogens Patterns in Pneumonia and Associated Pathogens

Pattern	Pathogen(s)
Lobar or segmental infiltrates	*Streptococcus pneumoniae, Haemophilus influenzae, Klebsiella, Escherichia coli, Legionella* spp.
Patchy or streaky opacities	*Mycoplasma pneumoniae,* viruses, *Legionella* spp., mixed anerobic/aerobic organisms
Diffuse homogeneous infiltrates	*Legionella* spp., viruses, *Pnemocystis carinii*
Nodular opacities	*Mycobacterium* spp., *Aspergillus, Candida,* organisms involved in hematogenous spread
Cavitary lesion	*Staphylococcus aureus, Klebsiella, H. influenzae,* anaerobes, *Mycobacterium tuberculosis, Aspergillus, S. pneumoniae*
Lower lobe	*Mycoplasma, Pseudomonas,* other gram-negatives

TREATMENT

General

Adequate hydration is essential. Control pleuritic chest pain with non-steroidal anti-inflammatory drugs (NSAIDs) or analgesics.

Oxygen when indicated (titrated to keep O_2 saturation greater than 90%).

Antitussives may be necessary if cough is continuous. Benzonatate 200 mg three times a day or dextromethorphan 15 mg two or three times a day may be given.

Guiafenesin 200-600 mg every 4 to 8 hours as needed may help to mobilize sputum.

Empirical Therapy

Community-Acquired Pneumonia

Patient Older Than 18 Years, Not Hospitalized
- Primary regimen:
  Azithromycin 0.5 g PO for initial dose, then 0.25 g/day OR
  Clarithromycin 500 mg twice daily OR
  Clarithromycin extended-release formulation 1 g daily
- Alternative regimen:
  Gatofloxacin 400 mg daily OR
  Levofloxacin 500 mg daily OR
  Moxifloxacin 400 mg daily OR
  Second-generation oral cephalosporin—cefdinir 300 mg OR cefpodoxime 300 mg OR cefprozil 500 mg OR cefuroxime 250-500 mg—every 12 hours OR
  Augmentin 875/125 twice daily OR
  Doxyclycline 100 mg twice daily

Note: Consider hospitalization and/or intravenous antibiotics if patient is still febrile after 72 hours of antibiotics. If patient becomes afebrile, drug course should be continued for 7 to 14 days total course.

Patient Older Than 18 Years, Hospitalized
- Primary regimen: Differs depending on whether patient is in intensive care unit (ICU).
  NON-ICU PATIENTS
  Third-generation cephalosporin—cefotaxime 2 g IV every 8 hours (2 g IV every 4 hours for severe infection) OR ceftriaxone 2 g IV daily (*in persons older than 60 years:* reduce to 1 g IV daily)—PLUS erythromycin 15-20 mg/kg/day IV in divided doses every 6 hours OR
  Azithromycin 500 mg IV on day 1, then 500 mg PO daily for 5 to 7 days OR
  Cefuroxime PLUS erythromycin OR
  Fluoroquinolone with enhanced activity against *S. pneumoniae*—alatrofloxacin 200 mg IV daily OR gatifloxacin 400 mg IV/PO

daily OR levofloxacin 500 mg IV/PO daily OR moxifloxacin 400 mg PO daily

ICU PATIENTS

Third-generation cephalosporin—cefotaxime 2 g IV every 8 hours (2 g IV every 4 hours for severe infection) OR ceftriaxone 2 g IV daily (*in persons older than 60 years*: reduce to 1 g IV daily)—PLUS azithromycin 500 mg IV daily OR

Fluoroquinolone with enhanced activity against *S. pneumoniae*—alatrofloxacin 200 mg IV daily OR gatifloxacin 400 mg IV/PO daily OR levofloxacin 500 mg IV/PO daily OR moxifloxacin 400 mg PO daily

Hospital-Acquired Pneumonia

Patient Older Than 18 Years

- Primary regimen:
  Imipenem 0.5 g IV every 6 hours OR
  Meropenem 1.0 g IV every 8 hours OR
  Piperacillin-tazobactam 3.375-4.5 g IV every 6 to 8 hours PLUS ciprofloxacin 400 mg IV every 8 hours OR
  Ticarcillin-clavulanate 3.1 g IV every 6 hours PLUS ciprofloxacin 400 mg IV every 8 hours OR
  Piperacillin-tazobactam 3.375-4.5g IV every 6 to 8 hours PLUS gentamicin 1-1.7 mg/kg IV every 8 hours OR
  Ticarcillin-clavulanate 3.1g IV every 6 hours PLUS gentamicin 1-1.7 mg/kg IV every 8 hours OR
  Cefepime, ceftazidime, OR cefoperazone PLUS an aminoglycoside (gentamicin, tobramycin, amikacin, netilmicin), with or without clindamycin or vancomycin, 1 g IV every 12 hours PLUS a fluoroquinolone

Aspiration Pneumonia

- Primary regimen:
  Clindamycin 300-900 mg IV every 6-12 hours
- Alternative regimen:
  Cefoxitin 2.0 g IV every 8 hours OR
  Ticarcillin-clavulanate 3.1 g IV every 6 hours OR
  Piperacillin-tazobactam 3.375-4.5 g IV every 6 to 8 hours OR
  Fluoroquinolone PLUS clindamycin OR high-dose penicillin G—has been effective historically

Chronic Pneumonia

Specific antibiotic therapy is determined by mechanism of infection and likely causative organism.
- Recommended regimens:

Viral

> Zanamivir 10 mg twice daily by inhalation for 5 days OR
> Oseltamivir 75 mg twice daily for 5 days

Influenza A Virus

> Rimantadine 100 mg twice daily for 3 to 5 days OR
> Amantadine 100 mg twice daily for 3 to 5 days OR
> Ribavirin aerosol treatment, with reservoir concentration 20 mg/mL: 12 to 18 hours/day for 3 to 7 days

Streptococcus Pneumoniae

> From 60% to 80% of strains are susceptible to clindamycin:
> Clindamycin 150-450 mg PO four times a day, or 300-600 mg IM or 300-900 mg IV every 6 to 12 hours
> ALTERNATIVE THERAPY: INPATIENT
> Penicillin G 1 million–2 million U IV every 4 hours for 14 days OR continuous infusion: *loading dose*: 3 million U, *then* 10 million–12 million U over 12 hours OR
> Ampicillin 2 g IV every 4 hours for 14 days OR
> Vancomycin 1 g IV every 12 hours for 14 days OR
> Fluoroquinolone for 14 days
> ALTERNATIVE THERAPY: OUTPATIENT
> Amoxicillin 500-1000 mg three times a day for 14 days OR
> Penicillin V potassium (Pen-Vee K) 500 mg four times a day for 14 days OR
> Fluoroquinolone for 14 days OR
> Cefuroxime 500 mg twice daily for 14 days

Haemophilus Influenzae

> About 35% of strains are beta-lactamase positive, with increasing resistance to trimethoprim-sulfamethoxazole (TMP-SMX) and doxycycline.
> INPATIENT THERAPY
> Cefuroxime 750 mg IV every 8 hours for 10 to 14 days OR
> Ceftriaxone 1 g IV daily for 10 to 14 days
> OUTPATIENT THERAPY
> Amoxicillin-clavulanate 875/125 mg twice daily for 10 to 14 days OR
> Macrolide—azithromycin, clarithromycin—for 10 to 14 days OR
> Oral second- or third-generation cephalosporin—cefaclor, cefprozil, cefuroxime, cefixime, ceftibutin—for 10 to 14 days OR
> Fluoroquinolone for 10 to 14 days
> *Note*: If beta-lactamase negative: Ampicillin IV, amoxicillin PO, TMP-SMX, macrolides, or doxycycline often effective.

Mycoplasma Pneumoniae

> INPATIENT THERAPY
> Macrolide treatment OR
> Doxycycline 100 mg PO/IV every 12 hours for 10 to 14 days OR
> Fluoroquinolone treatment for 10 to 14 days

OUTPATIENT THERAPY
Doxycycline 100 mg twice daily for 14 days OR
Macrolide treatment OR
Fluoroquinolone treatment

Chlamydia Pneumoniae

INPATIENT THERAPY
Macrolide treatment OR
Doxycycline 100 mg PO/IV every 12 hours for 10 to 14 days OR
Fluoroquinolone treatment for 10 to 14 days
OUTPATIENT THERAPY
Doxycycline 100 mg twice daily for 14 days OR
Macrolide treatment OR
Fluoroquinolone treatment

Legionella Pneumophila

INPATIENT THERAPY
Macrolide treatment OR
Doxycycline 100 mg PO/IV every 12 hours for 21 days OR
Fluoroquinolone treatment for 10 to 14 days
OUTPATIENT THERAPY
Macrolide treatment OR
Doxycycline 100 mg twice daily for 21 days OR
Fluoroquinolone treatment

Moraxella Catarrhalis

Approximately 93% of strains are beta-lactamase positive.
Amoxicillin-clavulanate 875/125 mg twice daily for 10 to 14 days
    OR
Macrolide—azithromycin, clarithromycin—for 10 to 14 days OR
Oral second- or third-generation cephalosporin—cefaclor, cef-
    prozil, cefuroxime, cefixime, ceftibutin—for 10 to 14 days OR
Fluoroquinolone for 10 to 14 days OR
TMP-SMX for 10 to 14 days OR
Doxycycline 100 mg twice daily for 10 to 14 days

Staphylococcus Aureus

INPATIENT THERAPY
Nafcillin 0.5-2 g IV every 4 hours for 14 days OR
Vancomycin 1 g IV every 12 hours for 14 days
OUTPATIENT THERAPY
Not recommended

HIV-infected (immunocompromised) Patients

TMP-SMX 15-20 mg/kg/day IV daily OR
Pentamadine 4 mg/kg/day IV or IM

Bacillus Anthracis

Mortality rate greater than 80% if treatment is not initiated until
    after the onset of clinical symptoms.
• Primary regimen:

Ciprofloxacin 400 mg IV every 12 hours OR levofloxacin 500 mg
IV daily; *children*: 20-30 mg/kg/day in two divided doses
- Alternative regimen:
Penicillin G 4 million U IV every 4 hours OR
Doxycycline 100 mg IV every 12 hours
Children younger than 12 years: 50,000 U/kg penicillin G IV every
6 hours
Note: Treatment is continued for 60 days.

PEDIATRIC CONSIDERATIONS

Special consideration must be given to those children with underlying pulmonary pathology (e.g., cystic fibrosis) and those with a propensity for gastroesophageal reflux. Infections in neonates and other patients with less effective immunologic defenses are decidedly different from infections occurring in otherwise healthy children. Consider the possibility of foreign body aspiration in an otherwise healthy child with recurrent lower respiratory infections.

Signs and symptoms of lower respiratory infections in infants and younger children are often nonspecific. Respiratory distress in the very young may be manifested by grunting, nasal flaring, intercostal retractions, and/or tachypnea. Cough is an unusual initial presentation but may occur later. Physical examination may be normal or reveal diminished breath sounds and crackles over the affected area. Radiographic studies do not always correspond with the clinical picture. Older children often present with symptoms similar to those more typically seen in adults.

Respiratory viruses (RSV, influenza viruses, parainfluenza virus, or adenovirus) are the most common cause of pneumonia during the first several years of life. In general, viral pneumonias are more prevalent during the winter months. Whereas bronchiolitis is the most common lower respiratory infection during the first year of life, peak incidence of viral pneumonia is between the ages of 2 and 3 years. Viral pneumonias are often preceded by upper respiratory symptoms, and frequently with associated rhinitis. Viral pneumonias are characterized by nonproductive cough and fever with temperature lower than expected with a bacterial etiology. Tachypnea and the use of accessory muscles are common, but may be normal. Chest radiographs most frequently show diffuse infiltrates but may show a more lobar pattern. Leukocytosis (greater than 20,000 cells/mm^3) may be present, with a predominance of lymphocytes on peripheral smear. Viral antigen tests are required to establish the diagnosis. Treatment includes oral amantadine or rimantadine (*age younger than 10*: 5 mg/kg/day, maximum 150 mg/day; *age 10 and older*: 100 mg twice daily) in the treatment of influenza A. Aerosolized ribavirin for 2 to 5 days is used in the treatment of RSV infection.

RSV prophylaxis for children less than 2 years of age with chronic pulmonary disease and/or born prematurely (earlier than 28 weeks' gestation) includes: RSV immune globulin (RespiGam) IV monthly over 6 hours at 750 mg/kg IV infusion OR palivizumab (Synagis) 15 mg/kg IM monthly; start either drug at the beginning of RSV season. May continue for up to one year.

Mycoplasma pneumoniae is the most common pathogen in school-aged and older children. Infection due to this organism is rarely seen in infants but occasionally seen in pre–school-aged children. Peak incidence occurs autumn to early winter. Onset of symptoms is gradual; the infection usually is characterized by headache, scratchy sore throat, and low-grade fever with progression to lower respiratory symptoms including hoarseness and a dry cough. The cough frequently worsens over 1 to 2 weeks and then gradually diminishes over the next 3 to 4 weeks. The fever intensifies, cough becomes worse, and dyspnea may occur as the disease worsens. Physical examination most frequently reveals fine crackles. Radiographic findings are often non-specific but most frequently include interstitial involvement of the lower lobes. Treatment is with clarithromycin (15 mg/kg/24 hours in two divided doses for 10 days) or azithromycin (10 mg/kg on day 1, then 5 mg/kg/24 hours on days 2 to 5).

Although bacteria are less frequent pathogens, they are responsible for more severe infections than those caused by the nonbacterial agents. Pneumococci account for over 90% of childhood cases of bacterial pneumonia, followed by *Streptococcus pyogenes*, and *S. aureus*. Incidence of *H. influenzae* infection has decreased with the availability of effective vaccines. Often there is a 3- to 5-day history of an upper respiratory illness followed by abrupt onset of high fever, restlessness, apprehension, and respiratory distress. Children may splint movement on the affected side to minimize pleuritic pain and improve ventilation. Physical examination findings are variable, with dullness to percussion, diminished vocal and tactile fremitus, and bronchial breath sounds, wheezing, or crackles. Diagnosis is by appropriate bacteriologic studies. A leukocytosis (15,000-40,000 cells/mm^3) with a preponderance of polymorphonuclear cells is usually found. Radiographic findings most often include a lobar consolidation in older children, but are variable in younger children. Treatment is with penicillin G (100,000 units/kg/24 hours), cefotaxime (50 mg/kg every 6 to 8 hours IV or IM), or ceftriaxone (50 to 75 mg/kg/day divided every 12-24 hours). If the organism is found to be resistant to penicillin and cephalosporins, vancomycin (10 mg/kg IV every 6 hours) should be used.

Neonates and infants should be hospitalized for fluid resuscitation and intravenous antibiotics. Most children beyond infancy can be managed as outpatients. Most children recover rapidly and completely. From 30% to 50% of infants will have recurrent wheezing throughout their infancy following an infection with RSV. Premature infants and those with underlying lung disease may be candidates for prophylactic ribavirin.

OBSTETRIC CONSIDERATIONS

Pneumonia is the most common nonobstetric infection to cause maternal mortality in the peripartum period. Pneumonia can complicate pregnancy at

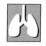

any time during gestation and may be associated with preterm birth, poor fetal growth, and perinatal loss. Although usually no pathogen is identified, the pneumococcus is the most frequently identified causative agent, followed by *H. influenzae*. Viral pneumonias may be complicated by a superimposed bacterial infection.

The antibiotic of choice is intravenous penicillin G until the patient is afebrile for 48 hours and demonstrates signs of clinical improvement. At that point an oral cephalosporin can be started and continued for a total treatment time of 10 to 14 days. Oxygen supplementation should be considered to maintain the Po_2 at 90 mm Hg to ensure adequate fetal oxygenation. Positioning the patient in the left lateral recumbent position may also improve uteroplacental perfusion and thus fetal oxygenation.

Viral pneumonias are common in pregnancy; therefore, influenza vaccine should be routinely given to pregnant patients beyond their first trimester. Once a viral infection is established, use of antiviral agents such as amantadine and ribavirin can be considered. Of special note is varicella pneumonia in pregnancy. Women in their third trimester are at increased risk of developing this pneumonia following a skin infection with the same virus. Varicella pneumonia carries an increased mortality rate (up to 40%) in pregnant patients; early and aggressive treatment with acyclovir is indicated.

GERIATRIC CONSIDERATIONS

Both an increased incidence and higher mortality rate are seen with pneumonia in elderly patients. These patients often do not present with typical symptoms; they may be afebrile and often have no cough on presentation as a result of the immunocompromised state that is associated with advanced age. Older patients develop dyspnea significantly later in their disease process than do younger patients.

Consider the age of the patient when initiating empirical drug therapy. Elderly patients are at increased risk for pneumococcal pneumonia and aspiration pneumonia. Fourteen percent of new tuberculosis cases occur in the over-65 population.

Patients who are older than 65 who received pneumococcal vaccination 6 or more years earlier should be considered for re-vaccination.

PREVENTIVE CONSIDERATIONS

Pneumococcal vaccine should be considered for all patients who are immunocompromised, who have underlying lung pathology, or who have comorbid conditions that may be affected by the development of pneumonia.

PEARLS FOR THE PA

Administration of monovalent pneumococcal vaccine may prevent or decrease the severity of pneumococcal infections in immunocompromised patients. Vaccination is recommended in the following groups of adult patients:

1. *Patients with chronic illnesses that lead to increased morbidity from respiratory infections*

2. *Patients with underlying illnesses or conditions associated with increased risk of pneumococcal disease (e.g., asplenism, Hodgkin disease)*

3. *Patients older than 65 years of age*

4. *Patients older than 65 whose last vaccination was received 6 or more years previously; "booster" vaccination recommended*

Pneumothorax

Judith E. Colver, MMS, PA-C

DEFINITION

Pneumothorax (PTX) is defined as the accumulation of air in the pleural space. It is present in up to half of all patients with transpleural penetrating injuries. It may also occur spontaneously or in concert with underlying pulmonary disease. Iatrogenic PTX occurs as a complication of therapeutic or diagnostic procedures.

PTX can be divided into three classifications: simple, communicating, and tension. *Simple* PTX occurs when there is no communication with the outside atmosphere and there is no shift in the mediastinum or hemidiaphragm. Simple PTXs can be further classified by the degree of collapse as either small (15% or less), moderate (15% to 60%), or large (greater than 60%). *Communicating* PTX is most often associated with a penetrating injury of the chest wall. The loss of chest wall integrity results in lung collapse on inspiration and slight expansion on expiration. This produces a significant loss of ventilation of the involved lung and often results in a severe ventilatory disturbance.

A *tension* PTX follows pulmonary injury in which there is progressive accumulation of air within the pleural cavity, causing a shift of the mediastinum away from the involved lung, with compression of the contralateral lung and vasculature. It occurs when the injured tissue acts as a one-way valve, allowing air to enter the pleural cavity on inspiration but preventing it from leaving on expiration. Tension PTX is a medical emergency and leads to rapid onset of hypoxia and shock.

HISTORY

Symptoms. Dyspnea and chest pain on the affected side are the most common complaints. Pain may radiate to the ipsilateral scapular area or shoulder. Cough may be present.

General. Patient appearance is highly variable ranging from acutely ill with cyanosis and tachypnea to misleadingly healthy. Patients prone to spontaneous PTX tend to be tall and thin. History of smoking is common. Patients may have a history of trauma, underlying pulmonary disease (e.g., asthma, chronic obstructive pulmonary disease [COPD]), prior invasive procedure, or infection.

Age. Spontaneous PTX is more common in persons older than 20 years of age. Traumatic PTX may occur at any age.

Onset. Usually acute, but may be gradual.

Duration. Usually short.

Intensity. Often severe to life-threatening. May be mild and slowly progressive.

Aggravating Factors. Smoking and ectomorphic body habitus, primarily in spontaneous PTX. There is some familial occurrence, and a history of spontaneous PTX puts a patient at increased risk of subsequent PTX.

Alleviating Factors. None.

Associated Factors. Obstructive lung disease, interstitial lung disease, neoplasm, infectious disease, penetrating chest trauma.

PHYSICAL EXAMINATION

General. Patient may be febrile, is frequently anxious and tachypneic. Hypotension or cyanosis may indicate a tension PTX.

Cardiovascular. Tachycardia (heart rate greater than 100 beats/minute); suspect tension pneumothorax with heart rate greater than 140 beats/minute.

Head, Eyes, Ears, Nose, Throat. Jugular venous distention indicates compromised venous return to the right side of the heart. Trachea may be deviated (away from the affected side) in tension PTX.

Pulmonary. Tachypnea, with reduced respiratory excursion on the affected side. Hyperresonant to percussion with absent tactile fremitus and decreased to absent breath sounds. Occasionally a pleural friction rub may be present. With smaller PTXs, examination may be normal.

Skin. Cyanosis is late finding. Occasionally, subcutaneous emphysema may be present.

PATHOPHYSIOLOGY

Any condition that results in rupture or tear of the visceral pleura with the subsequent accumulation of air in the pleural space. In primary spontaneous PTX, the most common mechanism is rupture of pleural blebs, allowing air to escape from the lung parenchyma into the pleural space. Secondary spontaneous PTX occurs when air dissects in a retrograde fashion along the bronchovascular structures to the hilum, where a rupture occurs or pneumomediastinum forms.

Tension PTX occurs most frequently following penetrating thoracic trauma. Occasionally, a unidirectional valve forms at the interface of the parenchymal air space and the pleural air space, allowing air to enter the pleural cavity on inspiration and prohibiting it from being removed on expiration.

DIAGNOSTIC STUDIES

Laboratory
Arterial Blood Gas Analysis.   Often reveals hypoxia (Pao_2 less than 55 mm Hg).

Radiology
Chest Film.   Presence of a visceral pleural line on chest radiograph is diagnostic. In equivocal cases, lateral decubitus films obtained with the patient placed on the contralateral side may facilitate the diagnosis. Expiratory films are no more sensitive than inspiratory films and are not recommended. Occasionally a small pleural effusion is present on the ipsilateral side.

DIFFERENTIAL DIAGNOSIS

Traumatic
Chest Wall Injury.   History of trauma or evidence of trauma will be obtained.

Infectious
Tuberculosis or Lung Abscess.   Chest film and chest CT appearances differ.

Neoplastic
Primary or Metastatic Neoplasm.   Mass seen on chest film or chest CT.

Vascular
Pulmonary Embolism.   Acute onset of dyspnea and chest pain (often pleuritic) with a normal chest film.

Metabolic
Congenital.   Not applicable.
Acquired.   Not applicable.

TREATMENT

Treatment is determined by the size of the PTX and clinical symptoms.

Tension PTX is a medical emergency. Insertion of a large-bore needle (18 gauge or larger) in the second anterior intercostal space at the midclavicular line on the side opposite the tracheal deviation may provide relief of dyspnea and time to perform a tube thoracostomy.

With small PTX, if few symptoms are apparent, the patient can be observed. Spontaneous resolution is common. In some cases, the pleural air can be aspirated using a large-bore needle and syringe.

With large PTX or significant symptoms, the pleural air is aspirated with a needle, catheter, or thoracostomy tube.

With recurrent spontaneous PTX, pleurodesis may be accomplished via tube thoracostomy by instillation of a sclerosing agent (most commonly tetracycline) to induce adhesions between the visceral and parietal pleura. In some cases, open thoracostomy and oversewing or stapling of the pulmonary blebs and/or pleural abrasion may be required.

PEDIATRIC CONSIDERATIONS

PTX in the pediatric population is uncommon beyond the neonatal period. Asymptomatic PTX occurs in a small number of newborns (1% to 2%) and is more common in males and in term or post-term infants. Incidence is increased in those infants with underlying lung disease (hyaline membrane disease, meconium aspiration) and following vigorous resuscitation or assisted ventilation. The most common cause is over-inflation, with resultant rupture of alveoli. The findings in asymptomatic PTX are hyperresonance over the affected lung and decreased breath sounds.

Irritability and restlessness or apnea may be the earliest signs of symptomatic PTX. The chest may appear asymmetrical with increased anteroposterior diameter on the affected side and occasionally with bulging of the intercostal spaces. Bilateral PTX occurs in up to 10% of cases, so findings of a symmetrical chest do not rule out PTX. Twenty-five percent of infants with PTX will have a coexisting pneumomediastinum, but it is usually asymptomatic. PTX should be suspected in any infant who shows signs of respiratory distress, who is restless or irritable, or who has a sudden change in condition. Transillumination of the thorax may provide clues, with the affected side transmitting excessive light. Diagnosis is by characteristic radiographic findings.

In older children, pneumothorax is most often associated with thoracic trauma or surgical procedures but can occur with underlying lung disease (asthma, cystic fibrosis, pneumonia), bronchopleural fistula, foreign bodies in the lung, or rupture of a pseudocyst. PTX may also occur in patients with lymphoma or other malignancy. Spontaneous PTX may occur in teenagers and young adults with ectomorphic body habitus.

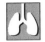

OBSTETRIC CONSIDERATIONS

Management of PTX in the obstetric patient is the same as in the nonobstetric patient.

GERIATRIC CONSIDERATIONS

Emphysematous patients are at increased risk of developing spontaneous pneumothorax when blebs rupture.

PREVENTIVE CONSIDERATIONS

Observing the usual precautions with insertion of a central line will reduce the incidence of iatrogenic pneumothorax.

PEARLS FOR THE PA

The classic patient presenting with a primary spontaneous pneumothorax is a tall, thin, white male smoker.

Chest film is the key to diagnosis.

Pulmonary Embolism

Judith E. Colver, MMS, PA-C

DEFINITION

Obstruction of the pulmonary arterial circulation by thrombus or embolus of foreign material that usually has traveled from a systemic vein. Pulmonary embolism (PE) is the most common acute pulmonary disorder among hospitalized patients in the United States.

HISTORY

Symptoms. Acute onset of severe dyspnea and pleuritic chest pain, with or without hemoptysis, cough, fever, diaphoresis, or syncope.

General. Must be considered in the differential diagnosis in any patient with acute onset of chest pain, dyspnea, tachycardia, or tachypnea. Patient may have a history or physical finding of calf pain or swelling.

Age. Any, more common in adulthood.

Onset. Abrupt.

Duration. Usually of short duration, may become chronic.

Intensity. Mild to rapidly fatal.

Aggravating Factors. Limb immobilization, recent surgery, obesity, trauma, coagulopathies, pregnancy, underlying malignancy, cardiac disease, age older than 60 years, use of estrogen or oral contraceptives, smoking.

Alleviating Factors. Prophylactic treatment is indicated in selected patients.

Associated Factors. High-risk patients include those with chronic obstructive pulmonary disease (COPD), diabetes mellitus, hematologic disease, or traumatic injury to or recent surgery involving the lower extremities or pelvis. Persons with deficiencies in protein C or protein S also are at high risk.

PHYSICAL EXAMINATION

General. Wide range of presentations, from mild dyspnea to severe distress with diaphoresis. Hemoptysis is often present.

Cardiovascular. Tachycardia is common. Auscultation may reveal an increased pulmonic component of the second heart sound (P_2), right-sided S_4, or right ventricular heave suggesting acute right ventricular overload. Fixed splitting of the second heart sound is an ominous finding.

Extremities. May reveal evidence of thrombophlebitis including tenderness, swelling, or a venous cord. Homan sign (calf pain with flexion of the knee and dorsiflexion of the ankle) or Moses sign (pain with calf compression against the tibia), may be present, but these are nonspecific findings.

Head, Eyes, Ears, Nose, Throat. Jugular venous distention if right-sided heart failure is present.

Pulmonary. Tachypnea is most common finding. Findings on auscultation are usually normal but may include a transient pleural friction rub or localized wheezing or fine crackles.

Skin. Often diaphoretic acutely; may become cyanotic with significant ventilation-perfusion abnormality.

PATHOPHYSIOLOGY

Under normal conditions, tiny aggregates of red cells, platelets, and fibrin (also known as microthrombi) are continually formed and lysed within the venous system. Under pathologic conditions, microthrombi may escape the normal fibrinolytic activity and propagate larger thrombi. When fragments of a thrombus break loose and lodge in the pulmonary arterial tree, perfusion defects occur. If a significantly large fraction of the vasculature is occluded, right-sided heart failure and hemodynamic collapse will ensue.

Embolic obstruction of a pulmonary artery is followed by three primary events: alveolar dead space is created; pneumoconstriction occurs in the lung

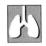

distal to the obstruction, further reducing the size of the ventilated area; and alveolar surfactant activity declines, resulting in the collapse of the alveoli and regional atelectasis. As a consequence of these events, arterial hypoxemia occurs. Ventilation-perfusion mismatch, intrapulmonary shunting of mixed venous blood, alveolar hypoventilation, and preexistent cardiopulmonary disease further contribute to the hypoxemia. A rare consequence of the embolic event is infarction of the pulmonary parenchyma.

DIAGNOSTIC STUDIES

Laboratory
Complete Blood Count.   Hemoglobin and hematocrit are usually normal, but the presence of polycythemia puts the patient at high risk of embolism. Clotting function is normal in most cases.

Screening Tests for Protein C, Protein S, Lupus Anticoagulant, Antithrombin III Deficiency, and Factor V Leiden.   May be helpful in identifying important risk factors if coagulopathy is suspected.

Arterial Blood Gas Analysis.   This study has no predictive value regarding clinical outcome. However, most patients will exhibit a respiratory alkalosis, and PaO_2 is 80 mm Hg or less in most cases.

Alveolar-Arterial (A–a) Gradient.   Value greater than 10 mmHg is suggestive but not diagnostic of PE.

Radiology
Chest Film.   Frequently normal. Atelectasis or elevation of a hemidiaphragm may occur. Pleural effusion may also be seen. Although rare, the classic wedge-shaped density of pulmonary infarction (Hampton hump) and the hypovascularity distal to the embolus (Westermark sign) may be seen. When found, these may be the earliest radiographic manifestations of PE.

Other
ECG.   The most common ECG abnormalities seen in PE are tachycardia and nonspecific ST segment and T wave abnormalities. ECG abnormalities for PE are related to right-sided heart strain: tall peaked P wave in lead II (P pulmonale), right axis deviation, right bundle branch block, atrial fibrillation, and S_1-Q_3-T_3 pattern (large S wave in lead I, deep Q wave in lead III, inverted T wave in lead III).

Echocardiography.   Should be considered in patients with suspected PE. The presence of right-sided heart strain from PE is a strong predictor of mortality. Early fibrinolysis can reduce the mortality rate by 50%; therefore, positive echocardiographic findings should prompt consideration for immediate fibrinolysis.

Transesophageal Echocardiography (TEE).   Can reveal thrombus in the central pulmonary arteries. Although TEE is specific, it is too insensitive to use as a screening tool.

Radionuclide Lung Scan (Ventilation-Perfusion [V|Q] Scan). V/Q scans remain in the diagnostic tree despite the fact that most patients will have nondiagnostic scans. A normal perfusion pattern means that the patient has less than a 5% chance that PE will be identified if angiography is performed. An abnormal but nondiagnostic pattern means that the patient has a 15% to 85% likelihood that PE will be found on angiography. A high-probability pattern means that the patient has an 85% or greater likelihood that PE will be found at angiography.

Pulmonary Angiography. The "gold standard" diagnostic test for PE. Finding of an intraluminal defect or arterial cutoff is diagnostic. Angiography may falsely diagnose PE in the presence of an intraluminal tumor or an extrinsic mass, and it may be falsely negative when thrombus is small and distal. It is indicated for patients with contraindications to anticoagulation, patients being considered for embolectomy, and patients with suspected recurrent PE despite adequate anticoagulation.

Chest CT/MRI. Spiral (helical) CT scans, CT angiography (CTA), and MRI are growing in use and popularity. As interpretation is refined, it seems likely that they will replace the V/Q scan and angiography in the diagnosis of PE.

Lower Extremity Venous Studies. Because the most common source of PE is the deep veins of the lower extremities, venous studies may reveal the source of the thrombus. Doppler ultrasound is currently the study of choice. However, lower extremity venograms are still in use in some institutions.

DIFFERENTIAL DIAGNOSIS

Traumatic
Pneumothorax. Collapsed lung on chest film.

Infectious
Pneumonia. Usually with productive cough, leukocytosis, and infiltrate on chest film.

Pleuritis. Usually without dyspnea of acute onset; may have fever and other systemic signs. Frequently pulmonary effusion seen on chest film.

Neoplastic
Primary or Metastatic Lung Neoplasm. Usually mass is evident on chest film or chest CT scan.

Vascular
Acute Myocardial Infarction. Usually with diagnostic ECG changes; elevated cardiac enzymes.

Valvular Heart Disease. Rarely, acute onset; echocardiogram is diagnostic test of choice.

Acquired
Chronic Obstructive Pulmonary Disease (COPD). Usually a more chronic presentation with acute exacerbations. May coexist with or be complicated by PE.

Metabolic
Not applicable.

Congenital
Not applicable.

TREATMENT

Treatment is largely supportive and symptomatic initially. Morphine (10-15 mg IV or IM every 4 hours) can be given for pain control and relief of apprehension. Oxygen (titrate to keep O_2 saturation greater than 90%) is given to prevent worsening hypoxemia and may be helpful as a pulmonary vasodilator. Shock must be managed with inotropic or pressor agents and with fluid resuscitation (if indicated) until fibrinolytic therapy is instituted or surgical intervention can be done.

Anticoagulation with heparin by continuous intravenous infusion for at least 5 days, starting with 5000 U bolus followed by hourly dose of approximately 1000 U adjusted to keep activated partial thromboplastin time (PTT) at 1.5 to 2.0 times the control is the regimen of choice. Heparin does not dissolve the thrombus; it inhibits the action of thrombin and decreases the formation of new thrombi. After initial anticoagulation with heparin, long-term therapy may be changed to oral warfarin. Therapy with warfarin should be started on day 1 or 2 and given in doses to prolong the prothrombin time to 1.3 to 1.5 times the control or to achieve an international normalized ratio (INR) of 2.0 to 3.0. Therapy should be maintained for 6 months or longer; chronic therapy may be required in patients with recurrent episodes.

Low-molecular-weight heparin (LMWH) is rapidly replacing unfractionated heparin. It is easier to administer and is more effective for prophylaxis of deep vein thrombosis (DVT) and in the treatment of PE. LMWH has the added advantage of a lower incidence of bleeding complications. It is not necessary to monitor the PTT with use of LMWH, as even patients with full anticoagulation may have a normal PTT level. Enoxaparin is administered by subcutaneous injection. The adult dose is 1 mg/kg subcutaneously every 12 hours or 1.5 mg/kg as a single subcutaneous injection every 24 hours. Dalteparin and ardeparin are indicated for DVT prophylaxis.

Thrombolytic agents are the treatment of choice in massive PE that leaves the patient hemodynamically unstable and when there are no contraindications to their use. Compared with anticoagulation alone, lytic therapy produces more rapid and complete clot resolution, relieves symptoms better, and is more effective in reducing recurrence of DVT and PE. Alteplase is administered as 100 mg intravenously as a continuous infusion over 2 hours. Heparin is then initiated immediately following completion of lytic therapy. Streptokinase may be used in a loading dose of 250,000 U intravenously over 30 minutes with a maintenance dose of 100,000 U/hour for 24 to 72 hours.

Vena cava interruption may be indicated to limit reembolization in patients who have contraindications to anticoagulation or in patients with recurrent emboli despite adequate anticoagulation.

Surgical embolectomy is reserved for patients with severe cardiac or pulmonary compromise who are not candidates for fibrinolysis, or in whom fibrinolytic therapy has failed.

PEDIATRIC CONSIDERATIONS

Pulmonary embolism is rare in infants and children. Most often, thrombi arise from the femoral or pelvic veins in response to venous stasis or trauma. Thrombus formation is occasionally seen in the postoperative patient, and embolization may occur following spinal cord injury or in the case of severe burns. Emboli can occur in newborns with congenital heart defects or in those born to diabetic mothers. Asphyxia and subsequent respiratory distress may also predispose the neonate to formation of pulmonary emboli.

Pulmonary emboli can occasionally occur as a complication of sickle cell anemia, rheumatic fever, bacterial endocarditis, cyanotic heart disease, ventriculoatrial shunts used in the treatment of hydrocephalus, severe dehydration in acute diarrheal disease, and in longstanding nutritional deficiencies. Fat embolism from the fracture of a long bone may also cause PE.

OBSTETRIC CONSIDERATIONS

Pulmonary embolism is the leading cause of maternal mortality and is usually the result of amniotic fluid embolism or, less frequently, thromboembolic events. The risk for thromboembolism is increased during pregnancy. There is an increased risk in the puerperal period, particularly after delivery by cesarean section. Thrombophlebitis in pregnancy is treated with LMWH (enoxaparin) and continued after delivery. Enoxaparin is cleared more rapidly during pregnancy, so twice-daily dosing may be needed. Heparin still has some use in pregnancy; dosage is 5000 units subcutaneously every 8 to 12 hours. Warfarin is contraindicated in pregnancy owing to its teratogenic effects.

GERIATRIC CONSIDERATIONS

Elderly patients are at increased risk of developing pulmonary embolism because of underlying arrhythmias, congestive heart failure, sedentary lifestyle, and venous stasis. There is increasing evidence that some elderly people may have a hypercoagulable state.

PREVENTIVE CONSIDERATIONS

Early identification and treatment of thrombophlebitis may reduce the incidence of pulmonary embolism.

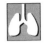

PEARLS FOR THE PA

Perioperative prophylaxis of deep vein thrombosis is helpful in preventing PE.

Intermittent pneumatic compression boots or gradient elastic stockings used intraoperatively may help reduce thrombus formation. LMWH has become the agent of choice for prophylaxis of PE (enoxaparin 30 mg given subcutaneously) and should be started no later than 12 to 24 hours postoperatively and continued for 12 to 14 days.

Sleep Apnea

Judith E. Colver, MMS, PA-C

DEFINITION

Sleep apnea is the cessation of airflow at the nose and mouth during sleep. There are two main kinds of sleep apnea: obstructive and central. In *obstructive sleep apnea* (OSA) *syndrome*, airflow ceases because of an occlusion of the upper airway. Often, respiratory effort is present without airflow. *Central sleep apnea* (CSA) *syndrome* occurs when the central drive to the respiratory muscles is temporarily abolished. In this case, there is no airflow and no respiratory effort. Other disorders that are considered subtypes of OSA include obesity hypoventilation syndrome (OHS), an overlap syndrome of OSA with chronic obstructive pulmonary disease (COPD), and upper airway resistance syndrome (UARS).

HISTORY

Symptoms. May be present during sleep or in the waking state. Often with a history of nasal obstruction or congestion, hypertension, or recent weight gain.

Nocturnal. Snoring that is irregular and interrupted by silences and/or snorting, restless sleep, choking or gasping, somnambulism, enuresis, night sweats, or nocturia.

Waking. Excessive sleepiness, personality changes (e.g. depression), impotence, morning headaches, impaired cognitive skills, especially memory.

General. Predisposing factors include male gender, advancing age, alcohol or sedative-hypnotic use, obesity, hypothyroidism, and acromegaly. Sleep apnea affects 1% to 4% of the adult population.

Age. Onset during the fourth decade of life, with increasing incidence with age.

Onset. Gradual over months to years.

Duration. Slowly progressive.

Intensity. Can become life-threatening.

Aggravating Factors. Alcohol, sedative-hypnotics.

Alleviating Factors. Treatment of the underlying cause, if applicable.

Associated Factors. Obesity, advancing age.

PHYSICAL EXAMINATION

General. Sixty percent of patients with OAS are overweight (body mass index [BMI] greater than 20% over ideal). May have systemic hypertension. May be cyanotic with severe apnea.

Cardiovascular. Evaluate for congestive heart failure (CHF). Nocturnal hypoxia may cause CHF, or underlying CHF can be worsened with the onset of apnea.

Head, Eyes, Ears, Nose, Throat. Careful examination of the nares for evidence of polyps, deviated septum, or other obstruction. Inspect the oral cavity for redundant pharyngeal tissue, retrognathia, micrognathia, or macroglossia. Affected patients often have short, thick necks. Evaluate the thyroid gland for goiter. Auscultate for carotid bruit. Evaluate for jugular venous distention (JVD), which may be present if there is associated CHF.

Genitourinary. Usually not involved, although nocturia and enuresis are a part of the sleep apnea syndrome.

Neurologic. Neuropsychiatric manifestations include intellectual impairment, memory loss, poor judgment, and personality changes. Patients may also have mental "fogginess" or disorientation and early morning headache. Depression is common.

Pulmonary. Auscultate for rhonchi or crackles that might indicate an underlying pulmonary disease.

Skin. Occasionally cyanotic with severe apnea.

PATHOPHYSIOLOGY

Asphyxia develops as a result of the apnea. Chronic, intermittent asphyxia is responsible for cardiovascular changes. Systemic blood pressure rises during the apneic period as a result of sympathetic activation and reflex vasoconstriction. Chronic hypertension is found in 50% of sleep apnea patients, probably related to excessive sympathetic activation and elevated plasma norepinephrine concentrations. There is also evidence that sleep apnea may affect left ventricular function. Acutely, the increased negative intrathoracic pressure reduces stroke volume and cardiac output by increasing left ventricular afterload and reducing preload. Intermittent hypoxia during apnea may impede right ventricular emptying and lower the relaxation rate of both ventricles. Hypoxia may also contribute to the elevation of systemic blood pressure by stimulating the sympathetic nervous system. In OSA, 10% to 15% of patients develop persistent pulmonary hypertension and right-sided heart failure, usually the result of daytime hypoxemia and hypercapnia along with severe nocturnal desaturation.

From 10% to 15% of patients with OSA will develop chronic hypercapnia. The combination of obesity, right-sided heart failure, and daytime sleepiness used to be termed "pickwickian syndrome." This pathologic condition is now more appropriately referred to as OHS.

DIAGNOSTIC STUDIES

Laboratory
Complete Blood Count. May help rule out polycythemia secondary to hypoxia.

Thyroid Function Tests. As indicated to rule out underlying hypothyroidism.

Arterial Blood Gas (ABG) Analysis. Most patients have will exhibit hypoxia during sleep but have normal ABG values during waking hours. The exception is the patient with OHS, who may have daytime hypoxia and hypercarbia. Daytime hypoxia alone is usually only seen in those patients who have daytime pulmonary hypertension and right-sided heart failure.

Radiology
Chest Film. Usually normal; some patients will have cardiomegaly.

CT of the Upper Airway. May reveal reductions in oropharyngeal size.

Other
ECG. Persistent arrhythmias (sinus, atrial, or ventricular) and heart block (all types) are common with sleep apnea.

Sleep Logs. A log of daily wake and sleep activities divided into 30- or 60-minute intervals over a 2-week period. Inexpensive screening tool, but may be unreliable, as it is dependent on self-reporting by the patient.

Overnight Oxygen Saturation. Arterial oxygen saturation (SaO_2) with or without transcutaneous CO_2 monitoring is helpful as a screening test, but nondiagnostic.

Overnight Holter Monitoring. Helpful in assessing arrhythmias associated with apnea.

Polysomnography (PSG). Overnight sleep studies provide a recording of sleep patterns, electroencephalogram (EEG), eye movements, chin muscle tone, limb muscle activity, ECG, respiratory effort, nasal airflow, and arterial oxygen saturation (SaO_2).

Multiple Sleep Latency Test (MSLT). Used in conjunction with PSG. Patients are allowed five 20-minute sleep opportunities, separated by 2 hours of wakefulness.

DIFFERENTIAL DIAGNOSIS

Traumatic
Head Injury. May lead to excessive somnolence. Accurate history is imperative.

Infectious
Central Nervous System (CNS) Infection. May lead to depression of the respiratory centers of the brain. CT/MRI may show brain abscess; cerebrospinal fluid examination may show white blood cells in meningitis.

Metabolic
Hypothyroidism. Differentiated by thyroid-stimulating hormone level.
Diabetes Mellitus. Differentiated by serum glucose level. *Note*: Whereas hyperglycemia merits concern, nocturnal hypoglycemia may be fatal.

Neoplastic
CNS Neoplasm. CT/MRI of brain should show mass.

Vascular
Anemia. Decreased hemoglobin and hematocrit.
Congestive Heart Failure. Decreased ventricular function on echocardiogram; patient is often dyspneic.

Congenital
Multiple Congenital Anomalies and Diseases. Interfere with respiratory drive.

Acquired
Depression, insomnia, narcolepsy, alcohol, drugs, periodic leg movements of sleep. May interfere with sleep.

TREATMENT

Treat underlying medical condition as applicable (e.g., hypothyroidism). Weight loss of 10% to 15% of body weight can result in up to 50% reduction in apneic episodes.

Modify sleep position by elevating the head of the bed and/or inhibiting supine position. Inhibiting supine position can be accomplished simply by sewing a pouch on the middle back of a pajama top and placing a tennis ball in the pouch.

Avoid the use of alcohol, sedatives, and hypnotics.

Patients with CSAS/OHS may benefit from the use of respiratory stimulants, the most common of which is medroxyprogesterone. However, the side effects of this medicine (impotence, hair loss, hypertriglyceridemia) often limit its use.

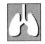
Oral appliances may be used that are designed to move the mandible forward and/or keep the tongue in a forward position.

Nasal continuous positive airway pressure (nasal CPAP) will help most snorers but is often poorly tolerated. Its use should be instituted in a sleep laboratory with supervision. CPAP is the treatment of choice for patients with OSA (or CSA) and cardiac disease.

Uvulopalatopharyngoplasty (UPPP) is reserved for more severe cases. In extreme cases, tracheostomy may be performed.

In patients who do not tolerate any of the foregoing treatments, supplemental nocturnal oxygen may reduce CO_2 retention in selected cases. Because supplemental oxygen may result in more severe hypoventilation and prolonged episodes of apnea, it should be used with extreme caution.

Electrophrenic pacing of the diaphragm during sleep or mechanical ventilation by either a positive-pressure ventilator applied through a tracheostomy or nose mask or a negative-pressure ventilator applied to the chest wall is reserved for a very few CSA patients in whom no other treatment has been effective.

PEDIATRIC CONSIDERATIONS

During the first months of life, normal full-term infants may have occasional episodes in which normal breathing is interrupted with short pauses during sleep. This breathing pattern is known as *periodic breathing* and is more common in premature infants until they reach approximately 36 weeks of gestational age. Infants rarely exhibit cyanosis or change in heart rate, and this periodic breathing usually ceases spontaneously.

Occasionally, an infant will develop prolonged apneic pauses as a result of depression of CNS control of respiration from a variety of causes. In the premature infant without identifiable predisposing causes, apneic pauses constitute *idiopathic apnea of prematurity*. Although most infants have a mixed form of apnea, some will have a purely obstructive form and others pure central apnea. Apnea of short duration is most often central, whereas longer episodes are more often mixed. The number of apneic episodes appears to be inversely proportional to the degree of immaturity.

Apnea monitors should be used for all infants at risk. Infants with mild intermittent apnea often respond to gentle cutaneous stimulation. Infants with recurrent, prolonged apnea who become hypoxic should be treated urgently with bag and mask ventilation. Packed red blood cells (RBCs) may be helpful in reducing apnea in a severely anemic infant. CPAP is also useful in the obstructive form.

Pharmacologic management with methylxanthines or caffeine is reserved for those infants with apnea of prematurity in whom a precipitating identifiable cause cannot be determined. Doses are as follows:

Aminophylline: *loading dose*: 5 mg/kg IV; *then* 1-2 mg/kg IV every 6 to 8 hours. Adjust to blood levels of 6-13 µg/mL. Switch to oral dosing every 12 hours when stable.

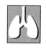

Caffeine: *loading dose*: 10 mg/kg IV over 30 minutes; *then* begin 2.5 to 5 mg/kg/day PO 24 hours later.

OBSTETRIC CONSIDERATIONS

No specific considerations in the obstetric patient.

GERIATRIC CONSIDERATIONS

Snoring is more common in the elderly, and the prevalence of apnea appears to increase with age.

PREVENTIVE CONSIDERATIONS

Obesity is one of the major etiologic factors in the development of sleep apnea; weight reduction of even a modest amount may significantly decrease symptoms.

PEARLS FOR THE PA

The telltale signs of OSA are stentorian snoring and severe daytime hypersomnolence.

Consider underlying OSA in hypertensive patients.

Further Reading

Pulmonary

Gilbert DM, Moellering RC, Sande MA (eds): The Sanford Guide to Antimicrobial Therapy, 14th ed. Hyde Park, VT, Antimicrobial Therapy Inc. 2001.

George RB, Light RW, Matthay MA, Matthay RA: Chest Medicine: Essentials of Pulmonary and Critical Care Medicine, 4th ed. Philadelphia, Lippincott Williams & Wilkins, 2000.

Goetz CG, Pappert EJ: Textbook of Clinical Neurology. Philadelphia, WB Saunders, 1999.

Goldman L, Ausiello D (eds): Cecil Textbook of Medicine, 22nd ed. Philadelphia, Saunders, 2004.

Goroll AH, Mulley AG: Primary Care Medicine, 4th ed. Philadelphia, Lippincott Williams & Wilkins, 2000.

Guidelines for the Diagnosis and Management of Asthma: NAEPP Expert Panel Report 2. Bethesda, MD, National Heart, Lung, and Blood Institute, National Institutes of Health, 1998.

Mandell GL, Bennett JE, Dolin R (eds): Principles and Practice of Infectious Diseases, 5th ed. Philadelphia, Churchill Livingstone, 2000.

Marx JA, Hockberger RS, Walls RM (eds): Rosen's Emergency Medicine: Concepts and Clinical Practice, 5th ed. St. Louis, Mosby, 2002.

Murray JF, Nadel JA (eds): Textbook of Respiratory Medicine, 3rd ed. Philadelphia, WB Saunders, 2000.

www.epocrates.com, ID 1.0 software program for Palm OS handhelds. ePocrates, Inc, 2002.

Pediatric Considerations

Behrman RE, Kliegman RM, Jenson HB (eds): Nelson Textbook of Pediatrics, 16th ed. Philadelphia, WB Saunders, 2000.

AAP 2000 Red Book: Report of the Committee on Infectious Diseases, 25th ed. Elk Grove Village, IL, American Academy of Pediatrics, 2000.

Obstetric Considerations

Beckmann CRB, Ling FW, Laub DW, et al (eds): Obstetrics and Gynecology, 4th ed. Philadelphia, Lippincott Williams & Wilkins, 2002.

Cunningham FG, MacDonald PC, Gant NF, et al (eds): Williams Obstetrics, 20th ed. East Norwalk, CT, Appleton & Lange, 1997.

Gabbe SG, Niebyl JR, Simpson JL: Obstetrics—Normal and Problem Pregnancies, 4th ed. Philadelphia, Churchill Livingstone, 2002.

Geriatric Considerations

Duthie EH Jr, Katz PR: Practice of Geriatrics, 3rd ed. Philadelphia, WB Saunders, 1998.

RHEUMATOLOGY/ ORTHOPEDICS

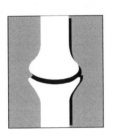

16

Ankylosing Spondylitis

Roderick S. Hooker, PhD, PA

DEFINITION

Ankylosing spondylitis (AS) is a chronic inflammatory disease that primarily affects the axial skeleton and large joints. It is characterized by progressive fusion of the spine.

HISTORY

Symptoms.   Low back pain relieved by rest; often, improvement with exercise. The patient may have a sense of "gelling" or stiffening up of the joints of the back and knees after sitting for 30 to 60 minutes.

General.   Men tend to have a more classic presentation, whereas women have an atypical presentation of "skipped" spinal lesions on radiographs and symphysis pubis involvement. Diagnosed in men and women in a ratio of 5:1.

Age.   Most commonly affects persons in their late teens to early 30s.

Onset.   Usually insidious and progressive.

Duration.   Progressive.

Intensity.   Variable, but because some patients have few complaints, diagnosis may be delayed. Severe back pain is rarely a presentation.

Aggravating Factors.   Physically demanding labor.

Alleviating Factors.   High-potency nonsteroidal anti-inflammatory drugs (NSAIDs) and rheumatologic drugs (e.g., sulfasalazine, methotrexate, corticosteroids).

Associated Factors.   Family history of seronegative spondyloarthropathy.

PHYSICAL EXAMINATION

General.   Loss of spinal motion and neck rotation; inability to gaze upward. Rheumatoid nodules are notably *absent*. Extra-articular manifestations such as aortic regurgitation and pulmonary upper lobe fibrosis are rare.

Chest.   Limited chest expansion reflects costovertebral involvement. Chest measurements are made at rest and on inspiration. Less than 5 cm of chest expansion is considered reduced.

Extremities.   Proximal joint involvement (of hips, knees, shoulders) is often asymmetrical. Enthesopathies (tendinitis, epicondylitis, fasciitis) are common.

Head, Eyes, Ears, Nose, Throat.   Acute anterior uveitis (iritis) may be seen in 40% of patients.

Spine.   Tenderness of the sacroiliac (SI) joints and lumbosacral muscles. Also, positive result on *Schober test*: With the patient standing erect, marks are made connecting the dimples over the SI joints (dimples of Venus) and also 10 cm above these marks on the spine. The distance between the marks (the measure of expansion of the spine) is measured in maximum forward flexion. Less than 5 cm of distraction is abnormal.

PATHOPHYSIOLOGY

Fibrocartilage is the primary site of inflammation in articular and ligamentous tissue. The synovitis of AS can mimic rheumatoid arthritis (RA). The initial cellular inflammatory changes are followed by fibrosis and often calcification of the spinal ligaments, which leads to characteristic bony ankylosis. Changes are seen in the SI joints, intervertebral disk spaces, apophyseal and costrovertebral joints of the axial skeleton, manubriosternal and sternoclavicular joints, and symphysis pubis.

DIAGNOSTIC STUDIES

Laboratory
Complete Blood Count. Mild normocytic anemia is seen in severe cases; consistent with anemia of chronic disease.

Acute-Phase Reactants: Erythrocyte Sedimentation Rate, Platelets, Alpha$_1$-Globulins and Alpha$_2$-Globulins in Serum Protein Electrophoresis, C-Reactive Protein. May reveal elevations. Findings do not correlate with disease activity.

Synovial Fluid. Mildly elevated white blood cell (WBC) count with a slight preponderance of polymorphonuclear leukocytes. Positive in greater than 50% of patients.

HLA-B27 Tissue Typing. HLA-B27 present in 95% of white patients with AS; also present in at least 8% of all North Americans.

Radiology
Single View of SI Joint. Usually diagnostic for sclerosis of the joint margins.
CT/MRI. More sensitive for joint involvement, but rarely necessary.
Radionuclide Scan. In rare cases in which the diagnosis is uncertain, a technetium bone/joint scan will reveal increased uptake at the SI joint.

Other
Pulmonary Function Tests. Mild to moderately diminished total lung capacity when the thoracic spine is involved.

DIFFERENTIAL DIAGNOSIS

Traumatic
Lumbar Strain. Myofascial pain syndrome. Relieved by rest and exacerbated by exercise.

Infectious
Diskitis/Osteomyelitis. History of sepsis or invasive bony procedure.

Metabolic
Osteoarthritis (OA). Facet OA and other degenerative conditions of the spine or large joints are represented by a loss of cartilage. Well differentiated on radiograph; rarely involves the SI joint.
Diffuse Idiopathic Skeletal Hyperostosis (DISH) (Forester disease). Proliferative OA; does not involve the sacroiliac joint.
Osteitis Condensans Ilii. Asymptomatic sclerosis of the iliac side of the SI joint seen as a radiographic anomaly in parous women.

Neoplastic
Metastatic Disease of Bone. Differentiated on radiographs; patient may have a history of a primary cancer.

Vascular
Osteonecrosis of Hips. Does not involve the SI joint; confined to the hip femoral head joint. May have a history of chronic steroid use.

Congenital. Not applicable.
Acquired. Not applicable.

TREATMENT

Treatment is primarily pharmacologic. Agents and regimens are as follows:

- Nonsteroidal anti-inflammatory drugs (NSAIDs)
    Indomethacin 25-50 mg three times a day as required; this high-potency NSAID may put the patient at higher risk for a gastrointestinal bleed
    Phenylbutazone 100 mg three or four times a day; monitor complete blood count every 3 months for leukopenia
    Naproxen 500 mg twice daily
    Others: sulindac, meclofenamate, tolmetin, various cyclooxygenase-2 (COX-2) inhibitors
- Disease-modifying antirheumatic drugs (DMARDs)
    Sulfasalazine 500 mg 2 to 6 tablets daily
    Methotrexate 10-50 mg IM/SC/PO 1 day/week
- Corticosteroids
    Intra-articular triamcinolone hexacetonide (Aristospan) 20-40 mg/dL PLUS bupivacaine 1-2 mL (in same syringe)
    Methylprednisolone 125 mg IV as a single dose for acute flare-ups
    Prednisone 10-25 mg PO in divided doses for a few days to a few months; not generally recommended for long-term use

PEDIATRIC CONSIDERATIONS

AS is typically a disease of young and middle-aged adults, but it may begin in childhood, most commonly affecting male patients older than 8 years of age. AS should be considered in any child with persistent pain in the hips, thighs, or lower back, with or without peripheral arthritis.

OBSTETRIC CONSIDERATIONS

Methotrexate should be avoided in women considering becoming pregnant. NSAIDs also should be avoided, especially during the third trimester of pregnancy. These medications are implicated in premature closure of the fetal ductus arteriosus and may interfere with labor.

GERIATRIC CONSIDERATIONS

Osteoarthritis increases in incidence with advancing age and may manifest with similar symptoms. Radiographs may be necessary to differentiate.

PREVENTIVE CONSIDERATIONS

None specific.

PEARLS FOR THE PA

The diagnosis of AS is made by history, Schober test, and single radiographic view of the SI joint.

Rarely is HLA-B27 tissue typing necessary if the radiograph is diagnostic.

AS should not be confused with rheumatoid arthritis, which is a symmetrical disease of the wrists and MCP joints.

Rheumatoid factor and antinuclear antibody (ANA) assays are not indicated and, if positive, will only cloud the clinical picture.

Fibromyalgia

Roderick S. Hooker, PhD, PA

DEFINITION

Fibromyalgia is a soft tissue, nonarticular pain disorder characterized by chronic, generalized musculoskeletal aches and pains and stiffness that occurs primarily in muscles and their attachments. It is associated with specific sites of tenderness.

HISTORY

Symptoms. Widespread chronic pain, stiffness, nonrestorative sleep, and aggravated by modulating factors such as weather, depression, and stress. Subjective swelling of the fingers, fatigue, irritable bowel syndrome, and exacerbation of symptoms with repetitive use of extremities (e.g., vacuuming, reaching overhead). Depression and anxiety are other common symptoms.

General. Generally affects otherwise healthy women nine times more often than men. Impaired function may be a complaint related to pain and fatigue, despite the absence of neuromuscular abnormalities. No specific fibromyalgia personality profile has been identified.

Age. From 8 to 70 years, but more frequent in persons 30 to 55 years of age.

Onset. Insidious in most cases. Some patients can identify an inciting event.

Duration. Lifetime, although may go into remission for long periods.

Intensity. Deep, ache-like pain that is widespread from the neck to the heels.

Aggravating Factors. Cold and humid weather, anxiety/stress, sleep deprivation, and mental/physical fatigue.

Alleviating Factors. Vacation from home or work. Temporary relief with heat, hot showers, and baths. Stretching exercises are mildly beneficial.

Associated Factors. Fibromyalgia is sometimes erroneously considered an associated or concomitant condition if it occurs in patients with other rheumatologic conditions. However, the other rhematologic condition may remit with no relief from the fibromyalgia symptoms.

PHYSICAL EXAMINATION

General. The patient may present in acute or chronic pain and distress.

Extremities. Joints and muscle strength are normal. Palpation of the upper edge of the trapezius muscles, neck muscle insertion at the occiput, deltoids, infrascapularis, second costochondral junction, inferior to the lateral (elbow) epicondyles, trochanters, lower lumbar area, medial fat pads of the knees, and the medial and lateral insertions of the Achilles tendons will reveal 12 or more tender points. Circumferential squeeze of the distal arm or leg is often painful.

Neurologic.   General examination is normal.

PATHOPHYSIOLOGY

Fibromyalgia may be part of a post-traumatic stress syndrome, although only one-third of patients identify a precipitating event. Etiology is unknown, but it is postulated that the origin is either neurochemical or behavioral.

Neurochemical evidence includes decreased serotonin, abnormalities in other neurochemicals, and abnormalities in central pain pathways.

The behavioral theory suggests patients with fibromyalgia tend to disproportionately seek treatment for pain syndromes. This is not based on the degree of pain but rather due to previous abuse, psychiatric illnesses, or the perception of physical or emotional trauma.

DIAGNOSTIC STUDIES

Laboratory
The diagnosis of fibromyalgia is made on clinical findings, excluding other disorders. There are no characteristic laboratory tests to make the diagnosis.

Complete Blood Count.   As indicated to rule out infectious diseases.

Erythrocyte Sedimentation Rate.   Nonspecific, may be mildly elevated.

Thyroid Function Studies.   Thyroid-stimulating hormone assay to rule out hyperthyroidism/hypothyroidism.

Rheumatoid Factor/Antinuclear Antibody (RF/ANA) Assays.   Not indicated and should not be considered, as this pain is not characteristic of connective tissue diseases.

Radiology.   Not applicable.
Other.   Not applicable.

DIFFERENTIAL DIAGNOSIS

Traumatic
Tendinitis/Epicondylitis.   Tends to be acute and responds to treatment.

Infectious
Chronic Fatigue Syndrome.   Considerable overlap with fibromyalgia; however, the profound fatigue and episodic pharyngitis of chronic fatigue syndrome are not part of the fibromyalgia syndrome.

Metabolic

Polymyalgia Rheumatica (PMR). Tends to be abrupt and affect persons older than 60 years of age.

Polymyositis/Dermatomyositis. Patients present with an elevated creatine kinase and exhibit proximal weakness.

Hypothyroidism/Hyperthyroidism. Abnormal thyroid stimulating hormone.

Hypoparathyroidism/Hyperparathyroidism. Abnormal calcium.

Adrenal Insufficiency. Patients present with anorexia/weight loss.

Parkinson Disease: Dyskinetic Phase. Slow, painful gait.

Neoplastic

Metastatic Carcinoma. Progressive illness. Tumor seen on radiographs.

Vascular

Vasculitis. Elevated erythrocyte sedimentation rate.

Congenital

Not applicable.

Acquired

Alcoholic myopathy. History of alcohol abuse.

Depression. Anhedonia, labile affect, weight gain or loss, early morning awakening or hypersomnia.

TREATMENT

Education of the patient about the condition is the cornerstone of management. The Arthritis Foundation is the best source for literature. In addition, the following agents and measures may be useful:

- Soporifics: Tricyclic antidepressants (e.g., doxepin 10 mg or imipramine 10 mg, given in the early evening, once to three times daily) can be tried. Benzodiazepines should be avoided.
- Conditioning program: High- or low-impact aerobic exercises for a minimum of 10 minutes every 48 hours. After this regimen is established, gradually increase the duration until 20 to 30 minutes every 48 hours is sustained.
- Narcotics and nonsteroidal anti-inflammatory drugs (NSAIDs): Narcotics should be avoided if possible, but some patients benefit from NSAIDs for a while.
- Muscle relaxants: They have little efficacy for chronic pain and may be habit-forming (especially carisoprodol). The exception is cyclobenzaprine HCl, which is similar in structure to amitriptyline.
- Acupuncture and chiropractic manipulations may be of benefit in a small number of patients and usually not sustained.

Note: Patients in chronic pain are at risk for gimmicks and special curative treatments. Special diets, massages, manipulations, and promises of cure are tempting to the uninformed.

PEDIATRIC CONSIDERATIONS

The diagnosis of fibromyalgia in children is rarely made by pediatricians. It should be suspected in a child with generalized pain of more than 3 months' duration after inflammatory disease has been excluded.

OBSTETRIC CONSIDERATIONS

The use of NSAIDs should be avoided, especially during the third trimester of pregnancy. These medications are implicated in premature closure of the fetal ductus arteriosus and may interfere with labor.

Chronic aspirin use has been associated with decreased fetal birth weight, increased incidence of stillbirth, neonatal mortality, antepartum and postpartum bleeding, delivery complications, and prolonged gestation.

Fibromyalgia is neither exacerbated nor relieved by pregnancy.

GERIATRIC CONSIDERATIONS

Polymyalgia rheumatica may mimic some fibromyalgia symptoms if it occurs in an elderly person. The prevalence does not increase with age.

PREVENTIVE CONSIDERATIONS

Educate the patient regarding the benign nature of the disease. Attempt to identify any underlying emotional or psychiatric contributor to the patient's complaint.

PEARLS FOR THE PA

The diagnosis of fibromyalgia is made by history and physical examination and not by laboratory and imaging inclusion or exclusion criteria.

The pain described by patients is dramatic, affecting many sites, and is not characteristic of most rheumatologic conditions.

Gout

Roderick S. Hooker, PhD, PA

DEFINITION

A heterogeneous group of diseases in which the most common manifestation is an increased serum uric acid.

HISTORY

Symptoms. Overt gout is manifested by recurrent episodes of acute arthritis in a characteristic pattern. The classic presentation is one of acute monoarticular arthritis of sudden onset in a middle-aged man (more than 70% of episodes involve the first metatarsophalangeal [MTP] joint). The first episode often begins at night. The pain is exquisite, and will often suggest an infection by the presence of cellulitis (from the uric acid in the skin). Polyarticular gout can occur in 30% of patients with recurrent gout, usually involving 2 to 4 joints, and has a predisposition for the feet and legs.

General. Acute gouty arthritis occurs most commonly in males (95%). Women may develop gouty arthritis in the perimenopausal phase, as estrogen levels drop. In many cases, if the disorder is left untreated, urate crystals are deposited, usually in and around the joints of the extremities and occasionally the viscera. In some patients, deposits of uric acid form within the urinary collecting tubules.

Age. Initial attack usually occurs in the fourth to fifth decade.

Onset. Sudden and acute.

Duration. The acute phase, left untreated, lasts 3 to 5 days. Symptoms of arthritis may last 3 to 6 weeks.

Intensity. Can be quite severe. The patient may not be able to tolerate even a sheet on the feet at night. Weight bearing and wearing footwear may be impossible. Some patients may experience fever and chills with an acute attack.

Aggravating Factors. Diuretic therapy, weight loss, renal failure, lead nephropathy (saturnine gout), daily or excessive alcohol consumption, shellfish or organ meat ingestion (e.g., brain, liver, kidney).

Alleviating Factors. Appropriate medical treatment and avoidance or discontinuance of aggravating factors.

Associated Factors. Ninety percent of patients with gout are undersecretors of serum uric acid. The remainder are overproducers of urate.

PHYSICAL EXAMINATION

General. A patient who presents during an acute attack may have difficulty ambulating and be in significant distress secondary to pain.

Extremities.   The involved joint is swollen, tender, red, and warm.
Neurologic.   No deficits.
Renal.   Patients may have costovertebral angle tenderness as a result of calculus formation with chronic hyperuricemia.

PATHOPHYSIOLOGY

Monosodium urate crystals precipitate in the joints and bursa in a manner that is not completely understood. It occurs in a state of supersaturated or prolonged and hyperuricemia. The crystals accumulate in the avascular articular space, where they act as a nidus for inflammation, which provokes the release of inflammatory mediators.

DIAGNOSTIC STUDIES

Laboratory
Synovial Fluid.   For cell count and urate crystals. Positive in 85% of patients with acute gout.
Serum Uric Acid.   Elevated in 90% of patients with gout but not diagnostic.

Radiology
Radiograph of Affected Joint.   Soft tissue swelling during an acute attack. Soft tissue tophi may be present if the condition is present for more than 3 years. Punched-out, sharply marginated areas of bone destruction may be present in chronic cases.
Intravenous Pyelography.   From 80% to 90% of patients with gout who develop urolithiasis have pure urate stones, which are radiolucent and require intravenous pyelography for diagnosis.

Other
Not applicable.

DIFFERENTIAL DIAGNOSIS

Traumatic
Fracture.   Differentiated by history and radiograph.

Infectious
Osteomyelitis.   Differentiated by complete blood count and differential.
Cellulitis.   Presence of serosanguineous fluid, positive bacterial cultures.

Metabolic
Rheumatoid Arthritis (RA).   Polyarticular, symmetrical, rheumatoid factor (RF) positive.
Osteoarthritis.   Acute flare is atypical.

Pseudogout. Serum uric acid is normal. Radiograph reveals chondrocalcinosis.

Paget Disease, Hemolytic Anemia, Glycogen Storage Disease, Psoriasis, Sarcoidosis. All may cause secondary gout as a result of high cell turnover.

Neoplastic
Metastatic Disease of Bone. History of primary cancer; tumor seen on radiographs.

Vascular
Not applicable.

Congenital
Congenital Gout. Associated Lesch-Nyhan syndrome, a dysmorphology.

Acquired
Renal Insufficiency, Antineoplastic Drug Use. Causing an inability to excrete uric acid.

TREATMENT

Patient education regarding the maintenance of ideal weight, purine-restricted diet, and avoidance of alcohol and aspirin.

Drug Therapy
- Acute attacks:
    Indomethacin 50 mg four times a day OR prednisone 50 mg/day for
    5 days
- Recurrent attacks (after 3 years):
    Sulfinpyrazone 100 mg three times a day OR probenecid 500 to
    2000 mg daily
- Prophylactic:
    Colchicine 0.6 mg twice a day (side effect of diarrhea)
- Tophaceous gout and renal calculi:
    Allopurinol 100-600 mg daily depending on creatinine levels. The
    goal is to reduce the serum uric acid to less than 7.0 mg/dL

PEDIATRIC CONSIDERATIONS

Gout is exceptionally rare in children and, if present, is due to congenital factors.

OBSTETRIC CONSIDERATIONS

Rare in women taking or producing estrogen. Almost never seen in pregnancy.

GERIATRIC CONSIDERATIONS

In women, gout may develop in the perimenopausal phase owing to decreased estrogen levels. Comorbid conditions such as disorders requiring diuretic therapy, renal failure, and alcohol abuse contribute to gout.

PREVENTIVE CONSIDERATIONS

Gout can be prevented by avoidance of purine-rich foods (e.g., organ meats, shellfish, nuts), weight reduction, and reduction in thiazide diuretics.

Untreated gout can progress to deposition of urate crystals in and around the joints of the extremities and occasionally the viscera or within the renal collecting tubules. It can also progress to a destructive arthropathy.

PEARLS FOR THE PA

Gout is manifested by recurrent episodes of acute monoarticular arthritis (classically affecting the first MTP joint).

Rare in women taking or producing estrogen. Almost never seen in pregnancy.

Osteoarthritis/Osteoarthrosis

Roderick S. Hooker, PhD, PA

DEFINITION

Osteoarthritis (OA), also called *osteoarthrosis* and hypertrophic or degenerative joint disease, is the most common rheumatic condition. It is characterized by progressive loss of articular cartilage and by reactive changes at the margins of the joints (producing osteophytes) and in subchondral bones. OA is classified into idiopathic (primary) and secondary forms. Joint capsules are little affected, so adhesions are not formed. Although joint motion is restricted, ankylosis does not result.

HISTORY

Symptoms. Usually local. Pain may occur early in the course of the disease, especially in the fingers, with joint use and is relieved by rest. The pain of OA arises from the intra-articular and periarticular structures.

General. If symptoms are more general and bodywide, a systemic form of connective tissue disease or myofascial pain syndrome should be suspected. Generally, there is little correlation between joint symptoms and pathologic findings. Females, especially whites and Asians, are more likely to develop OA of the fingers. Incidence of OA is lower in blacks than in whites.

Age. Incidence increases with age: OA usually occurs after age 40 and is almost universal, from a radiographic standpoint, in persons older than 65.

Onset. Gradual over months to years.

Duration. Usually slow and progressive.

Intensity. Initially mild, but may be incapacitating at times. The extent of the disease does not correlate as well with pain as with function.

Aggravating Factors. The combination of age along with deterioration of the cartilage (accumulated microtrauma) contributes to the vast number of cases of OA. Occupations that require heavy lifting or repetitive use contribute to the development of OA.

Alleviating Factors. Joint protection (e.g., use of cane or crutches) and avoidance of overuse are beneficial.

Associated Factors. Secondary OA can arise from congenital and developmental disorders such as hip dysplasia, trauma (especially repetitive), neuropathic joint disease, and inflammatory joint diseases (e.g., rheumatoid arthritis, gout, pseudogout), which contribute to the structural breakdown of the cartilage. Genetic factors (especially with OA of the fingers) and biochemical factors are implicated.

PHYSICAL EXAMINATION

General. Joints may be tender, especially if swelling and warmth (synovitis) are present.

Extremities

Hands. Commonly affects the distal interphalangeal (DIP) joints, resulting in bone enlargement (Heberden nodes). Less commonly affects the proximal interphalangeal (PIP) joints, resulting in Bouchard nodes.

Knees. Involvement may lead to severe disability owing to the weight-bearing nature of the joint. Pain and bone enlargement are common, with or without effusion. Crepitus may be prominent. Instability and deformity may develop, resulting in a varus angulation.

Hips. OA of the hip (malum coxae) may be bilateral and is frequently disabling. Condition is worsened with weight bearing. Pain is usually in the inguinal or lateral areas and may radiate to the knee. Gait is antalgic. Internal and external rotation of the hips may be blocked by osteophytes. Sitting or rising from sitting may be difficult.

Other Joints. OA of the first metatarsophalangeal (MTP) joint causes pain and bony enlargement. Other joints at risk for OA include subtalar, acromioclavicular, elbow, glenohumeral, and temporomandibular joints (Costen syndrome). Involvement of any of these joints produces pain and crepitance with movement.

Neurologic

A careful neurologic evaluation for absence of reflexes or long tract signs. A radicular pattern of weakness and sensory abnormalities is important. Cord compression may result from intervertebral osteophytes at cervical levels. This in turn may result in progressive myelopathy with minimal or no radicular pain.

Spine

May involve the intervertebral synchrondroses, causing degeneration of the fibrocartilaginous intervertebral disk and changes in the vertebral bodies or facets. Changes are most significant in the middle to lower cervical spine (cervical spondylosis) and the lower lumbar area.

PATHOPHYSIOLOGY

OA results from the breakdown of cartilage that occurs with abnormal stresses on the normal cartilage or normal stresses on diseased cartilage. The phagocytosis of tissue breakdown products and crystals can activate inflammatory responses, resulting in further breakdown of cartilage and activation of bone remodeling.

DIAGNOSTIC STUDIES

Laboratory

Routine Chemistry and Complete Blood Count. Normal findings. Anemia of chronic disease should not be present.

Erythrocyte Sedimentation Rate. Should not be elevated.

Examination of Synovial Fluid from Involved Joints. Typically does not reveal evidence of inflammation. Synovial fluid cell counts are low, almost always less than 3000/mm^3. Mononuclear cells are predominant. Levels of protein, glucose, and complement components are normal.

Radiology

Radiograph of the Affected Joint. Severe degenerative changes are seen. They are usually graded from I to IV in severity of osteophyte formation and destruction of the joint. Oblique films are necessary to evaluate the neural foramina of the spine.

CT of the Spine. When neurologic symptoms are present, may be helpful.

DIFFERENTIAL DIAGNOSIS

Traumatic

Sprain. An acute condition.

Infectious

Septic Joint. Monoarticular and acute condition.

Osteomyelitis. A consideration in the elderly. Usually asymmetrical.

Metabolic
Rheumatoid Arthritis. Heberden and Bouchard nodes are hypertrophic bone formations and should not be confused with rheumatoid nodules.
Gout. Acute onset with elevated serum uric acid levels.
Pseudogout. Usually manifests like gout. Radiograph reveals chondrocalcinosis.
Psoriatic Arthritis. Tends to occur in younger patients and is associated with psoriasis.

Neoplastic
Bone Tumor. Seen on radiograph.

Vascular
Osteonecrosis. In advanced stages, tends to show collapse of the femoral head.

Congenital
Hip Dysplasia in Childhood. Predisposes the patient to develop OA of the hip.

Acquired
Joint Injuries. If significant, will predispose the patient to develop OA of the affected joint.

TREATMENT

There is no treatment to retard or reverse the pathologic process in OA. Therapy is empirical and symptomatic.

Initial nonpharmacologic management includes regular exercise, joint protection with wraps or supports, ergonomic evaluations and adjustments, heat (chronic) and ice (acute), moisture, ultrasound, and physical and occupational therapy. Other potentially beneficial therapies can be added as indicated.

Medical/Pharmacologic Therapies
- Nonsteroidal anti-inflammatory drugs (NSAIDs): Agents such as naproxen have been shown to be of some benefit in OA but appear to be no better than aspirin (acetylsalicyclic acid [ASA]) or acetaminophen for analgesia. Therefore, ASA and acetaminophen are preferred. The choice of an NSAID should take into account such factors as efficacy, cost, adverse reactions, compliance, and past treatment.

  Enteric-coated aspirin: Enteric-coated ASA (e.g., Ecotrin) is the drug of choice in most patients with OA. Sustained-release

ASAs (e.g., Easprin, ZORprin) are good alternatives. Dosage is 325-1000 mg four times a day or 975 mg twice a day in sustained-release form.

Acetaminophen: Studies have demonstrated that acetaminophen is comparable to ibuprofen in low and moderate doses for OA. Dosage is 500-650 mg three times a day.

Salicylate: Salsalate (Dilsalcid) is a nonacetylated salicylate with minimal gastrointestinal toxicity that does not affect platelet function. Salsalate is supplied in 500- and 750-mg tablets. Usual dosage is 750-1000 mg twice to four times a day. Other drugs in this family include choline salicylate, choline magnesium trisalicylate, and diflunisal.

Cox-2 inhibitors: These newer drugs may be comparable to the older NSAIDs and acetaminophen in effectiveness but are considerably more expensive.

- Most over-the-counter (OTC) topical emollients and rubefacients contain oil of wintergreen (salicylate). Their benefit is in increasing circulation and producing warmth. Capsaicin (Zostrix) 0.025% to 0.075% cream blocks substance P, a component in the pain cascade. This topical prescription may be effective in up to 50% of patients with OA. Used four times a day.
- Steroids: Systemic corticosteroids have no role in the treatment of OA. This is not an inflammatory systemic disease. Intra-articular injections may be of benefit in large joints if used selectively; they work best in shoulders, elbows, and knees. Limit use to no more than 3 or 4 times/year because of the adverse effect on local cartilage. Only the following agents are recommended (all other corticosteroids are immediately absorbed from the joint and do not provide long-lasting effect):

  Triamcinolone hexacetonide (Aristospan) OR betamethasone (Celestone) 1-2 mL PLUS bupivacaine 1-2 mL (in same syringe)

Surgical Management

A number of surgical procedures are beneficial in selected patients. These include arthroscopic debridement, osteotomy, arthrodesis, and total knee or hip replacement. Nerve roots or the spinal cord may require decompression owing to bone overgrowth (spinal stenosis).

Occupational and Physical Therapy

The concept of joint protection is the mainstay of OA therapy for all patients. This includes reducing use and avoiding overuse of the hands when Heberden and Bouchard nodes are present. Wrist supports are available OTC, and custom-made thumb splints can be crafted by occupational therapy personnel. In OA of the hip or knee, cane or crutch use coupled with muscle strengthening is an important component of management; these devices act to off-load weight-bearing joints. Foot orthotics can be beneficial in valgus deformities of the ankles and pes planus.

PEDIATRIC CONSIDERATIONS

OA in children is rare and usually secondary to congenital deformities such as hip dysplasia or severe trauma.

OBSTETRIC CONSIDERATIONS

OA is unusual in gravid women. In women so affected, the use of NSAIDs should be avoided, especially during the third trimester of pregnancy. These medications are implicated in premature closure of the fetal ductus arteriosus, and may interfere with labor. Chronic aspirin use has been associated with decreased fetal birth weight, increased incidence of stillbirth, neonatal mortality, antepartum and postpartum bleeding, delivery complications, and prolonged gestation.

GERIATRIC CONSIDERATIONS

Incidence increases with advancing age. Quality of life and mobility can be affected by joint pain or by neurologic compromise. The history must address self-care issues, and treatment must be individualized.

PREVENTIVE CONSIDERATIONS

Weight loss, routine exercise, decreased weight-bearing activity, avoidance of contact sports (e.g., football), and ergonomic adjustments all may help to retard the development of OA and to assist in maintaining function with OA.

PEARLS FOR THE PA

Joint pain, the symptom that most often leads patients with OA to seek treatment, may originate from stretching of the joint capsule or ligaments, periosteal irritation due to osteophyte formation, trabecular microfractures, interosseous hypertension, or muscle pain. It is rarely due to inflammation.

Pain at rest that keeps the patient with OA of the knee from sleeping needs to be investigated for infection (e.g., osteomyelitis) or osteonecrosis.

Polymyalgia Rheumatica

Roderick S. Hooker, PhD, PA

DEFINITION

Polymyalgia rheumatica (PMR) is a clinical syndrome of unknown cause that rarely occurs in persons younger than 60 years of age. It is characterized by aching and morning stiffness in the torso and proximal limbs. PMR is an inflammatory condition that is sometimes manifested by malaise, weight loss, fever, and anemia.

HISTORY

Symptoms.   Stiffness of the proximal limb muscles and shoulder and hip girdles. Classically, the patient presents with morning stiffness lasting more than 2 hours and of more than 2 weeks' duration.

General.   PMR should be considered in patients older than 60 years of age who experience the onset of diffuse pain. Because the diagnosis of PMR is essentially clinical, it becomes important to consider the different symptoms in relation to the symptoms of other arthritides that might cause diagnostic confusion.

Age.   Typically affects persons between 60 and 80 years of age. Another diagnosis should be suspected in a younger person.

Onset.   Insidious or acute.

Duration.   If PMR is left untreated, most patients recover in 2 to 3 years.

Intensity.   May be debilitating; often prevents self-care activities.

Aggravating Factors.   None.

Alleviating Factors.   None.

Associated Factors.   PMR may be a prodrome for rheumatoid arthritis.

PHYSICAL EXAMINATION

General.   Examination provides little explanation for symptoms for the majority of patients. There may be poorly localized tenderness over joints, especially prominent over shoulders and hips.

Neurologic.   Neuropsychiatric manifestations such as depression, dementia, acute disorientation, and amnesia (without focal neurologic disease) may be seen. Occasionally these are the presenting manifestations of PMR.

PATHOPHYSIOLOGY

The etiology of PMR is unknown, and no specific antibody is associated with this disease. The abnormal laboratory results usually found are elevated

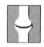

erythrocyte sedimentation rate (ESR), hypergammaglobulinemia, and increased alpha-globulinemia. These findings are consistent with chronic inflammatory disease and do not offer any evidence of a specific underlying disorder.

DIAGNOSTIC STUDIES

Laboratory
Westergren Erythrocyte Sedimentation Rate. ESR greater than 50 mm/hour is the laboratory hallmark of PMR.

Complete Blood Count. Reveals a normocytic, normochromic anemia in at least 50% of patients.

Serum Protein Electrophoresis. Reveals elevations of the proteins gammaglobulin and alpha$_1$-globulin. These are nonspecific indicators of inflammation.

Creatine Kinase (CK). Normal.

Rheumatoid Factor (RF) Assay. RF may be present but at low titers is nonspecific.

Antinuclear Antibody (ANA) Assay. Not necessary.

Thyroid-Stimulating Hormone Assay. Usually normal.

Radiology
Chest Film. Should be normal.

Joint Radiographs. Unnecessary.

Other
Electromyography. Normal findings.

DIFFERENTIAL DIAGNOSIS

Infectious
Bacterial Endocarditis. Positive blood cultures. Patient may have a prosthetic heart valve with septic emboli to the extremities.

Osteomyelitis. Elevated white blood cell count. May see bone destruction on radiograph.

Tuberculosis. Positive skin test.

Acquired Immunodeficiency Syndrome. Human immunodeficiency virus positive.

Hepatitis. Positive hepatitis profile.

Metabolic
Rheumatoid Arthritis Prodrome. Positive RF assay.

Hypothyroidism. Approximately 10% of PMR patients will eventually develop hypothyroidism.

Polymyositis, Dermatomyositis, Inclusion Body Myositis.   Elevated CK.
Fibromyalgia.   Not associated with an elevated ESR.

Neoplastic
Neoplasm.   Tumor seen on radiographs.

Vascular
Giant Cell Arteritis (Temporal Arteritis, Cranial Arteritis).   Will occur in
approximately 5% of people with PMR.

Traumatic.   Not applicable.
Congenital.   Not applicable.
Acquired.   Not applicable.

TREATMENT

In PMR, the patient's response to prednisone 10-15 mg/day (in divided
doses) within 48 hours is so dramatic that some experts consider this to be
diagnostic, and further testing other than chest film, complete blood count,
and ESR is unnecessary.

Aspirin and nonsteroidal anti-inflammatory drugs (NSAIDs) are used to
supplement and lower the dose of corticosteroids.

PEDIATRIC CONSIDERATIONS

Not a consideration.

OBSTETRIC CONSIDERATIONS

Not a consideration.

GERIATRIC CONSIDERATIONS

This is primarily a disorder of the elderly (older than 60 years of age).

PREVENTIVE CONSIDERATIONS

None specific.

PEARLS FOR THE PA

PMR should be suspected in patients older than 60 who experience aching and morning stiffness in the torso and proximal limbs and difficulty rolling over in bed.

The diagnosis is essentially clinical, with a nonspecific elevation in erythrocyte sedimentation rate. A chest film helps to rule out intrathoracic disease.

There is often a dramatic response to prednisone, which helps to confirm the diagnosis.

Rheumatoid Arthritis

Roderick S. Hooker, PhD, PA

DEFINITION

Rheumatoid arthritis (RA) is a systemic disease of unknown etiology. It typically affects the synovial membrane of peripheral joints in a symmetrical fashion. RA occurs in 1% to 2% of the population; more frequently in women than in men (gender ratio 3:1).

HISTORY

Symptoms. The chief pain of RA is likely to be a continuous nagging, perhaps throbbing pain in the wrists, metacarpophalangeal (MCP) joints, and sometimes proximal interphalangeal (PIP) joints. It is usually worst on arising (morning) and may ease somewhat with daily activities and worsen with joint abuse and fatigue. Pain can be severe and limit sleep but is not as severe as in gout. Hands are typically stiff in the morning, often with improvement after immersion in hot water.

General. Patients will typically volunteer that their hands are stiff on awakening (early morning stiffness), with duration of stiffness of longer than 1 hour. Finger flexion is limited, as evidenced by inability to touch the distal palmar pad with fingertips, and patients are unable to lift a pan or coffee pot or open a jar. RA does not involve the axial skeleton. Polymyalgia rheumatica (PMR)-type complaints sometimes accompany RA. Malaise, weight loss, and anemia of chronic disease may be accompanying signs and symptoms.

Age. Can affect any age but is most prevalent in the 35- to 50-year-old age group. Incidence increases with each decade.

Onset.   It can be insidious, over weeks or months, or sudden with an abrupt onset.

Duration.   Usually slow and progressive, over a lifetime. At least 10% of patients will experience spontaneous remission, but the rest will have symptoms for perhaps 25 years.

Intensity.   Initially may be mild, but in one-third of patients may progress to advanced stages in later life, which can be incapacitating.

Aggravating Factors.   Certain physical activities that unnecessarily stress the affected joints (e.g., carpentry or tennis will affect the hand joints).

Alleviating Factors.   Rest provides the most relief, and joint protection should always be emphasized. Medications are usually beneficial.

Associated Factors.   People with RA often have a large number of underlying systemic conditions that make prescribing medication and managing their care a challenge. The *HLADR4* gene confers a genetic predisposition. Extra-articular manifestations include rheumatoid lung disease, pulmonary nodules, osteoporosis (due to steroids or the primary disease), pericarditis, vasculitis, episcleritis, pancreatic insufficiency, and scleromalacia perforans (which can result in perforation of the globe.) The presence of splenomegaly and neutropenia accompanying RA defines a subset of RA termed Felty syndrome, which is associated with myelosuppressive manifestations.

PHYSICAL EXAMINATION

General.   General observation of the patient is important, because valuable clues can often be obtained by watching the patient walk across the office, take off a coat, sit, get up, or climb onto the examining table. Does the patient limp or favor one limb? Is the patient stiff or slow in moving? Does the patient struggle or use the arms when getting up from a chair? Does the patient wince when shaking hands or taking off a jacket? Does the patient fumble with buttons? These observations may help to define, for example, the location and severity of pain, identify stiffness and muscle weakness, and demonstrate any functional disability.

Extremities.   The cardinal signs of inflammation characterize RA: pain, redness, swelling, tenderness, and loss of function. RA almost always affects the MCP joints, and usually the wrists and PIP joints, sparing the thumb and distal interphalangeal (DIP) joints. Elbows may be involved but less frequently. The toes are also involved in a similar distribution to that of the hands. The axial skeleton is not involved in RA. Hips are rarely involved, but knees are involved at least 50% of the time. In the vast majority of cases, after a few months, the joints will be involved in a symmetrical fashion.

PATHOPHYSIOLOGY

The pathophysiologic mechanism in RA is a malignant (nonmetastatic) hypertrophy of the synovial membrane surrounding the joints. Susceptibility to RA is an inherited trait, determined by the gene for the B lymphocyte

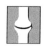

alloantigen HLA-DR4. This gene is present in 60% to 80% of white patients with adult seropositive nodular RA. The source and character of the stimulus for the immunologic abnormalities are not known, but atypical infectious agents have been of research interest. The terminal events of the pathogenesis of RA involve the generation of enzymes that cause tissue injury.

DIAGNOSTIC STUDIES

The diagnosis of RA should be made clinically, with confirmation by laboratory or imaging procedures. Diagnostic criteria include the following:

1. Persistent (for longer than 3 months), symmetrical polyarthritis (involvement of more than 5 joints) affecting the small joints of the hands and feet (excluding DIP joints)
2. The presence of systemic features such as fatigue, weight loss, and anemia
3. The presence of rheumatoid nodules (found in 20% of RA patients)
4. The exclusion of other systemic disorders such as systemic lupus erythematosus, Reiter syndrome, psoriatic arthritis, ankylosing spondylitis, ulcerative colitis, and other synovial diseases

Laboratory
Rheumatoid Factor (RF) Assay. RF is found in approximately 70% of all people with RA (and in 5% of all non-RA patients). A latex fixation titer of 1:160 or greater is considered specific but not diagnostic for RA. Repeating this assay is not clinically useful because it does not correlate with symptoms.

Erythrocyte Sedimentation Rate. Three tests are available: the Westergren method, the Wintrobe method, and the zeta sedimentation ratio. All are nonspecific reflections of the amount of inflammation and are sensitive but nonspecific.

Other Tests for Acute Phase Reactants. Platelet count, C-reactive protein, serum protein electrophoresis

Complete Blood Count, Urinalysis, Creatinine, Serum Uric Acid, Thyroid-Stimulating Hormone, Aspartate Aminotransferase (AST)/Alanine Aminotransferase (ALT) (Formerly Serum Glutamic-Oxaloacetic Transaminase [SGOT]/Serum Glutamate-Pyruvate Transaminase [SGPT]). Other tests that should be performed at the time of diagnosis to rule out coexisting or contributing disorders. Anemia of chronic disease may be present.

Antinuclear Antibody (ANA) Assay. Not a good screening test. A positive result probably will not change the diagnosis.

Radiology
Radiographs of the Hands (Single View). May be helpful in diagnosing this condition if present for more than 2 years. In an acute first phase

of RA, a radiograph serves only to document the swelling of the joints. In nodular RA, erosions of the MCP and MTP joints often develop within the first 1 to 2 years.

Technetium Bone Scan.   Can quantify the inflammation and distribution of the joint disease, and occasionally used to determine if inflammatory disease is present. Generally not necessary; not recommended.

Other
Nerve Conduction Studies.   Occasionally employed when carpal tunnel syndrome is suspected.

DIFFERENTIAL DIAGNOSIS

Traumatic
Myofascial Pain Syndromes.   Absence of joint involvement.

Infectious
Septic Joint.   Usually acute, monoarticular; large joints affected.
Arthritis from Other Causes.   Arthritis due to systemic lupus erythematosus (in acute stage) can mimic RA in young women for a few weeks, but rarely develops into a chronic arthritis.
Systemic Sclerosis.   Psoriatic arthritis, polyarticular gout may mimic RA.

Neoplastic
Bone Tumor/Metastasis.   Tumor seen on radiographs.

Acquired
Carpal Tunnel Syndrome.   Median nerve distribution of symptoms. Frequently occurs with repetitive use. Neurodiagnostic tests positive.

Vascular.   Not applicable.
Congenital.   Not applicable.

TREATMENT

Pharmacologic
The following may be beneficial:
- Salicylates:
    Enteric-coated aspirin 3000-4000 mg/24 hours
    Alternatives: extended-release aspirin (Easprin, ZORprin), choline
        magnesium trisalicylate (Trilisate), salsalate (Disalcid)
- Newer nonsteroidal anti-inflammatory drugs (NSAIDs): ibuprofen, naproxen, cyclooxygenase-2 (COX-2) inhibitors
- Antimalarial drugs: hydroxychloroquine
- Disease-modifying antirheumatic drugs (DMARDs): methotrexate, gold sodium thiomalate, penicillamine, azathioprine, sulfasalazine,

leflunomide, etanercept, infliximab, and others. At the time of this writing there are 8 new drugs in clinical trials or coming to market.
- Intra-articular or systemic corticosteroids: prednisone
- Prosorba Column: Used in patients in whom RA is refractory to other treatments. It requires a setup similar to that for hemodialysis.

Surgical

Surgical treatment includes joint replacement or stabilization procedures (e.g., for C1-C2 atlantoaxial subluxation).

Other

Referral to physical or occupational therapy can be considered for home exercise instruction and to maximize self-care and activity function.

PEDIATRIC CONSIDERATIONS

At least 60% of all pediatric patients with juvenile RA will improve without use of DMARDs. Patients should be referred for specialty care to practitioners with experience in management of juvenile RA.

OBSTETRIC CONSIDERATIONS

RA does not have an effect on pregnancy; in fact, 75% of patients with RA experience an alleviation of their symptoms during pregnancy. Unfortunately, 90% of these patients will experience an exacerbation of their RA disease within a few months post partum.

Many RA treatments are contraindicated in pregnancy, and some agents are teratogenic. Contraception should be urged in women taking routine medications for RA. Medications may be modified or discontinued in those wishing to become pregnant.

The use of NSAIDs should be avoided, especially during the third trimester of pregnancy. These medications are implicated in premature closure of the fetal ductus arteriosus and may interfere with labor. Chronic aspirin use has been associated with decreased fetal birth weight, increased incidence of stillbirth, neonatal mortality, antepartum and postpartum bleeding, delivery complications, and prolonged gestation.

GERIATRIC CONSIDERATIONS

PMR may precede or coexist with RA in patients older than 60.

PREVENTIVE CONSIDERATIONS

Isotonic exercise is recommended. Abrupt, forceful exercise may exacerbate symptoms.

PEARLS FOR THE PA

The rheumatoid factor assay may be falsely positive, so the diagnosis of RA should be made on clinical grounds first, using this test only to confirm the diagnosis.

Morning stiffness of the hands for more than 1 hour is the critical clue to a possible diagnosis of RA. Without prompting for specifics, ask patients to describe what it is like for them to use their hands in the morning.

If possible, all patients with RA should see a rheumatologist. A chest film helps to exclude intrathoracic disease.

Sprains, Strains, and Fractures

Leith Audrey Fitch, BMS, PA-C

DEFINITION

A *sprain* is acute trauma to a joint that causes pain and disability; it classically involves a tear of the tissue, usually a ligament. A *strain* is excessive repetitive use of a body part that stretches fibers at a frequency beyond their inherent capacity to regenerate/recover. It usually involves a musculotendinous unit. A *fracture* is the loss of the structural integrity of a bone.

HISTORY

Symptoms. The affected area is swollen, painful, and tender; ecchymosis with possible deformity. The patient may refrain from using the affected area. If there is associated nerve, muscle, or vascular injury, the patient may experience weakness or numbness distal to the injury.

General. Take a full history regarding the mechanism of injury. Determine what body part(s) are affected; the force (amount, weight, height, and direction); position of the injured area; time after injury to symptom onset; and other relevant information. Assess sensory and motor function distal to the injury. Inquire about the presence of underlying medical conditions (e.g., liver, ulcer, kidney, or reflux disease) that may affect medical management.

The most likely area for sprain is the ankle, followed by the knees, shoulders, wrists, fingers, and occasionally the hip or elbow.

A fracture usually requires a significant force to create a break in the bone. Fractures happen most often when the body is falling or when something falling strikes a body part. Radiographs usually reveal the fracture. Navicular wrist and stress fractures may not be seen on initial film, necessitating repeat x-ray study depending on symptoms at 2 to 3 weeks after injury.

The most commonly missed fracture is the second one. Do not focus on only the most obvious injury.

Age.   In children, injury to the tendon-bone connection is more common. This predisposition changes to the muscle-tendon connection in adults. Young adults complain more often of overuse injuries. Beyond age 40, degenerative conditions affecting tendons, joints, and intraspinal disks are more common. Elderly persons have less compliant tissues, so less force is required to sprain or tear tissue.

Onset.   Acute with fractures and sprains. Strains make take weeks to months to become manifest.

Duration.   Variable, depending on the mechanism of injury, underlying illness, secondary gain, smoking, and duration between injury and treatment.

Intensity.   Can be mild with an early strain to severe and life- or limb-threatening with significant fracture.

Aggravating Factors.   Continued significant activity aggravates the underlying sprain, strain, or fracture. Smoking will increase time required for healing; poor physical conditioning can predispose a patient to injury.

Alleviating Factors.   Regimen of rest, ice, compression, and elevation (RICE) for sprain and strain. Immobilization for fracture.

Associated Factors.   Intoxication, risk-taking behavior, work-related injury, metabolic bone disease (e.g., osteoporosis).

PHYSICAL EXAMINATION

General.   Observe the patient when the patient is unaware of the observation (e.g., in the waiting room, during transfer to the examination room) to note the degree of disability.

Musculoskeletal.   Observe the area of pain and compare with the contralateral body part when possible.

Note any deformity, skin discoloration, focal and distal swelling, tenting of the skin, and the underside or backside of the injured part, as gravity-dependent swelling or ecchymosis can be missed.

Gently press distal to the wound on the skin or nails to assess capillary refill. Assess sensory function for sharp and dull sensation. Palpate for point tenderness, deformity, or crepitus, which may signify a fracture.

Consider performing an x-ray study before testing joint mobility if there is a possibility of a fracture. Test the active and passive range of motion of the affected area. Include the joints above and below the injured area. Test laxity of ligamentous tendon structures that may have been involved in the injury. Test muscle strength of the extremity to assess for neurologic or muscular injury.

PATHOPHYSIOLOGY

Ligaments attach bones to bones, and tendons are those tissues that attach muscles to bones.

Sprains are injuries in which the involved tissue stretches to an extent that some, many, or all of the fibers tear. The tears are called micro or grade I if only some of the tissue fibers tear; they are associated with minimal swelling and mild pain. In partial or grade II injuries, much of the ligament tears but is still attached; this grade of tear accounts for most clinical injuries. In complete or grade III injuries, the entire ligament is torn, resulting in instability of the joint or joint space widening.

Fractures usually require significant force, but examples of fractures that do not require significant force include stress fractures, fractures associated with metabolic disease (e.g., osteoporosis, osteomalacia, osteopenia, parathyroid disturbances), and pathologic fractures from osteoclastic action of neoplasms or multiple myeloma.

Open fractures may lead to osteomyelitis, which will appear on radiographs as diffuseness or vagueness of the periosteum.

Types of fractures include the following:

Open fracture: A break in the bone that is accompanied by a break in the skin, through which the bone may or may not extrude.

Transverse fracture: A break that is horizontal to the longest measurement of the bone.

Oblique fracture: A break that is both longitudinal and horizontal along the bone.

Compression fracture: A fracture caused by axial pressure against a bone in which the matrix is crushed onto itself. Unlike most fractures, it appears as density and not as opacity of the bones on radiographs. Occurs often in vertebrae and at the distal radius as a result of fall onto the hand or wrist.

Articular fracture: A break that crosses the articular cartilage and involves the joint.

Displaced fracture: A break in which one or more fracture fragments are displaced from their natural position and have no contact with the other broken surface. Such displacement lessens the opportunity for natural healing/repair processes, and surgical fixation will probably be required.

Angulated fracture: An angulated break in which a broken bone piece is not in line with the bone from which it broke. Stated differently, the displacement of the bone is not equidistant at all points of displacement, so that a turn of the broken piece must have occurred during the injury.

Comminuted fracture: A break in which the bone is crushed or splintered.

SPECIFIC INJURIES

Ankle Injuries

Ankle sprains are the most commonly seen sprains. The mechanism of injury is usually an inversion: The ankle is typically swollen laterally, but some patients have medial pain.

Point tenderness at the lateral malleolus (distal fibula) or base of the fifth metatarsal suggests fracture of these areas. Some forceful injuries cause an avulsion of the fibula at the lateral knee joint. Stability is determined as follows: The examiner pulls forward on the back of the heel (calcaneus) while holding the front of the lower leg (the distal tibia-fibula) with the other hand. If the joint slides forward more than 4 mm, creating a ridge, it is unstable.

Treatment for sprain includes RICE, immobilization to minimize inversion and eversion, and crutches for ambulation if weight bearing is too painful or if the joint is unstable. Nonsteroidal anti-inflammatory drugs (NSAIDs) can be given for pain and swelling. Fractures require non–weight-bearing status and referral to orthopedics.

Achilles Tendon Tear

A sudden fall onto a dorsiflexed foot may cause an Achilles tendon tear. Palpate for lumps, tenderness, and deformity. Preservation of plantar flexion, even minimal, means that the Achilles is at least partially intact. On squeezing the calf, the gastrocnemius muscles will plantar flex the foot passively. If there is no movement, then Achilles tendon tear is present and the patient is referred for surgery.

Foot/Toe Injuries

For nondisplaced toe fractures, "buddy tape" with anatomic supportive padding between the toes. An orthopedic (postoperative) shoe may be used for immobilization of the great toe. A few days of elevation when the patient is seated and limited standing and walking to less than 10% to 50% of the time will reduce swelling and throbbing.

If the fifth metatarsal (key to balance) is fractured, the patient must be kept non–weight bearing. Repeat film is obtained in these injuries if symptoms persist, as the thickness and radiograph overlay of the foot bones make some fractures difficult to visualize. Nontraumatic pain at the sole of the foot is often plantar fasciitis and responds to a regimen of ice, stretching, anti-inflammatories, and weight reduction.

Knee Injuries

Mechanism of injury should be ascertained. Determine if the injury was sudden, if the patient is able to bear weight, if there is locking, or if the pain onset was gradual.

A sudden severe onset of pain with anterior laxity, tested by supporting the femur and pulling behind the superior tibia (anterior drawer or Lachman test), suggests an anterior cruciate ligament (ACL) tear. Locking of the knee and pain with passive twisting of the foot with the knee flexed (McMurray test) suggest meniscus tear. Consider an MRI study for diagnosis.

Lateral or medial longitudinal ligament injuries may be revealed by a varus or valgus laxity, respectively.

An effusion causes swelling above the patella; bursitis is usually present below the patella. In bursitis, the affected bursa looks like a marshmallow beneath the skin. Long-standing effusion often is a sign of internal derangement, although sometimes it resolves without further problems.

Observe the knee for swelling, ecchymosis, skin integrity, warmth, erythema. Check for posterior tibia or dorsalis pedis pulses. Test function with deep knee bend, and test strength with heel and toe walking. Weight bearing and any limp can also be clues to the diagnosis.

A hot, red, swollen knee that develops over 2 days is a septic joint until proven otherwise by an orthopedist.

Radiographs do not show the most common acute injuries of the knee, which are ligamentous and meniscal. Tibial plateau fractures may be seen on radiographs.

Treatment is with knee support with rigid sides if there are any signs of instability. Soft knee support is used for strains and sprains with no sign of ligamentous laxity or meniscal tear. Immobilization is used only for fractures. Add ice, physical therapy, NSAIDs; limit kneeling, squatting, and climbing stairs and ladders.

Hip Injuries
Palpate both trochanters and posterior superior and anterior superior iliac spine (PSIS and ASIS). Check range of motion, reflexes, and pulses, and assess function and strength of muscles of abduction, adduction, flexion, extension, and rotation.

On radiograph, check the femoral head and neck and the acetabulum of the ileus. Sometimes the force is transferred to the sacroiliac joints, so evaluate for symmetry. An abducted femur view should be obtained to reveal compression fractures.

Lumbar and/or Sacral Region Injuries
Low back strain is an exceedingly common injury, occurring most often between the ages of 30 and 50 years. At some point in life, 78% of all people will have a back injury.

Determine the mechanism of injury. Direct trauma, motor vehicle accident, and heavy/incorrect lifting all suggest different injuries. Inquire about the presence of radicular pain (lower extremity/dermatomal numbness, tingling, pain, myotomal weakness). Examine the extremities for motor strength, sensation, and deep tendon reflexes. It is imperative to ask about bowel, bladder, or sexual dysfunction as well as paresthesias in the "saddle" area or perineum, which may indicate a cauda equina syndrome that is a surgical emergency.

Consider x-ray studies, especially if the patient is older than 50 years, has a history of multiple back injuries, was involved in a high-impact injury, or has radicular symptoms, or if the pain was of insidious onset.

Thoracic Injuries
The thorax is easy to sprain and strain. Thoracic pain may also be related to visceral pain, which must always be a consideration. Injury to the shoulder (scapula/rhomboids) may manifest as a thoracic injury, as can chest wall

strains and rib fractures. X-ray studies should be performed to evaluate the spine and internal organs.

Cervical Injuries

With all high-velocity injuries and with low-velocity injuries in the elderly, the patient should be immobilized and radiographs obtained (possibly with CT scanning) before any range of motion testing. Inquire about the presence of radicular pain (upper extremity/dermatomal numbness, tingling, pain, myotomal weakness). Examine the extremities for motor strength, sensation, and deep tendon reflexes. It is imperative to ask about bowel, bladder, or sexual dysfunction. Lower extremity greater than upper extremity weakness suggests a central cord syndrome, which may be encountered in the elderly patient.

Key elements to look for on radiograph are the odontoid fracture, facet fractures, vertebral body fractures (these require great force or specifically applied force), and any discontinuity of three gently curving lines on lateral view (representing anterior portion of vertebral bodies, posterior portion of vertebral bodies, and posterior spinous processes) Note any arthritic changes, bone bridging between vertebrae, loss of disk space, loss of natural lordotic curve (although loss of lordosis is present in 20% to 30% of uninjured persons).

Once spine films have ruled out overt injury and the neurologic examination has confirmed that function is intact, test range of motion. Spurling test for radicular signs is simultaneous rotation and extension of the neck, which elicits pain radiating into the ipsilateral upper extremity. There is a loss of radial pulse on abduction in cases of thoracic outlet syndrome and in some cervical nerve compression injuries.

Shoulder Injuries

This joint can move in almost any direction, so any trauma occurring in any plane has the potential of tearing soft tissue. Examiner must look for signs of impingement (adduction across the chest), dislocation (tenderness or gap at the acromioclavicular [AC] joint), rotator cuff tears (positive *drop arm test*: arm cannot be held out to the side).

X-ray studies are performed to evaluate for AC separation and dislocation. Contralateral films can be very useful.

Early physical therapy should be instituted for sprains and strains to avoid development of a "frozen shoulder." Reduce anterior shoulder dislocation and obtain repeat films to ensure correct positioning and rule out avulsion fractures.

Elbow Injuries

Usually the injury results when the patient falls, landing on the elbow, or when the elbow is struck by something.

Examine the olecranon, ulnar groove, medial and lateral epicondyles, and radial head for tenderness. Test range of motion, as inability to fully extend or flex and pain with supination and pronation are clinical signs of occult fracture. Squeeze the radius and ulna together at the forearm gently to elicit complaint of pain in the elbow.

On radiograph, check for *fat pad sign* on lateral view, suggesting radial head fracture. This is seen as an oval or a circular opacity, representing the marrow from a break bleeding into the space of least resistance, medial to the distal humerus. "Tennis elbow" is pain in the lateral epicondyle. Medial epicondylitis is termed "golfer's elbow." A tennis elbow support or strap may be used to reduce pressure on the epicondyle.

Wrist Injuries

Determine the mechanism of injury. A fall on the outstretched hand can cause a fracture. The wrist is frequently the site of repetitive joint injury.

Examination includes palpation of the scaphoid, snuffbox (navicular), and flexor and extensor ligaments; testing range of motion in all planes; palpation of pulses; testing of grip strength, interosseous muscle strength; *Finklestein test*: ulnar deviation of the wrist with the thumb abducted elicits pain, suggesting a de Quervain tendinitis.

There are special tests for carpal tunnel syndrome—*Phalen maneuver*: holding wrists in full flexion or extension for 60 seconds causes reproduction of symptoms; *Tinel sign*: percussion of the ventral aspect of the wrist causes tingling in the first, second, and third digits.

X-ray studies are performed to check for scaphoid fracture (obtain repeat radiograph at 2 to 3 weeks if snuffbox pain persists, as a missed fracture can result in avascular necrosis). Also check the distal radius for fracture (Colles fracture), and look for the Terry-Thomas (gap tooth) sign between the lunate and triquetrum bones as an indication of ligament tear or injury.

Carpal tunnel syndrome is confirmed via electromyography (EMG).

Wrist splint is used during activity and possibly at night for most sprains and strains. NSAIDs may be added.

Hand/Finger Injuries

In the hand, dislocation of a joint is a result of opposing forces hitting on opposite sides of the digit, disrupting the joint between the adjacent bones. Distal interphalangeal (DIP) and proximal interphalangeal (PIP) joints are most often affected.

Ligamentous laxity can indicate ligament injury, which may necessitate surgical referral. Tendon function must be tested in both flexors and extensors.

Refer for any open fracture, tendon or nerve injury, articular fracture, or persistent symptoms.

Digital tendon sheath infection (felon) necessitates immediate referral. The patient presents with a "sausage finger" and painful inability to flex the digital tendons, associated with a recent open wound involving the palmar aspect of the digits or metacarpals.

DIAGNOSTIC STUDIES

Laboratory

Complete Blood Count. Elevated white blood cell (WBC) count with infection (e.g., osteomyelitis).

Erythrocyte Sedimentation Rate (ESR). Elevated in arthritides, inflammatory processes, and other acute processes (e.g., metastatic cancer).

Radiology
Plain Films: Anteroposterior, Lateral, and (Often) Oblique Views. Imperative for any musculoskeletal injury involving any force. If the cause of injury was routine lifting or repetitive motion, radiographs are not as useful, as these hold a low yield of bone pathology. Radiographs are more important in patients who have a history of prior injury to the same body part, are older than 50 years of age, are in poor health, or have a history of cancer.

In previously injured patients, arthritic changes such as extra bone deposits at the joint or loss of joint space in degeneration are often found.

Examine for dark lines in the bone, wider spaces than usual, avulsions at the attachment of a tendon or ligament. Avulsed bone will be rough-edged and not smooth like many normal sesamoid bones.

Consider obtaining a film of the contralateral body part for comparison.

If significant symptoms persist for 3 weeks or longer and the first films were negative, consider obtaining repeat radiographs, especially with navicular wrist injuries and stress fractures.

Other
Not applicable.

DIFFERENTIAL DIAGNOSIS

Traumatic
Contusion. X-ray studies are negative.

Infectious
Bone Infection (e.g., Osteomyelitis, Diskitis). Fever, elevated WBC count, elevated ESR. May have radiographic changes.

Metabolic
Gout. Negative radiograph. Reddened joint, usually great toe. No history of trauma. May have elevated serum uric acid and elevated ESR.
Rheumatoid Arthritis. See "Rheumatoid Arthritis" in this chapter.
Lupus. More diffuse symptoms. ESR elevated.
Visceral Pathology. May cause pain that is referred to the back and mimic a sprain/strain. A full history and complete physical examination should differentiate.

Neoplastic
Metastatic Cancer. May have a history of cancer, especially lymph, blood, liver, lung, breast, colorectal, or prostate cancer.
Primary Bone Tumor. Night pain is more characteristic of tumor.

Vascular
Aortic Dissection or Aneurysm. Should be a consideration with intrascapular pain.
Myocardial Infarction. May cause extremity pain.

Congenital
See Pediatric Considerations section.

Acquired
Long-Term Steroid Use. Can weaken connective tissue.
Fluoroquinolone Use. Even short-term use has been implicated in increased likelihood of tendon injury and dysfunction.

TREATMENT

Sprains/Strains

Splint
Protect the joint by immobilization or support.

Rest, Ice, Compression, Elevation (RICE)
In the acute phase, or the first 72 hours after the injury, this regimen will help minimize dead cells and blood collection in injured tissue. Ice the area at least four times per day. Compress with an Ace wrap or orthotic. Elevate the involved area above the level of the heart as much as possible.

Immobilization for 2 or 3 days is indicated with mild injuries and in well-conditioned patients. With more severe injuries and in poorly conditioned persons, 2 to 3 weeks of splinting may be indicated. Beyond that, risk of prolonged weakness and stiffness markedly increases. Occasionally, strains of a chronic nature or tendinitis may be well served by a more prolonged use of orthotics for stabilization until strength is regained. The patient should be instructed to perform range of motion exercises to keep the tissues mobile during the healing process. Limitations should be as few as possible, to discourage development of dependence syndrome, but generous enough to keep the patient safe. No activity and/or bedrest should be reserved for only the most serious and completely debilitating injuries

Medication
NSAIDs are given for pain and swelling. Narcotic analgesics may be used for severe pain in the short term.

Duration
Most sprains and strains require 2 to 3 weeks for essentially complete recovery . Mild injuries can resolve in 2 to 3 days, and severe or complete tears may require surgery and/or 2 to 3 months to heal completely.

Weight Bearing

If there is instability, report of giving out, or marked limp, advise the patient to maintain non–weight-bearing status and prescribe crutches.

Fracture

Initial treatment is reduction of the fracture to align distal to proximal fragments to allow for healing and prevent nerve, muscle, or vascular compromise. Displaced fractures will usually require surgery. This is followed by immobilization using a splint, cast, pins, traction, or open reduction and internal fixation (ORIF).

Ice approximately 15 minutes per hour for 72 hours or more.

For pain management, narcotics should be prescribed far more generously than in sprains. Avoid aspirin if surgery is indicated.

In pregnant patients with a fracture, avoid analgesics except acetaminophen unless prescribed or cleared by the obstetrician.

Potential complications of fracture include delayed union, nonunion, malunion, shortening of a limb, and compartment syndrome.

PEDIATRIC CONSIDERATIONS

A child with a fracture may present with a refusal to use a limb or may have a limp, pain, and swelling. Fractures in children differ from those in adults because their bones are less brittle. A fracture may involve only one cortex (torus fracture). A *greenstick fracture* occurs when one cortex is fractured and the opposite cortex bends significantly. The most common area of injury in the child is the bone-tendon insertion (in adults the injury occurs more often at the muscle-tendon insertion). Bone healing is much more rapid in children.

Ligamentous injuries are less common in children.

Open epiphyses (growth plates) may be present up to age 25 years. From 15% to 20% of fractures involve the epiphysis; these injuries are successfully treated with closed reduction and casting.

Any child who presents with bone pain should have a full evaluation with consideration for referral to an orthopedist. Significant disease manifesting as bone pain is more common in children. Pain worse on awaking may represent juvenile rheumatoid arthritis; night pain may signify a tumor. Consider neurologic disorders, growth abnormalities, and injuries. Always consider child abuse if the history does not make sense, if there are conflicting reports of how injury occurred, or if there are multiple injuries in various stages of healing.

OBSTETRIC CONSIDERATIONS

X-rays are to be avoided in pregnant patients. When radiographs are unavoidable, the patient should be draped with a lead apron to minimize exposure to radiation. No pelvic/abdominal films should be obtained.

GERIATRIC CONSIDERATIONS

The elderly patient is more prone to have metabolic bone disease (e.g., osteoporosis), underlying medical problems (e.g., metastatic disease), unsteadiness, and falls. The bones are more brittle, so fractures may occur more readily. Morbidity and mortality are increased in the elderly patient. Assess gait and activities of daily living, and recommend accommodations such as a walker, evenly spaced furniture, frequent checks, or even assisted living.

Elder abuse must be considered if the history does not make sense, if there are conflicting reports of how injuries occurred, or if there are multiple injuries in various stages of healing. If the patient is able to participate, take a private history from the patient and from family members separately.

PREVENTIVE CONSIDERATIONS

For the younger person, appropriate conditioning and stretching should be encouraged before participation in athletics, strenuous physical activity, or work involving physical exertion.

With advancing age, modifications can be made to prevent falls and injury. Continued conditioning, use of orthotics or walkers, attention to walking surfaces, and assistance in the home can be considered. Appropriate measures to prevent metabolic bone disease should be employed (see "Metabolic Bone Disorders" in Chapter 4, Endocrinology).

PEARLS FOR THE PA

Ligaments attach bones to bones, and tendons are those tissues that attach muscles to bones.

Pain worse on awaking may represent juvenile rheumatoid arthritis; night pain may signify a tumor.

Consider child or elder abuse if the history is inconsistent with nature of the injury.

Tendinitis/Bursitis

Roderick S. Hooker, PhD, PA

DEFINITION

Tendinitis is an inflammation of the tendon tissue or the tendon sheath (tenosynovitis). *Bursitis* is an inflammation of the bursa. A bursa is a closed sac containing a small amount of synovial fluid (usually less than 1 cm³). There are approximately 160 formed bursae in areas where tendons and muscles move over bony prominences. Unfortunately, both terms are often used interchangeably, but in a true bursitis, the bursa contains fluid that can be aspirated. Tendinitis is often mislabeled as bursitis.

HISTORY

Symptoms. Edema of the affected area is common, and occasionally there will be a fluctuant mass suggesting bursitis.

General. Strenuous, repetitive motion or direct injury is the most common etiologic mechanism. Further questioning often reveals that this is an activity in which the patient seldom participates in, such as painting or hoeing. Replication of the repetitive motion will be painful or the condition may sometimes be manifested as blocking of the normal motion of the tendon.

Age. Most common in adults.

Onset. Usually acute, within 1 to 3 days of activity.

Duration. Weeks to months.

Intensity. Moderate; severe with activity.

Aggravating Factors. Use of the extremity in activities in which the tendon overrides the involved bursa.

Alleviating Factors. Ice, rest, protection.

Associated Factors. None.

PHYSICAL EXAMINATION

General

The patient will be observed avoiding the use/overuse of the affected area.

Extremities

Shoulder

The *Yergason maneuver* tests for the presence of the biceps tendon in the groove. The patient flexes the elbow 90 degrees and holds it alongside the body. The examiner grasps the flexed elbow in one hand while holding the patient's wrist with the other hand. The examiner externally rotates the grasped arm as the patient resists. Pain is replicated in the shoulder if there is tendinitis or a slippage of the bicipital tendon out of the groove.

The *drop arm test* detects whether or not there are any tears in the rotator cuff. The patient fully abducts the arm (straight out laterally from the side). Then the patient is asked to slowly lower it to the side. If there are tears in the rotator cuff or supraspinatus tendon, the arm will drop to the side from a position of 90 degrees. The patient will not be able to lower it smoothly in rotator cuff tear and will not be able to raise it to 90 degrees in tendinitis.

Subacromial bursa lies between the acromion and the rotator cuff. Subdeltoid bursa lies between the deltoid muscle and the rotator cuff.

Subcoracoid bursa lies at the attachments of the biceps, coracobrachialis, and pectoralis minor tendons to the coracoid process.

Elbow

Olecranon bursitis is palpable or inspissated (thickened) over the olecranon process.

Tennis elbow test reproduces the pain of lateral epicondylitis. The examiner stabilizes the patient's forearm and instructs him or her to make a fist and extend the wrist. The examiner applies pressure with the other hand to the dorsum of the patient's fist in an attempt to force the wrist into flexion. If epicondylitis (tennis elbow) is present, the patient will experience a sudden severe pain at the site of the wrist's common extensor origin, the lateral epicondyle.

Hip

Trochanteric tendinitis, usually known as "trochanteric bursitis," involves the hip in gait and often arises from the imbalanced stresses incurred with limping on the contralateral side. The soft tissues that cross the bone portion of the greater trochanter are protected by the trochanteric bursa. Tenderness indicates trochanteric tendinitis. If the bursa is inflamed, the area feels boggy.

Groin tendinitis may involve the sartorius or adductor longus muscle. Palpation of these tendons is with the leg flexed and the ankle placed across the opposite knee, with the hip abducted.

Ischiogluteal bursa separates the gluteus maximus muscle from the ischial tuberosity.

Wrists

Stenosing tenosynovitis of the wrist (de Quervain disease) is chronic pain in the anatomic snuffbox when the tendon sheath of the extensor hallucis pollicis brevis tendon is involved. In long-standing cases, orange seed–sized swellings may be palpable near the radial styloid process. In the *Finkelstein test*, the fist is clenched over the thumb; forceful ulnar deviation of the hand by the examiner elicits pain in the radial styloid process area.

Fingers

Stenosing tenosynovitis of the finger flexors ("trigger finger") is the sudden and sometimes audible snapping that occurs on flexion or extension of the finger. The snapping results when a nodule in the flexor tendon catches on a narrower annular sheath or pulley opposite the metacarpal head. It may take place either in flexion or in extension. The thumb may also be involved.

Knee

Bursitis is a rather common ailment around the knee joint; tendinitis is less common. Most of the bursitides are situated in the anterior portion of the knee.

Osgood-Schlatter disease is epicondylitis (or enthesitis) resulting from swelling and inflammation of the infrapatellar tendon insertion into the tibial tubercule in young persons.

The prepatellar bursa lies between the skin and the prepatellar tendon, and bursitis in this area of the knee is known as "housemaid's knee." This condition differs from presence of fluid in the joint cavity, which produces swelling on either side of the patella and the patellar ligament and the quadriceps tendon.

Infrapatellar bursitis, involvement of the bursa that lies deep under the insertion of the patellar ligament, is known as "clergyman's knee." Swelling occurs on both sides of the patellar ligament, near the tibial tuberosity. Fluctuation can be demonstrated from one side of the ligament to the other.

Popliteal bursae are numerous. The largest lies between the semimembranosus muscle and the medial head of the gastrocnemius muscle.

Pes Anserine Tendinitis/Bursitis.   On the posteromedial side of the knee, the sartorius, gracilis, and semitendinosus muscles converge to create the pes anserinus insertion into the lower portion of the medial tibial plateau. At the common insertion lies the pes anserine bursa, which may become inflamed, resulting in pain during motion.

Foot

Achilles tendinitis usually occurs at the medial or lateral insertion of this tendon. A thickened distal portion suggests tendinitis. A fluctuant mass just above the calcaneus where the tendon inserts into the posterior aspect of the calcaneus suggests calcaneus bursitis.

Subcalcaneal bursitis occurs at the insertion of the plantar fascia into the medial tuberosity of the calcaneus.

Plantar fasciitis is a type of tendinitis that occurs on the plantar aspect of the foot, may lead to toe walking behavior, and is a common injury in long-distance runners.

PATHOPHYSIOLOGY

Tendinitis/tenosynovitis is an inflammation of the cellular lining of the membrane of the fibrous tube (vagina) through which a tendon moves.

Stenosing tenovaginitis is primarily a disorder of the fibrous wall of the tendon sheath, particularly at locations where the tendon passes through a fibrous ring or pulley.

Bursitis occurs when the bursal sac, otherwise thinly lined with synovial tissue, fills with inflammatory fluid as a result of friction or trauma.

DIAGNOSTIC STUDIES

Laboratory

Aspiration of Bursal Fluid.   Will demonstrate inflammatory fluid with white blood cell (WBC) counts ranging from 1000 to 10,000/mm³. Usually the polymorphonuclear leukocytes will exceed 50%.

Radiology
Plain Radiographs of Affected Area. Depending on the primary disease, may demonstrate bone changes, calcific deposits of the tendon or bursa, or actual enlargement of the bursa.

Arthrography or MRI. May show a communication with the gleno-humeral joint capsule when bursitis is caused by a complete rupture of the rotator cuff.

Bursography. May be useful in demonstrating the impingement syndrome, adhesive capsulitis, or rotator cuff tears. Rarely performed.

Other
Ultrasound Examination. Depending on the site of the lesion, may help to visualize the extent of the tendinitis or bursitis. Helpful in rotator cuff tears.

DIFFERENTIAL DIAGNOSIS

Traumatic
Rotator Cuff Tear. Positive drop arm test.

Infectious
Septic Bursitis. Warm and red, and the aspirate will be purulent.
Intra-articular Effusions. Will cause loss of joint motion, either passive or active, whereas tendinitis still allows the joint to be flexed or extended.

Metabolic. Not applicable.
Neoplastic. Not applicable.
Vascular. Not applicable.
Congenital. Not applicable.
Acquired. Not applicable.

TREATMENT

Treatment of tendinitis or bursitis is directed at pain relief, maintenance of maximal joint function, and prevention of complications such as adhesive capsulitis or the reflex sympathetic dystrophy syndrome. Early rehabilitation and education constitute the mainstay of treatment.

Limit the use of the extremity during acute painful periods. Immobilize the affected area with an adduction sling for shoulder, wrist support for hand and wrist, or Unna boot or elastic wrap for ankle. Physical therapy includes cold for acute conditions, heat for subacute and chronic conditions. Ultrasound and diathermic and hydrocollator packs are sometimes helpful. Active exercise with resistance or assistance is recommended.

Nonsteroidal anti-inflammatory drugs (NSAIDs) are frequently prescribed, but generally the anti-inflammatory levels are not adequate for substantial penetration of the bursae and tendons. Analgesics include codeine, propoxyphene, and hydrocodone. Muscle relaxants are not recommended.

Corticosteroid injections are employed if these basic measures fail to control symptoms and restore movement. In bursitis, the first step is aspiration of the bursal fluid. Then intra-articular instillation is performed using the following:

In *bursitis*:

Prednisolone tebutate (Hydeltra-T.B.A.) 5-30 mg PLUS bupivacaine 0.5-10 mL (in same syringe)

In *tendinitis*:

Triamcinolone hexacetonide (Aristospan) 5-30 mg PLUS bupivacaine 0.5-10 mL (in same syringe)

In addition to the possible complications of systemic absorption and the risk of infection (remote), corticosteroids may reduce the tensile strength of the tendon, ultimately causing tendon rupture. This is especially true with the Achilles tendon.

Surgery is the final (albeit rare) option, sometimes required for refractory cases of flexor tendinitis or chronic elbow bursitis.

PEDIATRIC CONSIDERATIONS

Tendinitis and bursitis from trauma and repetitive use is unusual in preadolescents. Look for systemic forms of rheumatism such as juvenile rheumatoid arthritis.

OBSTETRIC CONSIDERATIONS

The use of NSAIDs should be avoided, especially during the third trimester of pregnancy. These medications are implicated in premature closure of the fetal ductus arteriosus and may interfere with labor. Chronic aspirin use has been associated with decreased fetal birth weight, increased incidence of stillbirth, neonatal mortality, antepartum and postpartum bleeding, delivery complications, and prolonged gestation.

A specific type of tendinitis that has had increasing incidence in pregnancy and the postpartum period is de Quervain disease (a type of wrist tendinitis). Women who are having their first pregnancy after the age of 30 years are at the greatest risk. Cortisone injections and wrist splinting have proved to be effective and safe for treatment of this disease entity during pregnancy.

GERIATRIC CONSIDERATIONS

None specific.

PREVENTIVE CONSIDERATIONS

Decrease weight bearing and repetitive motion activities. Ergonomic evaluation and modification may be of benefit. Referral to physical or occupational therapy for acute treatment and to develop home exercise program also is indicated.

PEARLS FOR THE PA

The physical examination is the key to the diagnosis of tendinitis or bursitis, not radiographs or laboratory tests.

If you can palpate a fluctuant mass, it is probably bursitis; otherwise, the diagnosis is probably tendinitis.

Further Reading

American Academy of Orthopaedic Surgeons: Essentials of Musculoskeletal Care. Rosemont, IL, American Academy of Orthopaedic Surgeons, 1997.

Baldry P: Myofascial Pain and Fibromyalgia Syndromes: A Clinical Guide to Diagnosis and Management. New York, Churchill Livingstone, 2001.

Koopman WJ: Arthritis and Allied Conditions: A Textbook of Rheumatology. Philadelphia, Lea & Febiger, 2001.

Labus JB, Lauber AA (eds): Patient Education and Preventive Medicine. Philadelphia, WB Saunders, 2001.

Moskowitz RW, Howell DS, Altman RD, et al (eds): Osteoarthritis: Diagnosis and Medical/Surgical Management, 3rd ed. Philadelphia, WB Saunders, 2001.

Ruddy S, Harris ED, Sledge CB (eds): Kelly's Textbook of Rheumatology, 6th ed. Philadelphia, WB Saunders, 2001.

Schumacher HR, Klippel JH, Koopman WJ: Primer on the Rheumatic Diseases. Atlanta, Arthritis Foundation, 2001.

UROLOGY

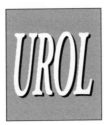

17

Benign Prostatic Hyperplasia

Robert J. McNellis, MPH, PA-C

DEFINITION

Benign prostatic hyperplasia (BPH) is nonmalignant growth of the prostate gland resulting in enlargement. May lead to bladder outlet obstruction and hydronephrosis.

HISTORY

Symptoms
Obstructive Symptoms. Hesitancy and straining to begin urination, decrease in caliber and force of stream, inability to empty bladder completely, difficulty in stopping urination, double voiding, dribbling.

Irritative Symptoms. Frequency, urgency, nocturia.

General. Patients commonly present with complaints related to quality of life due to changes in urination patterns. Commonly, the patient is frustrated because of frequency of urination, nocturia, incontinence, or postvoid dribbling. Patients with untreated BPH can present with acute urinary retention. Quantifying symptoms by use of the American Urological Association Symptom Score questionnaire is an important component of evaluation.

Age. Typically affects men in their mid-40s to 80s. More common with each decade. Mean age at onset 60 to 65 years.

Onset. Gradually progresses over the course of many years.

Duration. Up to 80% to 90% of patients have symptoms that remain unchanged or improve; 10% to 20% will require treatment.

Intensity. Symptoms increase in severity with increase in degree of obstruction. Severity often subjective, related to impact on patient's quality of life, but chronic obstruction may progress to renal insufficiency in 10% of patients.

Aggravating Factors. Intake of caffeine or alcohol, use of some medications (anticholinergics, antidepressants, tranquilizers, nasal decongestants), prolonged delay in voiding.

Alleviating Factors. None known.

Associated Factors. Recurrent urinary tract infections (UTIs), prostatitis, renal insufficiency.

PHYSICAL EXAMINATION

General. Patients appear very uncomfortable if experiencing acute urinary retention. Cardiovascular and pulmonary examinations should always be included in this patient age group to identify renal disease; screen for hypertension.

Gastrointestinal. Examine kidneys for enlargement (hydronephrosis), bladder for distention, flanks for costovertebral angle (CVA) tenderness, renal arteries for bruits. Digital rectal examination should be performed to evaluate tone, mucosa, and contents. Palpate prostate for normal size, symmetrical and smooth shape, distinct median sulcus and lateral margins, firm consistency. Tenderness and induration suggest prostatitis. Asymmetry and presence of nodule suggest prostate carcinoma. Crepitus with calculi may be found with chronic prostatitis. Size of prostate is not always related to severity of symptoms or degree of obstruction.

Genitourinary. Examine penis and foreskin for urethral meatal stenosis, urethra for calculi, corpora cavernosa for Peyronie disease (presence of penile curvature and firm penile plaques), perineal area for inflammation and tenderness. Examine scrotum and testes.

PATHOPHYSIOLOGY

Exact etiology is unclear, but BPH is possibly related to advancing age and hormonal influence. Mechanism is hyperplastic proliferation of the periurethral glandular portion of the prostate, often in combination with constriction of fibromuscular stroma of prostate. This causes compression of the prostatic urethra and obstruction of the bladder outlet. The detrusor muscles of the bladder then undergo a compensatory hypertrophy to overcome increased pressures needed to void. Long-term obstruction can lead to secondary ureteral obstruction and renal insufficiency.

DIAGNOSTIC STUDIES

Laboratory
Urinalysis. Performed to exclude UTI and identify hematuria.

Blood Urea Nitrogen (BUN)/Serum Creatinine Levels. Elevated, with decreased renal function from chronic obstruction.

Prostate-Specific Antigen (PSA). Interpret increased PSA with caution, as it may be elevated in both BPH and prostate cancer.

Radiology
Intravenous Pyelography. Recommended in the presence of other urinary tract disease. Examine upper urinary tract for ureteral dilatation, hydronephrosis, or stones, lower urinary tract for postvoid residual, bladder trabeculation, large prostatic impression in bladder, or bladder stones or diverticula.

Ultrasound Examination. Optional. Abdominal examination of kidneys for enlargement and bladder for determining capacity and postvoid residual volume. Transrectal examination of prostate for size and consistency.

Other

Uroflowmetry. Optional. Used to measure voiding urinary flow rates; greater obstruction produces decreased flow rates.

Cystometrography. Reserved for patients with suspected neurologic disease. Measures urine volumes and voiding pressures in the bladder to evaluate level of detrusor muscle contraction; pressures usually elevated.

Cystoscopy. Useful evaluation for patients requiring surgical intervention. Visualization of lower urinary tract will reveal prostatic enlargement and secondary bladder changes such as trabeculation and diverticula. Inflammation or bladder stones may be seen.

DIFFERENTIAL DIAGNOSIS

Traumatic

Urethral Instrumentation or Foreign Body Insertion. Historical or physical evidence.

Infectious

Cystitis, Prostatitis, Urethritis. Positive urinalysis and culture without prostatic enlargement.

Metabolic

Renal Failure. Increased BUN/creatinine; signs and symptoms of renal failure are present (edema, ecchymosis, pruritus, nutritional deficiencies, anemia).

Bladder Calculus. Visible during cystoscopy.

Polyuria Due to Diabetes Mellitus or Insipidus. Increased volume of urine without obstructive symptoms.

Neoplastic

Prostate Carcinoma. Prostate asymmetrical or nodular, elevated PSA, hypoechoic lesions on transrectal ultrasound study.

Bladder Carcinoma. Gross hematuria, visible lesions on cystoscopy.

Vascular

Renal Vascular Insufficiency. Presence of renal bruits, anemia, uremia, and other signs of atherosclerotic disease.

Congenital

Bladder Neck Contracture, Anterior or Posterior Urethral Valves, Müllerian Duct Cysts. Positive findings on cystoscopy.

Acquired

Neurogenic Bladder. History of diabetes mellitus, spinal cord injury, decreased pressures on cystometrogram.

Urethral Stricture, Bladder Neck Contracture. Visible on cystoscopy.

Meatal Stenosis. Visible with inspection of urethral meatus.

Detrusor Muscle Failure. History of myogenic disease.
Medication Side Effects. History of intake of diuretics, sympathomimetics, parasympatholytics.

TREATMENT

Medical/Pharmacologic

"Watchful waiting" is conservative management involving frequent follow-up and monitoring of renal function. Appropriate for men with mild symptom scores.

Pharmacologic agents that may be beneficial include:

- Alpha-adrenergic blockers: Useful because they decrease tone of prostate and bladder musculature/tissue. Begin with the lowest possible dose and titrate to the most effective dose while observing for side effects (commonly, orthostatic hypotension, dizziness, tiredness, headache). Agents include phenoxybenzamine, prazosin, terazosin, doxazosin, and tamsulosin. Dosage is drug specific, once or twice daily.
- 5α-Reductase inhibitors: Finasteride blocks conversion of testosterone to dihydrotestosterone, resulting in decreased size of prostate. Six months of therapy required for maximum effect. Reduces serum PSA, lessening effectiveness of prostate cancer screening.

Surgical

Transurethral resection of prostate (TURP) is treatment for progressive disease unresponsive to medical treatment. Open simple prostatectomy is often preferred technique for very large glands weighing more than 100 g. Transurethral incision of the prostate (TUIP) is effective in well-selected patients.

Other

Transurethral balloon dilatation, microwave hyperthermia, transurethral laser incision of prostate (TULIP), intraurethral stent placement, and transurethral needle ablation of the prostate are other minimally invasive modes of management.

PEDIATRIC CONSIDERATIONS

BPH is not a cause of obstruction in the pediatric population; other causes for obstruction should be sought.

OBSTETRIC CONSIDERATIONS

Not applicable.

GERIATRIC CONSIDERATIONS

A majority of men over age 65 will have this disorder. All treatment options are available, but it is important to evaluate for concomitant diseases that will affect renal or bladder function.

PREVENTIVE CONSIDERATIONS

No prevention techniques have proved effective; however, zinc supplements and saw palmetto have been claimed to improve prostate health.

PEARLS FOR THE PA

BPH is a very common disease in men in their mid-40s to 80s; eventually nearly all men will have the condition.

The treatment must be individualized.

The primary goal of treatment is reduction of potential for renal damage and improvement in quality of life.

Severity of the symptoms can be unrelated to the size of the gland.

Epididymitis

Timothy F. Quigley, MPH, PA-C

DEFINITION

Infectious and noninfectious inflammation of the epididymis.

HISTORY

Symptoms. Scrotal pain, possibly radiating up the spermatic cord to the groin or flank. Associated with frequency, urgency, and dysuria. Fever with temperatures up to 104° F (40° C).

General. The patient may have a recent history of heavy lifting or trauma, or the sexual history may include recent intense sexual activity, multiple partners, new partner, or unprotected anal intercourse.

Age. Puberty to old age.

Onset. Acute. In 3 to 4 hours the scrotum may double in size.

Duration. Patients usually seek medical attention within 24 hours of onset.

Intensity. Severe.

Aggravating Factors. Walking, movement, lack of scrotal support.

Alleviating Factors. Elevation of the scrotum.

Associated Factors. May be associated with sexually transmitted diseases (STDs), especially urethritis in younger men. In older men, may be associated with urinary tract infections and prostatitis. Uncircumcised adolescent boys have a threefold higher risk. Commonly coexists with orchitis.

PHYSICAL EXAMINATION

General. The patient may have fever with temperatures up to 104° F (40° C).

Genitourinary. Scrotum may be "heavy," enlarged, red, and flaky. The epididymis and testis are swollen and, within 3 to 4 hours of onset, may double in size. Later in the course of the disease, the epididymis and testis may appear as one enlarged, tender mass. The spermatic cord is enlarged, thick, and tender. The prostate may be tender to palpation. Prehn sign—diminished pain on elevation of the scrotum—can be elicited. Reactive hydrocele is common.

PATHOPHYSIOLOGY

The route of infection is usually ascending—from the urethra to the ejaculatory duct, to the vas deferens, and then to the epididymis. Infection of the epididymis may be caused by sexually transmitted organisms (*Neisseria gonorrhoeae*, *Chlamydia trachomatis*) or enteric organisms (members of family Enterobacteriaceae, *Pseudomonas*). Vesicoureteral reflux caused by increased hydrostatic pressure may allow for invasion by the causative organism.

Noninfectious epididymitis is a chemical inflammation caused by the reflux of urine into the ejaculatory ducts occurring with heavy physical straining. This type of epididymitis is usually self-limited.

DIAGNOSTIC STUDIES

Laboratory

Urinalysis with Culture and Sensitivity Testing. Positive if there is greater than 3 to 5 white blood cells (WBCs)/high-power field (hpf), greater than 0 to 2 red blood cells (RBCs)/hpf, presence of nitrate, or bacteriuria. Presence of white cells without visible organisms probably represents nongonococcal urethritis, especially that due to *Chlamydia trachomatis*. Gram stain of urethral discharge smear may demonstrate *N. gonorrhoeae*. If the epididymitis is not of sexually transmitted origin, urinalysis will show pyuria, hematuria, and bacteriuria, and urine cultures will demonstrate the offending pathogen.

Complete Blood Count. May show a leukocytosis with a left shift.

Radiology
Not applicable.

Other
Nuclear Scan. Will differentiate from testicular torsion.

Scrotal Ultrasound Examination. May be helpful in differentiating scrotal contents, especially if there is a reactive hydrocele. Essential to rule out testicular torsion.

DIFFERENTIAL DIAGNOSIS

Traumatic
Orchitis, Testicular Torsion. Prehn sign absent as there is increased pain on scrotal elevation; negative nuclear scan. Torsion typically has acute onset.

Infectious
Orchitis. Differentiated on nuclear scan by increased uptake on unhealed structure. Clinical diagnosis by exclusion.

Metabolic
Fournier Gangrene. Associated with diabetes mellitus. Definitive diagnosis made on exploration.

Neoplastic
Testicular Tumor. Usually nontender and discrete, with normal urinalysis.

Vascular
Varicocele. Nontender and easily diagnosed clinically by palpation of a "bag of worms."

Congenital
Congenital Hydrocele. Transilluminable.

Incarcerated Indirect Hernia. Easily diagnosed clinically, by a palpable mass entering the peritoneal cavity.

Acquired
Spermatocele. Nontender and discrete.

TREATMENT

Pharmacologic
Sexually transmitted:

If causative agent is *Neisseria gonorrhoeae*, treat according to Centers for Disease Control and Prevention (CDC) 2002 Guidelines:

Cefixime (Suprax) 400 mg PO in a single dose OR ceftriaxone (Rocephin) 125 mg IM in a single dose OR ciprofloxacin (Cipro)

500 mg PO in a single dose OR ofloxacin 400 mg OR levofloxacin 250 mg orally in a single dose PLUS

Chlamydial treatment as listed below if chlamydia is not ruled out.

If causative agent is *Chlamydia trachomatis*, treat with:

Azithromycin 1 g PO (single dose) or doxycycline 100 mg twice daily for 7 days OR

Erythromycin base 500 mg four times daily for 7 days OR

Erythromycin ethylsuccinate 800 mg four times daily for 7 days OR

Ofloxacin 300 mg twice daily for 7 days OR

Levofloxacin 500 mg once daily for 7 days

Non–sexually transmitted:

Ciprofloxacin 250-500 mg PO every 12 hours for 3 weeks OR ofloxacin 200-400 mg PO every 12 hours for 3 weeks OR trimethoprim-sulfamethoxazole (TMP-SMX) 160/800 mg PO every 12 hours for 3 weeks

Other Measures

Analgesics. Rest; no strenuous physical activity. Scrotal support, with ice packs to scrotum as necessary.

Abstinence from intercourse. Treat sexual partners if STD present.

May inject lidocaine into spermatic cord for symptomatic relief.

Consider hospitalization with persistent high fever; comorbid conditions such as diabetes mellitus, immunosuppression, or advanced age; urosepsis; acute urinary retention. If tenderness and swelling persist after 3 days of treatment, diagnosis and treatment should be reevaluated.

PEDIATRIC CONSIDERATIONS

Epididymitis should be considered in the differential diagnosis of acute scrotal pain and swelling, especially in children older than 13 years of age (acute painful and swollen testes should suggest testicular torsion until proven otherwise). Epididymitis is rare before puberty, and the possibility of congenital abnormality of the wolffian duct (ectopic ureter entering the vas) should be raised. Urinalysis often abnormal, may suggest antecedent history of sexual activity or urinary tract infection. Also may be associated with orchitis in adolescents secondary to mumps.

OBSTETRIC CONSIDERATIONS

Not applicable.

GERIATRIC CONSIDERATIONS

Epididymitis in the older man is usually caused by *Escherichia coli* infection. Look for underlying cause such as obstruction, acute urinary retention, prostatitis, urinary tract infection, indwelling catheter, history of genitourinary surgery.

PREVENTIVE CONSIDERATIONS

Prevention of STDs through safer sexual practices including condom use would prevent many cases of epididymitis.

PEARLS FOR THE PA

Always rule out testicular torsion in evaluation for epididymitis.

Prehn sign is diminished pain on elevation of the scrotum.

Erectile Dysfunction

Robert J. McNellis, MPH, PA-C

DEFINITION

An inability to obtain or sustain an erection that is satisfactory for sexual intercourse. Erectile dysfunction (impotence) should be viewed within the broad scope of male sexual dysfunction involving disorders of desire, arousal, sensation, orgasm, ejaculation, and relationship.

HISTORY

Symptoms. Difficulty obtaining an erection when desired, decreased duration of erections, decreased rigidity of erection, inability to have satisfactory penetration for sexual intercourse.

General. Transient periods of impotence may be experienced in about 50% of men, and such disturbances are not considered dysfunctional. Symptoms are dependent on the cause. Sexual history is very important to determine pattern, frequency, duration, and rigidity of erections, and to identify absence or presence of morning or nocturnal erections; strength of libido; drug and alcohol use; presence of concomitant medical diseases (e.g., peripheral vascular disease, coronary artery disease, hypertension, dyslipidemia, diabetes mellitus); medication use; and history of pelvic trauma or surgery.

Age.   Sexually active males of any age, most commonly 40 to 70 years of age.

Onset.   Can be gradual or sudden; also may be situational or partner specific.

Duration.   Generally, 6 to 12 months between onset and seeking of medical treatment.

Intensity.   May begin intermittently and become constant.

Aggravating Factors.   Alcohol use, medications (antihypertensives, psychotropics, hormonal agents, histamine H_2 blockers), relationship conflicts.

Alleviating Factors.   New sexual partner, changes in patterns of sexual relations.

Associated Factors.   Other psychogenic events such as stress or depression, hormonal imbalances, neurologic dysfunctions, vascular diseases, or pelvic surgery.

PHYSICAL EXAMINATION

General.   Vital signs, including orthostatic blood pressure (hypotension), presence of skin striae.

Cardiovascular.   Evaluate for signs of cardiac and peripheral or vascular disease, palpation of carotid, brachial, femoral, and penile arteries.

Endocrine.   Thyromegaly (thyroid dysfunction), loss of beard or body hair, gynecomastia, testicular atrophy (hypogonadism). Atrophic changes in extremities or central obesity (endocrine dysfunction).

Genitourinary.   Examine for deformed or curved penis (Peyronie disease), testicular atrophy or absence (hypogonadism or orchiectomy).

Neurologic.   Examine for decreased sensation to pinprick, light touch, and vibratory sensation in external genitalia, perineum, and lower extremities, and evaluate the bulbocavernosus reflex (to detect central or peripheral neuropathy).

PATHOPHYSIOLOGY

An erection is a complex event involving vascular, hormonal, neurologic, and psychologic factors. Psychogenic causes (performance anxiety, stress, or depression) used to be considered the most common reason for impotence but now are thought to be the primary reason in few cases. A secondary psychologic component can be expected in all cases of impotence. Diabetes is the most common hormonal cause, but impotence usually is due to vascular, neurologic, or psychogenic factors.

Organic causes include:

- Vascular causes of poor inflow due to arterial insufficiency or enhanced outflow due to venous leakage
- Endocrine causes due to low testosterone levels following orchiectomy or with hypothalamic or pituitary tumors

- Neurologic causes including diabetic neuropathy, multiple sclerosis, and spinal cord injury
- End-organ causes including priapism or Peyronie disease can cause cavernosa injury, resulting in erectile dysfunction

DIAGNOSTIC STUDIES

Laboratory
Serum Testosterone.   Low testosterone level may lead to decreased libido.
Serum Prolactin.   High levels may indicate prolactinoma.
Fasting Blood Glucose.   Elevated in diabetes mellitus.

Radiology
Doppler Studies.   Used to analyze arterial response to intracavernosal agents.
Arteriography.   Will visualize localized arterial disease.
Penile Cavernosography.   Used to measure venous outflow.

Other
Snap Gauge Test.   Measures nocturnal penile tumescence (circumference).
Rigiscan.   Measures nocturnal penile tumescence and rigidity.
Intracavernosal injection.   Injection of papaverine HCl or prostaglandin E_1 will produce erection in males without organic dysfunction.
Neurologic Evaluation.   Assessment of pudendal nerve pathways by somatosensory evoked potentials if neurologic findings in physical examination are abnormal.

DIFFERENTIAL DIAGNOSIS

Traumatic
Penile Injury or Vascular Trauma.   Historical or physical evidence.
Spinal Cord Injury.   History and physical findings present.

Infectious
Not applicable.

Metabolic
Diabetes Mellitus.   Elevated fasting blood glucose, associated with peripheral neuropathy, retinopathy.
Thyroid Dysfunction.   Thyromegaly, elevated thyroxine levels.
Renal Failure.   Pallor, peripheral edema, pruritus, nutritional deficiencies, uremia.
Primary Testicular Failure.   Decreased testosterone levels and testicular atrophy.

Neoplastic
Prolactinoma. Elevated prolactin levels, decreased libido.

Vascular
Arterial Insufficiency. Usually systemic disease associated with atherosclerosis, hypertension, or coronary artery disease.

Venous Insufficiency. Pattern of gradual loss of erectile function beginning with decreased duration and increasing loss of rigidity during intercourse. Cavernosography reveals incompetent venous constriction.

Congenital
Microphallus, Hypospadias. Corresponding findings on physical examination.

Acquired
Peyronie Disease. Presence of penile curvature and firm penile plaques.

Priapism. Use of intracavernosal agents for impotence, history of event.

Phimosis. Characteristic of inflamed prepuce.

Depression, Schizophrenia, Relationship Disorders, Personality Disorders, Anxiety. Evidence from history.

Medications. Use of antihypertensive agents (especially sympatholytics, alpha-adrenergic blockers, or beta blockers) or other drugs that inhibit libido or erections, such as antidepressants, tranquilizers, hypnotics, antiandrogens, estrogens, marijuana, alcohol, or narcotics; cigarette smoking.

TREATMENT

A unified conservative approach to management will provide the best opportunity for successful treatment of impotence. Counseling is important in nearly all cases. Involvement of urologist, endocrinologist, neurologist, and psychologist should be considered. Any discovered organic cause should be treated.

Psychologic treatment should provide sexual counseling for individual patients and couples that includes sensate focus therapy and efforts to improve communication between partners.

Medical
The following pharmacologic agents may be of benefit:

Sildenafil citrate (Viagra), an oral phosphodiesterase inhibitor, 50-100 mg taken 1 hour before sexual activity (carefully assess patient for underlying cardiovascular disease prior to treatment) once daily

Yohimbine, an oral alpha-adrenergic 5.4 mg, 1 tablet three times a day

Testosterone cypionate injections (in men with decreased levels): 200 mg IM every 2 to 3 weeks

Constriction ring is useful to prevent venous outflow.

Transurethral alprostadil is an effective treatment, especially when combined with a constriction device. A condom should be used if the female partner is pregnant.

Intracavernosal injections will provide satisfactory erections in most men. A small test dose is given initially to minimize the risk of the priapism. Thereafter, the usual dose is:

Papaverine 15-60 mg OR papaverine with phentolamine or prostaglandin E_1 5-15 mg

Use of a vacuum suction device combined with venous constriction and sometimes intracavernosal injection is a very effective means to provide a satisfactory erection.

Surgical treatments include ligation of penile veins (which has given mixed results) and insertion of penile prosthesis.

PEDIATRIC CONSIDERATIONS

Impotence is not a problem in pediatric patients who are not sexually active.

OBSTETRIC CONSIDERATIONS

Not applicable.

GERIATRIC CONSIDERATIONS

Many older men feel that reduced potency is a normal part of aging. However, appropriate evaluation and treatment of organic causes of impotence can restore a satisfying sex life.

PREVENTIVE CONSIDERATIONS

Detection and treatment of cardiovascular disease and diabetes mellitus and cessation of tobacco use can prevent erectile dysfunction in those men with highest risk.

PEARLS FOR THE PA

Important to ask about erectile dysfunction, as men are often ashamed or embarrassed to discuss this problem. A nonjudgmental attitude with detailed discussion of sexual history is the key.

Important to consider all possible causes. Psychogenic causes are usually secondary but almost always present.

Treatment should begin conservatively; surgery should be the last possible option.

Orchitis

Timothy F. Quigley, MPH, PA-C

DEFINITION

Infectious inflammation of the testicle, frequently seen in conjunction with epididymitis.

HISTORY

Symptoms.   Severe pain that may radiate into groin, fever, and general malaise. Usually absent are urinary frequency, urgency, and dysuria.

General.   Inquire about history of adult-onset mumps infection, recent intense sexual contacts, sexually transmitted disease (STD) history.

Age.   Any.

Onset.   Acute, over several hours. Onset of mumps orchitis associated with parotitis occurs approximately 7 to 10 days after onset of parotitis in the postpubertal patient.

Duration.   Patients usually seek medical attention very soon after the onset of symptoms.

Intensity.   Severe.

Aggravating Factors.   Walking, movement.

Alleviating Factors.   Elevation of the scrotum may relieve pain.

Associated Factors.   Epididymitis, history of mumps infection.

PHYSICAL EXAMINATION

General.   Fever with temperatures up to 104° F (40° C). Parotitis may or may not be present in mumps orchitis.

Genitourinary.   The scrotum is typically enlarged, erythematous, and edematous. The testis and epididymis are swollen and within 3 to 4 hours of onset may double in size and become indistinguishable on palpation. Reactive hydrocele may be seen.

PATHOPHYSIOLOGY

Orchitis may occur from direct extension (if it occurs in conjunction with epididymitis) or via hematologic spread (without epididymitis), or may be due to a syphilitic gumma or be secondary to mumps (paramyxovirus) orchitis. Infection can be caused by sexually transmitted organisms (*Neisseria gonorrhoeae, Chlamydia trachomatis*) or enteric organisms (*Escherichia coli*) or may be a manifestation of tuberculosis.

DIAGNOSTIC STUDIES

Laboratory
Urinalysis. May show bacteriuria or microhematuria, but results are usually normal.
Complete Blood Count. Will show a leukocytosis.

Radiology
Not applicable.

Other
Nuclear Scan. Will help differentiate orchitis from torsion and epididymitis.
Scrotal Ultrasound Examination. May be helpful in distinguishing scrotal contents.

DIFFERENTIAL DIAGNOSIS

Traumatic
Testicular Torsion. Radionuclide scan will show an avascular "cold spot."

Infectious
Tuberculosis, Epididymitis and Urethritis, Mumps, Syphilitic Gumma. Differentiated through appropriate cultures (e.g., Venereal Disease Research Laboratory [VDRL] test, fluorescent treponemal antibody [FTA] test).

Metabolic
Not applicable.

Neoplastic
Testicular Tumor. Usually nontender.

Vascular
Varicocele. Nontender and easily diagnosed clinically by palpating a "bag of worms."

Congenital. Not applicable.
Acquired. Not applicable.

TREATMENT

For mumps orchitis, treatment is primarily supportive. Treat gonorrhea and/or *Chlamydia* infection, if present, according to Centers for Disease

Control and Prevention (CDC) 2002 Guidelines for Treatment of Sexually Transmitted Diseases.

If causative agent is *Neisseria gonorrhoeae*, treat with:

Cefixime (Suprax) 400 mg PO in a single dose OR ceftriaxone (Rocephin) 125 mg IM in a single dose OR ciprofloxacin (Cipro) 500 mg PO in a single dose OR ofloxacin 400 mg or levofloxacin 250 mg PO in a single dose PLUS

Chlamydia treatment as listed below if chlamydia not ruled out.

If causative agent is *Chlamydia trachomatis*, treat with:

Azithromycin 1 g PO in a single dose OR doxycycline 100 mg PO twice daily for 7 days OR

Erythromycin base 500 mg four times daily for 7 days OR

Erythromycin ethylsuccinate 800 mg four times daily for 7 days OR

Ofloxacin 300 mg twice daily for 7 days OR

Levofloxacin 500 mg once daily for 7 days

In orchitis of any cause, other measures often beneficial include:

Rest, local heat

Scrotal support by suspension with a toweling "bridge"; ice packs

Pain relief with codeine or meperidine as necessary

Local infiltration of lidocaine into spermatic cord to decrease swelling and pain, thereby improving circulation and decreasing the chance of infertility

PEDIATRIC CONSIDERATIONS

In postpubescent boys and young men, rule out a recent history of parotitis. One-third of infected testes atrophy, but bilateral involvement and sterility are rare.

OBSTETRIC CONSIDERATIONS

Not applicable.

GERIATRIC CONSIDERATIONS

In absence of mumps orchitis, consider coexisting epididymitis-orchitis.

PREVENTIVE CONSIDERATIONS

Mumps immunization is highly efficacious, and clinical disease is rare in immunized children and adults.

Safer sex practices, including condom use and avoidance of anal intercourse, will help prevent orchitis in the sexually active male.

PEARLS FOR THE PA

Always rule out testicular torsion in a patient presenting with acute scrotal symptoms.

Prostatitis

Robert J. McNellis, MPH, PA-C

DEFINITION

Prostatitis is inflammation of the prostate gland from any of various causes and may be acute or chronic, bacterial or nonbacterial, inflammatory or noninflammatory, and symptomatic or asymptomatic. Categories include acute bacterial prostatitis, chronic bacterial prostatitis, chronic pelvic pain syndrome (CPPS) (comprising inflammatory and noninflammatory types), and asymptomatic prostatitis.

HISTORY

Symptoms. Frequent and urgent urination, dysuria, and low back, scrotal, pelvic, or perineal pain are common to all presentations. Pain is the predominant feature. Acute bacterial prostatitis manifests with sudden onset of chills and fever. Chronic bacterial prostatitis manifests with some pain, usually without fever or chills. Chronic pelvic pain syndrome manifests similarly to chronic prostatitis. Painful ejaculation or hematospermia may be present in any type.

General. Acute presentation with symptoms of a urinary tract infection (UTI) that may resolve with antibiotic treatment but can frequently recur following completion of treatment. Asymptomatic patients have prostatic inflammation found incidentally during evaluation for other prostatic diseases.

Age. Rarely occurs in prepubescent boys but common in sexually active men aged 30 to 50 years. Chronic prostatitis more common in men older than 50.

Onset. Dramatically sudden in acute prostatitis, gradual in chronic prostatitis.

Duration. Days to months. CPPS is most common presentation of prostatitis.

Intensity. Acute prostatitis is associated with moderate to severe symptoms; chronic prostatitis, with mild to moderate symptoms.

Aggravating Factors. Benign prostatic hypertrophy (BPH), lower UTI, prostatic calculi, urethral instrumentation.

Alleviating Factors. None known.
Associated Factors. Cystitis, urethritis, BPH.

PHYSICAL EXAMINATION

General. Pyrexia, tachycardia, chills in acute presentation.

Genitourinary. Acutely inflamed prostate is warm, boggy, exquisitely tender, and enlarged; crepitus may be present from prostatic calculi; fluctuance is present only if there is a prostatic abscess; gentle palpation may produce purulent urethral discharge. In chronic cases, presentation may be normal or milder.

PATHOPHYSIOLOGY

Acute bacterial prostatitis is most commonly due to invasion by *Escherichia coli* and sometimes other aerobic gram-negative bacteria. Possible modes of spread of infection are via ascending urethral infection, reflux of urine into prostatic ducts, direct or lymphatic spread of rectal bacteria, or hematogenous spread.

Chronic bacterial prostatitis generally results from long-term colonization of prostatic tissue with one organism that has been subclinical or unresponsive to treatment. Predominant organism is similar to that in acute prostatitis. Often a prostatic calculus will serve as a nidus for infection.

Chronic pelvic pain syndrome is poorly understood but may be associated with *Chlamydia trachomatis*, anaerobes, and some aerobes (e.g., staphylococci). Possible role for mycoplasmal, ureaplasmal, and other chlamydial species.

DIAGNOSTIC STUDIES

Laboratory

Fractional Urine Examination. First 10 mL for urethral specimen, midstream urine for bladder specimen, prostatic massage for expressed prostate secretion, then final urine specimen. In prostatitis, will show 10 to 15 white blood cells (WBCs)/high-power field (hpf) or positive culture of prostatic or final urine specimen with urethral and bladder specimens negative. In chronic prostatitis, will show lower bacterial count. In CPPS, will show white cells with negative culture. Not recommended in acute prostatitis.

Urinalysis. Acute bacterial specimen shows pyuria, hematuria, and bacteriuria.

Culture. Most common organism is *E. coli.* Chronic bacterial prostatitis shows reinfection with same organism.

Radiology. Not applicable.
Other. Not applicable.

DIFFERENTIAL DIAGNOSIS

Traumatic
Foreign Body. Historical or physical evidence.

Infectious
Cystitis. Positive bladder specimen culture.
Urethritis. Positive urethral specimen culture.
Pyelonephritis. Severe systemic signs and symptoms and WBC casts in urine.
Prostatic Abscess. Fluctuant prostate.
Epididymitis. Scrotal pain and enlargement, testicular tenderness.

Metabolic
Obstructive Bladder Calculus. Negative urinalysis and culture, seen on intravenous pyelography.

Neoplastic
Prostate Carcinoma. Prostate is nodular and asymmetrical, rarely tender or inflamed.
Benign Prostatic Hypertrophy. Urinalysis and culture are rarely positive. Prostate is nontender; no systemic symptoms.

Vascular. Not applicable.
Congenital. Not applicable.
Acquired. Not applicable.

TREATMENT

General
Measures include analgesics, antipyretics, stool softeners, hydration, sitz baths for pain and spasm. In acute cases, avoid transurethral procedures and prostatic massage.
Acute Bacterial. Effectively treated with fluoroquinolones or trimethoprim/sulfamethoxazole (TMP/SMX) given orally for 4 to 6 weeks.
Chronic Bacterial. Fluoroquinolones have most favorable penetration. Other agents include TMP/SMX, doxycycline, and carbenecillin. Treatment is required for 3 to 4 months. Suppressive therapy for relapses is with TMP/SMX, nitrofurantoin, or ciprofloxacin. Presence of infected calculi or bacterial microcolonies may require prostatectomy.
Nonbacterial (CPPS). Antibiotics frequently not effective, but may try doxycycline or erythromycin for several weeks. Alpha-adrenergic blockers have some usefulness. Pelvic floor relaxation techniques, biofeedback, prostate massage, and muscle relaxants may lead to relief of symptoms.

PEDIATRIC CONSIDERATIONS

Rarely a problem in young males.

OBSTETRIC CONSIDERATIONS

Not applicable.

GERIATRIC CONSIDERATIONS

Older men may present with less dramatic symptoms. It is important to recognize and treat the infection to prevent systemic spread.

PREVENTIVE CONSIDERATIONS

Condom use will decrease risk of infection. Some believe that regular sexual activity or prostatic massage may also decrease risk of prostatitis.

PEARLS FOR THE PA

Recognition of acute bacterial prostatitis is based on the finding of a tender prostate.

Important to treat bacterial prostatitis with adequate duration of antibiotic therapy.

Recurrent urinary tract infection is hallmark of chronic prostatitis.

Urethritis

Timothy F. Quigley, MPH, PA-C

DEFINITION

Inflammation of the urethra, usually infectious. Classified as gonococcal (GCU) or nongonococcal urethritis (NGU).

HISTORY

Symptoms.   Urethral discharge, dysuria, pruritus, and occasional hematuria. Associated symptoms of prostatitis/epididymitis. GCU discharge typically is purulent; NGU discharge typically is thin, clear. Many patients have no discharge.

General. Complete sexual history necessary. The patient may have a history of recent intercourse within 3 days to 2 weeks.

Age. Usually sexually active adult.

Onset

GCU. From 2 to 5 days after sexual contact.

NGU. From 7 to 21 days after exposure.

Duration. Progressive with complications if left untreated (see Associated Factors).

Intensity. Dysuria and pruritus can be severe.

Aggravating Factors. Urination (painful).

Alleviating Factors. Appropriate treatment, rest, time.

Associated Factors. Other sexually transmitted disease (STD). Monoarticular septic arthritis may be seen with GCU. The disorder may progress to involve prostate and epididymis in men and may cause sterility. In women, chronic cervicitis may follow untreated urethritis and may evolve into pelvic inflammatory disease, ectopic pregnancy, and sterility. Coexisting anal and pharyngeal infections are common.

PHYSICAL EXAMINATION

General. The patient usually appears generally healthy.

Skin. Disseminated gonococcal infections may manifest as skin rash on soles, palms, trunk, and perineum.

Genitourinary

GCU. Yellow/brown/green purulent discharge, meatal erythema and edema.

NGU. Typically clear to yellow discharge, which may be thick and less purulent. Inguinal and femoral areas should be inspected for adenopathy.

Head, Eyes, Ears, Nose, Throat/Gastrointestinal. As indicated by the sexual history, oropharyngeal and proctoscopic examinations with cultures should be performed. Pharyngitis may be asymptomatic. Inspection of perianal region and rectal examination.

PATHOPHYSIOLOGY

Causative organisms are *Neisseria gonorrheae* for GCU and *Chlamydia trachomatis* or *Ureaplasma urealyticum* (in males with more than 3 to 5 partners) for NGU.

Other, rarer causes of NGU include human papillomavirus, *Trichomonas*, and *Mycoplasma genitalium*.

DIAGNOSTIC STUDIES

Laboratory
Culture and Sensitivity Testing, Direct Immunofluorescence Assay, Enzyme-Linked Immunoassay, DNA Amplification Probe Test of Urethral Discharge Specimen.   Use of calcium gluconate swab is preferred, as a cotton swab may be bactericidal. Obtain endourethral swab to diagnose chlamydial infection.

Gram Stain of Urethral Discharge.   May show gram-negative diplococci. Culture confirms diagnosis.

Ligase Chain Reaction Assay of Urine.   Detects *N. gonorrhoeae* and *C. trachomatis.*

Culture of the Oropharynx and Rectum.   As indicated by the sexual history.

Urinalysis.   Positive if greater than 3 to 5 white blood cells (WBCs)/high-power field (hpf), greater than 0 to 2 red blood cells (RBCs)/hpf, nitrate-positive, bacteriuria. Urinalysis frequently shows only pyuria, but may be entirely normal.

Radiology.   Not applicable.
Other.   Not applicable.

DIFFERENTIAL DIAGNOSIS

Traumatic
Foreign Body.   Quite rare. May cause urethral discharge.

Infectious
Epididymitis, Prostatitis.   Rarely are associated with urethral discharge.

Metabolic
Reiter Syndrome.   Associated with conjunctivitis, arthritis, and positive HLA-B27 assay.

Neoplastic
Penile Carcinoma.   Patients with a discharge refractory to treatment should undergo a full evaluation, as a rare presentation of penile carcinoma is urethral discharge.

Vascular.   Not applicable.
Congenital.   Not applicable.
Acquired.   Not applicable.

TREATMENT

Treatment is pharmacologic. All sexual partners should also be treated.

If causative agent is *N. gonorrhoeae*, treat according to Centers for Disease Control and Prevention (CDC) 2002 Guidelines:

Cefixime (Suprax) 400 mg PO in a single dose OR ceftriaxone (Rocephin) 125 mg IM in a single dose OR ciprofloxacin (Cipro) 500 mg PO in a single dose OR ofloxacin 400 mg OR levofloxacin 250 mg PO in a single dose

If the causative agent is nongonococcal, treat with:

Azithromycin 1 g PO in a single dose OR doxycycline 100 mg twice daily for 7 days OR

Erythromycin base 500 mg four times daily for 7 days OR

Erythromycin ethylsuccinate 800 mg four times daily for 7 days OR

Ofloxacin 300 mg twice daily for 7 days OR

Levofloxacin 500 mg once daily for 7 days

If the causative agent is human papillomavirus, therapy is aimed at eradication of lesion.

Trichomonal urethritis is treated with metronidazole PLUS erythromycin.

PEDIATRIC CONSIDERATIONS

In a child with urethritis, *always* suspect child abuse.

OBSTETRIC CONSIDERATIONS

Ceftriaxone or spectinomycin are the drugs recommended by the CDC for treatment of urogenital gonorrhea. Only ceftriaxone should be given for pharyngeal gonorrhea.

GERIATRIC CONSIDERATIONS

Not otherwise applicable.

PREVENTIVE CONSIDERATIONS

Patient education regarding safer sexual practices, including condom use, is an important part of management. Early diagnosis and treatment can prevent complications and transmission. Treatment of sexual partners prevents reinfection.

PEARLS FOR THE PA

Nongonococcal urethritis is a chlamydial infection until proven otherwise.

Monoarticular arthritis is a frequent complication of (or presenting complaint in) GCU.

Urinary Tract Infection

Timothy F. Quigley, MPH, PA-C

DEFINITION

Infection of the urinary bladder and kidney caused by a variety of organisms. The causative agent in 80% of cases is *Escherichia coli*.

HISTORY

Symptoms. Dysuria, urgency, and urinary frequency are the classic symptoms. Hematuria and voiding small amounts of urine may be present. Occasionally there may be fever and gross pyuria. Rarely, there is suprapubic pain and pressure.

General. The most common presenting complaints are dysuria and gross hematuria. More common in females (owing to shorter length of urethra) but may also be seen in males. In children (especially boys), underlying congenital abnormality must be ruled out. In men, all urinary tract infections (UTIs) should be investigated for underlying disease process or anatomic factors predisposing to infection (e.g., diabetes mellitus, bladder outlet obstruction, benign prostatic hyperplasia, prostate cancer). Insertive anal intercourse is another risk factor for men.

Age. Any.

Onset. Acute.

Duration. Usually self-limited, even without treatment. Can progress to pyelonephritis.

Intensity. Mild to severe dysuria.

Aggravating Factors. Poor hygiene, intercourse, use of diaphragm, pregnancy, lack of estrogen. Urinary tract pathology.

Alleviating Factors. Hydration, time, and appropriate antimicrobial therapy.

Associated Factors. Diabetes mellitus, pregnancy. With recurrent infections, congenital anomalies and urolithiasis (possible source of obstruction and persistent bacteriuria) must be ruled out.

PHYSICAL EXAMINATION

General. Occasionally, fever and chills are seen with uncomplicated cystitis. Marked fever (with temperatures to greater than 104°F [40° C]), chills, and rigors are seen with upper tract infection such as pyelonephritis.

Genitourinary. Suprapubic tenderness to palpation. Tenderness to percussion over the costovertebral angle if there is renal involvement.

PATHOPHYSIOLOGY

UTIs usually ascend from the lower to the upper tract.

In *female patients*, pathogenic mechanisms include retrograde inoculation of enteric bacteria from the rectum to the urethra and sexual intercourse–induced urethral trauma or introduction of enteric bacteria.

In *male patients*, mechanisms include sexual contact, compromised defenses, infection-induced ureteral reflux, abnormal ureterovesical valve function, blood-borne infection (gastrointestinal, colitis), urethral stenosis, and bladder neck obstruction.

Common pathogens are *E. coli* (accounting for 80% of cases), *Staphlococcus saprophyticus* (5% to 15%), *Proteus mirabilis*, *Klebsiella pneumoniae*, *Chlamydia trachomatis*, and *Candida albicans* (especially in debilitated and/or immunosuppressed persons).

DIAGNOSTIC STUDIES

Laboratory

Urinalysis. Urinalysis of clean-catch midstream specimen should demonstrate greater than 3 to 5 white blood cells (WBCs)/high-power field (hpf), greater than 0 to 2 red blood cells (RBCs)/hpf. Dipstick test is nitrate-positive for breakdown of bacteria and leukocyte esterase–positive for neutrophils. WBC casts indicate pyelonephritis. Abundance of epithelial cells indicates contamination.

Complete Blood Count. Leukocytosis with renal involvement.

Urine Culture and Sensitivity Testing. As indicated to identify the causative pathogen. Presence of greater than 10^3 colony-forming units defines infection.

Radiology

Radiologic studies rarely performed in uncomplicated UTI.

Pelvic Ultrasound Examination. Used to identify bladder neck obstruction, urinary retention, bladder tumor.

Renal Ultrasound Examination. Used to identify renal mass, nephrolithiasis, abscess.

Intravenous pyelography. Used to evaluate for urolithiasis, tumors, or congenital abnormalities.

Other
Cystoscopy.   Offers direct visualization of the bladder mucosa. Biopsy samples can be taken to evaluate for chronic cystitis.

DIFFERENTIAL DIAGNOSIS

Traumatic
Pelvic or Urethral Trauma.   May manifest with hematuria without bacteriuria.

Infectious
Tuberculous Infection.   May manifest with hematuria.

Metabolic
Diabetes Mellitus/Insipidus, Syndrome of Inappropriate Antidiuretic Hormone Secretion (SIADH).   All may manifest with polyuria.

Neoplastic
Bladder Tumors, Prostate Carcinoma, Urolithiasis.   All may manifest with hematuria.

Vascular
Not applicable.

Congenital
Urethral Valves, Fistulas.   Must be ruled out.

Acquired
Prostatism, Bladder Outlet Obstruction Due to Other Causes, Congestive Heart Failure, Ingestion of Large Amounts of Fluid.   All may manifest with polyuria and/or nocturia.

TREATMENT

Antibiotics may be instituted prior to culture and sensitivity testing results, but antibiotic therapy may need to be changed on the basis of the results.
  Cephalexin, 250-500 mg PO every 6 hours for 7 to 14 days
  Ciprofloxacin, 250-500 mg PO every 12 hours for 7 to 14 days
  Nitrofurantoin macrocrystals 100 mg PO four times a day
  Norfloxacin 400 mg PO every 12 hours for 3 to 7 days
  Ofloxacin 300 mg PO every 12 hours for 7 days
  Trimethoprim-sulfamethoxazole 160/800 mg PO two tablets in a
    single dose for 10 to 14 days

PEDIATRIC CONSIDERATIONS

Neonatal

Overall incidence is 0.1% of newborns. UTI is three times more common in boys than in girls, with a higher incidence in low-birth-weight infants. The responsible pathogen in 75% of cases is *Escherichia coli*; the remainder of cases are caused by other gram-negative enteric bacilli and gram-positive cocci. Signs are varied and nonspecific. UTI may be secondary to sepsis or a primary source of infection. Urine culture should be included in the evaluation for sepsis of a febrile or septic-appearing infant 72 hours of age or older. Urine specimen obtained by catheterization or suprapubic aspiration is advised.

General Pediatrics

Beyond the newborn age group, UTIs are much more common in girls, most commonly in the 7- to 11-year-old age group. Infections are quite rare in boys of similar age. In children with fever of unknown origin, urine culture specimens should be obtained. In infancy, fever, weight loss, failure to thrive, nausea, vomiting, diarrhea, and jaundice are common. Later, urinary frequency, dysuria, urgency, bedwetting in a previously "dry" child, abdominal pain, and foul-smelling urine are common manifestations.

OBSTETRIC CONSIDERATIONS

Urinary stasis during pregnancy and overdistention (due to oxytocin or genital hematoma) and bladder catheterization during the puerperium predispose the patient to develop UTIs.

Asymptomatic bacteriuria is present in 2% to 7% of pregnant patients and should be treated to prevent the development of symptomatic infections.

Treatment should be based on culture and sensitivity, but empirical treatment with nitrofurantoin (pregnancy class B) 100 mg daily for 10 days or ampicillin or a cephalosporin (class B) four times a day may be effective. Isolated, uncomplicated UTIs may be treated with a 3-day course, but recurrent infection or bacteriuria require a 7-day course.

Symptomatic UTI (cystitis) is manifested by frequency, urgency, and dysuria. These infections may ascend and involve the kidney (pyelonephritis). Treatment should be based on results of culture and sensitivity testing. Ampicillin, sulfonamides, nitrofurantoin, or a cephalosporin may be used for 10 days. UTI symptoms associated with a sterile urine culture may be due to infection caused by *C. trachomatis*. These cases should be treated with erythromycin.

Fluoroquinolones and tetracycline are contraindicated. Trimethoprim is teratogenic during the first trimester, and sulfamethoxazole may cause hyperbilirubinemia in the third trimester.

GERIATRIC CONSIDERATIONS

UTIs are the most common bacterial infections in the geriatric population. Risk factors in the elderly that predispose to UTI include significant postvoid residual urine, vaginal and urethral atrophy, stones, tumors, strictures, reduced mobility, cognitive decline, and indwelling catheters. Older patients, especially in nursing homes, may present with new-onset incontinence, confusion, lethargy, anorexia, or delirium.

Consider the age-related decrease in renal and hepatic function when prescribing antibiotics.

PREVENTIVE CONSIDERATIONS

Frequent urination, increasing fluid intake, voiding before and after sexual intercourse, using alternatives to diaphragm and spermicides for contraception. Prevent perineal-vaginal contamination by wiping anterior to posterior after voiding. Cranberry juice may inhibit the adherence of *E. coli* to uroepithelial cells. Cultured yogurt with *Lactobacillus* may be of some preventive benefit. Prophylactic antibiotic therapy is often given to prevent recurrence.

PEARLS FOR THE PA

Remember classic triad of symptoms: frequency, urgency, dysuria.

Further Reading

Centers for Disease Control and Prevention. Sexually Transmitted Disease Treatment Guidelines 2002. MMWR 51 (RR-6):1-80.

Murphy JL (ed): Physician Assistant's Prescribing Reference, Summer 2003. New York, Prescribing Reference Inc., 2003.

Tierney LM, McPhee SJ, Papadakis MA (eds): Current Medical Diagnosis and Treatment: Adult Ambulatory and Inpatient Management, 41st ed. New York, Lange Medical Books/McGraw-Hill, 2002.

Nseyo UO, Weinman E, Lamm DL: Urology for Primary Care Physicians. Philadelphia, WB Saunders, 1999.

Teichman JMH: Twenty Common Problems in Urology for Primary Care Clinicians. New York, McGraw-Hill, 2001.

ANESTHESIA

Rhea Sumpter, MMSc, PA, AA-C

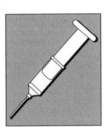

18

Improvements in the delivery of anesthesia over the past several decades have been remarkable. Technologic advances such as pulse oximetry, capnography, and hemodynamic and neurologic monitoring have resulted in greater safety for a more diverse patient population, as well as accommodating more demanding surgical procedures.

In 1969, specialty-trained physician assistants (PAs) employed under the supervision of an anesthesiologist became part of the anesthesia care team. As anesthesiologist assistants (AAs), PAs are valuable participants in anesthetic procedures using both general and specialized techniques. In today's operating room, the PA anesthetist plays a vital role in this exciting and challenging aspect of patient care.

DEFINITION

Anesthesia is that condition in which a person is rendered insensitive to a painful stimulus.

BASICS OF ANESTHESIA

The following overview of the *anesthesia machine, anesthesia monitors, airway management techniques*, and *pharmacologic agents* describes how the anesthetic is delivered to the patient.

ANESTHESIA MACHINE

The primary function of the anesthesia machine is to deliver, with safety and precision, variable concentrations of oxygen and anesthetic gases. Oxygen, air, and nitrous oxide (N_2O) may be supplied to the anesthesia machine either through the hospital gas inlet supply system or by gas cylinders directly attached to the machine. The anesthesia machine has a fail-safe system that is designed to prevent the administration of a hypoxic gas mixture if the oxygen supply pressure drops below a certain level and also incorporates flowmeters to prevent the inadvertent delivery of a hypoxic O_2-N_2O combination. All anesthesia machines must have an oxygen analyzer that continuously monitors the fraction of inspired oxygen concentration (FiO_2), an audible low-level oxygen alarm, and apnea and ventilator disconnect alarms.

Administration of the volatile anesthetic agents halothane, isoflurane, desflurane, and sevoflurane is accomplished with use of agent-specific, calibrated vaporizers mounted on the anesthesia machine. The most common method of delivering anesthetic gases to the patient is through a semiclosed circle breathing system. This system allows for the partial rebreathing of expired gases after the elimination of CO_2 via the CO_2 absorber.

A collapsible 3-liter rebreathing bag is integrated within the circle system. This bag can be used to allow the patient to breathe spontaneously, or by adjusting a pressure-limiting valve, the bag can be manually operated to assist or control ventilations. A mechanical ventilator is also available. For the safety of all personnel, anesthetic gas waste is scavenged into the hospital's vacuum system. All anesthesia machines have an oxygen flush button that when activated delivers 100% oxygen at a very high flow rate to the circle system. The oxygen flush button may be repeatedly depressed to rapidly reinflate the rebreathing bag if there is a significant leak during control of an airway. Another use of the oxygen flush button is to rapidly displace any residual anesthetic gases from the breathing system and quickly replace the breathing circuit with 100% oxygen.

For practicality and convenience, a suction apparatus and patient monitors have been incorporated within some machines. Additional patient monitors and gas analyzers typically are secured on the top of the anesthesia machine. Having everything in one central location makes visual scanning easier for the anesthetist and safer for the patient, as attention is divided among observing the patient, the surgical field, the anesthesia machine, and the patient monitors. Before each procedure, a detailed anesthesia machine check is performed following a standard protocol established by the American Society of Anesthesiologists (ASA).

ANESTHESIA MONITORS

Technologic advances in monitoring have been a major contributing factor in decreasing the morbidity and mortality associated with the administration of an anesthetic. Even so, the practice of "a hand on the pulse and an ear on the chest" should never be abandoned. Visual, tactile, and auditory senses are continually used to evaluate the patient's condition. These observations are enhanced by adherence to basic monitoring standards, which have been set forth by the ASA.

Basic monitoring for all patients includes evaluation of oxygenation, circulation, ventilation, and body temperature. For all general anesthetic procedures, basic monitoring includes ECG and evaluation of blood pressure, pulse, respirations, inspired oxygen concentration, oxygen saturation (using pulse oximetry), end-tidal CO_2 ($ETCO_2$) using capnography, and temperature. If muscle relaxants are given, the level of neuromuscular blockade is monitored with a peripheral nerve stimulator (PNS).

The decision to use more advanced monitoring is dependent on the patient's physical status and the extent of the surgical procedure. These monitoring devices may include an arterial line, central venous pressure or pulmonary artery (PA) catheter, transesophageal echocardiography (TEE) probe, precordial Doppler, electroencephalography (EEG), cerebral oximeter, intracranial pressure (ICP) catheter, cerebrospinal fluid (CSF) catheter, or evoked potential (EP) monitor. Even with these sophisticated monitors, the importance of physical observation should not be overlooked.

AIRWAY MANAGEMENT TECHNIQUES

Routine Airway Management

Management of the patient's airway is one of the most demanding of responsibilities. Regardless of whether the patient is receiving a local or a general anesthetic, untoward events such as partial or complete upper airway obstruction, laryngospasm, bronchospasm, or pulmonary aspiration may occur. The efficiency of airway management is constantly monitored by pulse oximetry, capnography, observation of chest excursions, auscultation of breath sounds, and arterial blood gas analysis, as indicated.

During a regional or local anesthetic procedure, or monitored anesthesia care (MAC), supplemental oxygen is administered to the patient. This is done because these patients are usually sedated before entering the operating room, and with the addition of intraoperative sedation, a decrease in alveolar ventilation is expected. Delivery of oxygen may be by either insufflation through a face shield, face mask, or O_2 delivery–CO_2 sampling nasal cannula.

As intraoperative intravenous sedation is given, there may be brief episodes of hypoventilation or upper airway obstruction as the soft tissues relax. Verbally or physically arousing the patient and having him or her take deep breaths may resolve this problem. If a partial airway obstruction persists, a simple head tilt–chin lift maneuver is done to regain airway patency.

During a general anesthetic procedure, the administration of intravenous induction agents produces profound relaxation of the upper airway soft tissues and a decrease in alveolar ventilation, usually to the point of apnea. The following adjunctive devices are used for managing the patient's airway.

Anesthesia Face Mask
With the proper application of the anesthesia face mask and the head tilt–chin lift maneuver, ventilations often can be controlled or assisted until efficient spontaneous breathing returns. If partial or complete airway obstruction persists, an oral or nasal airway may be placed. If the obstruction is relieved, face mask delivery of oxygen or anesthetic gases may be continued. If the airway cannot be secured with any of these methods, the patient may be awoken or more advanced adjuncts employed.

Laryngeal Mask Airway
The laryngeal mask airway (LMA) is a cuffed tube that is blindly positioned in the hypopharynx. After confirmation of proper LMA positioning by auscultation, observing chest excursions, and $ETCO_2$ monitoring, the anesthetist either controls, assists, or allows the patient to resume spontaneous ventilations. Because the LMA is positioned in the supraglottic region, the trachea is not isolated. Consequently, elective use of the LMA is contraindicated on patients with increased risk of aspiration or with low pulmonary compliance requiring excessive peak inspiratory pressure.

Endotracheal Tube
The endotracheal tube (ETT) typically is inserted into the trachea under direct visualization using a laryngoscope. The choice of using a cuffed ETT is to help ensure a patent airway, allow positive-pressure ventilations, and protect the airway from aspiration. An ETT is generally used in patients who are in surgical positions other than supine, in head and neck surgery, in procedures of long duration requiring positive-pressure ventilation, in

patients suspected of having a full stomach or bowel obstruction, in morbidly obese patients, and in patients in whom face mask or LMA management is unsatisfactory.

Double-Lumen Endotracheal Tube

The double-lumen endotracheal tube (DLT) is used to periodically administer unilateral lung ventilation during intrathoracic surgery. Collapsing the surgical field lung greatly enhances surgical exposure. Left- and right-sided DLTs are commercially available. The following description of placement refers to the left-sided DLT.

Correct placement of the DLT is critical for proper functioning. Position is confirmed by auscultation, fiberoptic bronchoscopy (FOB), and observation of chest excursions. If the tube is properly positioned, the left lumen should be in the left main bronchus with its cuff just below the carina. The right lumen should be in the trachea just above the carina. When the bronchial and tracheal cuffs are inflated, each lung should be isolated. To check for proper placement, the chest is auscultated for the presence or absence of breath sounds as alternating lumens are clamped off. FOB via the tracheal lumen is used to confirm that the inflated bronchial cuff is visible in the left main bronchus just below the carina, and that the right main bronchus is patent. With one-lung ventilation techniques, 100% oxygen is used for ventilation. It is essential to recheck the position of the tube any time the patient is repositioned or any time there is a surgical event that may affect the proper functioning of the DLT. If there are dramatic or unsatisfactory changes in Sao_2 or $ETco_2$ levels, immediate attention is mandatory. If proper tube placement is reconfirmed by FOB and auscultation, and appropriate respiratory care has failed to improve the situation, continuous positive airway pressure (CPAP) may be added to the collapsed lung, or the collapsed lung may be periodically reinflated during the surgical procedure.

Endobronchial Blocker

One-lung ventilation may also be achieved by using an endobronchial blocker. After routine single-lumen ETT placement, a specially designed wire-guided balloon-tipped catheter is selectively positioned into the left or right main bronchus using a flexible fiberoptic bronchoscope. When the balloon is properly inflated, the selected lung will be isolated during ventilations. Proper positioning is confirmed by auscultations, observation of chest excursions, and FOB.

Difficult Airway Management

A difficult airway may be encountered in (1) the patient with a known history of a difficult airway or intubation, (2) the patient who is suspected of having a difficult airway when evaluated during the physical examination, or (3) the patient with an unsuspected difficult airway.

With a known or suspected difficult airway, there is some advance warning, and an elective "awake" intubation should be considered. In the patient with an unsuspected difficult airway, problems may not be recognized until after induction or attempted intubation.

The elective awake intubation procedure begins with preoxygenation. Because the objective is to let the patient maintain the airway until tracheal intubation is successful, caution must be used not to oversedate the patient. As the patient becomes sedated, topical anesthesia is applied to the nasopharynx or the oropharynx, depending on the selected route of intubation. If a nasotracheal tube is to be used, a vasoconstrictive agent such as cocaine or phenylephrine may be topically applied intranasally to prevent or minimize bleeding. A superior laryngeal nerve block or transtracheal administration of lidocaine may also be used to provide localized airway anesthesia. When a satisfactory level of block has been achieved, any of several methods may be used to intubate the patient's trachea:

- A flexible *fiberoptic scope* over which an endotracheal tube has been placed may be visually directed either orally or nasally down into the trachea. Once the trachea has been entered, the ETT is advanced over the scope into position.
- Another option may be the use of a *light wand* over which an endotracheal tube has been placed. After the operating room has been darkened, the light wand is inserted orally into the posterior pharynx. While observing changes in light intensity upon the surface of the patient's neck, the light wand and ETT are manipulated and advanced into the trachea.
- A special-design *LMA* through which an endotracheal tube may be inserted is also useful in facilitating tracheal intubation.
- A *blind approach* through the nasal or oral route may be used; as the tracheal tube is advanced and enters the trachea, the operator listens for changes in the intensity of breath sounds.
- The *retrograde wire technique* begins with placing a needle through the cricothyroid membrane. A long wire is passed through the needle and threaded in retrograde fashion into the hypopharynx. The wire is then retrieved from the mouth and an ETT tube is threaded over the wire and into the trachea.

Regardless of which method is chosen, once the tube has entered the trachea, the cuff is inflated. Tracheal intubation is confirmed by $ETCO_2$ monitoring, FOB, and watching the patient breathe through the anesthesia reservoir bag. Because the patient is still breathing spontaneously, confirmation by auscultation is not a guarantee that the tube is correctly positioned, so auscultation alone should not be the only source of confirmation. Observing the capnograph for the presence of a CO_2 waveform is the best assurance. Once correct tube placement has been confirmed, general anesthesia can commence. If the trachea cannot be intubated, elective surgery may be canceled.

For the patient with the unsuspected difficult airway, problems are not apparent until induction or attempted intubation. For these patients, the "difficult airway algorithm" is initiated as established by the ASA.

If at any point control of airway management is lost and the situation becomes life-threatening, *jet ventilation* through the cricothyroid membrane or a surgical airway created by emergency *cricothyroidotomy* or *tracheostomy* must be performed. The two key components of difficult airway management are to be prepared and to immediately call for assistance.

PHARMACOLOGIC AGENTS

The anesthetist administers many drugs during surgery. Most of the drugs are chosen because they are fast-acting and have a relatively short duration of action. The anesthetist must have an appreciation of how surgical stress and anesthetic agents alter homeostasis, and of potential effects of these factors on the sympathetic and parasympathetic nervous system. The pharmacokinetics and pharmacodynamics of all the drugs administered must be known, as well as the potential for their interaction with any unscheduled or scheduled medications. The surgical patient will be exposed to multiple and diverse pharmacologic agents. A healthy patient who is to receive a regional or local anesthetic with MAC typically may receive an analgesic, sedative, O_2, local anesthetic, and perhaps an antibiotic. On the other extreme, a patient scheduled for an open abdominal aortic aneurysm repair can easily receive more than 10 different drugs.

Anesthetic Agents

The objective of any anesthetic procedure is to ensure patient safety, provide analgesia and sedation, and maintain homeostasis with the judicious use of drugs and the adequate replacement of fluids.

Anesthetic agents are administered during surgery to provide analgesia, amnesia, and sedation. The anesthetist will typically use a combination of drugs to achieve the desired effect:

- Selected *anesthetic agents* may be applied topically; injected intravenously into the central circulation; instilled into the epidural space, into the subarachnoid space, or adjacent to nerve tissues; or inhaled from the anesthesia machine.
- For analgesia, the *intravenous narcotics* morphine, meperidine, fentanyl, sufentanil, alfentanil, and remifentanil and the nonsteroidal anti-inflammatory drug (NSAID) ketorolac may be used.
- For their *sedative-hypnotic* effect, the benzodiazepines diazepam, midazolam, and lorazepam or the alkylphenol propofol may be used.
- The *local anesthetics* cocaine, benzocaine, lidocaine, bupivacaine, tetracaine, etidocaine, mepivacaine, and chloroprocaine are used to produce a temporary regional block. Depending on the agent, administration may be used to achieve a topical, local, peripheral, or central neural block.
- The ultra-short-acting *induction agents* propofol, etomidate, thiopental, and ketamine may be used to produce unconsciousness if a general anesthetic procedure is planned. During MAC procedures, a continuous infusion of propofol may be used to provide conscious sedation.

- *Oxygen* and the *inhalational anesthetic agents* N_2O, halothane, isoflurane, desflurane, and sevoflurane are delivered from the anesthesia machine to the patient. These inhalational anesthetic agents are used to achieve or maintain varying depths of general anesthesia.

Cardiovascular Agents

The stress of surgery and the administration of anesthetics disrupt homeostasis. The anesthetist is responsible for controlling blood pressure and heart rate and optimizing cardiac function. A wide variety of *vasopressors*, *vasodilators*, and *chronotropic* and *inotropic drugs* may be administered during surgery to achieve this goal. Many of these agents have mixed effects, and the best agent must be selected to appropriately treat hypertension, hypotension, abnormal heart rate, or low cardiac index.

Antiarrhythmics also must be available. Malignant arrhythmias may result from cardiac ischemia, electrolyte imbalance, hypothermia, malignant hyperthermia (MH), drug overdose, or cardiac catheter insertion, or may be a result of intense vagal stimulation induced by surgical retraction or manipulation.

Neuromuscular Blocking Agents (Muscle Relaxants)

Muscle relaxants are given to facilitate tracheal intubation and to provide a relaxed surgical field when indicated. Muscle relaxation during certain surgical procedures is mandatory. Choice of a muscle relaxant generally depends on the drug's duration of action, the length of the surgical procedure, and the patient's ability to metabolize or excrete the drug.

The depolarizing muscle relaxant succinylcholine is similar to the neurotransmitter acetylcholine and produces skeletal muscle paralysis of reliably rapid onset and short duration. When this agent is given in a sufficient dose to help facilitate tracheal intubation, the patient's muscles will fasciculate prior to total paralysis. The fasciculations may appear as mild to severe spasmodic muscle contractions that may result in postoperative myalgia. To prevent or minimize fasciculations, a small dose of a nondepolarizing muscle relaxant is administered a few minutes before administration of succinylcholine. However, the pretreatment is not always successful.

The nondepolarizing muscle relaxants atracurium, cisatracurium, mivacurium, pancuronium, vecuronium, pipecuronium, and rocuronium produce skeletal muscle paralysis by competing for and blocking acetylcholine receptor sites on skeletal muscle motor end plates. This competitive blockade prevents the neurotransmitter acetylcholine from binding with its receptor site. The resulting skeletal muscle paralysis is of moderate to long duration, depending on the choice of agent and the patient's response to the drug. Some of these agents may require reversal with an anticholinesterase before extubation.

Adjunctive Agents

The anesthetist is also responsible for the administration of a wide variety of nonanesthetic drugs during surgery. These may include antibiotics, antiemetics, steroids, histamine H_1 and H_2 receptor blockers, diuretics, bronchodilators, electrolytes, acidifiers, anticoagulants, procoagulants, insulin, and drug reversal agents, as well as various crystalloid, colloid, and fluid volume expanders.

THE ANESTHETIC PLAN

Prior to surgery, an anesthesiologist interviews the patient and an anesthetic plan is formulated. To determine the best anesthetic plan for elective surgery, several factors must be considered: the patient's age, ASA class (I [healthy] to V [critically ill]) as determined from the history and physical examination, type and duration of the proposed surgical procedure, airway anatomy, required positioning during the procedure, and if appropriate, the patient's preference for a general, regional, or local anesthetic procedure with MAC and sedation. The anesthetic plan encompasses the preoperative, intraoperative, and postoperative care of the patient.

Once an anesthetic plan has been devised, the patient is informed about what to expect. If a regional or local anesthetic procedure is selected, the patient is forewarned of the possibility of having to convert it to a general anesthetic procedure if the regional or local anesthetic fails or becomes unsatisfactory. The patient is instructed not to eat or drink after midnight for surgery scheduled for early morning and is informed that he or she will be given preoperative medications that will cause drowsiness and relaxation. The need for intravenous line placement is discussed, as well as the requirement for monitoring of blood pressure, pulse, respirations, temperatures, and oxygen saturation. If invasive monitoring procedures are necessary, these also are explained. It is also very important to tell the patient what to expect in the postanesthesia care unit (PACU) or intensive care unit (ICU), especially if the patient is to remain intubated. Postoperative pain management options, such as patient-controlled analgesia (PCA), are also discussed with the patient.

The patient is assured that the anesthesia care team will be with him or her throughout the operative procedure, and that the team will be responsible for his or her care until the effects of the anesthetic have worn off. The risks and benefits of the proposed anesthetic plan are explained, and questions or concerns regarding the anesthetic plan are solicited and addressed as appropriate.

During the surgical procedure, a detailed anesthesia record is maintained, which is a chronologic documentation of procedures, events, and patient data. The information collected on the anesthesia record is interpreted and used in management decisions.

The anesthesia and surgical care teams are responsible for safely positioning the patient for surgery. To avoid paresthesias or other patient injury, periodic checks of the patient position are performed.

PREOPERATIVE CARE

On the day of surgery, preoperative medications are usually given 1 to 2 hours before transport of the patient to the operating room. The preoperative medications may include an analgesic, a sedative, an H₂ antagonist, and an anti-cholinergic. The anticholinergic may be prescribed for its vagolytic properties or its antisialagogue effect, although dry mouth is a major patient complaint. Because narcotics and sedatives may decrease alveolar ventilation, supplemental oxygen may be ordered for the patient with cardiac or pulmonary disease.

When the patient is brought to the surgical area, he or she may first be admitted to the presurgical care unit (PSCU). After proper patient identification and procedure confirmation, the anesthesia consultation record and the patient's chart are rechecked to see if there are any recent changes in the patient's status or new data from additional consultations that may affect the proposed anesthetic plan. If the anesthetic plan needs to be changed, consent from the unpremedicated patient or the family of the premedicated patient must be obtained.

For the patient who appears to be inadequately sedated on arrival to the PSCU, reassurance or additional sedation may be given (once intravenous access has been established). To minimize operating room time, insertion of additional invasive monitoring devices (e.g., arterial line, CVP catheter, PA catheter, continuous epidural catheter) may be performed in the PSCU.

PATIENT CARE IN THE OPERATING ROOM

When the operating room team is ready, the patient is accompanied from the PSCU to the operating room. Even though the patient may appear to be well sedated, entering the operating room may be a frightening experience. Extraneous noise should be kept to a minimum and reassurance provided. The operating room bed should be kept warm or a warm blanket provided to prevent shivering. If the patient is to be supine, he or she is assisted onto the operating table and comfortably positioned before being anesthetized. The patient who is to be prone or is in too much pain to be moved may be anesthetized on the stretcher before being positioned on the table.

Before the anesthetic procedure is begun, the patient is connected to the ECG monitor, blood pressure cuff, and pulse oximeter, and a precordial stethoscope is positioned. If the patient has invasive monitoring lines (e.g., arterial line, CVP catheter, PA catheter), they are connected to the hemodynamic monitor, calibrated, and displayed. The patient who is to receive a regional or peripheral nerve block may need to be temporarily repositioned to facilitate administration of the block.

GENERAL ANESTHESIA

General anesthesia is a method of surgical anesthesia in which the patient is rendered unconscious and insensitive to pain. Key determinants in choosing a general anesthetic are the type and duration of surgery, body position, patient's preference to be "put to sleep," and presence of a contraindication to alternative anesthetic techniques.

Preinduction

As the patient is being made comfortable on the operating room table and the monitors are being applied, important preinduction procedures are performed. Ideally, the patient should be preoxygenated for several minutes by breathing 100% oxygen through the anesthesia face mask or by taking three or four vital capacity breaths through the mask. This nitrogen washout procedure fills the lungs with approximately 100% oxygen, which adds a margin of safety if difficulty is encountered during subsequent airway management.

During this time, a small dose of a nondepolarizing muscle relaxant may be administered if the depolarizing muscle relaxant succinylcholine is to be given. This pretreatment will prevent or minimize the fasciculations caused by succinylcholine.

The course of a general anesthetic procedure may be divided into three major parts: induction, maintenance, and emergence.

Induction

After satisfactory preoxygenation, the patient is again afforded reassurance as he or she is rendered unconscious. Pulse oximetry tones should be audible.

The most commonly used intravenous induction agents are propofol, etomidate, and barbiturates (e.g., thiopental). When one of these agents is administered as a bolus dose, loss of consciousness usually occurs within 30 to 60 seconds. The patient becomes unresponsive to simple commands such as "Open your eyes." For confirmation, the patient's eyelid may be stroked to check for the absence of the lid reflex.

After the patient becomes unconscious, the patient's eyes may be taped closed to prevent drying of the cornea or an inadvertent corneal abrasion. Because of patient positioning or inaccessibility preventing continual monitoring of eye care, special goggles may be applied for additional protection.

As the patient loses consciousness, rapid respiratory and cardiovascular changes must be anticipated. Depending on the dosage of the intravenous induction agent, there is usually a significant decrease in ventilations, generally to the point of apnea. This is attributed to the drug's depressant effect on the cerebellar respiratory center.

This anticipated decrease in or absence of ventilations requires immediate attention. At this point, the patient's ventilations are assisted or controlled via face mask by hand-squeezing the reservoir bag on the anesthesia machine. In procedures of short duration, the face mask may be used throughout the procedure to administer O_2 and inhalational anesthetics.

In most procedures, an LMA or ETT is used. If an ETT is used, a muscle relaxant is commonly given to help facilitate intubation. To help determine when the patient is sufficiently paralyzed so that a laryngoscopy can be performed, a PNS may be used to monitor twitch responses as electrical shocks are applied to the side of the face or the forearm.

After intubation and confirmation of correct tube placement, the ETT is taped securely into place. A temperature-monitoring esophageal stethoscope may be inserted into a position that maximizes heart and breath sounds. While the patient is still relaxed, a soft bite block may be positioned to prevent dental damage or occlusion of the ETT incurred if the patient bites down when muscle tone returns.

After administration of the induction agents, a drop in blood pressure is anticipated. This drop is caused by a decrease in sympathetic tone or by the myocardial depressant effect of some intravenous induction agents. The decrease in blood pressure may be more dramatic in the patient who has not been adequately rehydrated preoperatively after being NPO. The hypotensive episode may be treated by giving additional intravenous fluids, by placing the patient in Trendelenburg position, or by administering a vasopressor or cardiotonic agent. If instrumentation of the airway or surgical stimulation is about to occur, the resulting stimulus may be sufficient to increase the blood pressure.

As the airway is secured and hemodynamics are stabilized, the anesthetic effect of the ultra-short-acting induction agent is rapidly dissipating and the patient will begin to wake up if additional anesthetics are not given. To achieve a surgical depth of anesthesia, additional intravenous analgesics, sedative-hypnotics, and inhalational agents are generally administered. If indicated, nondepolarizing muscle relaxants are administered after recovery of neuromuscular function from succinylcholine is evident. Usually a combination of the foregoing techniques is employed to maintain general anesthesia.

Maintenance

During the maintenance phase, the depth of anesthesia is continuously assessed. The patient's blood pressure, oxygen saturation, $ETCO_2$, heart rate, respirations, temperature, skeletal muscle function, intravascular volume status, urine output, glucose, electrolytes, blood gases, and acid-base status are measured and managed. The most common method for maintenance in a general anesthetic procedure is the use of inhalational agents along with the administration of preemptive intravenous analgesics. Inhalational anesthetics have the advantage of a quick onset and a rapid rate of elimination. The volatile inhalational agents isoflurane, desflurane, and sevoflurane are administered with either 100% O_2 or an N_2O-O_2 or O_2-air mixture. Halothane rarely is used in adults. The inhalational agents in sufficient concentrations cause unconsciousness, analgesia, and amnesia. They are also dose-dependent myocardial and respiratory depressants.

The administration of these volatile inhalational agents may be started as soon as loss of consciousness occurs. Most volatile inhalational agents, except sevoflurane, are upper airway irritants and may cause breath holding, coughing, laryngospasm, or bronchospasm if an excessive initial concentration is delivered. The concentration of the inhalational agent is frequently adjusted to achieve or maintain a surgical depth of anesthesia. The depth of anesthesia is assessed by evaluating changes in blood pressure, heart rate, pupil size, and ventilation patterns (assisted or spontaneous) and by observing for tearing, sweating, or skeletal muscle movement in response to noxious stimuli.

Because the volatile inhalational agents are dose-dependent myocardial depressants and potent vasodilators, blood pressure tends to drop during the waiting period between induction of anesthesia and the surgical incision.

This period of decreasing blood pressure usually coincides with the time during which the surgical team is scrubbing. During this period, providing adequate anesthesia while maintaining an adequate blood pressure may prove difficult. If the patient becomes hypotensive, the anesthetist may elect to increase the blood pressure by placing the patient in a Trendelenburg position, administering additional intravenous fluids, or administering a vasopressor. If the results are unsatisfactory, the inhalational agent may be decreased or discontinued until blood pressure is restored. Procedures such as prepping the site for the incision or inserting a urinary catheter may be enough to raise the blood pressure.

If the incision is made during the light stage of anesthesia, the stimulus may result in a significant increase in blood pressure, heart rate, and respiratory rate, as well as possible skeletal muscle movement.

Although not as dramatic as during induction or emergence, moderate fluctuations in blood pressure and heart rate are expected throughout the surgical procedure. These changes typically occur in response to the varying degrees of noxious stimuli and fluid volume shifts. The depth of anesthesia is increased or decreased in anticipation of or in response to these hemodynamic changes.

Ventilations during maintenance may be either controlled, assisted, or spontaneous. If the patient is paralyzed, breathing is controlled either by using a ventilator or by manually squeezing the anesthesia reservoir bag. If the patient is breathing but is unable to maintain acceptable respiratory function, squeezing the reservoir bag during inspiration is performed to assist patient respirations. During spontaneous ventilations, the patient is able to self-maintain adequate respiratory functions.

Depth of anesthesia may be judged by observing ventilatory rate and pattern in patients with assisted or spontaneous respirations. Unexpected, abrupt changes may be indicative of a mechanical airway problem or an untoward pulmonary or neurologic event.

Adequacy of ventilation and respiration is assessed by monitoring Sao_2, $ETco_2$, respiratory rate, and tidal volume; listening to breath sounds; and, if indicated, analysis of arterial blood gases. Intraoperatively, the Fio_2 and minute ventilation (tidal volume × respiratory rate) may be adjusted to optimize pulmonary function. If mechanical ventilation will be used, available options include volume or pressure control mode, inspiratory-expiratory ratio, and positive end-expiratory pressure (PEEP) adjustments.

Temperature is monitored throughout the procedure. General anesthetics are known to inhibit the thermoregulatory response (shivering and peripheral vasoconstriction). When this effect is combined with the cold environment typically encountered within the operating room, mild hypothermia is expected.

Heat loss is greatest during procedures involving exposure of a large surface area of cutaneous or surgical tissue. The goal is to prevent hypothermia-induced intraoperative complications such as myocardial depression, arrhythmias, or coagulopathies. To keep the patient warm, all nonsurgical cutaneous areas are covered, and the patient may be actively rewarmed by using circulating water or a forced-air heating blanket. Intravenous fluids are warmed, especially for use during rapid, large-volume fluid replacement. Because the delivered anesthetic gases are cool and dry, a heat-moisture exchanger is placed in the breathing circuit to retain airway humidity.

Conversely, hyperthermia may result from sepsis, thyrotoxicosis, or over-aggressive rewarming or during a malignant hyperthermia (MH) crisis. In these situations, the circulating water or air blanket may be used in the cooling mode; intravenous and surgical field fluids are not warmed, and more skin surface area is exposed. MH is a rare but potentially fatal condition that requires special considerations. If the patient is suspected of having MH, a standard MH protocol for management is initiated.

Muscle relaxants may be used as part of the anesthetic plan or administered to provide profound muscle relaxation for special surgical considerations. A PNS is used to assess the degree of neuromuscular blockade (NMB). Sufficient NMB may be maintained by a continuous infusion or repeat bolus doses of the muscle relaxant. If the surgical team notes that the patient is "too tight" or "pushing," the surgical field is evaluated and findings on use of the PNS help determine if additional muscle relaxant is required. An overdose of nondepolarizing muscle relaxants near the end of the surgical procedure may be difficult to pharmacologically reverse, and the patient may require postoperative ventilatory support. For this reason, long-acting muscle relaxants are given judiciously toward the end of a surgical procedure.

During maintenance, the volume and rate of intravenous fluid administration are determined by the type of procedure and by the amount of blood loss during surgery. For example, during minor surgery on an extremity, 1-2 mL/kg/hour of crystalloid may be administered as maintenance. For major abdominal surgery, 10-20 mL/kg/hour of crystalloid may be necessary to maintain sufficient intravascular volume.

For each milliliter of blood lost, 3 mL of crystalloid is used as replacement in addition to the calculated maintenance volume. If there has been major blood loss, blood product replacement must be considered. If appropriate, recovery of red blood cells (RBCs) into a cell saver for reinfusion should be considered. Adjustments to these basic guidelines for crystalloid infusion are made if the patient receives colloids and/or blood products. Moderation of fluid volumes is also considered for the patient with significant renal or cardiac impairment, in whom a volume overload may not be tolerated.

The adequacy of volume replacement is constantly evaluated by interpreting the blood pressure and heart rate changes in response to the administration of intravenous fluids, administration of anesthetic agents, or changes in table positioning (e.g., Trendelenburg or reverse Trendelenburg position).

If a urinary catheter is inserted, measurement of urine output is an excellent monitor for assessing renal function and intravascular volume status in the patient with normal renal function. Urine output should be between 0.5 and 1.0 mL/kg/hour. If oliguria develops, intravascular volume status and hemodynamics are reassessed. Polyuria develops from overhydration or the administration of a diuretic. If anuria suddenly develops, evaluation is made for mechanical problems (kinked or disconnected urinary catheter) before institution of aggressive fluid and/or diuretic therapy.

CVP measurements or data derived from the use of a multipurpose PA catheter provide important data in determining intravascular volume status. The CVP and the PA occlusion pressure (wedge pressure) are representative of the filling pressures (preload) of the heart. Additional data derived with the PA catheter are used to assess heart function and temperature.

To help maintain homeostasis, blood gas specimens may be drawn to assess oxygenation, ventilation, and acid-base status, as well as glucose, electrolyte, and hemoglobin values. Intraoperative coagulation studies may also be performed in patients with suspected coagulopathy.

Emergence

Emergence from a general anesthetic procedure involves the patient's return to consciousness. The proper timing of emergence is crucial. Early emergence is disruptive to the surgical team and may be detrimental to the outcome. Delayed awakening increases operating room time, delays subsequent surgeries, and raises the possibility of an adverse intraoperative neurologic event.

As emergence progresses, the central nervous system (CNS) and peripheral autonomic system become more sensitive to external stimuli. As analgesic effects begin to dissipate, the blood pressure and heart rate tend to increase. Timely administration of preemptive analgesics will minimize this response. Antiemetics may also be administered prior to emergence to prevent or minimize postoperative nausea and vomiting.

Plans are made for the return of muscle and respiratory function to a level sufficient to maintain spontaneous ventilations. If the patient is intubated, any residual neuromuscular block must be pharmacologically reversed prior to extubation. The reversal of muscle paralysis is generally timed to occur toward the end of the surgical procedure so that the return of muscle tone does not interfere with surgery. Testing with a PNS must demonstrate a strong, equal in intensity response to a "train of four" and no fade during the sustained tetanus test.

If sufficient pulmonary function has returned, either a deep or an "awake" extubation technique may be used. The *deep extubation technique* is used to prevent the patient from coughing or straining on the ETT as the tube is removed. This technique is selected for use in patients in whom a transient increase in pressure caused by coughing and bucking on the ETT could adversely affect surgical outcome. This technique may also be used in the asthmatic patient in the hope of preventing bronchospasm. Because airway reflexes remain obtunded, the patient should not cough during manipulation of the ETT as it is removed.

For use of the *awake extubation technique*, the patient must demonstrate the ability to self-maintain and protect the airway after the ETT is removed. The awake technique is used in patients in whom there is a potential for aspiration of gastric contents, in patients who experienced a difficult intubation, or in patients with a potentially compromised airway (secondary to trauma or a surgical procedure that alters airway anatomy). During an awake extubation, coughing during removal of the ETT generally occurs because the airway reflexes are intact. Extubation may be delayed until the patient is able to demonstrate the cough reflex, because this indicates that the patient is able to protect the airway if emesis does occur. If laryngospasm occurs immediately after extubation, the airway must be actively managed by applying CPAP and 100% O_2 through the face mask until the spasm subsides. If hypoxemia or hemodynamic instability develops, more aggressive maneuvers may become necessary.

Before a deep or an awake extubation is performed, it must be established that the patient is capable of maintaining adequate pulmonary function while breathing spontaneously after the ETT is removed. To make this determination, multiple parameters are measured and monitored prior to extubation. The Sao_2, $ETco_2$, respiratory rate, tidal volume, and maximal inspiratory pressure are evaluated. In the cooperative awakening patient, measuring vital capacity and having the patient demonstrate a sustained head lift are additional tests used in judging the patient's ability to maintain adequate ventilations after extubation. In patients who have received neuromuscular blocking agents, response to the PNS as described previously also is evaluated. If indicated, arterial blood gas analysis may be helpful. If the anesthetist believes that the patient is not ready for extubation, the ETT is left in place until recovery is sufficient for extubation.

Transport

After surgery, the anesthetist and the anesthesiologist must determine when the patient can safely be transported from the operating room to the PSCU or postanesthesia care unit (PACU). Criteria for transport readiness include hemodynamic stability, satisfactory Sao_2, and the patient's physical comfort.

When stable, the patient is moved from the operating table onto the stretcher or bed. After the move, cardiopulmonary status is reassessed, especially if the patient has been in a position other than supine, because intravascular volume shifts may dramatically alter the blood pressure. If not contraindicated, the head of the stretcher or bed is elevated to help improve functional residual capacity (FRC) and reduce the work of breathing. If the patient is at potential risk for aspiration, he or she is placed in a lateral decubitus position to help control emesis. To prevent and minimize shivering, warm blankets are applied. Supplemental O_2 is administered during transport to help maintain a satisfactory Sao_2. Continued ECG, Sao_2, and hemodynamic monitoring during transport is advisable in critically ill patients, especially if their disposition is to another floor or remote recovery area.

On arrival to the PACU or ICU, a pulse oximeter is applied and vital signs are taken as monitoring is reestablished. A thorough report is then given to members of the team who will be caring for the patient. The anesthesia care team maintains responsibility for the patient until the effects of the anesthetics have worn off and remains immediately available for bedside care.

REGIONAL ANESTHESIA

Regional anesthesia involves selectively anesthetizing a region of the patient's body. A regional anesthetic procedure is accomplished with deposition of a local anesthetic agent adjacent to neuronal membranes. Neural blockade results from penetration of the neuronal membrane by local anesthetic, temporarily interrupting the transmission of nerve impulses. The term "regional anesthetic" refers to the centroneuraxis blocks (spinal, epidural, and caudal), the peripheral nerve blocks, and the head and neck blocks.

The choice of a regional anesthetic technique is made during the preoperative anesthesia consultation. If a regional anesthetic is suitable for the proposed surgical procedure and there are no contraindications, the risks and benefits are discussed with and agreed on by the patient for consent. The patient is also informed that if the block fails or becomes inadequate during the procedure, the administration of a general anesthetic may become necessary.

The patient is informed that he or she will be sedated, will be continuously monitored, and will receive supplemental O_2. The goal is to keep the patient safe, comfortable, hemodynamically stable, and sedated (yet responsive) while providing a quiet surgical field.

As part of preparation for a regional anesthetic procedure, the patient is appropriately sedated. Oversedation should be avoided because communication with a cooperative patient is crucial for the administration of safe, effective regional anesthesia. The responsive patient can help with positioning, voice discomfort from paresthesia during needle or catheter placement, announce warning signs of drug-induced toxicity, help describe the degree of neural blockade, or alert operating room personnel to any other problems (e.g., angina pectoris may occur in the patient with coronary artery disease who becomes hypotensive).

Centroneuraxis Blocks: Spinal, Epidural, and Caudal

The administration of a spinal, epidural, or caudal anesthetic procedure requires knowledge of the CNS, spinal column, spinal cord, and neural structures. Selection of the appropriate neural blocking agent requires understanding of the pharmacology of local anesthetic agents and adjuvants that may be used to alter the block. Management of a centroneuraxis anesthetic procedure requires knowledge of the dermatomal distribution of the spinal nerves, as well as the autonomic, sensory, and motor responses to central neural blockade.

Contraindications to the administration of these blocks include patient refusal, infection at the puncture site, sepsis, coagulopathy, increased intracranial pressure (ICP), uncorrected severe hypovolemia, demyelinating CNS disease, and allergy to the specific class of local anesthetic agent.

Spinal Block

Spinal anesthesia is most suitable for procedures on the lower half of the body and is accomplished by injecting a small volume of a local anesthetic solution through a spinal needle into the subarachnoid space, which contains CSF, the spinal cord (which in adults usually terminates at L1), and spinal nerves. To avoid inadvertent needle trauma to the spinal cord, the spinal needle is introduced into the lumbar region at or below the L2-L3 interspace into the subarachnoid space. Proper placement is confirmed by the return of clear CSF. If the patient complains of paresthesia during needle placement or during injection of local anesthetic, the needle must be withdrawn or redirected in order to avoid nerve injury.

The injected local anesthetic mixes with the CSF and bathes the nerve roots, dorsal root ganglia, and possibly the periphery of the spinal cord. The agent causes temporary neural blockade by penetrating the neural membrane and inhibiting the transmission of nerve impulses. The spread of the local anesthetic depends on the amount of agent injected, the baricity of the anesthetic solution, and the position of the patient during and immediately after the injection. *Baricity* is determined by comparing the specific gravity of the anesthetic solution with the specific gravity of the CSF. A hyperbaric solution is heavier than CSF, a hypobaric one is lighter, and an isobaric solution has the same specific gravity as that of CSF. A hyperbaric solution flows downward toward the most dependent portion of the CSF column, a hypobaric solution ascends toward the higher portion of the CSF column, and the isobaric solution remains within the approximate zone of injection. As the agent spreads, the concentration decreases while the drug is absorbed.

Appropriately positioning the patient during and immediately after the injection is crucial for proper distribution of the anesthetic agent. With the patient in the sitting, lateral decubitus, or prone position, a spinal anesthetic is commonly administered as a single-shot technique (some operators elect to temporarily place an indwelling subarachnoid catheter for repeated intraoperative dosing). Depending on the intended distribution of anesthetic agent, the patient may remain in the original position for several minutes after injection or be immediately repositioned after injection to achieve the desired effect.

The duration of action of the anesthetic agent is an important consideration. The most commonly used preservative-free agents are tetracaine, lidocaine, and bupivacaine. Each possesses a different duration of action. The anticipated length of time required to complete a procedure also influences the selection of a particular agent. Except for bupivacaine, the duration of action may be extended further by mixing epinephrine or phenylephrine with the local anesthetic prior to injection.

Once the anesthetic agent has been injected into the subarachnoid space, the onset of action is very rapid, and evidence of neural blockade may be manifested within 1 to 2 minutes. Because the onset of action is so rapid, the lumbar puncture usually is performed in the operating room. The level of the block should be well established within 15 to 20 minutes.

Because of the differences in nerve size, fiber type, and myelination, some nerves are blocked more easily than others. Consequently, differential zones of neural blockade are expected. The smaller myelinated fibers (sympathetic, pain) are more easily blocked than the larger motor fibers. As a result, the sympathetic block occurs first and is generally two dermatome levels above the sensory block. Motor blockade occurs last and is typically two dermatome levels below the level of sensory blockade.

A dermatome's sensory level corresponds to the vertebrae from which the spinal nerve exits the intervertebral foramen. Sensory levels T4 (nipple line) and T10 (umbilicus) are good reference points. Immediately after the administration of the local anesthetic, the progression of neural blockade is evaluated by testing successive dermatome levels for a response (or lack of a response) to a stimulus. Touching the skin with an alcohol wipe for sympathetic blockade and pricking the skin with a dull needle for sensory blockade may be used as testing methods. After the block has been established, asking the patient to move the lower extremities may be used to assess the degree of motor blockade.

Tracking the level of sensory blockade is very important to ensure adequate anesthesia for the surgical procedure. The level of sympathetic block must be known, because resulting cardiovascular effects are proportionate to the degree of neural block. The sympathetic fibers from the T5-L1 distribution help maintain vascular tone (e.g., blood pressure). The cardioaccelerator fibers from T1-T4 help maintain heart rate.

Within the first few minutes after injection of the local anesthetic, a decrease in blood pressure is anticipated. The higher the level of sympathetic block, the greater the drop in blood pressure. A partial sympathectomy at T8-T10 may be well tolerated in the normovolemic patient, because intact baroreceptor activity and the cardiac accelerator fibers provide sufficient input to maintain blood pressure and heart rate. If the sensory level is at or above the T3 level, the patient is considered to have a total sympathectomy. Support of the cardiovascular system with pharmacologic agents, increased intravenous fluid administration, or Trendelenburg positioning is often necessary to help maintain an acceptable blood pressure and heart rate. If these functions are not corrected, hypoperfusion to the respiratory center in the brain may result in apnea.

The respiratory effect is dependent on the height of the motor block. Effective ventilation results from adequate use of the diaphragm, intercostal, and abdominal muscles. For patients with normal respiratory mechanics, lower-level blocks that paralyze the abdominal muscles should have no effect on ventilation. With higher-level thoracic blocks, the intercostal muscles become paralyzed. Because the diaphragm is still functional, these patients should still be able to maintain a normal tidal volume, Sao_2, and $ETco_2$. With a high-level thoracic block, patients may complain of dyspnea because of the loss of chest wall sensation. These patients may need to be reassured that they are being monitored and are breathing adequately. The phrenic nerve, which controls the diaphragm, is a large nerve that originates mainly from C4 (with small communicating branches from C3 and C5) and is rarely affected by the administration of a standard spinal anesthetic. If the phrenic nerve does become paralyzed, the result is a "total spinal," and ventilatory support will be necessary.

The urologic effects may include an atonic bladder and urinary retention. If the patient has been given a large volume of intravenous fluids or is unable to void within a reasonable time after the block has worn off, urinary catheterization should be considered.

The gastrointestinal effect may be beneficial for the surgical team. A sympathetic block of T5-L1 results in unopposed vagal stimulation of the intestine. This results in contracted intestines with active peristalsis. This level of blockade also provides excellent skeletal muscle relaxation, an advantage for the surgical team. A feeling of nausea may be secondary to the increased vagal tone or hypotension. Administration of an anticholinergic and increasing the blood pressure are standard treatments.

As the surgery progresses, regression of the neural blockade is expected. This regression occurs in the opposite order relative to progression of the neural blockade. Although the patient may be able to move the legs toward the end of the procedure, there still may be sufficient sensory blockade to complete the procedure. If the spinal block becomes inadequate, injection of a local anesthetic into the surgical site, a field block, or administration of a general anesthetic may be necessary. If a subarachnoid catheter was placed for continuous spinal anesthesia, a sufficient level of block can be maintained throughout surgery.

Complications attributed to the administration of a spinal anesthetic are uncommon, and permanent neurologic deficits are rare. The two most common complications are back pain and spinal headache. The back pain is usually the result of needle instrumentation and should resolve with time. A spinal headache results from the loss of CSF through the dural puncture site. The intensity of the headache is increased when the patient is in the upright position. Conservative management includes keeping the patient supine, aggressive hydration, and administration of intravenous analgesics and caffeine. If this therapy is unsuccessful after 24 hours, an epidural blood patch procedure may be performed. A blood patch procedure involves withdrawing 10 to 15 mL of the patient's blood and immediately administering the blood into the epidural space at the level of the original lumbar puncture. The resulting hemostatic plug should seal the hole in the dura, preventing further leakage of CSF.

Epidural Block

Epidural anesthesia is also indicated for procedures on the lower half of the body and is more versatile than a spinal anesthetic. A significant advantage is that an epidural catheter may be placed within the epidural space to deliver a continuous infusion of anesthetic agents. This catheter is used during obstetric or surgical procedures to maintain a sufficient level of anesthesia and then may be used postoperatively for pain control with a continuous infusion of a local anesthetic agent or narcotic through the catheter.

An epidural anesthetic is accomplished by injecting a local anesthetic agent into the epidural space. The epidural space extends the length of the vertebral column and contains loose connective tissue, fat, and epidural veins. For surgical procedures, an epidural needle may be placed through the lumbar or thoracic interlaminar space. The needle is advanced midline (to avoid epidural veins) into the firm ligamentum flavum. Needle entrance into the epidural space may be identified by either the hanging drop technique or the loss of resistance technique.

For the *hanging drop technique*, the epidural needle is placed into the ligamentum flavum. A drop of saline is placed onto the needle hub. As the needle is advanced and enters the epidural space, negative pressure within this space draws the drop inside the needle, indicating proper placement.

For the *loss of resistance technique*, an air or saline-filled syringe is attached to the epidural needle after the needle has been positioned in the ligamentum flavum. As the needle is being advanced, continuous or intermittent pressure is applied to the plunger of the syringe. A sudden loss of resistance indicates entry of the needle tip into the epidural space.

Note: The epidural space is narrow, so continued advancement of the needle eventually will result in inadvertent dural puncture. Return of CSF or blood during needle placement indicates that the dura or an epidural vein has been punctured. If either occurs, the needle must be withdrawn or repositioned.

Regardless of which technique is employed, a 3-mL test dose of local anesthetic with 1:200,000 epinephrine first is injected through the epidural needle or epidural catheter. If the dura has been punctured and the local anesthetic enters the subarachnoid space, signs of a spinal anesthetic develop. If the injected dose enters an epidural vein, the epinephrine causes a notable increase in heart rate.

If there is no evidence of blood or CSF return, the same needle may be used for a single-dose injection, or an epidural catheter may be threaded 2 to 5 cm rostrally into the epidural space. The catheter may be used intraoperatively for anesthetic management as well as postoperatively for pain control.

If there are no adverse reactions to the test dose within 3 to 5 minutes, the calculated dose of local anesthetic is administered slowly in divided doses. After each 5-mL injection of local anesthetic, aspiration is performed to make certain that the epidural needle or indwelling catheter has not migrated into the subarachnoid space or epidural vein.

Because the volume of local anesthetic injected into the epidural space is much greater than that used for a spinal anesthetic procedure, there is a greater risk of systemic or CNS toxicity. Local anesthetic agents such as chloroprocaine, lidocaine, mepivacaine, prilocaine, etidocaine, and bupivacaine are selected on the basis of a specific onset of action, intensity of blockade, or duration of action.

After injection, the anesthetic effect results from the absorption of the agent through the dural sheath by the neural membranes located in the predural space, or possibly by diffusion through the dura into the subarachnoid space. The onset of action is not as rapid as with a spinal anesthetic, so patience must be exercised in waiting for the block to fully develop.

Adjunctive agents such as epinephrine, sodium bicarbonate ($NaHCO_3$), and narcotic may be combined with the local anesthetic solution to alter the onset of action and duration of the block. Adjusting the dosage or concentration of the local anesthetic results in varying degrees of sympathetic, sensory, and motor blockade, which can be tailored to match the demands of the surgical procedure. Dosage adjustments are made for patients who have spinal deformities or are morbidly obese, elderly patients, or pregnant women.

Once the epidural anesthetic agent has been administered, the level of the neural blockade must be monitored in the same manner as described for the spinal anesthetic. If motor blockade develops, it may be detected five dermatome levels below the level of the sensory block. Although the neural blockade occurs at a slower rate than in a spinal anesthetic procedure, preparations for untoward effects must be made.

Complications resulting from an epidural anesthetic are similar to those occurring with a spinal anesthetic. If dural puncture does occur, it is associated with a much greater incidence of spinal headache (with epidurals, a 16- to 18-gauge needle is used; with spinals, a 22- to 25-gauge needle is used). Unintentional injection of a large volume of local anesthetic into the subarachnoid space or an epidural vein results in drug overdosage, which may cause CNS or systemic toxicity.

Epidural hematoma is extremely rare. Use of intraoperative heparin or postoperative anticoagulants in patients with indwelling catheters increases the incidence of occurrence. For such patients, normalization of coagulation studies needs to be confirmed before the catheter is withdrawn. Documentation of an epidural hematoma (by MRI) necessitates immediate evacuation to relieve pressure on neural structures. Knotting, kinking, or breakage of indwelling epidural catheters has been reported. Also, as with any invasive procedure, infection is a potential risk.

Caudal Block

Caudal anesthesia is most useful during obstetric or surgical procedures involving the perineal region. A 1½- to 2-inch needle is placed through the sacral hiatus and advanced into the caudal canal until it enters the epidural space. An indwelling catheter may be inserted through the needle. As with an epidural anesthetic procedure, a test dose of local anesthetic is administered to rule out inadvertent subarachnoid space or epidural vein puncture. If no adverse effects are detected, the appropriate dosage of local anesthetic is injected into the epidural space using a single-dose technique or through the catheter for repeated dosing. Because the anesthetic agent is introduced into the epidural space, physiologic effects and complications similar to those associated with a lumbar epidural anesthetic procedure should be considered.

Peripheral Nerve Blocks

Peripheral nerve blocks are chosen for surgical procedures on the upper or lower extremity. The choice to use this block is made in agreement with the patient during the preoperative anesthesia consultation. As with all regional anesthetic procedures, the patient is monitored, provided with supplemental O_2, and appropriately sedated yet responsive.

Knowledge of neuroanatomy, the actions of the local anesthetic agents, the effects of the resulting neural blockade, and any associated complications resulting from the administration of a peripheral nerve blockade is essential. Contraindications to this procedure include patient refusal, infection at the proposed puncture site, coagulopathy, and preexisting neuropathy of the extremity.

An advantage of a peripheral nerve block is that it typically has minimal effect on the cardiovascular or pulmonary system. A disadvantage is that the block may not be completely successful, may take a prolonged period to become effective, or may require supplementation. To allow sufficient time for onset and to ensure the adequacy of the neural blockade, the administration of the nerve block may be performed in a "block room" or the PSCU.

Several techniques are employed to favorably position the needle adjacent to the nerve. Identification of bone landmarks and muscle groups and palpation of arteries are used in selecting the site of needle insertion.

The *nerve stimulator technique* is a relatively safe method for locating the nerve. With the patient electrically grounded, an insulated needle (except for the blunt tip) is connected to a nerve stimulator and directed toward the nerve. As the needle is advanced, motor or sensory response becomes pronounced. Ideal needle placement is achieved when the maximal neural response is obtained with the lowest current output.

The *elicitation of paresthesia technique* involves advancing the needle until it comes in direct contact with the nerve. There may be a higher incidence of postblock neuropathy with this procedure. Severe paresthesia during injection of the local anesthetic may indicate intraneural rather than perineural injection. If this occurs, the needle is withdrawn.

The loss of resistance technique takes advantage of the fact that some nerves used for neural blockade reside in neurovascular bundles surrounded by a fascial sheath. A blunt, beveled needle is advanced toward the nerve, and a loss of resistance is felt as the needle passes through the fascial sheath and enters the neurovascular bundle.

Regardless of the technique employed, a test dose of local anesthetic is injected to rule out inadvertent intravascular, intraneural, or subarachnoid needle placement. If there are no adverse reactions, the local anesthetic is administered in incremental doses with interval pauses. This method of injection is used for large-volume dosing because if any adverse effect is noted as a result of needle malposition, the injection can be terminated prior to administration of the full dose.

Upper Extremity Block

For the upper extremity, the brachial plexus block provides the greatest area of blockade. Depending on the proposed surgical site, the interscalene, supraclavicular, or axillary approach to the brachial plexus may be used. The intrascalene approach may provide adequate anesthesia for the shoulder; the supraclavicular approach, for the elbow, forearm, and hand; and the axillary approach, for procedures distal to the elbow. Selective blockade of the musculocutaneous, radial, median, ulnar, or digital nerve is employed for anesthetizing more specific regions, or it may be used to supplement a brachial plexus block.

Lower Extremity Block

For the lower extremity, the lumbar plexus, sacral plexus, and peripheral nerves are targeted for neural blockade. Because the major nerve plexuses are not in close proximity, multiple blocks are necessary to provide sufficient anesthesia for the entire lower extremity. The most commonly performed nerve blocks include lumbar plexus, femoral nerve, obturator nerve, lateral femoral cutaneous nerve, sciatic nerve, ilioinguinal/iliohypogastric nerve, and popliteal nerve blocks. For an ankle block, the deep peroneal, saphenous, superficial peroneal, posterior tibial, and sural nerves are targeted for blockade.

Complications associated with the administration of peripheral nerve blocks include drug reaction, toxicity, intravascular or subarachnoid injection, neuropathy from needle trauma or intraneural injection, hematoma, or pneumothorax from pleural puncture.

Intravenous Regional Block (Bier Block)

An intravenous regional anesthetic procedure provides an excellent sensory and motor block for upper or lower extremity surgical procedures of short duration. The technique for this block involves placing a double tourniquet (proximal cuff–distal cuff) around the proximal portion of the surgical extremity. A small-gauge intravenous line is inserted into the most distal vein. An Esmarch bandage is used to exsanguinate the limb, applied starting from the most distal portion and continuing up to the base of the double tourniquet. The proximal cuff of the tourniquet is then inflated to occlude blood flow. The Esmarch bandage is removed and the local anesthetic agent is injected through the intravenous catheter. The resulting block has a rapid onset and provides excellent anesthesia for approximately 45 to 60 minutes. If the patient begins to complain of tourniquet pain, the distal cuff is inflated. After confirmation that the distal cuff is inflated, the proximal cuff is deflated. The tourniquet pain should then subside. On completion of surgery, the tourniquet is deflated, reinflated, and deflated in timed sequence. This procedure minimizes the possibility of a systemic reaction to the remaining local anesthetic as it returns to the central circulation.

Regional Head and Neck Blocks

Contraindications to and complications associated with the administration of head and neck blocks are the same as those described for centroneuroaxis and peripheral nerve blocks.

Cervical Plexus Blocks

The cervical plexus blocks are used for procedures on the neck and occipital portion of the scalp. A superficial plexus block is accomplished by injecting a local anesthetic agent along the posterior border of the sternocleidomastoid muscle. A deep cervical block involves individual injections adjacent to the transverse process to access C2, C3, and C4 of the cervical plexus.

Superior Laryngeal Nerve Block

Superior laryngeal nerve block anesthetizes the airway between the epiglottis and vocal cords and is used to suppress airway reflexes during laryngoscopy. Bilateral nerve blocks are accomplished by injecting a local anesthetic agent below the greater cornu on each side of the hyoid bone.

Translaryngeal Nerve Block

Translarygeal nerve block anesthetizes the airway below the vocal cords and frequently is used in combination with the superior laryngeal nerve block during awake intubations. This block is accomplished by directing a needle through the cricothyroid membrane into the trachea, with subsequent injection of the local anesthetic agent.

Retrobulbar Nerve Block

A retrobulbar nerve block provides excellent anesthesia for corneal, lens, and anterior chamber ocular procedures. This block is accomplished by injecting a local anesthetic agent into the muscle cone behind the globe of the eye.

Facial Nerve Block

Facial nerve block frequently is given in combination with the retrobulbar block. Injection of a local anesthetic agent adjacent to the facial nerve causes akinesia of the eyelid and permits placement of the eyelid speculum.

Monitored Anesthesia Care

Some minor surgical procedures are suitable for MAC. In this technique, the anesthesia care team monitors the patient, provides intraoperative sedation, and is prepared to administer a general anesthetic if necessary.

Even with minor surgical procedures, the physical status of the patient may range from healthy ASA class I to critically ill ASA class V. The patient's instructions for the night before surgery are the same as if he or she were undergoing a general anesthetic procedure.

The patient is appropriately sedated before entering the operating room. Basic monitoring includes ECG, blood pressure, heart rate, respirations, Sao_2, $ETco_2$, and temperature. Supplemental oxygen is generally administered via a split O_2 delivery–CO_2 sampling nasal cannula. If electrocautery is used during head or neck surgery, a high concentration of O_2 must be avoided because of the danger of fire. Because MAC procedures often are conducted on an outpatient basis, intravenous sedation generally consists of a short-acting analgesic or an ultra-short-acting sedative-hypnotic.

After monitors have been placed and the patient has been effectively sedated, the surgeon infiltrates a local anesthetic agent around the surgical incision site (field block). Throughout the procedure, care is taken to ensure that the patient remains comfortable, proteced from injury, hemodynamically stable, and well oxygenated. If at any point the patient expresses discomfort, additional local anesthetic may be given to extend the field block.

To help avoid overdosage, a record is kept of the total amount of local anesthetic infiltrated.

The cooperative patient usually does very well with MAC. In occasional cases, the anesthetic plan needs to be changed during the surgical procedure. A general anesthetic procedure may become necessary if the surgeon is unable to provide or maintain a field block sufficient to keep the patient comfortable. Some patients under sedation become confused and uncooperative, and administration of additional intravenous sedative agent may exacerbate this problem. If the patient is oversedated, the airway may become difficult to manage. In this situation, pharmacologic reversal of the sedative agent or conversion to a general anesthetic procedure may become necessary.

In general, local MAC is an effective anesthetic approach for minor surgical procedures. The anesthetic agents used have a minimal effect on the autonomic nervous system, which is advantageous in the critically ill patient. The rapid recovery from the short-acting agents also allows for an earlier discharge from the hospital.

Further Reading

American Society of Anesthesiologists: www.asahq.org

Barash PG, Cullen BF, Stoelting RK (eds): Clinical Anesthesia, 4th ed. Philadelphia, Lippincott Williams & Wilkins, 2001.

Hurford WE, Bailin MT, Davison JK (eds): Clinical Anesthesia Procedures of the Massachusetts General Hospital, 6th ed. Philadelphia, Lippincott Williams & Wilkins, 2002.

Miller RD (ed): Anesthesia, 5th ed. New York, Churchill Livingstone, 2000.

Morgan GE, Mikhail MS: Clinical Anesthesiology. Norwalk, CT, Appleton & Lange, 1992.

Practice Guidelines for the Management of the Difficult Airway: A Report by the American Society of Anesthesiologists Task Force on Management of the Difficult Airway. Anesthesiology 78:597, 1993.

Stoelting RK, Dierdorf SF (eds): Handbook for Anesthesia and Co-Existing Disease, 4th ed. New York, Churchill Livingstone, 2002.

PROCEDURES

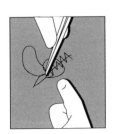

19

Casting/Splinting Techniques

Nancy Anderson, PA-C

DEFINITION

Immobilization of a body part following fracture or subluxation to allow realignment and healing.

TECHNIQUE

Casting

Casting is performed primarily by orthopedists and is not usually done in the acute situation owing to the potential for complications from edema. Support may be added to an existing, worn, or broken cast in the emergency department. Cast material is rolled over the existing cast for reinforcement. Casts that are too tight may be split to allow for edema. A cast is "bivalved" by cutting through the cast, padding the cut edges, and rewrapping with an elastic (Ace) bandage.

Splinting

General Instructions

Pad the limb well with cast padding for comfort, apply the splint material, cover the splint with an elastic bandage (allowing for expansion due to edema), and mold into desired position.

Or preformed splints may be used as appropriate.

Common Splints and Their Application

Jones Long-Leg Splint. Used for knee immobilization. Splints are applied from medial and lateral to the groin down to just proximal to the malleoli. The orientation of the cast is usually extended for weight bearing or flexed up to 45 degrees for non–weight bearing.

Sugar-Tong/Stirrup Splint. A continuous U-shaped splint used to prevent inversion/eversion of the foot. This splint runs medially and laterally from the level of the tibial tubercle and is continued across the plantar hindfoot.

Posterior Splint: Foot. Runs from the toes on the plantar foot surface, up the posterior lower leg, to the knee. Keep the foot at a 90-degree angle to the lower extremity (neutral). Used for foot or ankle injuries.

Posterior Splint: Arm. The position of function has the wrist dorsiflexed to 35 degrees with the fingers flexed (as if for holding a glass).

Posterior Splint: Elbow. Apply the splint on the dorsal forearm extending posteriorly on the upper arm and flex the elbow to 90 degrees. Extend the plaster to support the wrist.

Posterior Splint: Wrist. Apply the splint from the metacarpophalangeal (MCP) joints to just below the elbow. Allow the fingers and MCP joints to be free.

Volar Splint. Apply from the palmar crease to below the elbow. Keep the MCP joints free.

Sugar-Tong Splint. Runs from the palmar crease proximally on the volar surface, around the flexed elbow, and back on the dorsal forearm to just below the MCP joints. Used to decrease pronation and supination.

Gutter Splint. Runs from the palmar crease to just below the elbow on either the radial or ulnar aspect of the forearm. Used for radial or ulnar injuries.

Thumb Spica Splint. Circumferentially splint the thumb in full extension on the end of a radial gutter splint. Used for navicular injuries.

INDICATIONS

Necessity for immobilization due to fracture, dislocation, or significant soft tissue injury.

CONTRAINDICATIONS

Significant laceration necessitating frequent inspection, compartment syndrome.

COMPLICATIONS

If the cast or splint is applied too tightly, or if edema develops subsequent to the application of the cast or splint, the distal vascular supply may be interrupted, causing cyanosis, peripheral nerve injury, or necrosis of the affected area with tissue loss. Infection may occur within the casted or splinted area if an abrasion or laceration is unrecognized. Pressure sores may result if the cast or splint is incorrectly applied.

Chest Tube Thoracostomy

Deborah A. Opacic, EdD, PA-C

DEFINITION

Insertion of a tube into the pleural space for decompression.

TECHNIQUE

Materials
Thoracostomy tray, assorted chest tubes (usually No. 24, 28, 32), Pleurovac, chest catheter, povidone-iodine (Betadine) solution, gown, gloves.

Pre-Procedure Considerations
Explain the rationale and procedure to the patient.

Patient Positioning
For anterior tube placement, the patient is supine and the head of the bed is elevated 30 to 45 degrees. For lateral tube placement, the patient is placed into the lateral decubitus position with the involved side up.

Procedure
Determine the placement of the tube; prepare the operative site and drape the patient.

Plan the incision to be one interspace below the rib where the tube will actually be placed.

Anesthesize the skin along a line parallel to the rib. Using a long needle, extend the lidocaine infiltration superiorly in the direction that the tube will be tracked. The final area to be anesthetized will be the pleura where the tube will be placed. In anesthetization and placing the tube, avoid the intercostal neurovascular bundle that lies on the inferior aspect of each rib (see Fig. 19-1).

Incise the skin over the anesthetized wheal and then create a tunnel superiorly toward the intercostal space using a Kelly clamp.

Enter the pleural space, with the Kelly clamp over the superior aspect of the rib. Spread the clamp to create an opening where the tube will be placed.

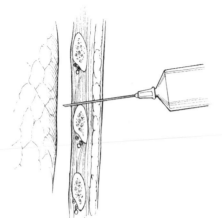

Figure 19–1. Insert the needle over the superior aspect of the rib to avoid the neurovascular bundle that lies on the inferior aspect of the rib. (From Rakel RE: Saunders Manual of Medical Practice, 2nd ed. Philadelphia, WB Saunders, 2000, p. 224.)

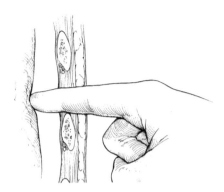

Figure 19–2. Place a finger into the pleural space to confirm that the chest has been entered and to check for adhesions. (From Rakel RE: Saunders Manual of Medical Practice, 2nd ed. Philadelphia, WB Saunders, 2000. p. 225.)

Place a finger into the pleural space to confirm that the chest has been entered and to check for adhesions (see Fig. 19-2). The chest tube is placed by either grasping the tip of the tube with the Kelly clamp and inserting it into the pleural space (see Fig. 19-3), withdrawing the clamp and directing the tube further into the pleural space, or by leaving the trocar in the chest tube, placing the tube in the same way as described, and removing the trocar after entering the pleural space. The clinician placing the tube must take care to control the trocar as it enters the pleural space, to avoid iatrogenic trauma.

After placing the tube and ensuring that all of the holes in the tube are within the pleural space, secure it to the chest wall with heavy suture material.

Cover with a sterile dressing of petroleum gauze and sponges.

Obtain a chest film to confirm tube position.

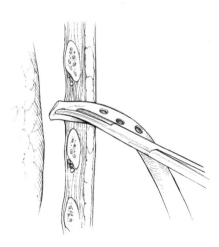

Figure 19–3. Grasp the chest tube with a Kelly clamp and insert the tube into the pleural space. (From Rakel RE: Saunders Manual of Medical Practice, 2nd ed. Philadelphia, WB Saunders, 2000, p. 225.)

INDICATIONS

Pneumothorax, hemothorax, empyema, hydrothorax or chylothorax, severe chest trauma with instability and unknown injuries, chemical pleural sclerosis for persistent pneumothoraces, recurrent effusions, and malignancy.

CONTRAINDICATIONS

Essentially none, but small pneumothoraces may spontaneously resolve without chest tube insertion; patients with bleeding dyscrasias need to be managed cautiously owing to the possibility of hemorrhage.

COMPLICATIONS

Hemorrhage, laceration of the lung, infection, cardiac injury, subcutaneous placement, subcutaneous/mediastinal emphysema, bronchopleural-cutaneous fistula.

Emergency Cricothyroidotomy

Jack Pike, BS, PA-C

DEFINITION

Urgent access to the airway through the cricothyroid cartilage indicated in acute respiratory compromise.

TECHNIQUE

Materials

Knife blade and handle, tracheostomy tube (or pediatric endotracheal tube or large-gauge angiocatheter), bag-valve ventilation unit, and oxygen.

Procedure

Anesthesia is not required, as, by definition, a patient requiring emergency cricothyroidotomy does not need local anesthesia.

The patient is positioned supine with head extended. Palpate the cricothyroid membrane between the thyroid and cricoid cartilages (see Fig. 19-4). Make a vertical incision in the midline over the cricothyroid membrane and incise the membrane horizontally. Place the blunt end of the knife handle, or an instrument such as a Delaborde dilator, through

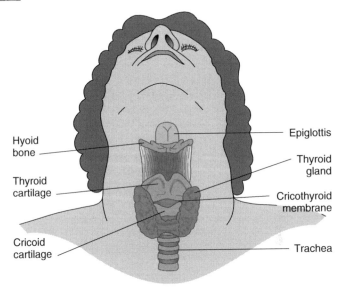

Figure 19–4. Anatomic landmarks used when palpating for the cricothyroid membrane. (From Bledsoe BE, Porter RS, Shade BR: Brady Paramedic Emergency Care, 3rd ed. Upper Saddle River, NJ, Prentice-Hall, 1996, p. 270.)

the cricothyroidotomy and enlarge the opening. Place the tracheostomy tube or endotracheal tube through the opening, inflate the cuff, and ventilate.

Secure the tracheostomy tube to the skin with suture and/or umbilical tapes.

INDICATIONS

Emergency tracheotomy is indicated when respiratory obstruction is too severe to allow time for an orderly tracheotomy, when an endotracheal tube and equipment are unavailable, or when risk of brain damage is increased by waiting even a few minutes.

CONTRAINDICATIONS

None.

COMPLICATIONS

Hemorrhage, esophageal perforation, failure to achieve tracheostomy.

Internal Jugular Vein Cannulation

Jack Pike, BS, PA-C

DEFINITION

Cannulation of the internal jugular (IJ) vein, often performed to establish means of central venous pressure (CVP) monitoring.

TECHNIQUE

Related Anatomy

The IJ vein arises from the base of the skull posterior to the internal carotid artery (ICA) and lateral to the common carotid. It lies medial to the sternocleidomastoid (SCM) muscle superiorly, crossing deep to the muscle, and emerges at the triangle between the two heads of the SCM.

Patient Positioning

Supine, Trendelenburg at 10 to 20 degrees from horizontal, head turned to the opposite side; roll placed between scapulae (see Fig. 19-5).

Procedure

There are three approaches to the IJ: central, anterior, and posterior.

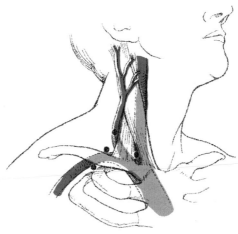

Figure 19–5. Correct patient positioning for internal jugular cannulation. (From Rakel RE: Saunders Manual of Medical Practice. Philadelphia, WB Saunders, 1996.)

Central Approach

After preoperative preparation and draping, locate the triangle formed by the two heads of the SCM (if possible, have patient lift the head to assist in localization of the triangle).

Insert a 22-gauge finder needle with syringe at the apex of the triangle formed by the two heads.

Aim the needle parallel to the clavicular head, toward the ipsilateral nipple at a 45-degree angle, until the vein is entered. If the needle is inserted more than 3 cm with no blood return, withdraw the needle and attempt a new angle. Be careful proceeding medially, because the carotid artery can be punctured.

When the IJ is located, use the 18-gauge needle with syringe to puncture the vein.

Remove the syringe and pass the guidewire. It should advance easily. If resistance is encountered, do NOT force it. Try again.

Withdraw the needle, leaving the guidewire. Nick the skin with a No.11 blade, slide a dilator over the wire to enlarge the tract, and remove the dilator.

Advance the catheter over the wire and into position; remove wire, flush and cap all ports, and suture catheter to skin. Place sterile dressing.

Obtain chest film to confirm catheter position.

Anterior Approach

Retract the carotid artery medially from anterior border of the SCM.

Introduce the needle at the midpoint of the anterior border of the SCM at the point halfway between mandible and clavicle.

Aim the needle at an angle of 30 to 45 degrees toward the ipsilateral nipple.

Use the technique described previously for the remainder of the venous access procedure.

Posterior Approach

Insert the needle under the SCM at the junction of the middle and lower thirds of the posterior border, aiming anteriorly to the suprasternal notch at a 45-degree angle to sagittal and horizontal planes. The vein should be entered within 5 cm.

If venous blood is encountered, follow the technique described previously for the remainder of the venous access procedure.

INDICATIONS

Vasopressor administration, CVP monitoring, emergency establishment of intravenous route, hyperalimentation.

CONTRAINDICATIONS

Thrombosis of veins, coagulopathy.

COMPLICATIONS

Arterial puncture, hemorrhage, pneumothorax, air embolus, thoracic duct injury (left-side approach), neural injury (brachial plexus), infection, thrombosis.

Intrauterine Devices: Insertion and Removal

Paul Taylor, BS, PA-C

DEFINITION

The two intrauterine contraceptive devices available in the United States are the ParaGard T 380A copper IUD (intrauterine device) and the Mirena levonorgestrel-releasing intrauterine system (IUS).

The *T 380A* (which is T-shaped) is made of radiopaque polyethylene, with two flexible arms that bend for insertion but open in situ to hold sleeves of solid copper against the fundus of the uterus. Fine copper wire also is wrapped around the stem of the IUD. The total surface area of copper is approximately 380 mm^2. Monofilament polyethylene tail string is threaded through and knotted below the blunt ball at the base. The T 380A works as a spermicide. Copper ions inhibit sperm motility and acrosomal enzyme activation, so that sperm rarely reach the tube and are unable to fertilize the ovum. The inflammatory reaction created in the endometrium causes phagocytosis of the sperm. This IUD is effective for 12 years of contraception. The typical user failure rate in the first year is 0.8%.

The *Mirena IUS* also is a T-shaped device that is placed within the uterine cavity. This IUS releases 20 µg/day of levonorgestrel from its vertical reservoir. This progesterone agent causes cervical mucus to become thicker, so that sperm cannot enter the upper reproductive tract. Changes in uterotubal fluid also impair sperm migration. Alteration of the endometrium prevents implantation of fertilized ovum. This device also has some anovulatory effect (in 5% to 15% of treatment cycles). It is approved for 5 years of contraception. The typical user failure rate in the first year is 0.1%.

TECHNIQUE

Pre-Procedure Considerations

Initially it is determined that the patient is:

- Not pregnant
- Interested in long-term contraception (for longer than 2 years)
- At low risk for sexually transmitted diseases (STDs) (typically is in a mutually monogamous relationship)

The device may be placed:
- Immediately post partum or prior to discharge
- At 6 weeks post partum in a patient who is exclusively breastfeeding
- At 6 weeks post partum in a patient who has not resumed menstruating, is not breastfeeding, and has a negative result on assay for human chorionic gonadotropin (HCG)
- After a first-trimester abortion (immediately or up to 3 weeks after the procedure)

Procedure

IUD Insertion

ParaGard T 380A Copper IUD

Insert speculum and view the cervix. Use an antiseptic solution (such as Betadine or Hibiclens) on cotton-tipped swabs to thoroughly clean the cervix.

Using a tenaculum, grasp the anterior lip of the cervix 1.5 to 2.0 cm from the os.

Using the tenaculum for gentle retraction, sound the uterus. A depth of 5 cm or greater is necessary for proper insertion. An endometrial biopsy curette is the most user-friendly; centimeters are well marked.

Load the IUD into the inserter barrel under sterile conditions. Do not bend the arms of the T earlier than 5 minutes prior to insertion.

Introduce the push rod from the opposite end of the insertion tube, being careful not to dislodge the IUD. Adjust the movable flange on the tube so that it matches the sounded depth of the uterus. This is best done by holding the endometrial biopsy curette parallel (without touching) to the insertion tube.

Introduce the insertion tube through the cervical canal into the uterine fundus. Again, gentle traction on the tenaculum aids in straightening the cervical canal. Insert the tube to the flange.

Note: Do NOT force the insertion or touch the vaginal side walls!

Insert/eject the IUD by holding the push rod in place and sliding the insertion tube away from the IUD. This releases the arms of the T.

Slowly withdraw the insertion tube and push the rod from the cervix and vagina.

Cut the IUD strings long so that they are inside the vagina but easily felt by the patient.

Schedule a follow-up visit 1 week after the next menstrual period to check IUD position and make sure strings are in place. Expulsion rate is higher with first menses following insertion.

Mirena IUS

Open the Mirena sterile package. Place sterile gloves on hands, or prepare IUS within package. Pick up the inserter containing the device. Carefully release the threads from behind the slider. Make sure the slider is the farthest position away from you (pushed all the way forward). Pull on both threads to draw the device into the insertion tube (the arms of the IUS should now be vertical, and the knobs at the ends of the arms now cover the end of the inserter). Gently secure the threads in the cleft at the end of the handle. Set the flange to the depth measured by the sound, use sterile technique. The IUD is now ready to be inserted.

Hold the inserter so that your thumb rests on the slider (blue). Retract the cervix with the tenaculum and apply gentle traction to align the cervical canal with the uterine cavity. Gently insert the plastic tube into the cervical canal until the flange is 1.5 to 2.0 cm from the cervical os. This allows room for the arms of the IUD to open. While holding the insertion device 2 cm from the os, release the arms of the device by pulling the slider back until the top of the slider is even with the mark (raised horizontal line on the handle). Wait 30 seconds to allow arms to fully extend, then push the inserter gently into the uterine cavity, until the flange touches the cervix; then push the T to the fundus. Holding the inserter firmly in position, release the threads by pulling the slider down all the way (the threads will be released automatically from the cleft). Remove the inserter from the uterus/cervix. Cut the threads to leave about 4 to 5 cm visible outside the cervix. Be careful not to pull on the device while retracting the inserter or while cutting the strings.

IUD Removal
Removing at the time of menses or at midcycle may be easiest.

Using forceps, always apply gentle, steady traction and remove slowly while grasping the string.

If necessary, a tenaculum may be used to steady the cervix or straighten the cervical canal. For difficult removals, use laminaria or cervical dilators.

If no strings are visible, probe the cervical canal with narrow forceps. If the strings are absent or entirely within the uterine canal, an ultrasound examination or radiograph may confirm the location of the IUD.

If the IUD is in the uterine cavity, alligator forceps, a hook, uterine packing forceps, or a Novak curette may be used to grasp the strings or the IUD itself.

INDICATIONS

Prevention of pregnancy (but not protection against STDs). Both types of IUD may be used for emergency contraception (up to 5 days following intercourse). Both IUDs are cost-effective if left in place for at least 2 years

Patients best suited for IUD placement are parous women in a monogamous relationship with no history of STDs. IUDs have a high level of effectiveness (98.5% to 99.2%) and are not associated with systemic/metabolic side effects. A single act (of insertion) leads to long-term use (10 years), they are less expensive than other methods in terms of yearly cost, and they may be placed on "the morning after" to prevent pregnancy.

The Copper T 380A is a good option for women who do not wish to use hormones and who desire longer than 5 years of contraception. The Mirena IUS is a good option for women who have heavy menses, cramps, or anemia. Amenorrhea occurs in 20% of users by 1 year. Dysmenorrhea generally lessens. A 70% reduction in menstrual blood loss can be expected (by 3 to 6 months).

Women who use IUDs may consider taking estrogen for menopause and to protect the endometrium (off-label indication).

CONTRAINDICATIONS

Pregnancy, high risk for STDs, multiple sexual partners, uterine depth less than 6 cm or greater than 9 cm, undiagnosed abnormal vaginal bleeding; cervicitis, pelvic inflammatory disease (PID), vaginitis, actinomycosis; recent endometritis (within past 3 months); AIDS or HIV-seropositive status. For Copper T 380A: allergy to copper, Wilson disease; severe anemia. For Mirena IUS: allergy to levonorgestrel.

COMPLICATIONS

The Copper T 380A is associated with increased bleeding and cramping. Removal rates for bleeding and pain the first year are 11.9%. The Mirena IUS initially may cause an increase in bleeding and cramping; however, by the third month there is a one-third reduction in bleeding and an overall decrease in dysmenorrhea.

Expulsion is most common during the first 3 months after placement. The device may be expelled overtly or silently. With obvious expulsion, increased cramping and bleeding may occur (the IUD may be in a blood clot). Silent expulsion increases the risk of pregnancy. Rate of expulsion declines over time. The 5-year cumulative expulsion rate is 11.3%; expulsion rate during the fifth year is 0.3%. Patients are instructed to feel for the threads each month (after menses or at another preferred time).

All uterine perforations begin at insertion. If perforation occurs at insertion (usually from the uterine sound, not the IUD), management depends on symptoms. If no bleeding is seen, blood pressure and pulse are stable, the patient is pain free, and hematocrit is stable for next several hours, she may be sent home. With persistent pain or signs of other organ damage, immediate surgical referral for laparoscopic evaluation is indicated. Incidence of PID is transiently increased after insertion.

Infections occurring while the IUD is in place may be treated without removal most of the time. With bacterial vaginosis, yeast vaginitis, or trichomoniasis, treat and reassess the patient. IUD removal is not necessary with PID and cervicitis unless no improvement is seen after antibiotic therapy.

Early IUD Warning Signs
P—Period late, pregnancy
A—Abdominal pain, pain with intercourse
I—Infection exposure, abnormal vaginal discharge
N—Not feeling well, fever, chills
S—Strings missing, shorter or longer?

Subclavian Line Insertion

Deborah A. Opacic, EdD, PA-C

DEFINITION

Insertion of a catheter into the subclavian vein for central venous access via the infraclavicular (IC) or supraclavicular (SC) approach. The supraclavicular approach is associated with less risk of pneumothorax and malposition of the catheter.

TECHNIQUE

Patient Positioning

The right side is preferred because it is the most direct route to the superior vena cava (SVC) and to avoid the thoracic duct on the left side. Place the patient in the Trendelenburg supine position. Place a towel between the patient's shoulders. Turn the patient's head away from the procedure.

Procedure

Identify the following landmarks:
- A point just lateral to the midclavicular line at the junction of the medial third of the clavicle
- 1 cm lateral to the insertion of the clavicular head of the sternocleidomastoid

Apply a local anesthetic (e.g., 1% lidocaine) from the skin to the clavicle.

Insert the central line needle (14-gauge) and advance the needle under the clavicle and aiming toward the midpoint, staying close to the undersurface of the clavicle, parallel to the floor. This is done while gentle aspiration is applied to a syringe to confirm venous return.

Remove the syringe with a hemostat (so that the needle does not torque), and have the patient perform the Valsalva maneuver while the hub is covered (to prevent influx of air), and introduce the J wire with the tip toward the heart, maintaining the needle in the same position. There should be minimal resistance with the advancement.

Remove the needle and enlarge the site with a scalpel.

Introduce the dilator over the wire for 3 to 4 cm while controlling the wire.

Remove the dilator and introduce the catheter over the wire to 15 cm on the right and 18 cm on the left.

Remove the wire and check for blood return through all ports; then flush with sterile saline.

Suture and dress the wound.

Obtain a chest film to rule out a pneumothorax and to ensure accurate positioning in the SVC.

INDICATIONS

Establishing emergency intravenous route, hyperalimentation, vasopressor administration, central venous pressure measurement, rapid volume resuscitation, transvenous pacemaker insertion, Swan-Ganz catheter placement, establishing intravenous access if a peripheral route cannot be used, infusion of hypertonic or irritative solutions, or hemodialysis.

CONTRAINDICATIONS

Vein thrombosis, coagulopathy, untreated sepsis, chest wall deformities.

COMPLICATIONS

Arterial puncture, pneumothorax, chylothorax, hemothorax, air embolus, malpositioning, dysrhythmias; with a posterior internal jugular vein approach, Horner syndrome.

Thoracentesis

Deborah A. Opacic, EdD, PA-C

DEFINITION

Puncture or intubation (using needle or catheter) of the pleural space for the purpose of decompressing the lung by removal of fluid or for diagnostic purposes.

TECHNIQUE

Materials

Usually done with sterile, disposable thoracentesis tray, gloves, povidone-iodine (Betadine) solution.

Pre-Procedure Considerations

Review current chest film for location of fluid. Then locate fluid level by clinical examination.

Explain procedure to patient.

Patient Positioning

Patient is sitting up with arms supported on a bedside table or tray and pillow (see Fig. 19-6).

Procedure

Insertion of needle/catheter is performed about one or two interspaces below the determined fluid level but not lower than the eighth intercostal space. Prepare and drape the area.

Anesthetize the skin using a 25-gauge needle and then insert needle perpendicularly into the deeper tissues to the rib. On finding the rib, walk the needle over the top of the rib and penetrate the pleura, keeping negative pressure with the syringe (see Fig. 19-7).

On penetration of the pleura and subsequent return of pleural fluid, inject anesthetic through the pleura as the needle is being withdrawn. Direct the bevel inferiorly into the pleural cavity.

Using the combination of a catheter-over-needle mounted on a syringe, reenter the pleura, again maintaining negative pressure. The needle is then removed and the catheter is advanced into the chest cavity and attached to a stopcock to allow for removal of the fluid into a container while air is prevented from entering (see Fig. 19-8).

After completion, place a small dressing on the entry wound and position the patient supine. Order a follow-up chest film to rule out any complications.

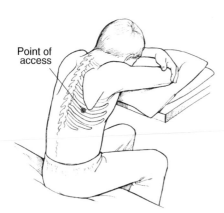

Point of access

Figure 19–6. Correct patient positioning for thoracentesis. (From Rakel RE: Saunders Manual of Medical Practice, 2nd ed. Philadelphia, WB Saunders, 2000, p. 230.)

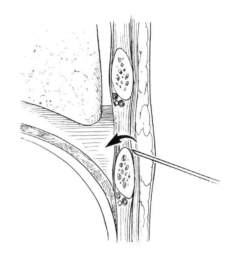

Figure 19–7. The needle is advanced over the superior aspect of the rib into the pleural space while negative pressure is applied to the syringe. (From Rakel RE: Saunders Manual of Medical Practice, 2nd ed. Philadelphia, WB Saunders, 2000, p. 230.)

INDICATIONS

Therapeutic indications include pneumothorax (tension or nontension) or effusions compromising respiratory or cardiovascular function. Pleural fluid can be assessed for infectious cause or malignancy.

CONTRAINDICATIONS

Pleural scarring, previous pleural ablation, bleeding dyscrasia.

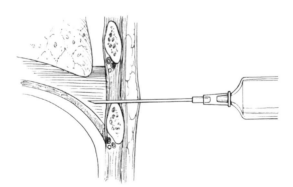

Figure 19–8. Pleural fluid is aspirated using a needle or catheter. (From Rakel RE: Saunders Manual of Medical Practice, 2nd ed. Philadelphia, WB Saunders, 2000, p. 230.)

COMPLICATIONS

Pneumothorax, hemothorax, lacerations/punctures of spleen and liver.

Wound Care

Deborah A. Opacic, EdD, PA-C

Local wound care is an integral part of the physician assistant (PA) practice. This topic focuses on wound care for the kinds of wounds more typically encountered by PAs; burns are covered in Chapter 3, Emergency Medicine.

A working knowledge of the principles of wound healing can lead to improved treatment results, is useful in patient and family counseling and education, and will allow for a deeper appreciation and interpretation of the pathophysiology of other diseases.

NORMAL WOUND HEALING

Wound healing is a complex process by which virtually all wounds heal in the same sequence, often with varying time frames, but always in the order that nature demands. As the clinician utilizes proper and timely treatment techniques, the process is facilitated to allow satisfactory outcomes.

Phases of Wound Healing

Wound healing is divided into three phases: substrate (or inflammatory), proliferative, and maturation.

Inflammatory Phase

Lasts up to 4 days. Immediately following injury, there is a short period of vasoconstriction followed by vasodilation that floods the wound with leukocytes, erythrocytes, and platelets. The leukocytes, mainly polymorphonuclear neutrophils (PMNs) and mononuclear cells, clean up the debris of dead cells and other foreign material to prepare the wound for fibroblast infiltration during the next phase. Additionally, a fibrin clot is formed as an initial barrier and to render a small amount of strength to the wound.

Proliferative Phase

Lasts 3 days to 3 weeks. The second phase of wound healing involves the continuing migration of epithelial cells into the wound to form a barrier that prevents further bacterial invasion into the wound. Fibroblasts, arising from the adventitia of the local capillaries and blood vessels in the area, infiltrate the wound, using the fibrin clot as a temporary buttress on which to build. Fibrinolysis is initiated to dissolve the fibrin clot as fibroblasts synthesize collagen.

Maturation Phase
Lasts 2 weeks to 18 months. In this final phase, the scar undergoes pronounced changes in bulk, form, color, and strength, which is often disconcerting to uninformed patients. Patients must understand that scar revision should not be carried out or planned until the maturation process is complete.

Factors in Wound Healing

Local Factors
Foreign Material. Proper débridement is necessary.
Infection. Prolongs the inflammatory phase.
Ischemia. Oxygen is needed for collagen synthesis and other cellular functions.
Temperature. Warm environments favor healing.

Systemic Factors
Diabetes Mellitus. Hyperglycemia inhibits PMN leukocyte phagocytosis and decreases collagen accumulation. Diabetic patients often have sensory deprivation, with inability to sense pressure changes and ischemic pain, which allows development of pressure sores.
Anemia. Decreases oxygen supply to wound.
Nutrition. Protein deficiency retards vascularization and healing, but not unless levels are significantly low.
Peripheral Vascular Disease. Impedes blood supply.

WOUND EVALUATION

It is imperative to take an adequate history from the patient to determine tetanus status, when the injury occurred, how it happened, where the injury took place, and so on. This information will help to determine the course of action to be taken at that time, as well as appropriate diagnostic studies needed.

The location of the injury on the body guides the clinician in performing the appropriate system examination and also helps to determine whether specialist consultations are needed. Assessment of neurovascular status is necessary, especially with wounds involving the hands, feet, and face.

Wounds may be classified as follows:
- *Clean*: typically elective surgical cases, not in the mouth, gut, or genitourinary or respiratory system; no foreign bodies or devitalized tissue
- *Clean contaminated*: clean wounds that involve mouth, gut, or genitourinary or respiratory system

- *Contaminated*: lacerations, open fractures, elective cases with spillage from gastrointestinal or other body systems
- *Dirty or infected*: perforated viscus, abscess, grossly contaminated wounds

TECHNIQUE

Providing Anesthesia

Local or regional anesthesia is essential for proper débridement and exploration of the wound but should not be used before sensory evaluation is performed.

Anesthetic Agents

Lidocaine without epinephrine has a rapid onset and low toxicity with amounts normally given. Maximum dose is 4.5 mg/kg.

Alternatively, procaine hydrochloride (Novocaine) can be used.

Lidocaine with epinephrine (a vasoconstrictor) prolongs anesthesia time; it is NEVER to be used on digits, nose, ear, or penis. Maximum dose is 7 mg/kg.

Marcaine, an alternative anesthetic, has a slower onset of action but lasts up to 10 hours.

Anesthetic Techniques

Local. The anesthetic is injected directly into the area where the procedure or repair will occur.

Field Block. Anesthetic is injected around the area to be worked on.

Digital Block. Used to numb an entire finger or toe.

Regional Block. Used to anesthetize a larger area, such as an arm or below the waist, than could be achieved with an epidural block.

Preparing the Wound

Clean the wound and irrigate with agent such as normal saline or dilute povidone-iodine (Betadine) solution.

Wound Closure

Materials

Sutures
- *Absorbable sutures*: Usually used for layers beneath the skin or mucosal surfaces.
    Chromic or *plain suture*: Absorbed rapidly (over 7 to 10 days); tensile strength is gone quickly.
    Synthetic sutures: Cause less inflammatory response; tensile strength lasts longer.
- *Nonabsorbable sutures*: Usually used for skin and subcutaneous pullout sutures. Silk is inexpensive but very tissue-reactive; holds

knots well. Monofilaments (nylon, propylene, steel wire) have prolonged tensile strength and low tissue reaction but require more "throws" to secure knot.

Needles
- *Taper-cut needle*: Has a round body with a sharp point; used on easily penetrated tissue.
- *Cutting needle*: A beveled needle with sharp cutting edges (can be forward cutting or reverse cutting); used on more dense tissue (e.g., skin, fascia).

Principles of Wound Closure
To achieve the best possible result for the patient, the wound is closed in layers, with care taken to ensure that each layer (e.g., peritoneum, fascia, fat, dermis, and epidermis) is matched to itself. Except for the scalp, hand, and feet, there exists little excuse for one-layer closures. Everting the skin edges or undermining the skin can be done to minimize tension on the wound.

As the wound heals in the initial period following injury, it will be virtually impossible to prevent some degree of stress being placed on the wound. The wound will naturally contract and loosen so that the edges are pulled down and away to flatten. If the edges are not everted in the initial closure, then it is likely that the wound will flatten and become concave, creating a depression.

Suturing Technique
There are advantages and disadvantages of both interrupted and continuous suturing techniques. Continuous (or running) sutures are less time-consuming, leave less foreign body in tissue overall, and may cause less tissue ischemia. A better cosmetic result may be obtained, but in the event of infection, the entire closure may be disrupted. Therefore, interrupted sutures, although more time-consuming, should be used if there is concern of infection.

Insert the needle perpendicular to the skin. Take equal bites on each side.

With skin sutures and a two-layer closure, skin sutures can be placed 1 to 2 mm from the wound edges. With a one-layer closure, sutures need to be 3 to 4 mm from wound edges.

Put the needle on the needle holder about three-fourths of the distance from the needle point. Use the needle holder in a manner that is best for you, but practice not getting your fingers locked into the needle holder holes, to gain better control for placing sutures.

Instrument Tie Technique.   Hold the needle holder parallel with the incision. With the long free end of the suture, make a loop around the end of the needle holder; grab the short end of the strand; pull through loop and bring end of strand to the opposite side of the wound. Repeat this maneuver three or four times alternating in the opposite direction. Always keep the instrument between the two ends of the suture while making loops; make square knots.

INDICATIONS

Primary repair can be performed in a clean, incised wound or in a clean contaminated wound if properly prepared. *Delayed primary repair* of contaminated wounds can proceed safely if the potential for infection has been eliminated; this approach allows open wounds to mount sufficient resistance to infection. *Secondary closure* (healing by *second intention*) is accomplished by allowing the wound to close by contraction rather than primary union. With this approach, the healing process is delayed and scar formation can be excessive, with weak union of tissues.

CONTRAINDICATIONS

Primary repair in a contaminated wound or a facial laceration older than 8 hours (because of the risk of infection) should be treated by a plastic surgeon; significant associated injuries may delay primary laceration repair.

COMPLICATIONS

Infection, injury to underlying tissue (vascular, nerve), poor cosmetic result, pain, keloid formation.

Further Reading

Ballweg R, Stolberg S, Sullivan EM: Physician Assistant: A Guide to Clinical Practice (2nd ed). Philadelphia, WB Saunders, 1999.
Bryant WM: Wound healing. Clin Symp 29(3):1-36, 1977.

APPENDIX

Symptoms and Treatment of Specific Poisons

Note: Chapters and tables referenced are in original source.

Poison	Symptoms	Treatment
ACE inhibitors	Vomiting, hypotension, seizures	Emesis, activated charcoal, and supportive therapy
Acephate: see Organophosphates		
Acetaminophen (see also ACETAMINOPHEN POISONING in Ch. 263)	Early: Often asymptomatic; mild nausea, vomiting, diaphoresis, pallor: beginning signs of hepatotoxicity; oliguria Later (at 24-48 h): Nausea and protracted vomiting, right upper quadrant pain, jaundice, coagulation defects, hypoglycemia, encephalopathy, hepatic failure, renal failure, possible myocardiopathy	Emesis: gastric lavage and/or activated charcoal; measurement of plasma drug levels at 4 h for prognosis: hepatic damage is possible if >160-200 µg/mL (>1060-1320 µmol/L) and is almost certain if >300 µg/mL (>1980 µmol/L); if before 18-48 h, acetylcysteine (Mucomyst) 140 mg/kg PO initially and 70 mg/kg PO q4h for 4-18 doses to prevent significant hepatotoxicity
Acetanilid Aniline (indelible) inks Aniline oil Chloroaniline Phenacetin (acetophenetidin)	Cyanosis due to formation of methemoglobin and sulfhemoglobin, dyspnea, weakness, vertigo, anginal pain, rashes and urticaria, vomiting, delirium, depression, respiratory and circulatory failure	Ingestion: Ipecac emesis: if this fails, gastric lavage and/or activated charcoal; then as for inhalation Skin contact: Clothing removed and area washed with copious soap and water; then as for inhalation Inhalation: O_2; respiratory support; blood transfusion; methylene blue 1-2 mg/kg IV for severe cyanosis
Acetic acid: see Acids and alkalis		
Acetone Ketones Model airplane glues, cements Nail polish remover	Ingestion: As below except direct pulmonary effect Inhalation: Bronchial irritation, pulmonary congestion and edema, decreased respirations, dyspnea, drunkenness, stupor, ketosis	Removal from source; stomach emptied except for small amounts; respiratory support; O_2 and fluids; correction of metabolic acidosis
Acetonitrile Cosmetic nail adhesive	Converted to cyanide, with usual symptoms and signs	See Cyanides

Acetophenetidin: see Acetaniild
Acetylene gas: see Carbon monoxide
Acetylsalicylic acid:* see ASPIRIN AND OTHER SALICYLATE POISONING in Ch. 263
Acids and alkalis (see also specific acids and alkalis and INGESTION OF CAUSTICS in Ch. 263)

Poison	Symptoms	Treatment
Acids Acetic Hydrochloric Nitric Phosphoric Sulfuric (some drain or toilet bowl cleaners, some dishwasher detergents) Alkalis Ammonia water (ammonium hydroxide) Ammonium, potassium, sodium carbonates Detergent powders Potassium hydroxide (potash) Sodium hydroxide (caustic soda, lye) Some drain or toilet bowl cleaners; some dishwasher detergents	Corrosive burns from ingestion, skin and eye contact, and inhalation; local pain; in general, greater GI tract damage with alkali; possible laryngeal damage	Ingestion: Water or milk to dilute: *do not induce vomiting:* possibly gastric lavage if amount of alkali granules ingested is large Skin or eye contact: Flushing with water for 15 min Hospitalization; opiates for pain; treatment of shock if present; possibly tracheostomy; antibiotics and dexamethasone 1 mg/m^2 BSA q6h or equivalent for 2-3 wk for verified esophageal burns, usually by nonemergency esophagoscopy (NOTE: Even in the absence of oral lesions, strong alkalis [pH >10.5-11.0] can burn the esophagus; esophagoscopy is advised.)

Airplane glues, cements (model-building): see Acetone; Benzene; Petroleum distillates

Poison	Symptoms	Treatment
Alcohol, ethyl (ethanol) Brandy Whiskey Other liquors	Emotional lability, impaired coordination, flushing, nausea and vomiting, stupor to coma, respiratory depression	Emesis; gastric lavage; respiratory support; IV glucose to prevent hypoglycemia, dialysis if blood levels >300-350 mg/dL (>65-76 mmol/L); generous fluid administration, because serum alcohol increases serum osmolarity
Alcohol, isopropyl Rubbing alcohol	Dizziness, incoordination, stupor to coma, gastroenteritis, hypotension	Emesis; gastric lavage; IV glucose; correction of dehydration and electrolyte changes; dialysis
Alcohol, methyl (methanol, wood alcohol) Paint solvent Solid canned fuel Varnish Windshield fluid	High toxicity with 60-250 mL (2-8 oz) in adults, 8-10 mL (2 tsp) in children: latency period 12-18 h; headache, weakness, leg cramps, vertigo, convulsions, dimmed vision, decreased respiration	IV sodium bicarbonate to combat acidosis; 10% ethanol/5% D/W IV: initial ethanol loading dose 0.7 g/kg infused over 1 h to impede methanol metabolism, followed by 0.1-0.2 g/kg/h to maintain a blood ethanol level of 100 mg/dL (22 mmol/L): possible use of fomepizole—see Ethylene glycol; hemodialysis

Continued

Poison	Symptoms	Treatment
Aldrin: see Chlorinated hydrocarbons		
Alkalis: see Acids and alkalis		
Aminophylline Caffeine Theophylline	Wakefulness, restlessness, anorexia, vomiting, dehydration, convulsions: with hypersensitivity, possible immediate vasomotor collapse; greater susceptibility in adults, especially after acute overdose on top of chronic intake	Ingestion: Emesis (avoid if seizures are imminent) or activated charcoal; medication stopped; measurement of theophylline blood level; phenobarbital or diazepam for convulsions: parenteral fluids; maintenance of **BP**: possibly dialysis if serum level >50-100 mg/L (>278-555 μmol/L): possibly β-blocker (e.g., esmolol) if patient is nonasthmatic
Amitriptyline: see Tricyclic antidepressants		
Ammonia gas	Irritation of eyes and respiratory tract; cough, choking; abdominal pain	Flushing of eyes for 15 min with tap water or saline; *no gastric lavage or emesis*: if severe toxicity, positive-pressure O_2 to manage pulmonary edema; respiratory support
Ammoniated mercury: see Mercury		
Ammonia water (ammonium hydroxide): see Acids and alkalis		
Ammonium carbonate: see Acids and alkalis		
Ammonium fluoride: see Fluorides		
Amobarbital: see Barbiturates		
Amphetamines Amphetamine sulfate, phosphate Dextroamphetamine Methamphetamine Phenmetrazine	Increased activity, exhilaration, talkativeness, insomnia, irritability, exaggerated reflexes, anorexia, dry mouth, arrhythmia, anginal chest pain, heart block, psychotic-like states, inability to concentrate or sit still	Emesis, lavage, or activated charcoal possibly effective long after ingestion because of recycling via gastric mucosa; sedation with chlorpromazine 0.5-1 mg/kg IM or PO q 30 min prn; external stimuli reduced; hypothermia; prevention of cerebral edema; hemodialysis; β-blockers possibly helpful in nonasthmatics
Amyl nitrite: see Nitrites		
Aniline: see Acetanilid		

Poison	Symptoms	Treatment
Anticoagulants Dicumarol Superwarfarins Warfarin	Prolonged prothrombin times after repeated doses	Observation for single ingestions in children; measurement of prothrombin time in adults for possible vitamin K treatment
Antidepressants: see Selective serotonin reuptake inhibitors, Tricyclic antidepressants		
Antifreeze: see Alcohol, methyl; Ethylene glycol		
Antihistamines	Excitation or depression, drowsiness, nervousness, disorientation, hallucinations, tachycardia, arrhythmias, hypotension, hyperpyrexia, delirium, convulsions	Ipecac emesis (avoid if seizures are imminent), gastric lavage, activated charcoal; respiratory/BP support; diazepam to control seizures; physostigmine 0.5-2.0 mg (adults). 0.02 mg/kg (children) IM or IV (slowly) only after all else fails (CAUTION: *Seizures*—see Physostigmine.)
Antimony: see Arsenic and antimony		
Antineoplastic drugs Methotrexate Mercaptopurine Vincristine >50 Others	Effects on hematopoiesis, nausea, vomiting; specific acute vs. chronic effects depending on drug	Emesis better than lavage; supportive care; leucovorin rescue; observation for postacute problems (>24-48 h)
Antipsychotic drugs Clozapine Haloperidol Risperidone	A wide range of symptoms (e.g., excitement, coma, hypotension)	Benzodiazepines and supportive treatment
Ant poison: see Chlorinated hydrocarbons (DDT): Thallium salts		
Arsenic and antimony Arsenic Donovan's solution Fowler's solution Herbicides Paris green Pesticides Antimony compounds Stibophen Tartar emetic	Throat constriction, dysphagia; burning GI pain, vomiting, diarrhea; dehydration; pulmonary edema: renal failure: liver failure	Emesis: gastric lavage, then a demulcent: chelation with penicillamine: dimercaprol if patient cannot take oral medication: hydration: treatment of shock and pain: sorbitol or saline cathartic (sodium sulfate 15-30 g in water)

Continued

Poison	Symptoms	Treatment
Arsine gas	Acute hemolytic anemia	Transfusions; diuresis
Aspirin*: see ASPIRIN AND OTHER SALICYLATE POISONING in Ch. 263		
Atropine: see Belladonna		
Automobile exhaust: see Carbon monoxide		
Barbiturates 　Amobarbital 　Meprobamate 　Pentobarbital 　Phenobarbital 　Secobarbital	Headache, confusion, ptosis, excitement, delirium, loss of corneal reflex, respiratory failure, coma	Stomach emptied up to 24 h after ingestion; if immediately after, ipecac emesis: if sedated, lavage and activated charcoal with cuffed endotracheal tube; good nursing care; respiratory support, O_2; correction of any dehydration; dialysis (rarely), especially for long-acting barbiturates when alkalization hastens excretion
Barium compounds (soluble) 　Barium acetate 　Barium carbonate 　Barium chloride 　Barium hydroxide 　Barium nitrate 　Barium sulfide 　Depilatories 　Fireworks 　Rat poisons	Vomiting, abdominal pain, diarrhea, tremors, convulsions, colic, hypertension, cardiac arrest, dyspnea and cyanosis, ventricular fibrillation, hypokalemia	Sodium or magnesium sulfate 60 g PO to precipitate barium in stomach, then emesis or gastric lavage; diazepam to control convulsions; atropine SC, IM, or IV 0.5-1.0 mg (adults), 0.01 mg/kg (children) for colic; sublingual nitroglycerin 1/100-1/50 for hypertension; O_2 for dyspnea and cyanosis; quinidine sulfate 100-300 mg PO (adults), 6 mg/kg PO (children) to prevent ventricular fibrillation; correction of hypokalemia
Belladonna 　Atropine 　Hyoscyamine 　Hyoscyamus 　Scopolamine (hyoscine) 　Stramonium	Dry skin and mucous membranes; dilated pupils; flushing, hyperpyrexia; tachycardia, restlessness; coma; respiratory failure: convulsions	Emesis or activated charcoal: respiratory support: possibly bladder catheterization: physostigmine 0.5-2.0 mg (adults). 0.02 mg/kg (children) IM or IV (slowly) to possibly reverse peripheral and CNS effects, but use only for severe problems (CAUTION: Seizures—see Physostigmine.)

Benzene Benzol Hydrocarbons Model airplane glue Toluene Toluol Xylene	Dizziness, weakness, headache, euphoria, nausea, vomiting, ventricular arrhythmia, paralysis, convulsions; with chronic poisoning, aplastic anemia, leukemia	Ingestion >0.5-1 mL/kg; emesis or cautious gastric lavage: O₂; respiratory support; ECG monitoring (ventricular fibrillation can occur early): diazepam to control seizures: blood transfusion for severe anemia: *do not give epinephrine*
γ-Benzene hexachloride Benzene hexachloride Hexachloro- cyclohexane Lindane	Irritability, CNS excitation, muscle spasms, atonia, clonic and tonic convulsions, respiratory failure, pulmonary edema	Emesis immediately after ingestion: gastric lavage: diazepam for convulsions avoidance of all oils, which promote absorption: activated charcoal hemoperfusion prn
Benzine (benzin): see Petroleum distillates		

Benzodiazepines
  Chlordiazepoxide
  Diazepam
  Flurazepam
	Sedation to coma, particularly if accompanied by alcohol	Emesis; lavage; supportive care; suicide precautions; IV flumazenil antidotes for overdose. (CAUTION: *If tricyclics are involved, seizures are a risk.*)

Benzol: see Benzene		
Bichloride of mercury: see Mercury		
Bichromates: see Chromic acid		
Bidrin: see Organophosphates		
Bifenthrin: see Pyrethroids		
Bishydroxycoumarin: see Warfarin		
Bismuth compounds	Poor absorption: ulcerative stomatitis, anorexia, headache, rash, renal tubular damage	Ipecac emesis; gastric lavage: respiratory support; dimercaprol† (see TABLE 307-2)
Bitter almond oil: see Cyanides		
Bitter almond oil, artificial: see Nitrobenzene		
Bleach, chlorine: see Hypochlorites		
β-Blockers	Hypotension, bradycardia, seizures, cardiac arrhythmias; several are also α₁ or α₂ agonists	Close monitoring, stomach emptied; if symptomatic, glucagon 3-5 mg IV or in saline; possibly cardiac pacing

Continued

Poison	Symptoms	Treatment
Borates Boric acid	Nausea, vomiting, diarrhea, hemorrhagic gastroenteritis, weakness, lethargy, CNS depression, convulsion, "boiled lobster" rash, shock	Ipecac emesis: gastric lavage; removal from skin; prevention or treatment of electrolyte changes and shock; control of convulsions; dialysis for severe poisoning
Boric acid: see Borates Brandy: see Alcohol, ethyl Bromates: see Chlorates		
Bromides	Nausea, vomiting, rash (may be acneiform), slurred speech, ataxia, confusion, psychotic behavior, coma, paralysis	Ipecac emesis, gastric lavage for acute ingestion; medication stopped; hydration and NaCl IV to promote mild diuresis; ethacrynic acid (specifically useful); hemodialysis only if severe
Bromine: see Chlorine Bulan: see Chlorinated hydrocarbons		
Bupropion HCl	Breathing problems, ataxia, seizures	Activated charcoal, benzodiazepines, supportive measures
Ca channel blockers Diltiazem Nifedipine Verapamil	Nausea, vomiting, confusion, bradycardia, hypotension, total collapse	Emesis or activated charcoal as soon as possible; atropine for bradycardia; calcium chloride (better than calcium gluconate) 1-2 g IV stat (in children, 100 mg/kg IV), repeated prn; BP support; consider pacemaker
Cadmium Solder	Severe gastric cramps, vomiting, diarrhea; dry throat, cough, dyspnea; headache; shock, coma; brown urine, renal failure	Ipecac emesis; gastric lavage with milk or albumin; respiratory support; hydration: intermittent positive pressure breathing for pulmonary edema; edetate calcium disodium (see TABLE 307-2); *do not give dimercaprol*
Caffeine: see Aminophylline Calomel: see Mercury		
Camphor Camphorated oils	Camphor odor on breath, headache, confusion, delirium, hallucinations, convulsions, coma	Ipecac emesis (avoid if seizures are imminent), activated charcoal, or gastric lavage; diazepam to prevent and treat convulsions: respiratory support: lipid dialysis is under study

Canned fuel, solid: see Alcohol, methyl

Cantharides Cantharidin Spanish fly	Irritated skin and mucous membranes, vesicles; nausea, vomiting, bloody diarrhea; burning pain in back and urethra; respiratory depression; convulsions, coma; abortion, menorrhagia	Avoidance of all oils; ipecac emesis: respiratory support; treatment of convulsions: maintenance of fluid balance; no specific antidote

Captan: see Chlorinated hydrocarbons

Carbamates Aldicarb Bendiocarb Benomyl Carbaryl Carbofuran Fenothiocarb Methiocarb Methomyl Oxamyl Propoxur	Slightly to highly toxic effects; similar to those for organophosphates	See Organophosphates, except for pralidoxime
Carbamazepine	Progressive CNS depression, occasional seizures: rarely cardiac arrhythmia	Supportive measures after decontamination; heart rate monitored

Carbolic acid: see Phenols

Carbonates (ammonium, potassium, sodium): see Acids and alkalis

Carbon bisulfide: see Carbon disulfide

Carbon dioxide	Dyspnea, weakness, tinnitus, palpitations	Respiratory support; O_2
Carbon disulfide Carbon bisulfide	Garlic breath odor, irritability, weakness, manic depression, narcosis, delirium, mydriasis, blindness, parkinsonism, convulsions, coma, paralysis, respiratory failure	Washing of skin; emesis; gastric lavage; O_2; diazepam sedation: respiratory and circulatory support

Continued

Poison	Symptoms	Treatment
Carbon monoxide Acetylene gas Automobile exhaust Carbonyl iron Coal gas Furnace gas Illuminating gas Marsh gas	Toxicity varies with length of exposure, concentration inhaled, respiratory and circulatory rates: symptoms vary with % carboxyhemoglobin in blood: headache, vertigo, dyspnea, confusion, dilated pupils, convulsions, coma	100% O_2 by mask; respiratory support if needed; immediate measurement of carboxyhemoglobin level: *avoid all stimulants*: hyperbaric O_2 (see Ch. 292) possibly effective if carboxyhemoglobin is $> \sim 25\%$; primary value possibly at the level of cytochrome
Carbon tetrachloride Cleaning fluids (nonflammable)	Nausea, vomiting, abdominal pain, headache, confusion, visual disturbances, CNS depression, ventricular fibrillation, renal injury, hepatic injury	Washing of skin; emesis or gastric lavage; O_2; cardiopulmonary support: monitoring of renal and hepatic function and appropriate treatment; *avoid alcohol, epinephrine, ephedrine, cimetidine*
Caustic soda: see Acids and alkalis (sodium hydroxide)		
Chloral hydrate Chloral amide	Drowsiness, confusion, shock, coma; respiratory depression; renal injury, hepatic injury	Ipecac emesis; gastric lavage; respiratory support; assessment of concomitant ingestions
Chlorates Bromates Nitrates Permanent wave neutralizers	Vomiting, nausea, diarrhea, cyanosis (methemoglobin), toxic nephritis, shock, convulsions, CNS depression, coma, jaundice	Ipecac emesis; gastric lavage; transfusion for severe cyanosis; *avoid methylene blue for chlorates or bromates*; ascorbic acid; treatment of shock; O_2; possibly dialysis for complex cases
Chlordane: see Chlorinated hydrocarbons		
Chlorethoxyfos: see Organophosphates		
Chlorinated hydrocarbons Aldrin Benzene hexachloride Bulan Captan Chlordane	Slightly toxic effects (e.g., methoxychlor) to highly toxic effects (eg. dieldrin); vomiting (early or delayed); paresthesias; malaise; coarse tremors, convulsions; pulmonary edema, ventricular fibrillation, respiratory failure	Emesis; gastric lavage, if no convulsions, or activated charcoal; diazepam or phenobarbital to prevent and control tremors and convulsions; epinephrine and sudden stimuli avoided; parenteral fluids; monitoring for renal and hepatic failure, cardiopulmonary support

Chlorothalonil
DDD (2-dichlorethane)
DDT (chlorophenothane)
Dicofol
Dieldrin
Dienochlor
Dilan
Endosulfan
Endrin
Heptachlor
Lindane
Methoxychlor
Perchlordecone
Prolan
Toxaphene
Other chlorinated organic insecticides and industrial compounds
Chlorinated lime: see Chlorine
Chlorine (see also Hypochlorites)

Bromine	Ingestion: Irritation, corrosion of mouth and GI tract, possible ulceration or perforation; abdominal pain, tachycardia prostration, circulatory collapse	Ingestion: Ipecac emesis; gastric lavage; treatment of shock
Chlorinated lime		Inhalation: O_2; respiratory support; observation for and treatment of pulmonary edema
Chlorine water		
Tear gas	Inhalation: Severe respiratory and ocular irritation, glottal spasm, cough, choking, vomiting; pulmonary edema; cyanosis	

Chloroaniline: see Acetanilid

Chloroform	Drowsiness, coma; with nitrous oxide, delirium	Ingestion: Ipecac emesis; gastric lavage; observation for renal and hepatic damage
Ether		Inhalation: Respiratory cardiac, and circulatory support
Nitrous oxide		
Trichloromethane		

Chlorothalonil: see Chlorinated hydrocarbons

Continued

Poison	Symptoms	Treatment
Chlorothion: see Organophosphates		
Chlorpromazine: see Phenothiazine		
Chlorpyrifos: see Organophosphates		
Chromates: see Chromic acid		
Chromic acid	Corrosive effects due to oxidation; ulcer and	Milk or water to dilute; dimercaprol (or penicillamine)
Bichromates	perforated nasal septum; severe gastroenteritis;	for severe symptoms; fluids and electrolytes, with
Chromates	shock, vertigo, coma; nephritis	caution, to support renal function
Chromium trioxide		
Chromium:† see TABLE 307-2		
Chromium trioxide: see Chromic acid		
Cimetidine; ranitidine	Slight dryness and drowsiness; possible altered	No specific antidote available; a focus on metabolism
	metabolism of concomitant drugs	of other drugs
Clonidine	Sedation; periodic apnea; hypotension	Emesis; lavage; supportive care; tolazoline IV and
		dopamine drip; naloxone 5 μg/kg up to 2-20 mg,
		repeated prn
Coal gas: see Carbon monoxide		
Cobalt:† see TABLE 307-2		
Cobaltous chloride: see Nitrogen oxides		
Cocaine	Stimulation, then depression; nausea and	Early emesis: activated charcoal or gastric lavage;
	vomiting; loss of self-control, anxiety,	diazepam for excitation (primary treatment); O₂,
	hallucinations; sweating; respiratory difficulty	respiratory and circulatory support; if needed,
	progressing to failure; cyanosis; circulatory	IV esmolol, with extreme caution, for arrhythmias;
	failure; convulsions; MI (rare); beware "stuffers"	observation for myocardial or pulmonary disorder
	and "packers" (i.e., those who smuggle	(usually before emergency room arrival)
	plastic bags of cocaine in the GI tract or vagina)	
Codeine: see Narcotics		
Copper:† see TABLE 307-2		

Copper salts
  Cupric sulfate,
    acetate, subacetate
  Cuprous chloride,
    oxide
Zinc salts
	Vomiting, burning sensation, metallic taste,
	diarrhea, pain, shock, jaundice, anuria,
	convulsions
		Emesis; gastric lavage; penicillamine or dimercaprol
		(see TABLE 307-2): electrolyte and fluid balance;
		respiratory support; monitoring of GI tract; treatment
		of shock, control of convulsions; monitoring for
		hepatic and renal failure

Corrosive sublimate: see Mercury

Coumaphos: see Organophosphates

Creosote: cresols: see Phenols

Cyanides
  Bitter almond oil
  Hydrocyanic acid
  Nitroprusside
  Potassium cyanide
  Prussic acid
  Sodium cyanide
  Wild cherry syrup
	Tachycardia, headache, drowsiness, hypotension,
	coma, rapid severe acidosis, convulsions;
	venous blood bright red; *very rapidly lethal*
	(1-15 min)
		Speed essential. Removal from source if inhaled;
		immediate emesis or lavage, amyl nitrite inhalation,
		0.2 mL (1 ampule) 30 sec of each min. 100% O_2;
		respiratory support; 10 mL 3% sodium nitrite 2.5-5
		mL/min IV (in child: 10 mg/kg), then 25-50 mL 25%
		sodium thiosulfate at 2.5-5 mL/min IV; treatment
		repeated if symptoms recur; Lilly cyanide kit

Cyfluthrin: see Pyrethroids

Cypermethrin: see Pyrethroids

DDD (2-dichlorethane): see Chlorinated hydrocarbons

DDT (chlorophenothane): see Chlorinated hydrocarbons

Deodorizers, household: see Naphthalene; Paradichlorobenzene

Depilatories: see Barium compounds

Desipramine: see Tricyclic antidepressants

Detergent powders: see Acids and alkalis

Dextroamphetamine: see Amphetamines

Diazinon: see Organophosphates

Dichlorvos: see Organophosphates

Dicofol: see Chlorinated hydrocarbons

Dicumarol: see Warfarin

Dieldrin: see Chlorinated hydrocarbons

Continued

Poison	Symptoms	Treatment
Diethylene glycol: see Ethylene glycol		
Digitalis, digitoxin, digoxin:‡ see discussion of digitalis under Drug treatment of systolic dysfunction in Ch. 203		
Dilan: see Chlorinated hydrocarbons		
Dimethoate: see Organophosphates		
Dinitrobenzene: see Nitrobenzene		
Dinitro-o-cresol Herbicides Pesticides	Fatigue, thirst, flushing; nausea, vomiting, abdominal pain; hyperpyrexia, tachycardia, loss of consciousness; dyspnea, respiratory arrest; skin absorption	Emesis; gastric lavage; fluid therapy; O_2; renal and hepatic toxicity anticipated; no specific antidote; detergents to rinse skin
Diphenoxylate with atropine	Lethargy, nystagmus, pinpoint pupils, tachycardia, coma, respiratory depression (NOTE: Toxicity may be delayed up to 12 h.)	Ipecac emesis, gastric lavage; activated charcoal; naloxone; all children closely followed for 12-18 h if ingestion is verified
Dishwasher detergents: see Acids and alkalis		
Disulfoton: see Organophosphates		
Diuretics, mercurial: see Mercury		
Doxepin: see Tricyclic antidepressants		
Drain cleaners: see Acids and alkalis		
Endosulfan: see Chlorinated hydrocarbons		
Endrin: see Chlorinated hydrocarbons		
Ergot derivatives	Thirst, diarrhea, vomiting, light-headedness, burning feet; convulsions, hypotension, coma, abortion; gangrene of feet; cataracts	Ipecac emesis; gastric lavage; cardiopulmonary support; benzodiazepine or short-acting barbiturate for convulsions; papaverine 60 mg IV (1-2 mg/kg IV for children)
Eserine: see Physostigmine		
Esfenvalerate: see Pyrethroids		
Ethanol: see Alcohol, ethyl		
Ether: see Chloroform		
Ethion: see Organophosphates		
Ethyl alcohol: see Alcohol, ethyl		
Ethyl biscoumacetate: see Warfarin		

Ethylene glycol
Diethylene glycol
Permanent antifreeze

Ingestion: Inebriation but no alcohol odor on breath; nausea, vomiting; later, carpopedal spasm, lumbar pain; oxalate crystalluria; oliguria progressing to anuria and acute renal failure; respiratory distress, convulsions, coma
Eye contact: Iridocyclitis

Ingestion: Emesis; gastric lavage, respiratory support, correction of electrolyte imbalance (anion gap); ethanol (see treatment of methyl alcohol); fomepizole 15 mg/kg IV stat, 10 mg/kg q 12 h × 4 plus dialysis for blood levels >50 mg/dL (to block alcohol dehydrogenase conversion of ethylene glycol to toxic metabolites); hemodialysis
Eye contact: Flushing of eyes

Explosives: see Barium compounds (fireworks); Nitrogen oxides
Famphur: see Organophosphates
Fava bean (favism§): see CHEMICAL FOOD POISONING in Ch. 28
Fenthion: see Organophosphates
Ferric salts: see Iron
Ferrous gluconate, ferrous sulfate: see Iron
Fireworks: see Barium compounds

Fluorides
Ammonium fluoride
Hydrofluoric acid
Rat poisons
Roach poisons
Sodium fluoride
Soluble fluorides generally

Ingestion: Salty or soapy taste; with large doses: tremors, convulsions. CNS depression; shock; renal failure
Skin and mucosal contact: Superficial or deep burns
Inhalation: Intense eye, nasal irritation; headache; dyspnea, sense of suffocation, glottal edema, pulmonary edema, bronchitis, pneumonia; mediastinal and subcutaneous emphysema from bleb rupture

Ingestion: Ipecac emesis; gastric lavage—leave aluminum hydroxide gel, calcium, or magnesium hydroxide or chloride in stomach; IV glucose and saline; 10% calcium gluconate, 10 mL IV (1 mL/kg in child); monitoring for cardiac irritability; treatment of shock and dehydration
Skin and mucosal contact: Copious flushing with cold water; débridement of white tissue; sometimes, injection of 10% calcium gluconate locally but, more often, intraarterially with application of magnesium oxide paste
Inhalation: O₂, respiratory support; prednisone for chemical pneumonitis (adults 30-80 mg/day in divided doses); management of pulmonary edema

Fluvalinate: see Pyrethroids

Continued

Poison	Symptoms	Treatment
Formaldehyde Formalin (NOTE: May contain methyl alcohol.)	Ingestion: Oral and gastric pain, nausea, vomiting, hematemesis, shock, hematuria, anuria, coma, respiratory failure Skin contact: Irritation, coagulation necrosis; dermatitis, hypersensitivity Inhalation: Eye, nose, respiratory tract irritation; laryngeal spasm and edema; dysphagia; bronchitis, pneumonia	Ingestion: Water or milk to dilute; treatment of shock; sodium bicarbonate to correct acidosis; respiratory support; observation for perforations Skin contact: Copious soap and water for washing Inhalation: Flushing of eyes with saline; O_2; respiratory support
Fowler's solution: see Arsenic and antimony		
Fuel, canned: see Alcohol, methyl		
Fuel oil: see Petroleum distillates		
Furnace gas: see Carbon monoxide		
Gas: see Ammonia gas; Carbon monoxide (acetylene gas, automobile, exhaust, coal gas, furnace gas, illuminating gas, marsh gas); Chlorine (tear gas); Hydrogen sulfide (sewer gas, volatile hydrides): Organophosphates (nerve gas agents)		
Gasoline: see Petroleum distillates		
Glues, model airplane: see Acetone; Benzene; Petroleum distillates		
Glutethimide	Drowsiness, areflexia, mydriasis, hypotension, respiratory depression, coma	Ipecac emesis; gastric lavage, activated charcoal; respiratory support, maintenance of fluid and electrolyte balance; hemodialysis possibly helpful; treatment of shock
Gold salts:† see gold in TABLE 307-2 and gold compounds under Treatment of rheumatoid arthritis in Ch. 50		
Guaiacol: see Phenols		
H_2 blockers	Minor GI problems: possibly altered concentration level of other drugs	Nonspecific supportive measures
Heptachlor: see Chlorinated hydrocarbons		
Herbicides: see Arsenic and antimony; Dinitro-*o*-cresol		
Heroin: see Narcotics		
Hexachlorocyclohexane: see γ-Benzene hexachloride		
Hexaethyltetraphosphate: see Organophosphates		
Hydrides, volatile: see Hydrogen sulfide		
Hydrocarbons: see Benzene		

Hydrocarbons, halogenated: see Chlorinated hydrocarbons		
Hydrochloric acid: see Acids and alkalis		
Hydrocyanic acid: see Cyanides		
Hydrogen chloride, fluoride: see Nitrogen oxides		
Hydrogen sulfide	"Gas eye" (subacute keratoconjunctivitis), lacrimation and burning; cough, dyspnea, pulmonary edema; caustic skin burns,	O_2, respiratory support; amyl nitrite and sodium nitrite as for cyanide (*do not give thiosulfate*)
Alkali sulfides	erythema, pain, profuse salivation, nausea,	
Phosphine	vomiting, diarrhea; confusion, vertigo;	
Sewer gas	sudden collapse and unconsciousness	
Volatile hydrides		
Hyoscine, hyoscyamine, hyoscyamus: see Belladonna		
Hypochlorites	Usually mild pain and inflammation of oral	Diluted milk for usual 6% household preparations
Bleach, chlorine	and GI mucosa; cough, dyspnea, vomiting;	(little else required); treatment of shock; esophagoscopy
Javelle water	skin vesicles	if concentrated forms have been ingested
Illuminating gas: see Carbon monoxide		
Imipramine: see Tricyclic antidepressants		
Insecticides: see Chlorinated hydrocarbons: Organophosphates; Paradichlorobenzene; Pyrethroids		
Iodine	Burning pain in mouth and esophagus; mucous membranes stained brown; laryngeal edema; vomiting; abdominal pain, diarrhea; shock; nephritis, circulatory collapse	Milk, starch, or flour PO: gastric lavage; fluid and electrolytes; treatment of shock; tracheostomy for laryngeal edema
Iodoform	Dermatitis; vomiting; cerebral depression,	Ingestion: Emesis or gastric lavage; respiratory support
Triiodomethane	excitation; coma: respiratory difficulty	Skin contact: Sodium bicarbonate or alcohol to wash
Iron	Vomiting, upper abdominal pain, pallor,	Ipecac emesis, gastric lavage; if serum iron
Carbonyl iron (see	cyanosis, diarrhea, drowsiness, shock;	>400–500 μg/dL (>72–90 μmol/L) at 3–6h (plus GI
Carbon monoxide)	concern if >40–70 mg/kg of elemental iron	symptoms), deferoxamine 1 g IV (maximal rate
Ferric salts	ingested	15 mg/kg/h) or 1–2 g IM q3-12h (urine turns red
Ferrous salts		within 2 h): for shock, deferoxamine 1 g IV (maximal
Ferrous gluconate		rate 15 mg/kg/h): chelation limited to 24 h: exchange
Ferrous sulfate		transfusion
Vitamins with iron		
(NOTE: Children's chewables with iron are remarkably safe)		

Continued

Poison	Symptoms	Treatment
Isofenfos: see Organophosphates		
Isoniazid	CNS stimulation, seizures, obtundation, coma	Emesis: lavage: diazepam sedation; pyridoxine (mg for mg ingested) up to 200 mg slowly IV for seizures, repeat prn; sodium bicarbonate for acidosis (rarely needed)
Isopropyl alcohol: see Alcohol, isopropyl		
Javelle water: see Hypochlorites		
Kerosene: see Petroleum distillates		
Ketones: see Acetone		
Lambda-cyhalothrin: see Pyrethroids		
Lead	Acute ingestion: Thirst, burning abdominal pain, vomiting, diarrhea, CNS symptoms as for acute inhalation	See LEAD POISONING in Ch. 263
Lead salts		
Solder	Acute inhalation: Insomnia, headache, ataxia, mania, convulsions	
Some paints and painted surfaces	Lead encephalopathy: see LEAD POISONING in Ch. 263	
Lead, tetraethyl	Vapor inhalation, skin absorption, ingestion: CNS symptoms—insomnia, restlessness, ataxia, delusions, mania, convulsions	Supportive treatment, e.g., diazepam, chlorpromazine, fluid and electrolytes; elimination of source
Lime, chlorinated: see Chlorine		
Lindane: see γ-Benzene hexachloride; Chlorinated hydrocarbons		
Liquor: see Alcohol, ethyl		
Lithium salts	Nausea, vomiting, diarrhea, tremors, drowsiness, renal failure, diabetes insipidus	Acute: Emesis: diazepam; possibly dialysis Chronic: Dose reduced: supportive therapy
Lye: see Acids and alkalis (sodium hydroxide)		
Lysergic acid diethylamide (LSD)	Confusion, hallucinations, hyperexcitability—coma, flashbacks	Supportive therapy; diazepam; chlorpromazine (50-100 mg IM in adults)
Malathion: see Organophosphates		
Manganese:† see TABLE 307-2		

Marsh gas: see Carbon monoxide
Meperidine: see Narcotics
Meprobamate: see Barbiturates

Mercury		Gastric lavage, activated charcoal; penicillamine (or succimer)—see TABLE 307-2: maintenance of fluid and electrolyte balance; hemodialysis for renal failure; observation for GI perforation
All mercury compounds	Acute: Severe gastroenteritis, burning mouth pain, salivation, abdominal pain, vomiting; colitis, nephrosis, anuria, uremia; skin burns from alkyl and phenyl mercurials	
Ammoniated mercury		
Bichloride of mercury	Chronic: Gingivitis, mental disturbance, neurologic deficits	Skin contact: Soap and water for scrubbing
Calomel		Lungs: Supportive care
Corrosive sublimate		
Diuretics		
Mercuric chloride		
Mercury vapor	Mercury vapor: severe pneumonitis	
Merthiolate		

Merthiolate: see Mercury—usually no problem

Metaldehyde	Nausea, vomiting, retching, abdominal pain, muscular rigidity, hyperventilation, convulsions, coma	Emesis, if not spontaneous; supportive therapy; diazepam
Slug bait		
Metals	See specific metals	See TABLE 307-2

Methadone: see Narcotics
Methamphetamine: see Amphetamines
Methanol: see Alcohol, methyl
Methidathion: see Organophosphates
Methoxychlor: see Chlorinated hydrocarbons
Methyl alcohol: see Alcohol, methyl
Methyl parathion: see Organophosphates
Methyl salicylate:* see ASPIRIN AND OTHER SALICYLATE POISONING in Ch. 263
Mineral spirits: see Petroleum distillates
Model airplane glues, solvents: see Acetone; Benzene; Petroleum distillates
Morphine: see Narcotics
Moth balls, crystals, repellent cakes: see Naphthalene: Paradichlorobenzene

Continued

Poison	Symptoms	Treatment
Mushrooms, poisonous:§ see CHEMICAL FOOD POISONING in Ch. 28		
Nail polish remover: see Acetone		
Naled: see Organophosphates		
Naphtha: see Petroleum distillates		
Naphthalene (see also Paradichlorobenzene) Deodorizer cakes Moth balls, crystals, repellent cakes	Ingestion: Abdominal cramps nausea, vomiting: headache, confusion; dysuria; intravascular hemolysis; convulsions; hemolytic anemia in persons with G6PD deficiency Skin contact: Dermatitis, corneal ulceration Inhalation: Headache, confusion, vomiting, dyspnea	Ingestion: Ipecac emesis, gastric lavage; blood transfusion for severe hemolysis; urine alkalization for hemoglobinuria; control of convulsions Skin contact: Clothing removed if formerly stored with naphthalene moth balls; flushing of skin and eyes
Naphthols: see Phenols		
Narcotics (see also OPIOID DEPENDENCE in Ch. 195) Alphaprodine Codeine Heroin Meperidine Methadone Morphine Opium Propoxyphene	Pinpoint pupils, drowsiness, shallow respirations, spasticity, respiratory failure	*Do not give emetics.* Gastric lavage, activated charcoal, respiratory support; naloxone 5 µg/kg IV to awaken and improve respiration; if patient does not respond, naloxone 2-20 mg (possibly repeated up to 10-20 times); IV fluids to support circulation
Neostigmine: see Physostigmine		
Nerve gas agents: see Organophosphates		
Nickel:† see TABLE 307-2		
Nicotine: see Tobacco		
Nitrates: see Chlorates		
Nitric acid: see Acids and alkalis		

Nitrites
  Amyl nitrite
  Butyl nitrite
  Nitroglycerin
  Potassium nitrite
  Sodium nitrite
	Methemoglobinemia, cyanosis, anoxia, GI disturbance, vomiting, headache, dizziness, hypotension, respiratory failure, coma	Ipecac emesis, gastric lavage: O_2; for methemoglobinemia, 1% methylene blue 1-2 mg/kg slowly IV; when >40% methemoglobin, transfusion with whole blood

Nitrobenzene
  Artificial bitter
    almond oil
  Dinitrobenzene
	Bitter almond odor (suggests cyanides), drowsiness, headache, vomiting, ataxia, nystagmus, brown urine, convulsive movements, delirium, cyanosis, coma, respiratory arrest	See Acetanilid

Nitrogen oxides (see also Chlorine, Hydrogen sulfide, Sulfur dioxide, and Ch. 75)		

Air contaminants
    that form
    atmospheric
    oxidants; liberated
    from missile fuels,
    explosives,
    agricultural wastes
	Delayed onset of symptoms with nitrogen oxides unless heavy concentration: other irritant gases give warnings—local burning in eye, nasal, pharyngeal mucous membranes: fatigue, cough, dyspnea, pulmonary edema; later, bronchitis, pneumonia	Bed rest: O_2 as soon as symptoms develop: for excessive pulmonary foam: suction, postural drainage, tracheostomy; prednisone 30-80 mg/day (adults) or dexamethasone 1 mg/m² BSA (children) to prevent pulmonary fibrosis

Cobaltous chloride
  Fluorine
  Hydrogen chloride
  Hydrogen fluoride		

Nitroglycerin: see Nitrites		
Nitrous oxide: see Chloroform		
NSAIDs Ibuprofen	Nausea, vomiting (for large overdoses, see discussion of acidosis under DISTURBANCES IN ACID-BASE METABOLISM in Ch. 12)	Emesis, gastric lavage, or activated charcoal in severe cases; clinical observations and supportive measures

Nortriptyline: see Tricyclic antidepressants
Octamethyl pyrophosphoramide: see Organophosphates
Oil of wintergreen:* see ASPIRIN AND OTHER SALICYLATE POISONING in Ch. 263
Oils: see Acetanilid (aniline oil); Petroleum distillates (fuel oil, lubricating oils)
Opium: see Narcotics

Continued

Poison	Symptoms	Treatment
Oral hypoglycemic drugs Chlorpropamide Glipizide	Most remain asymptomatic; hypoglycemia in a few, adults more often than children	Emesis, gastric lavage, or activated charcoal in severe cases; frequent feeding (not just sugar) plus close observation of behavior; for large overdoses, measurement of blood glucose
Organophosphates Acephate Bidrin Chlorethoxyfos Chlorothion Chlorpyrifos Coumaphos Demeton Diazinon Dichlorvos Dimethoate Disulfoton Ethion Famphur Fenthion Hexaethyl-tetraphosphate Isofenfos Malathion Methidathion Methyl parathion Naled Nerve gas agents Octamethyl pyrophosphoramide Oxydemeton-methyl Parathion Phorate	Nausea, vomiting, abdominal cramping, excessive salivation; increased pulmonary secretion, headache, rhinorrhea, blurred vision, miosis; slurred speech, mental confusion; breathing difficulty, frothing at mouth, coma; skin absorption via inhalation or PO	Removal of clothing, flushing and washing of skin; stomach emptied: atropine 2 mg (adults), 0.01-0.05 mg/kg (children) IV or IM q 15-60 min, if no signs of atropine toxicity, repeat prn; pralidoxime chloride 1-2 g (adults), 20-40 mg/kg (children) IV over 15-30 min, repeat in 1 h if needed; O₂; respiratory support; correction of dehydration. *Do not use morphine or aminophylline.* Attendant should avoid self-contamination

Phosdrin		
Phosmet		
Pirimiphos-methyl		
Temefos		
Terbufos		
Tetrachlorvinphos		
Trichlorfon		
Oxalic acid	Burning pain in throat, vomiting, intense pain; hypotension, tetany, shock; glottal and renal damage; oxaluria	Milk or calcium lactate; careful gastric lavage if at all; 10% calcium gluconate 10-20 mL IV; pain control, saline IV for shock; demulcents by mouth; observation for glottal edema and stricture
Ethylene glycol		
Oxalates		
Oxydemeton-methyl: see Organophosphates		
Paints: see Lead		
Paint solvents: see Petroleum distillates (mineral spirits); Turpentine		
Paradichlorobenzene	Abdominal pain, nausea, vomiting, diarrhea, seizures, tetany	Ipecac emesis, gastric lavage; fluid replacement; diazepam for seizure control
Insecticide		
Moth repellent		
Toilet bowl deodorant		
Paraldehyde	Paraldehyde odor on breath, incoherence, contracted pupils, depressed respirations, coma	Ingestion: Ipecac emesis, gastric lavage; O$_2$, respiratory support
Paraquat	Immediate: GI pain and vomiting	Emesis, fuller's earth PLUS sodium sulfate; limited O$_2$; consultation with poison control center or manufacturer
	Within 24 h: respiratory failure (Diquat causes no pulmonary problems.)	
Parathion: see Organophosphates		
Paris green: see Arsenic and antimony		
Pentobarbital: see Barbiturates		
Perchlordecone: see Chlorinated hydrocarbons		
Permanent wave neutralizers: see Chlorates		
Permethrin: see Pyrethroids		

Continued

Poison	Symptoms	Treatment
Pesticides: see Arsenic and antimony; Barium compounds; Chlorinated hydrocarbons; Dinitro-*o*-cresol; Fluorides; Organophosphates; Paradichlorobenzene; Phosphorus; Pyrethroids; Thallium salts; Warfarin		
Petroleum distillates (see also HYDROCARBON POISONING in Ch. 263)		
	Ingestion: Burning throat and stomach, vomiting, diarrhea; pneumonia, only if aspiration has occurred	Major problems consequential to aspiration (not GI absorption), thus, gastric evacuation usually not warranted; gastric lavage only with rapid onset
Asphalt	Vapor inhalation: Euphoria; burning in chest; headache, nausea, weakness; CNS depression, confusion; dyspnea, tachypnea, rales	depression from large amounts ingested; measurement of arterial blood gas levels to monitor care; supportive care for pulmonary edema; O_2, respiratory support
Benzine (benzin)		
Fuel oil		
Gasoline		
Kerosene	Aspiration: Early acute pulmonary changes	
Lubricating oils		
Mineral spirits		
Model airplane glue		
Naphtha		
Petroleum ether		
Tar		
Phenacetin: see Acetanilid		
Phencyclidine (PCP)	"Spaced-out" state, unconsciousness; hypertension	Quiet environment; prolonged gastric lavage; propranolol and diazepam
Phenmetrazine: see Amphetamines		
Phenobarbital: see Barbiturates		
Phenols	Corrosive effects; mucous membrane burns; pallor, weakness, shock; convulsions in children; pulmonary edema; smoky urine; respiratory, cardiac, and circulatory failure	Removal of clothing, washing of external burns with water, activated charcoal. *Do not use alcohol or mineral oil.* Demulcents: pain relief; O_2; cardiopulmonary support; correction of fluid imbalance; observation for esophageal stricture (rare)
Carbolic acid		
Creosote		
Cresols		
Guaiacol		
Naphthols		

Poison	Symptoms	Treatment
Phenothiazine Chlorpromazine Prochlorperazine Promazine Trifluoperazine	Extrapyramidal tract symptoms (ataxia, muscular and carpopedal spasms, torticollis), usually idiosyncratic; if overdose, dry mouth, drowsiness, coma, hypothermia, respiratory collapse: leukopenia, jaundice, coagulation defect, rashes	Ipecac emesis, activated charcoal, or gastric lavage; diphenhydramine 2-3 mg/kg IV or IM for extrapyramidal symptoms; diazepam for convulsions; warming of patient; levarterenol and epinephrine should be avoided; dialysis of no benefit (sodium bicarbonate for tachyarrhythmias)
Phenylpropanolamine	Nervousness, irritability, hypertension plus other sympathomimetic effects	Supportive therapy; diazepam; phentolamine (5 mg) or nitroprussides for hypertension
Phorate: see Organophosphates		
Phosdrin: see Organophosphates		
Phosmet: see Organophosphates		
Phosphoric acid: see Acids and alkalis		
Phosphorus (yellow or white) Rat poisons Roach powders (NOTE: Red phosphorus is unabsorbable and nontoxic)	1st stage—Garlicky taste; garlic breath odor: local irritation, skin and throat burns, nausea, vomiting, diarrhea 2nd stage—Symptom-free 8 h to several days 3rd stage—Nausea, vomiting, diarrhea, liver enlargement, jaundice, hemorrhages, renal damage, convulsions, coma Toxicity enhanced by alcohol, fats, digestible oils	Protection of patient and attendant from vomitus, gastric lavage, feces; if phosphorus is imbedded in skin, patient's body submerged in water; copious gastric lavage—potassium permanganate (1:5000) or cupric sulfate (250 mg in 250 mL water) recommended by some; mineral oil 100 mL (to prevent absorption), repeat in 2 h; prevention of shock; vitamin K_1 IV: transfusion with fresh blood
Physostigmine Eserine Neostigmine Pilocarpine *Pilocarpus*	Dizziness, weakness, vomiting, cramping pain; pupils dilated, then contracted; seizures	Atropine sulfate 0.6-1 mg (adults), 0.01 mg/kg (children) sc or IV repeated prn (CAUTION: *Using physostigmine to counter anticholinergics is associated with a 15% seizure rate*); benzodiazepine
Pilocarpine, *Pilocarpus*: see Physostigmine		
Pirimiphos-methyl: see Organophosphates		
Potash: see Acids and alkalis (potassium hydroxide)		
Potassium carbonate: see Acids and alkalis		
Potassium cyanide: see Cyanides		

Continued

Poison	Symptoms	Treatment
Potassium hydroxide: see Acids and alkalis		
Potassium nitrite: see Nitrites		
Potassium permanganate	Brown discoloration and burns of oral mucosa, glottal edema; hypotension; renal involvement	Gastric lavage, demulcents; maintenance of fluid balance
Prochlorperazine: see Phenothiazine		
Prolan: see Chlorinated hydrocarbons		
Promazine: see Phenothiazine		
Propoxyphene: see Narcotics		
Propranolol	Confusion and seizures	Emesis: lavage: supportive care: diazepam sedation: pacemakers and glucagon (0.05 mg/kg stat PLUS 2-5 mg/h)
Protriptyline: see Tricyclic antidepressants		
Prussic acid: see Cyanides		
Pyrethrin: see Pyrethroids		
Pyrethroids	Allergic response (including anaphylactic reactions, skin sensitivity) in sensitive persons: otherwise low toxicity, unless vehicle is a petroleum distillate	For sizable ingestion, emesis if patient is alert; otherwise, endotracheal tube and gastric lavage; thorough washing of skin
Bifenthrin		
Cyfluthrin		
Cypermethrin		
Esfenvalerate		
Fluvalinate		
Lambda-cyhalothrin		
Permethrin		
Pyrethrin		
Resmethrin		
Sumithrin		
Tefluthrin		
Tetramethrin		
Radium:† see Table 307-2		
Rat poisons: see Barium compounds; Fluorides; Phosphorus; Thallium salts; Warfarin		
Resmethrin: see Pyrethroids		

Poison	Symptoms	Treatment
Resorcinol (resorcin)	Vomiting, dizziness, tinnitus, chills, tremor, delirium, convulsions, respiratory depression, coma	Emetic or gastric lavage; respiratory support
Roach poisons: see Fluorides: Phosphorus: Thallium salts		
Rubbing alcohol: see Alcohol, isopropyl		
Salicylates:* see ASPIRIN AND OTHER SALICYLATE POISONING in Ch. 263		
Salicylic acid:* see ASPIRIN AND OTHER SALICYLATE POISONING in Ch. 263		
Scopolamine (hyoscine): see Belladonna		
Secobarbital: see Barbiturates		
Selective serotonin reuptake inhibitors Fluoxetine Paroxetine Sertraline	Drowsiness; interactions with alcohol, monoamine oxidase inhibitors, and other drugs	Emesis, gastric lavage, or activated charcoal in severe cases: supportive measures
Selenium:† see TABLE 307-2		
Sewer gas: see Hydrogen sulfide		
Silver salts Silver nitrate	Stain on lips (white, brown, then black); gastroenteritis, shock, vertigo, convulsions	Gastric lavage with saline (0.9% NaCl solution): control of pain; diazepam to control convulsions
Smog: see Sulfur dioxide		
Soda, caustic: see Acids and alkalis (sodium hydroxide)		
Sodium carbonate: see Acids and alkalis		
Sodium cyanide: see Cyanides		
Sodium fluoride: see Fluorides		
Sodium hydroxide: see Acids and alkalis		
Sodium nitrite: see Nitrites		
Sodium salicylate:* see ASPIRIN AND OTHER SALICYLATE POISONING in Ch. 263		
Solder: see Cadmium; Lead		
Stibophen: see Arsenic and antimony		
Stramonium: see Belladonna		

Continued

Poison	Symptoms	Treatment
Strychnine	Restlessness, hyperacuity of hearing, vision, and other problems: convulsions from minor stimuli, complete muscle relaxation between convulsions; perspiration; respiratory arrest	Isolation and restricted stimulation to prevent convulsions; activated charcoal PO: IV diazepam, curariform drugs to control convulsions: respiratory support: acid diuresis with ammonium chloride or ascorbic acid; gastric lavage *after* control of convulsions
Sulfur dioxide	Respiratory tract irritation; sneezing, cough, dyspnea, pulmonary edema	Removal from contaminated area: O_2; positive-pressure breathing, respiratory support
Smog		
Sulfuric acid: see Acids and alkalis		
Sumithrin: see Pyrethroids		
Syrup of wild cherry: see Cyanides		
Tar: see Petroleum distillates		
Tartar emetic: see Arsenic and antimony		
Tear gas: see Chlorine		
Tefluthrin: see Pyrethroids		
Temefos: see Organophosphates		
Terbufos: see Organophosphates		
Tetrachlorvinphos: see Organophosphates		
Tetraethyl lead: see Lead, tetraethyl		
Tetramethrin: see Pyrethroids		
Thallium salts (formerly used in ant, rat, and roach poisons)	Abdominal pain (colic), vomiting (may be bloody), diarrhea (may be bloody), stomatitis, excessive salivation; tremors, leg pains, paresthesias, polyneuritis, ocular and facial palsy; delirium, convulsions, respiratory failure; loss of hair about 3 wk after poisoning	Ipecac emesis, gastric lavage; treatment of shock, diazepam to control convulsions; chelation therapy is experimental; consultation with poison control center for latest information
Theophylline: see Aminophylline		
Thyroxine	Most are asymptomatic; rarely, increasing irritability progressing to thyroid storm in 5–7 days	Emesis; observation at home; diazepam; possibly antithyroid preparations and propranolol, *only* if symptoms occur

Tobacco	Excitement, confusion, muscular twitching, weakness, abdominal cramps, clonic convulsions, depression, rapid respirations, palpitations, collapse, coma, CNS paralysis, respiratory failure	Ipecac emesis, gastric lavage; activated charcoal; respiratory support; O₂; diazepam for convulsions; thorough washing of skin if contaminated
Nicotine		

Toilet bowl cleaners, deodorizers: see Acids and alkalis; Paradichlorobenzene
Toluene, toluol: see Benzene
Toxaphene: see Chlorinated hydrocarbons
Trichlorfon: see Organophosphates
Trichloromethane: see Chloroform

Tricyclic antidepressants	Anticholinergic effects (eg, blurred vision, urinary hesitation); CNS effects (eg, drowsiness, stupor, coma, ataxia, restlessness, agitation, hyperactive reflexes, muscle rigidity, convulsions); cardiovascular effects (tachycardia and other arrhythmias, bundle branch block, impaired conduction, congestive heart failure); respiratory depression, hypotension, shock, vomiting, hyperpyrexia, mydriasis, and diaphoresis also possible	Symptomatic and supportive treatment; emesis (avoid if seizures are imminent), activated charcoal, gastric lavage; vital signs and ECG monitored; maintenance of airway and fluid intake; sodium bicarbonate as a rapid IV injection (0.5–2 mEq/kg), repeat periodically to maintain blood pH > 7.45 and prevent arrhythmias; diazepam to control most CNS problems; physostigmine salicylate (slowly IV) only to reverse persistent CNS and cardiac manifestations of overdosage—adults: 2 mg with repeat of 1–4 mg prn q 20–60 min; children: 0.5 mg repeated prn q 5 min (maximum 2 mg)
Amitriptyline		
Desipramine		
Doxepin		
Imipramine		
Nortriptyline		
Protriptyline		

Trifluoperazine: see Phenothiazine
Triiodomethane: see Iodoform
Tungsten:† see TABLE 307–2

Turpentine	Turpentine odor: burning oral and abdominal pain, coughing, choking, respiratory failure; nephritis	Emesis (for alert patient) if > 1-4 oz ingested; gastric lavage; respiratory support: O₂; control of pain; monitoring of renal function
Paint solvent		
Varnish	Progressive CNS depression	Supportive measures; naloxone helpful

Valproic acid
Vanadium:† see TABLE 307-2
Varnish: see Alcohol, methyl; Turpentine

Continued

Poison	Symptoms	Treatment
Warfarin Bishydroxycoumarin Dicumarol Ethyl biscoumacetate Superwarfarins	Single ingestion not serious, multiple overdoses result in coagulopathy, but most overdoses are uneventful, even with "super" drugs	For hemorrhagic manifestations, vitamin K_1 see Ch. 3) until prothrombin time is normal, transfusion with fresh blood if necessary
Whiskey: see Alcohol, ethyl		
Wild cherry syrup: see Cyanides		
Wintergreen oil:* see ASPIRIN AND OTHER SALICYLATE POISONING in Ch. 263		
Wood alcohol: see Alcohol, methyl		
Xylene: see Benzene		
Zinc:† see TABLE 307-2		
Zinc salts: see Copper salts		

From The Merck Manual of Diagnosis and Therapy, Edition 17, pp. 2623-2644, edited by Mark H. Beers and Robert Berkow. Copyright 1999 by Merck & Co., Inc., Whitehouse Station, NJ, with permission.

*Aspirin and salicylate poisoning: Early symptoms include nausea and vomiting, tinnitus, hyperpnea, respiratory alkalosis, metabolic acidosis, hyperactivity, hyperthermia, and seizures. Later symptoms include hypoactivity, dehydration, significant loss of sodium and potassium, lethargy, and respiratory failure. Treatment includes ipecac syrup, activated charcoal up to several hours after ingestion, hydration, and bicarbonate.

†Metal poisonings: Toxicity can be caused by environmental, medical, or industrial exposure. Chromium and nickel have been implicated as a cause of cancer. Copper excess may be caused by Wilson's disease. All metal poisonings can be treated with chelation therapy.

‡Digitalis toxicity: Toxicity can result in fatal arrhythmias. Bidirectional ventricular tachycardia is pathognomonic of digitalis toxicity. Discontinue the drug and treat arrhythmias.

§Chemical food poisoning: Fava beans can cause hemolysis in persons with G6PD deficiency. Mushroom poisoning symptoms occur minutes to 24 hours after ingestion and include lacrimation, miosis, salivation, sweating, vomiting, abdominal cramps, diarrhea, vertigo, confusion, coma, or convulsions or anuria. Ingestion can be fatal. Treat with emesis, gastric lavage, and/or activated charcoal and hydration. Atropine (1 mg sc or IV q 1 to 2 h) is used for muscarine poisoning.

ACE, angiotensin-converting enzyme; BP, blood pressure; BSA, body surface area; CNS, central nervous system; D/W, dextrose in water; GI, gastrointestinal; G6PD, glucose 6-phosphate dehydrogenase; NSAIDs, nonsteroidal anti-inflammatory drugs.

Index

Note: Page numbers followed by "f" refer to figures; page numbers followed by "t" refer to tables; page numbers followed by "cpf" refer to color plate figures.

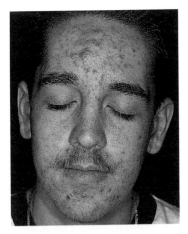

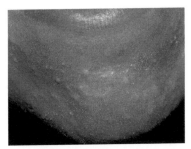

Figure 2–1. Acne vulgaris. (From Callen JP, Greer KE, Paller AS, Swinyer LJ: Color Atlas of Dermatology, 2nd ed. Philadelphia, WB Saunders, 2000, p 10).

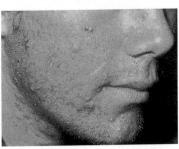

Figure 2–2. Acne: Open and closed comedones. (From Hooper BJ, Goldman MP: Primary Dermatologic Care. St. Louis, Mosby, 1999, p 12).

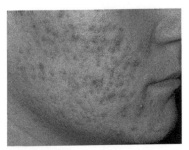

Figure 2–3. Acne: Closed comedones. (From White G: Levene's Color Atlas of Dermatology, 2nd ed. St. Louis, Mosby, 1997, p 75).

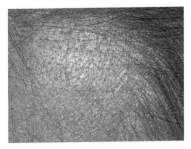

Figure 2–4. Acne: Scarring. (From White G, Cox N: Diseases of the Skin: A Color Atlas and Text. St. Louis, Mosby, 2000, p 93).

Figure 2–5. Hair appearance in alopecia. (From White G, Cox N: Diseases of the Skin: A Color Atlas and Text. St. Louis, Mosby, 2000, p 388).

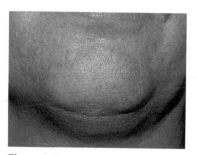

Figure 2–6. Alopecia: Beard. (From White G, Cox N: Diseases of the Skin: A Color Atlas and Text. St. Louis, Mosby, 2000, p 387).

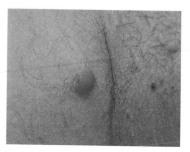

Figure 2–8. Dermatofibroma. (From White G, Cox N: Diseases of the Skin: A Color Atlas and Text. St. Louis, Mosby, 2000, p 417).

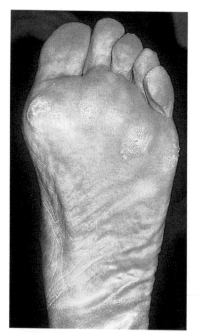

Figure 2–7. Callosities. (From Lawrence CM, Cox NH: Physical Signs in Dermatology, 2nd ed. St. Louis, Mosby, 2002, p 90).

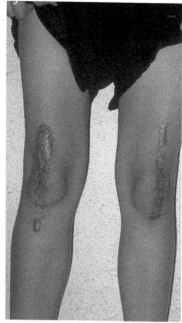

Figure 2–9. Keloid: Postoperative keloid scarring. (From White G, Cox N: Diseases of the Skin: A Color Atlas and Text. St. Louis, Mosby, 2000, p 300).

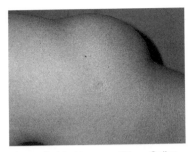

Figure 2–10. Lipomas. (From Callen JP, Greer KE, Paller AS, Swinyer LJ: Color Atlas of Dermatology, 2nd ed. Philadelphia, WB Saunders, 2000, p 106).

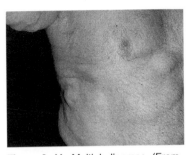

Figure 2–11. Multiple lipomas. (From Callen JP, Greer KE, Paller AS, Swinyer LJ: Color Atlas of Dermatology, 2nd ed. Philadelphia, WB Saunders, 2000, p 106).

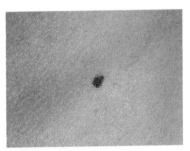

Figure 2–12. Junctional nevus. (From Callen JP, Greer KE, Paller AS, Swinyer LJ: Color Atlas of Dermatology, 2nd ed. Philadelphia, WB Saunders, 2000, p 32).

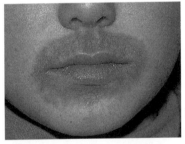

Figure 2–13. Contact dermatitis: Lip-licking dermatitis. (From White G, Cox N: Diseases of the Skin: A Color Atlas and Text. St. Louis, Mosby, 2000, p 34).

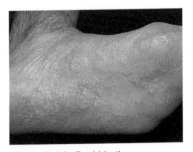

Figure 2–14. Dyshidrotic eczema. (From Callen JP, Greer KE, Paller AS, Swinyer LJ: Color Atlas of Dermatology, 2nd ed. Philadelphia, WB Saunders, 2000, p 318).

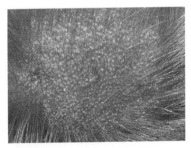

Figure 2–15. Tinea capitis. (From White G, Cox N: Diseases of the Skin: A Color Atlas and Text. St. Louis, Mosby, 2000, p 364).

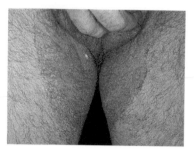

Figure 2–16. Tinea cruris. (From Callen JP, Greer KE, Paller AS, Swinyer LJ: Color Atlas of Dermatology, 2nd ed. Philadelphia, WB Saunders, 2000, p 303).

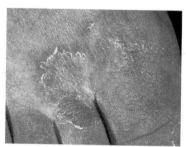

Figure 2–17. Tinea pedis. (From Lawrence CM, Cox NH: Physical Signs in Dermatology, 2nd ed. St. Louis, Mosby, 2002, p 123).

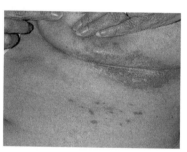

Figure 2–18. Cutaneous *Candida* infection. (From White G, Cox N: Diseases of the Skin: A Color Atlas and Text. St. Louis, Mosby, 2000, p 365).

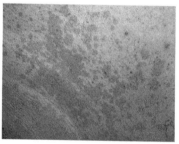

Figure 2–19. Tinea versicolor. (From Callen JP, Greer KE, Paller AS, Swinyer LJ: Color Atlas of Dermatology, 2nd ed. Philadelphia, WB Saunders, 2000, p 34).

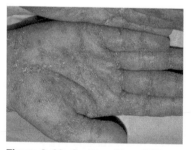

Figure 2–20. Scabies. (From White G, Cox N: Diseases of the Skin: A Color Atlas and Text. St. Louis, Mosby, 2000, p 371).

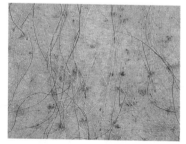

Figure 2–21. Pediculosis pubis. (From Callen JP, Greer KE, Paller AS, Swinyer LJ: Color Atlas of Dermatology, 2nd ed. Philadelphia, WB Saunders, 2000, p 309).

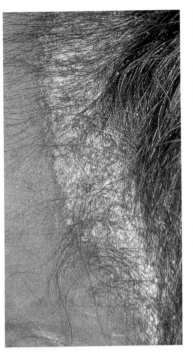

Figure 2–22. Psoriasis. (From White G, Cox N: Diseases of the Skin: A Color Atlas and Text. St. Louis, Mosby, 2000, p 54).

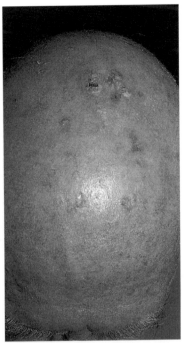

Figure 2–24. Actinic keratosis. (From Callen JP, Greer KE, Paller AS, Swinyer LJ: Color Atlas of Dermatology, 2nd ed. Philadelphia, WB Saunders, 2000, p 294).

Figure 2–23. Pityriasis rosea. (From Callen JP, Greer KE, Paller AS, Swinyer LJ: Color Atlas of Dermatology, 2nd ed. Philadelphia, WB Saunders, 2000, p 20).

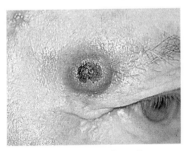

Figure 2–25. Basal cell carcinoma. (From Callen JP, Greer KE, Paller AS, Swinyer LJ: Color Atlas of Dermatology, 2nd ed. Philadelphia, WB Saunders, 2000, p 9).

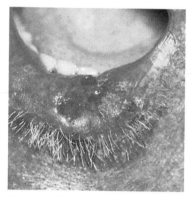

Figure 2–26. Squamous cell carcinoma. (From Lawrence CM, Cox NH: Physical Signs in Dermatology, 2nd ed. St. Louis, Mosby, 2002, p 184).

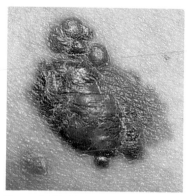

Figure 2–27. Malignant melanoma. (From Callen JP, Greer KE, Paller AS, Swinyer LJ: Color Atlas of Dermatology, 2nd ed. Philadelphia, WB Saunders, 2000, p 81).

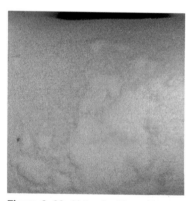

Figure 2–28. Urticaria. (From Hooper BJ, Goldman MP: Primary Dermatologic Care. St. Louis, Mosby, 1999, p 90).

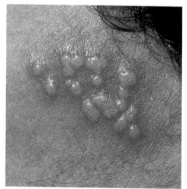

Figure 2–29. Herpes simplex. (From White G, Cox N: Diseases of the Skin: A Color Atlas and Text. St. Louis, Mosby, 2000, p 348).

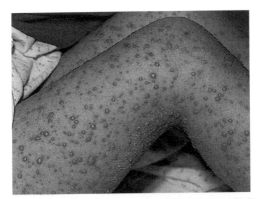

Figure 2–30. Varicella (chickenpox). (From Callen JP, Greer KE, Paller AS, Swinyer LJ: Color Atlas of Dermatology, 2nd ed. Philadelphia, WB Saunders, 2000, p 143).

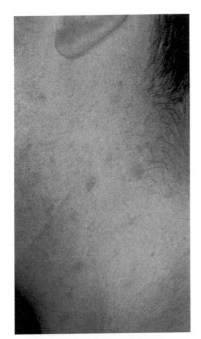

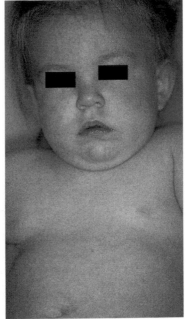

Figure 2–31. Measles (rubeola). (From Hooper BJ, Goldman MP: Primary Dermatologic Care. St. Louis, Mosby, 1999, p 166).

Figure 2–32. Roseola. (From Hooper BJ, Goldman MP: Primary Dermatologic Care. St. Louis, Mosby, 1999, p 173).

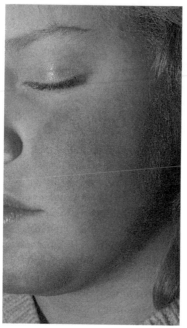

Figure 2–33. Erythema infectiosum. (From Hooper BJ, Goldman MP: Primary Dermatologic Care. St. Louis, Mosby, 1999, p 157).

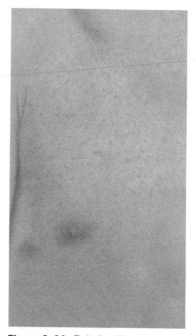

Figure 2–34. Rubella. (From Hooper BJ, Goldman MP: Primary Dermatologic Care. St. Louis, Mosby, 1999, p 57).

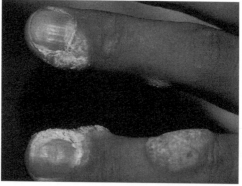

Figure 2–35. Warts. (From Hooper BJ, Goldman MP: Primary Dermatologic Care. St. Louis, Mosby, 1999, p 229).